Arthritis: A Growing Concern

Arthritis: A Growing Concern

Editor: Jerry Larson

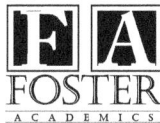

FOSTER
ACADEMICS

www.fosteracademics.com

www.fosteracademics.com

E A
FOSTER
ACADEMICS

Cataloging-in-Publication Data

Arthritis : a growing concern / edited by Jerry Larson.
     p. cm.
Includes bibliographical references and index.
ISBN 978-1-63242-764-9
1. Arthritis. 2. Joints--Diseases. I. Larson, Jerry.
RC933 .A784 2019
616.722--dc23

Foster Academics,
118-35 Queens Blvd., Suite 400,
Forest Hills, NY 11375, USA

ISBN 978-1-63242-764-9 (Hardback)

Contents

Preface

The purpose of the book is to provide a glimpse into the dynamics and to present opinions and studies of some of the scientists engaged in the development of new ideas in the field from very different standpoints. This book will prove useful to students and researchers owing to its high content quality.

Any disorder that affects the joints is called arthritis. There are over 100 different types of arthritis. Some common forms are osteoarthritis, rheumatoid arthritis, ankylosing spondylitis, gout, juvenile idiopathic arthritis, etc. The most common feature of all kinds of arthritis is pain. Joint stiffness, swelling and aching around the joints are other common symptoms. Decreased mobility combined with other symptoms, cause individuals to become obese and vulnerable to heart disease. Clinical examinations, X-rays and blood tests are performed for making a diagnosis. Based on the diagnosis of the arthritis, a treatment strategy is formed which may involve physical therapy, orthopedic bracing and medications. In eroding forms of arthritis, joint replacement surgery may be required. Disease-modifying antirheumatic drugs, non-steroidal anti-inflammatory drugs and pain relief medications offer a degree of relief to patients with arthritis. Exercises aimed at improving muscle strength, flexibility and endurance can be more effective than medications. The objective of this book is to give a general view of the different types of arthritis and their management strategies. It strives to provide a fair idea about this condition and to help develop a better understanding of the latest advances in this domain. This book on arthritis is a collective contribution of a renowned group of international experts.

At the end, I would like to appreciate all the efforts made by the authors in completing their chapters professionally. I express my deepest gratitude to all of them for contributing to this book by sharing their valuable works. A special thanks to my family and friends for their constant support in this journey.

Editor

Widespread pain in axial spondyloarthritis: clinical importance and gender differences

Thijs Willem Swinnen[1,2,3]* (iD), René Westhovens[1,2], Wim Dankaerts[3] and Kurt de Vlam[1,2]

Abstract

Background: There is a remarkable lack of detailed knowledge on pain areas in axial spondyloarthritis (axSpA), and their clinical relevance is largely unknown. Pain area may reflect local disease processes, but amplification of nervous system signalling may alter this relationship. Also, gender differences in pain area may exist in axSpA, possibly confounding disease activity outcomes. Therefore, we firstly detailed pain locations in axSpA and evaluated gender differences. Secondly, we explored the relationship of regional pain definitions with clinical outcomes. Finally, we explored the role of pain area in the assessment of disease activity.

Methods: Body charts informed on the presence of axial, peripheral articular and non-articular pain in 170 patients (108 men, 62 women) with axSpA. Multivariate Odds Ratios (ORs) were used to compare genders. General linear models were used to explore clinical differences in disease activity (Bath Ankylosing Spondylitis Disease Activity Index [BASDAI]), activity limitations (Bath Ankylosing Spondylitis Functional Index [BASFI]), fear of movement (Tampa Scale for Kinesiophobia 11-item version [TSK-11]), anxiety (Hospital Anxiety and Depression Scale subscale anxiety [HADS-A]) and depression (HADS subscale depression [HADS-D]) between four subgroups classified by widespread non-articular pain (WNAP+/−) and physician global assessment of disease activity (PGDA+/−) ($p < .05$). Principal Component Analysis (PCA) was performed to explore gender differences in the structure of disease activity.

Results: Axial thoracic pain was least prevalent (lumbar, 74.4%; cervical, 47.6%; cervicothoracic, 47.6%; thoracic, 32.4%), but it was about three times more likely in women (OR, 2.92; $p = .009$). Axial cervicothoracic junction pain spread more diffusely in women (OR, 2.48; $p = .018$). Women exhibited a two- to threefold increased likelihood of widespread axial (OR, 3.33; $p = .007$) and peripheral articular (OR, 2.34; $p = .023$) pain. A subgroup of WNAP+/PGDA− combined with low PGDA (27% of all patients) was associated with worse BASFI, BASDAI, HADS-A and HADS-D in men and worse TSK-11 and HADS-A in women ($p < .05$). Disease activity outcomes showed a two-factor structure in women but not in men.

Conclusions: In patients with axSpA, the location and spread of pain was different between genders and was related to worse clinical status. On the basis of pain area and PGDA, clinical subgroups exhibiting a remarkably distinct health status were identified. Outcome instruments such as BASDAI should acknowledge gender differences to ensure structural validity.

Keywords: Ankylosing spondylitis, Widespread pain, Anxiety, Disability, Inflammation, Depression, Body chart, Gender differences

* Correspondence: thijs.swinnen@uzleuven.be
Wim Dankaerts and Kurt de Vlam shared senior authorship.
[1]Division of Rheumatology, University Hospitals Leuven, Herestraat 49, 3000 Leuven, Belgium
[2]Skeletal Biology and Engineering Research Center, Department of Development and Regeneration, KU Leuven, Herestraat 49 box 7003/13, 3000 Leuven, Belgium
Full list of author information is available at the end of the article

Background

Disease processes in axial spondyloarthritis (axSpA) involve tissue inflammation seen as enthesitis, synovitis and bone marrow oedema, as well as structural damage in the form of erosion, fat metaplasia/backfill and bone formation (sclerosis, ankylosis) [1, 2]. Spinal articular features typically occur at intervertebral corners and end-plates, zygapophyseal, and costovertebral and costo-transverse joints, as well as at spinal ligament insertions [2, 3]. Asymmetrical mono- or oligoarthritis and enthesitis may add peripheral aspects to the predominant axial disease presentation [2]. Extra-articular features such as psoriasis, anterior uveitis or inflammatory bowel disease further illustrate the systemic nature of axSpA [2]. Although the exact aetiology of axSpA is largely unknown, a complex interplay between genetics (e.g., HLA-B27 [2]), biomechanical stress within the enthesis organ [4], gut bacterial dysbiosis [5] and several dysfunctional immune-competent cells (e.g., innate lymphoid group 3 cells [6]) may elicit auto-inflammation driven by key cytokines tumour necrosis factor (TNF)-α, interleukin (IL)-17 and IL-23 [7].

Cardinal clinical signs and symptoms of axSpA include inflammatory pain, stiffness and impaired mobility in the axial region and peripheral joints. To a large extent, these features are thought to reflect adaptive pain-motor mechanisms associated with inflammation and consequences of bone formation associated with the disease [8, 9]. To capture these local tissue processes, the Assessment in SpondyloArthritis international Society (ASAS) expert group endorsed classification and response (ASAS20, ASAS40, ASAS 4/5) criteria, as well as disease activity (Bath Ankylosing Spondylitis Disease Activity Index [BASDAI], Ankylosing Spondylitis Disease Activity Index [ASDAS]) and spinal mobility (Bath Ankylosing Spondylitis Metrology Index [BASMI]) scales in axSpA [2]. These mainly include self-reported numerical rating scales used to assess axial/peripheral pain intensity and spinal stiffness duration, but they also include clinical examination findings (e.g., joint effusion) and metrology using a tape measure [2].

Although useful for research, the mere focus on inflammation in the assessment of body structures and functions as proposed by ASAS may have pitfalls in clinical practice. Firstly, nociceptive/mechanical [10], neuropathic [11] or dysfunctional [12] pain mechanisms may complicate the clinical picture in axSpA and concurrently may influence pain intensity or stiffness duration scales. For example, ongoing low-grade or intense episodes of inflammation in axSpA likely induce a bottom-up amplification of neural signalling in the central nervous system that leads to pain hypersensitivity and to the spread of pain in a broader area, a process known as *central pain plasticity* (*central sensitization*) [13]. Also, psychological factors have been shown to exert top-down effects on disease activity estimates in axSpA [14]. Clinically, these pain mechanisms may translate to widespread pain, a feature seen in about 2–34% of patients with axSpA [12, 15, 16]. Secondly, ASAS outcome instruments including cut-offs for disease status or treatment response assume homogeneity in the axSpA population. Recently, gender differences in disease activity items such as higher reported pain intensity [17] or lower spinal mobility measures [18] have increasingly been observed in axSpA. Because cut-off levels might impact treatment decisions, this issue cannot be underestimated.

As a first step to improve the clinical assessment of pain in axSpA, the aim of this cross-sectional study was to explore the value of a more detailed pain area assessment as an adjunct to axial and peripheral articular pain intensity and stiffness. More specifically, the aims of this study were as follows:

1. To evaluate the prevalence of pain in anatomically distinct body regions and the body locations within these regions (topographical pain analysis)
2. To determine the association between the extent of axial, peripheral articular and peripheral non-articular pain areas and clinical variables (activity limitations, spinal mobility, disease activity, anxiety and depression)
3. To explore the role of assessing axial, peripheral articular and peripheral non-articular pain areas in the evaluation of the disease activity (using factor analysis)
4. To evaluate gender differences in all analyses.

Methods
Participants

Subjects ($n = 190$) with a definite diagnosis of axSpA according to the ASAS classification criteria [19], verified by an ASAS expert rheumatologist (KDV), were randomly included in this cross-sectional observational study. All patients were recruited from the outpatient spondyloarthritis clinic at the University Hospitals of Leuven, Belgium. Subjects with other inflammatory or systemic rheumatic conditions or who were unable to autonomously complete questionnaires in Dutch were excluded.

Outcome measures
Anthropometrics and demographics

Height was measured with a stadiometer (Holtain Ltd., Dyfed, UK) to the nearest 0.1 cm, and weight was measured with a digital scale (SECA, Birmingham, UK) to the nearest 0.1 kg. Age (in yr), gender (male = 1/female = 2), disease duration (in yr), work status (yes = 1/no = 0) and the use of medication (biologicals, NSAIDs, DMARDs, analgesics, psychopharmacologics, corticoids, yes = 1/no = 2) were assessed during an interview and verified via the patient's medical record.

Activity limitations

The ten-item BASFI numerical rating scale was used to assess patient-reported activity limitations [20]. The BASFI is an ASAS-endorsed instrument used to measure activity limitations with well-established psychometric properties in axSpA [2].

Spinal mobility

The BASMI was used to measure spinal mobility via five clinical tests, namely cervical rotation measured with a goniometer (accuracy 2 degrees; ORTEC Orthopedics, Leuven, Belgium) and a tape measure (accuracy 1 mm; Prym, Stolberg, Germany) of lumbar flexion, lumbar side flexion, tragus-to-wall distance and intermalleolar distance. For cervical rotation, lumbar side flexion and tragus-to-wall distance, the mean of the left and right measurements was taken, and all scores were converted according to the BASMI 10 scoring system [2]. The psychometric properties of the ASAS-endorsed BASMI in axSpA are well established [2, 21, 22].

Disease activity

The six-item BASDAI numerical rating scale was used to evaluate patient-reported disease activity. As recommended by ASAS, items 5 and 6 combined represented patient-reported inflammation [2]. The one-item Physician Global Assessment of Disease Activity (PGDA) numerical rating scale assessed during the routine rheumatology visit at inclusion represented physician-reported disease activity [2]. C-reactive protein (CRP, in mg/L) served as the laboratory-based disease activity marker [2]. The psychometric properties of the BASDAI, BASDAI inflammation, PGDA and CRP in axSpA are well established [2].

Fear of movement and (re)injury beliefs

The Tampa Scale for Kinesiophobia Dutch version with 11 items (TSK-11) was used to assess fearful beliefs regarding movement and (re)injury. Each item is provided with a 4-point Likert scale with scoring alternatives ranging from 'strongly disagree' to 'strongly agree' (range, 11–44). The psychometric properties of TSK-11 are well established in chronic pain populations [23] and recently in axSpA [24].

Anxiety and depression

The 14-item Hospital Anxiety and Depression Scale (HADS) was used to derive information on depression (7 items) and anxiety (7 items) using a 4-point Likert scale with higher values representing more depressed or anxious mood (range, 0–21 for each subscale). The

psychometric properties of HADS are well established in axSpA [25].

Pain area

An anterior and posterior body chart filled in by the patient during the intake interview determined the presence of pain (yes = 1/no = 0) during the past week in 80 body locations (LOC) from which 22 body regions were derived post hoc (Fig. 1). Articular peripheral body locations were modified from the 76/74-joint count in psoriatic arthritis [26]. Non-articular peripheral body locations were taken from the widespread pain index as applied in the preliminary diagnostic criteria for fibromyalgia [27]. Axial body locations and regions were defined according to the International Association for the Study of Pain [28] and known axial pain referral patterns [29]. A detailed numeric description of pain locations within different body regions is given in Table 2. Widespread axial pain was defined as pain present in the

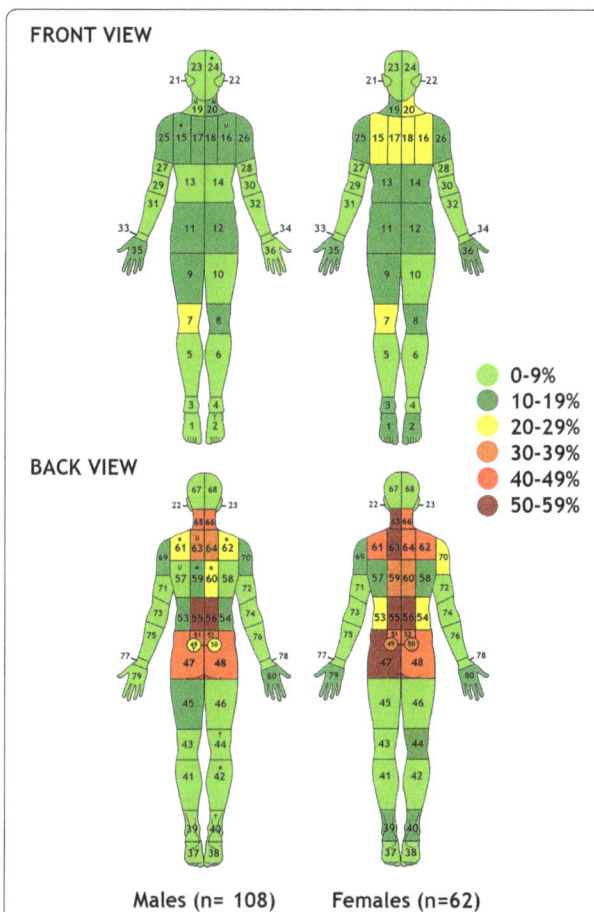

Fig. 1 Graphical illustration of pain locations displayed as prevalence estimates for the total group and by gender in patients with axial spondyloarthritis ($n = 170$). * $p < .05$ in both univariate chi-square and multivariate logistical regression analyses; U $p < .05$ only in univariate analysis; M $p < .05$ only multivariate analysis; T $p < .05$ in univariate but trend in multivariate analysis

lumbar (LX), thoracic (TX), cervicothoracic junction (CTJ) and cervical (CX) body regions. Widespread peripheral articular (WAP) and non-articular (WNAP) pain was considered present if the sum of painful (non-)articular peripheral body locations exceeded the median for this variable. Axial, peripheral articular and non-articular pain were also calculated as the sum of their respective body locations and expressed as percentages. Two blinded raters with a bachelor's-level degree in physical therapy independently scored the body charts showing good to excellent reliability of this procedure (kappa range, 0.742–1.00; percentage of agreement range, 94–100%) (Additional file 1: Table S1).

Data reduction and statistical analysis
Sample characteristics were presented as mean ± SD and median with IQR or frequencies as percentage. Normal distribution of all variables was evaluated with the Shapiro-Wilk test ($p < .05$). For each body region and location, prevalence with the corresponding 95% CI was calculated in the total group and for men and women separately. Cohen's kappa values and percentage of agreement were calculated as inter-rater reliability coefficients ($n = 170$), and thresholds for further use of body charts were set at minimally good (0.61–0.80), preferably excellent (> 0.80) [30].

Pain area between genders was univariate compared with an independent t test for continuous variables or chi-square test for frequencies ($p < .05$). In case of low cell counts (fewer than five) for the latter, the chi-square test was replaced by the phi coefficient to obtain valid p values. For each body region and location as dependent variables, BASDAI inflammation, gender, BASMI, disease duration, age and PGDA were entered as independent variables in a multivariate logistic regression model with ORs and their 95% CIs as output for the gender comparison. The same independent variables were entered into a multiple linear regression model for axial, articular and non-articular pain sum scores with (un)standardized beta (b, stß) values and their 95% CIs reported for gender effects.

Pearson product-moment correlation coefficients determined the univariate association between axial, peripheral non-articular and articular pain versus clinical variables ($p < .05$). Further, clinically relevant subgroups based on the median split of physician-reported disease activity and peripheral non-articular pain (PGDA–/WNAP–, PGDA–/WNAP+, PGDA+/WNAP–, PGDA+/WNAP+) were compared in a multivariate general linear model with subgroup and gender as between-subject factors; BASMI, BMI, disease duration and age as covariates; and BASDAI, BASFI, BASMI, HADS depression and HADS anxiety separately as dependent variables ($p < .05$). Results of post hoc tests were presented with uncorrected ($p < .05$) and Bonferroni-corrected p values.

PCA was performed to explore the contribution of all six items of BASDAI and axial, peripheral non-articular and articular pain sum scores in assessing disease activity. The covariance structure was analysed, and variables with an eigenvalue ≥ 1 were retained. Also, the scree plot was visually inspected to confirm the number of extracted factors. Factor loadings were varimax-rotated, and the variance explained per factor was reported. The magnitude of the rescaled rotated factor loadings determined factor membership for each variable and a large > 0.60 or smaller < 0.60 contribution to the total variance explained (Fig. 3). On the basis of this membership, the factor axial disease activity and peripheral disease activity were calculated as the arrhythmic mean of all items within the developed factor without weighting. PCA was repeated per gender to explore structural variability in disease activity outcomes. All analyses were performed with IBM SPSS Statistics version 20.0 software (IBM, Armonk, NY, USA).

Results
Demographic and anthropometrical data
Of all 190 patients invited, only 4 refused to participate, resulting in 186 included patients. The numbers of cases with missing data were 2 (1.1%) for the BASMI, 3 (1.6%) for the TSK-11, 3 (1.6%) for the HADS, 7 (3.8%) for the BASFI, 6 (3.2%) for the BASDAI, 26 for PGDA (14.0%), 31 for CRP (16.7%) and 9 for work status (4.8%). Full data across outcome measures were available for 170 patients (9.1% data loss) for analyses without PGDA and CRP. Analyses considering PGDA and CRP included 133 subjects (28.4% data loss). No statistically significant differences were found between groups with or without missing data ($p > .05$). Descriptive statistics for the total sample and per gender are given in Table 1.

Prevalence and gender differences for pain regions
Full prevalence data for all pain regions for the total group and per gender are presented in Table 2. Left (10.0% [9.7–10.3%]) and right (11.2% [10.8–11.6%]) whole-leg pain was a rare finding in this axSpA group for both men and women. In contrast, pain in the lumbar spine (LX) was highly prevalent (total group, 74.4% [74.2–75.2%]) and significantly more prevalent in women (83.9% [83.5–84.3%]) than in men (69.4% [68.9–69.9%]) in univariate analysis only (chi-square test, 4.338, $p = .037$; OR, 1.74 [0.73–4.14], $p = .210$). Pain in the thoracic spine (TX) was remarkably less prevalent overall (32.4% [31.9–32.9%]) and in men (25% [24.5–25.5%]), but about three times more likely in women (45.2% [44.6–45.8%], chi-square test, 7.315, $p = .007$; OR, 2.92 [1.30–6.55], $p = .009$). Cervicothoracic junction (CTJ) pain was moderately prevalent overall (47.6% [47–48.2%]) and in men (48.1% [47.5–48.7%]), but

Table 1 Descriptive statistics for all demographic, anthropometric and disease-related outcomes in patients with axial spondyloarthritis ($n = 170$)

Variables	Total group ($n = 170$)		Men ($n = 108$)		Women ($n = 62$)		
	Mean (SD)	Med (IQR)	Mean (SD)	Med (IQR)	Mean (SD)	Med (IQR)	p Value
Age, yr	42.9 (12.2)	42.7 (20.3)	43.8 (12.5)	43.2 (20.4)	41.3 (11.5)	42.1 (18.0)	.199
Disease duration, yr	13.1 (11.1)	10.7 (16.6)	14.0 (11.2)	11.9 (18.4)	11.5 (11.0)	8.8 (13.0)	.155
Height, cm	171.6 (9.4)	172.3 (12.9)	176.2 (7.1)	176.2 (9.1)	163.7 (7.4)	163.4 (9.5)	< .00
Weight, kg	77.0 (15.0)	76.6 (20.9)	81.7 (13.9)	80.5 (19.2)	69.7 (13.4)	67.0 (18.1)	< .00
BMI, kg/m^2	26.1 (4.4)	25.6 (6.4)	26.3 (4.4)	25.5 (6.1)	25.7 (4.4)	25.7 (7.1)	.408
BASDAI (0–10)	3.8 (2.1)	3.7 (3.3)	3.6 (2.2)	3.5 (3.5)	4.3 (2.0)	4.2 (3.1)	.027
PGDA (0–10) ($n = 146$)	1.4 (1.8)	1.0 (2.0)	1.4 (1.9)	0.9 (2.0)	1.4 (1.6)	1.0 (1.6)	.583
CRP, mg/L ($n = 141$)	8.3 (16.0)	2.9 (6.6)	8.9 (16.5)	3.0 (6.6)	7.4 (15.3)	2.2 (6.7)	.810
BASFI (0–10)	3.6 (2.4)	3.4 (3.8)	3.5 (2.4)	3.2 (4.0)	3.8 (2.3)	3.7 (3.7)	.459
BASMI (0–10)	3.0 (1.8)	2.8 (2.0)	3.3 (2.0)	2.8 (2.8)	2.6 (1.2)	2.6 (1.6)	.002
Cervical rotation, degrees	60.5 (19.6)	65.0 (25.0)	58.0 (21.3)	62.5 (27.8)	65.0 (15.6)	66.0 (20.5)	.015
Tragus to wall, cm	13.6 (4.6)	11.7 (4.5)	14.9 (5.0)	13.3 (6.2)	11.4 (2.3)	10.8 (1.8)	< .00
Lateral flexion, cm	12.4 (5.1)	12.7 (8.1)	11.7 (6.1)	12.1 (9.4)	13.5 (4.2)	13.1 (6.1)	.028
Intermalleolar distance, cm	99.0 (22.6)	103.3 (25.1)	101.0 (21.4)	105.2 (25.2)	95.5 (24.2)	100.7 (25.0)	.141
Modified Schober, cm	5.3 (2.1)	5.5 (2.5)	4.9 (2.3)	5.2 (3.1)	5.9 (1.7)	6.2 (2.0)	.002
TSK-11 (11–44)	24.8 (6.3)	25.0 (10.0)	27.8 (6.4)	25.0 (10.0)	24.9 (6.0)	25.0 (9.3)	.888
HADS depression (0–21)	4.6 (3.6)	4.0 (5.0)	4.8 (3.7)	4.0 (5.0)	4.4 (3.5)	3.0 (4.0)	.580
HADS anxiety (0–21)	7.1 (3.6)	7.0 (5.0)	6.7 (3.4)	7.0 (5.0)	7.8 (3.9)	7.5 (5.0)	.071
Frequencies (%)							
Gender, male/female	108/62 (64/36)		NA		NA		NA
NSAIDs, yes/no	87/83 (51/49)		56/52 (52/48)		31/31 (50/50)		.816
Biologicals, yes/no	67/103 (39/61)		45/63 (42/58)		22/40 (36/64)		.427
Corticosteroids, yes/no	12/158 (7/93)		6/102 (6/94)		6/56 (10/90)		.313[a]
DMARDs, yes/no	71/99 (42/58)		43/65 (40/60)		28/34 (45/55)		.496
Psychopharmacologic agents, yes/no	12/158 (7/93)		6/102 (6/94)		6/56 (10/90)		.313[a]
Analgesics, yes/no	73/97 (43/57)		33/75 (31/69)		40/22 (65/35)		< .00
Work status, yes/no[b]	99/64 (61/39)		64/38 (63/37)		35/26 (57/43)		.497

Abbreviations: BMI Body mass index, *BASDAI* Bath Ankylosing Spondylitis Disease Activity Index, *BASFI* Bath Ankylosing Spondylitis Functional Index, *BASMI* Bath Ankylosing Spondylitis Metrology Index, *CRP* C-reactive protein, normal value < 5 mg/L, *HADS* Hospital Anxiety and Depression Scale, *NSAIDs* Non-steroidal anti-inflammatory drugs, *DMARDs* Disease-modifying anti-rheumatic drugs, p<.05
[a] p Value based on phi coefficient instead of chi Square test
[b] $n = 163$ (9 males, 2 females missing)

about two and one-half times more likely in women (66.1% [65.6–66.6%], chi-square test, 5.139, $p = .023$; OR, 2.48 [1.17–5.26], $p = .018$). Pain in the cervical spine and head (CX and head) was also common overall (47.6% [47–48.2%]), but not significantly different between men (45.4% [44.8–46.0%]) and women (51.6% [51–52.2%]) ($p > .05$). Isolated occurrence of lumbar (LX only, 21.2% [20.7–21.7%]) and cervical (CX only, 10.6% [10.2–11.0%]) spine pain was common, but not in the thoracic spine (TX only, 2.4 [2.2–2.6%]). Also, no apparent gender differences existed ($p > .05$). Widespread axial pain was moderately prevalent (26.5% [26.0–27.0%]) and about three times more likely in women (38.7% [38.1–39.3%]) than in

men (19.4% [18.9–19.9%]) (chi-square test, 7.511, $p = .006$; OR, 3.33 [1.38–8.02], $p = .007$). Widespread articular peripheral pain also showed a twofold increased likelihood in women (56.5% [55.9–57.1%]) compared with men (40.7% [40.1–41.3%]; chi-square test, 3.908, $p = .048$; OR, 2.34 [1.12–4.88], $p = .023$), whereas for widespread non-articular peripheral pain, statistical significance was not met ($p = .079$). The sum score for axial pain locations (total group mean ± SD, 36.1 ± 21.1; median [IQR], 27.3 [28.4]) was significantly higher in women (mean ± SD, 37.5 ± 20.8; median [IQR], 36.4 [36.4]) than in men (mean ± SD, 28.3 ± 20.7; median [IQR], 27.3 [31.9]; t-test $p = .006$; b = 8.52 [1.42–15.63]; stß = .193; $p = .019$). No

Table 2 Prevalence estimates and gender differences in painful body regions in patients with axial spondyloarthritis ($n = 170$)

Body region	Location numbers	Total group	Males (n = 108)	Females (n = 62)	Chi-square value	p Value	OR[a]	p Value
Leg right	41, 43, 45, 47	11.2 (10.8–11.6)	10.2 (9.9–10.5)	12.9 (12.5–13.3)	0.293	.588	1.35 (0.43–4.30)	.588
Leg left	42, 44, 46, 48	10 (9.7–10.3)	9.3 (9–9.6)	11.3 (10.9–11.7)	0.181	.671	0.77 (0.21–2.77)	.687
SIJ	49, 50	32.9 (32.4–33.4)	26.9 (26.4–27.4)	43.5 (42.9–44.1)	4.971	**.026**	1.76 (0.82–3.81)	.149
LX	47–56	74.7 (74.2–75.2)	69.4 (68.9–69.9)	83.9 (83.5–84.3)	4.338	**.037**	1.74 (0.73–4.14)	.210
TX	57–60	32.4 (31.9–32.9)	25 (24.5–25.5)	45.2 (44.6–45.8)	7.315	**.007**	2.92 (1.30–6.55)	**.009**
CTJ	61–64	47.6 (47–48.2)	48.1 (47.5–48.7)	66.1 (65.6–66.6)	5.139	**.023**	2.48 (1.17–5.26)	**.018**
CX	65, 66	47.6 (47–48.2)	45.4 (44.8–46.0)	51.6 (51–52.2)	0.615	.433	1.55 (0.75–3.23)	.240
CX and head	19–24, 65–68	54.7 (54.1–55.3)	50.9 (50.3–51.5)	61.3 (60.7–61.9)	1.708	.191	1.71 (0.81–3.60)	.159
Sternum	17, 18	20.6 (20.1–21.1)	18.5 (18.1–18.9)	24.2 (23.7–24.7)	0.776	.378	0.98 (0.39–2.48)	.972
LX only	47–56	21.2 (20.7–21.7)	20.4 (19.9–20.9)	22.6 (22.1–23.1)	0.115	.734	0.97 (0.41–2.30)	.944
TX only	57–60	0.6 (1.5–0.7)	0.0 (0.0–0.0)	1.6 (1.5–1.7)	0.102[b]	.186	0.00 (0.00–0.00)	.999
CX only	61–68	10.6 (10.2–11.0)	12.0 (11.5–12.4)	8.1 (7.8–8.4)	0.657	.418	1.02 (0.31–3.34)	.999
Widespread axial pain	47–66[c]	26.5 (26.0–27.0)	19.4 (18.9–19.9)	38.7 (38.1–39.3)	7.511	**.006**	3.33 (1.38–8.02)	**.007**
Widespread peripheral articular pain	1–4, 7, 8, 25, 26, 29, 30, 33–36, 37–40, 43, 44, 73, 74, 77–80	46.5 (45.9–47.1)	40.7 (40.1–41.3)	56.5 (55.9–57.1)	3.908	**.048**	2.34 (1.12–4.88)	**.023**
Widespread peripheral non-articular pain	5, 6, 9–14, 25–28, 31, 32, 41, 42, 45, 46, 69–72, 75, 76	44.7 (44.1–45.3)	39.8 (39.2–40.4)	53.2 (52.6–53.8)	2.866	.090	1.97 (0.93–4.15)	.079

Abbreviations: SIJ Sacroiliac joint, *LX* Lumbar spine, *CX* Cervical spine, *TX* Thoracic spine, *CTJ* Cervicothoracic junction
[a]Multivariate OR ± 95% CI based on logistic regression analysis correcting for age, disease duration, spinal mobility (Bath Ankylosing Spondylitis Metrology Index), disease activity (Bath Ankylosing Spondylitis Disease Activity Index and physician global assessment of disease activity ($n = 146$)
[b]Phi value is given because of low cell frequency (fewer than cases); significant results in bold; $p < .05$
[c] Positive if pain is present in regions 47–56 and 57–60 and in regions 61–64 and 65–66

gender differences were found for articular (total group mean ± SD, 9.2 ± 12.3; median [IQR], 3.8 [15.4]) and non-articular (total group mean ± SD, 7.6 ± 10.0; median [IQR], 4.2 [12.5]) peripheral pain sum scores ($p > .05$).

Within-region prevalence and gender differences in pain locations
Full prevalence data for all 80 pain locations for the total group and per gender are presented in Additional file 2: Table S2 and graphically summarized in Fig. 1. Overall, the dominant axial involvement in axSpA was clearly confirmed for both genders. Of note was a higher prevalence of pain in the anterior right knee (LOC 7, 21.8% [21.3–22.3%]), regardless of gender. In addition to the predominance of regional CX and CTJ pain in women, the within-region results also confirmed the increased lateral spread of pain in the CTJ region in women (LOC 61, 45.2% [44.6–45.8%]; LOC 62, 41.9% [41.3–42.5%]) compared with men (LOC 61, 26.9% [26.4–27.4%]; chi-square test, 5.925, $p = .015$; OR, 2.23 [1.05–4.71], $p = .036$; LOC 62, 24.1% [23.6–24.6%]; chi-square test, 5.918, $p = .015$; OR, 2.48 [1.14–5.42], $p = .023$). A similar effect did not reach significance in the thoracic or lumbar region ($p > .05$).

Relationship of pain regions with disease-related outcomes
Univariate correlations between all variables for the total group and per gender can be found in Additional file 3: Table S3. General linear models (Fig. 2, Additional file 4: Table S4) revealed a graded relationship between subgroups combining non-articular peripheral pain and PGDA with BASFI, BASDAI, TSK-11 and HADS in men ($p < .05$). Of clinical interest was the subgroup of non-articular peripheral pain combined with low PGDA (WNAP+/PGDA–; 27% of all patients) that was associated with worse BASFI, BASDAI, and HADS anxiety and depression in men and worse TSK-11 and HADS anxiety in women ($p < .05$).

Role of pain area in disease activity
Factor analysis revealed a differential role for body regions in the assessment of disease activity (Fig. 3). Axial pain sum score loaded on an axial disease factor together with BASDAI items 1, 2 and 6 to explain 11% of the variance. Non-articular and articular peripheral pain sum score loaded on a peripheral disease activity factor explained 56% of the variance. Importantly, the factor structure did vary between genders with a single- and two-factor solution in men and women, respectively.

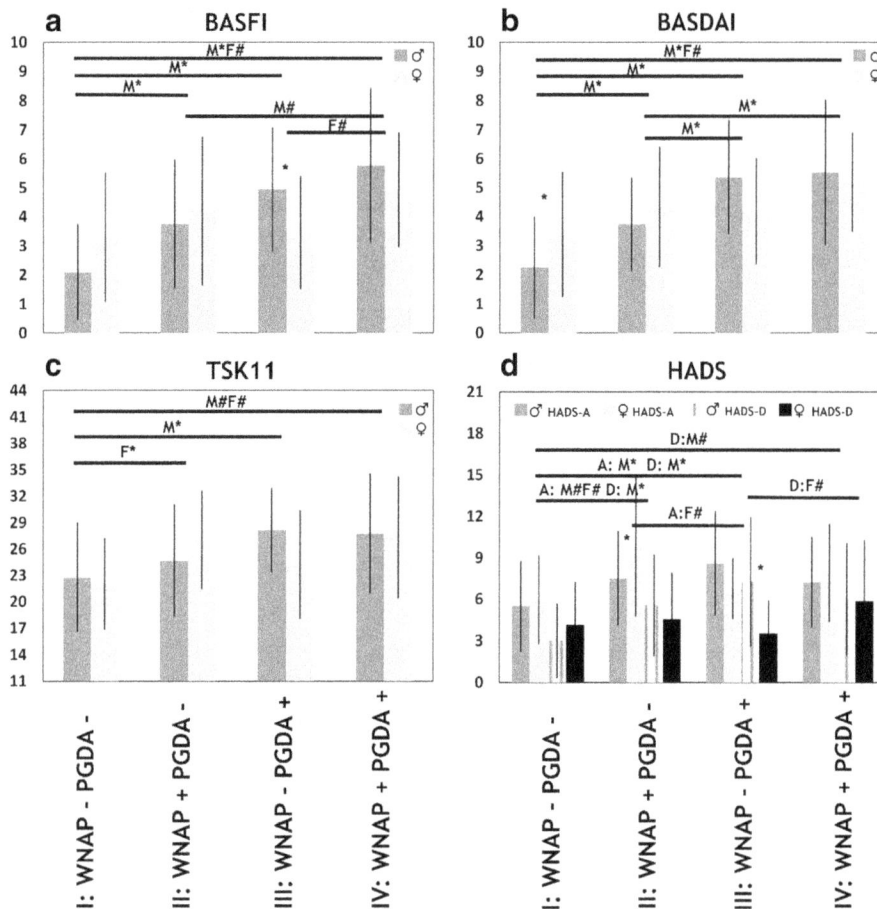

Fig. 2 Clinical subgroups based on the presence or absence of widespread non-articular pain (WNAP) and physician global assessment of disease activity (PGDA) and their relationship with clinical variables (panel **a-d**) in axial spondyloarthritis ($n = 146$). *BASFI* Bath Ankylosing Spondylitis Functional Index (0–10), *BASDAI* Bath Ankylosing Spondylitis Disease Activity Index (0–10), *TSK11* 11-item version of Tampa Scale for Kinesiophobia (11–44), *HADS-D/A* Hospital Anxiety and Depression Scale (HADS) subscale anxiety (A) or depression (D) (0–21), ♂/♀ and *M/F* Male/female, *n* (%) group I: 59 (40), group II: 40 (27), group III: 24 (16), group IV: 23 (16). *,# $p < .05$ indicating significant Bonferroni and uncorrected general linear model results between and within groups per gender, respectively

Discussion

To the best of our knowledge, this was the first study to detail the topography of pain in axSpA and to relate these findings to key clinical outcomes and the structural properties of BASDAI, the most commonly used self-reported method to assess disease activity. In the first part of the study, the prevalence of pain in clinically meaningful body regions was analysed. The observed dominant axial pain involvement likely confirmed axial disease, as enforced by the ASAS axSpA inclusion criteria [19]. The prevalence of pain was highest in the LX region (75%) when compared with the TX (34%), CTJ (48%) and CX (48%) regions. Indeed, the LX region was reported to be the first (LX: 67%, buttock: 40%, TX: 23.3%, CX/CTJ: 11.1%) and dominant (LX, 90%; buttock, 75%; TX, 55%) area affected in a large recent-onset inflammatory back pain cohort [31]. Comparable descriptions of axial pain locations in historic axSpA cohorts do not exist [32]; however, preferential thoracic inflammation and bone formation (thus discrepant with our dominant LX pain symptoms) have been reported [33]. We also found a strikingly low prevalence of unique pain involvement of the LX (20%), TX (1%) and CX (10%) regions. Blachier et al. [34] recently reported a similarly low TX (2%) but contrasting low LX (2%) with high SIJ (25%) prevalence of single inflammatory lesions visualised by magnetic resonance imaging (MRI). The mismatch at the lumbar level in our study can be explained by referral of pain in the LX region owing to SIJ inflammation [29, 35] or common local LX pain with a non-inflammatory origin, a differentiation that needs further study. For the peripheral joints, the more pronounced involvement of the right anterior knee may reflect increased loading of the dominant limb [36] and fits with the proposed link between biomechanics and disease processes in axSpA [37].

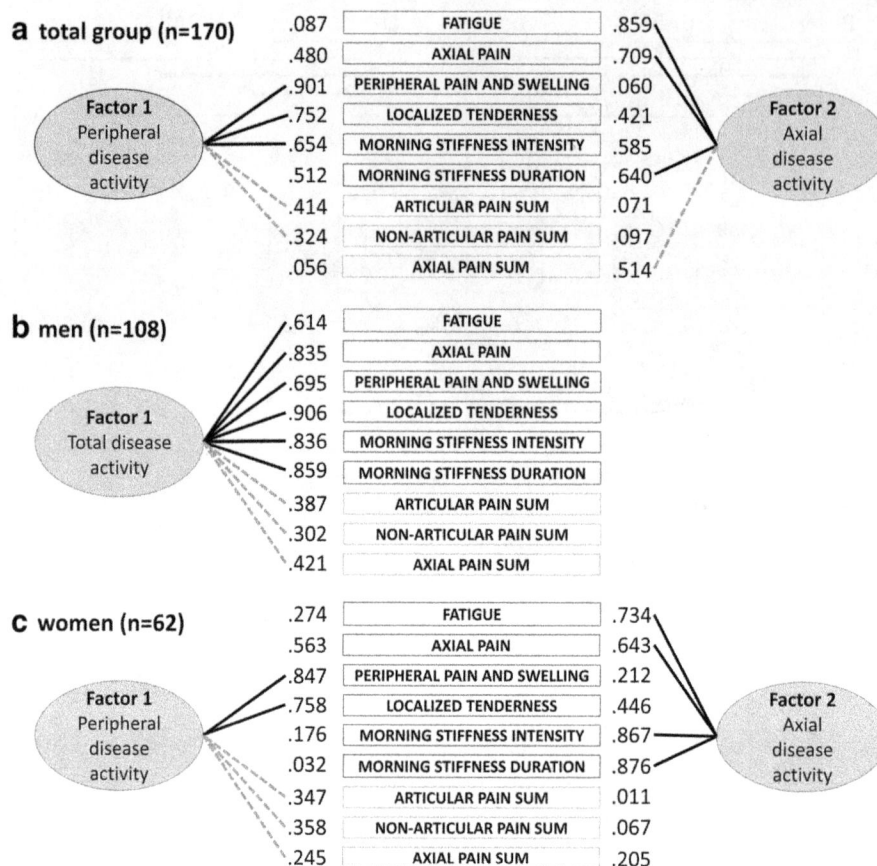

Fig. 3 Graphical illustration of the contribution of each Bath Ankylosing Spondylitis Disease Activity Index item and spinal, articular and non-articular pain sum scores to peripheral and axial disease activity factors* in men and women with axial spondyloarthritis (*n* = 170). BASDAI, Bath Ankylosing Spondylitis Disease Activity Index; (non)-articular and spinal pain sum of pain area estimates were based on body charts (0–100%). * PCA with varimax rotation in the total group (**a**), men (**b**) and women (**c**). Rescaled rotated factor loadings are presented. Level of statistical significance was set at $p < .05$. Lines connect items to the construct they represent. *Solid* or *dashed lines* represent larger (> .60) or smaller (< .60) contributions to the underlying construct, respectively

In the second part of the study, gender comparisons in regional pain prevalence revealed increased pain in the TX and CTJ, but not the CX region, in women. In the absence of other research on this topic, the observed gender differences in thoracic pain represent a novel finding. In contrast, the results of our study for the CTJ region probably coincided with the marked but ill-defined CX involvement in women that has been reported previously in both radiographic [32] and early axSpA cohorts [38]. Interestingly, and unique to this study, further within-region analysis revealed that the lateral spread of CTJ and sternal pain is more prevalent in women. On the basis of previous work on anterior chest pain, researchers have reported rather similar sternal pain occurrence between men and women, but focused on local joint pain only [39, 40].

In the third part of the study, on the widespread nature of pain and its clinical correlates, this cohort showed a fairly high occurrence of widespread spinal pain (27%) and spinal pain sum scores (35%), regardless of disease status and being even more pronounced in women (39% and 38%, respectively). Although rooted in different criteria definitions, these numbers mimic the prevalence of fibromyalgia in women with axSpA (39% versus range 11–34%) typically reported in the literature, but they were higher than expected in men (19% versus range 2–9%) [12, 15, 16, 27]. The latter may indicate incomplete correction for pain caused by partial bone formation via BASMI, a process known to affect the spine more in men [17]. These findings need careful interpretation, however, because multiple mechanisms may lead to a wider spread of spinal pain. Commonly involved anterior (e.g., anterior vertebral corner) versus posterior (e.g., zygapophyseal joint) spinal structures in axSpA have been shown to exhibit multisegmental/bilateral to unisegmental/unilateral innervation, respectively [41]. Consequently, the amount of disease processes, as well as the innervation pattern of the specific local tissues involved, likely results in a variable pain extent via local mechanisms of nociceptor activation and peripheral sensitization (primary hyperalgesia) [29, 35]. Also, central neural plasticity likely augments pain area and intensity in axSpA, especially in women [42], owing to activity- and transcription-dependent long-term potentiation (mono- and heterosynaptic) recruiting nearby receptive fields, a changed neural membrane excitability, the disinhibition of anti-nociceptive and facilitation of pro-nociceptive top-down pathways, all strongly influenced by immune-competent cells such as microglia (secondary hyperalgesia and widespread pain) [13].

To date, researchers in the few preliminary studies on pain physiology in axSpA have reported normal [43] (also in response to anti-TNF treatment [44]) to even elevated [45] pain pressure thresholds compared with control subjects and a moderate relationship with depression [46], non-superiority of algometry over manual palpation in the evaluation of entheseal pain [47] and pain-related brain morphology changes in response to anti-TNF treatment [11, 44], but all studies lacked proper gender comparisons. (For a recent mechanistic overview of gender differences in clinical and experimental non-axSpA pain research, see [42].) The observed increased widespread articular pain and trend for non-articular pain in women have been reported inconsistently in the literature [17, 32] and require a conclusive differentiation of local disease versus pain mechanisms. Further characterisation of the subgroup 'low disease activity but high spread of pain' (PGDA −/WPIP+) in this study, exhibiting a large burden of disease and association with anxiety in both genders and with depression in males, may help in this respect. Future work should concurrently include state-of-the-art assessment of inflammation/bone formation, pain mechanisms (including fibromyalgia criteria), psychosocial variables and clinical outcomes to unravel the spread of pain by gender, especially in clinically relevant subgroups of axSpA.

In the last part of the study, we revealed a two-factor structure of BASDAI that was linked to female gender and suggests the importance of considering axial and peripheral disease activity separately in women. Only one study reported a one-factor structure of BASDAI in both ankylosing spondylitis ($n = 211$, 82% men) and early spondyloarthritis ($n = 86$, 56% men), results that likely diverge from those of our study owing to lesser representation of women and small sample size [48]. Screening existing disease activity instruments in axSpA for gender compatibility is urgently needed. The impact of gender on cut-offs to define disease activity using the recently developed ASDAS in women has been reported [49] and may add to explanation of the lower response to biological therapy in women [50].

This study has a few limitations. First, we corrected all pain area estimates for differences in clinical outcome but were not able to include the ASDAS (missing patient global assessment) or MRI (feasibility and cost) to study local inflammation. In the absence of a gold standard [2], it is a strength, however, that objective and valid surrogate measures PGDA and CRP were included [51]. Similarly, plain radiographs were not available to evaluate bone formation, which was reflected by the reliable and valid BASMI [21]. Second, although this is the largest study reported to date on detailed topographical pain analysis axSpA, it must be recognized that our subgroup analysis is (for sample size reasons) exploratory. As a consequence, relevant differences between subgroups may have been missed. To tackle this power issue, we presented the uncorrected and corrected p values.

Conclusions

This study describes the topography of pain in axSpA in detail. Apart from the dominant axial prevalence of pain, especially in the LX region, women more frequently exhibited TX and CTJ pain with a wider lateral spread, regardless of disease status. Our finding of widespread (non-articular) peripheral pain in combination with low PGDA questions current clinical decision-making using disease activity measures in a subgroup of axSpA. Also, the two-factor structure of disease activity found in women should be considered in the development of outcome instruments in axSpA.

Abbreviations
+/−: Is/is not present; ASAS: Assessment in SpondyloArthritis international Society; ASDAS: Ankylosing Spondylitis Disease Activity Index; axSpA: Axial spondyloarthritis; β: Standardized β-value; b: Unstandardized β-value; BASDAI: Bath Ankylosing Spondylitis Disease Activity Index; BASFI: Bath Ankylosing Spondylitis Functional Index; BASMI: Bath Ankylosing Spondylitis Metrology Index; CRP: C-reactive protein; CTJ: Cervicothoracic junction body region; CX: Cervical body region; DMARDs: Disease-modifying anti-rheumatic drugs; HADS: Hospital Anxiety and Depression Scale; HLA: Human leucocyte antigen; IL: Interleukin; LOC: Body location(s); LX: Lumbar body region; MRI: Magnetic resonance imaging; NSAIDs: Non-steroidal anti-inflammatory drugs; ORs: Odds Ratios; PCA: Principal Component Analysis; PGDA: Physician global assessment of disease activity; SIJ: Sacroiliac joint region; TNF: Tumour necrosis factor; TSK-11: Tampa Scale for Kinesiophobia 11-item version; TX: Thoracic body region; WAP: Widespread peripheral articular; WNAP: Widespread non-articular pain

Acknowledgements
We thank all participants and staff members of UZ Leuven who operationally contributed to this study. In particular, we thank Evelyne Raddoux and Tim Van Rietvelde for their help in scoring the body charts for reliability purposes.

Funding
Funding for this study was provided by the Division of Rheumatology, University Hospitals Leuven, and Fonds voor Wetenschappelijk Reuma Onderzoek (FWRO), Brussels.

Authors' contributions
TWS, RW, WD and KdV were involved in the conception and design of the study; the acquisition, analysis and interpretation of data; and finalizing the manuscript. All authors read and approved the manuscript.

Competing interests

The authors declare that they have no competing interests.

Author details

[1]Division of Rheumatology, University Hospitals Leuven, Herestraat 49, 3000 Leuven, Belgium. [2]Skeletal Biology and Engineering Research Center, Department of Development and Regeneration, KU Leuven, Herestraat 49 box 7003/13, 3000 Leuven, Belgium. [3]Musculoskeletal Rehabilitation Research Unit, Department of Rehabilitation Sciences, KU Leuven, Tervuursevest 101 box 1501, 3001 Leuven, Belgium.

References

1. Pedersen SJ, Poddubnyy D, Sørensen IJ, Loft AG, Hindrup JS, Thamsborg G, et al. Course of magnetic resonance imaging-detected inflammation and structural lesions in the sacroiliac joints of patients in the randomized, double-blind, placebo-controlled Danish multicenter study of adalimumab in spondyloarthritis, as assessed by the Berlin and Spondyloarthritis Research Consortium of Canada methods. Arthritis Rheumatol. 2016;68(2):418–29.
2. Sieper J, Rudwaleit M, Baraliakos X, Brandt J, Braun J, Burgos-Vargas R, et al. The Assessment of SpondyloArthritis international Society (ASAS) handbook: a guide to assess spondyloarthritis. Ann Rheum Dis. 2009;68(Suppl 2):ii1–44.
3. Maksymowych WP, Crowther SM, Dhillon SS, Conner-Spady B, Lambert RG. Systematic assessment of inflammation by magnetic resonance imaging in the posterior elements of the spine in ankylosing spondylitis. Arthritis Care Res (Hoboken). 2010;62(1):4–10.
4. Jacques P, McGonagle D. The role of mechanical stress in the pathogenesis of spondyloarthritis and how to combat it. Best Pract Res Clin Rheumatol. 2014;28(5):703–10.
5. Tito RY, Cypers H, Joossens M, Varkas G, Van Praet L, Glorieus E, et al. Dialister as a microbial marker of disease activity in spondyloarthritis. Arthritis Rheumatol. 2017;69(1):114–21.
6. Venken K, Elewaut D. New immune cells in spondyloarthritis: key players or innocent bystanders? Best Pract Res Clin Rheumatol. 2015;29(6):706–14.
7. Ambarus C, Yeremenko N, Tak PP, Baeten D. Pathogenesis of spondyloarthritis: autoimmune or autoinflammatory? Curr Opin Rheumatol. 2012;24(4):351–8.
8. Woolf CJ. What is this thing called pain? J Clin Invest. 2010;120(11):3742–4.
9. Hodges PW, Smeets RJ. Interaction between pain, movement, and physical activity: short-term benefits, long-term consequences, and targets for treatment. Clin J Pain. 2015;31(2):97–107.
10. Rudwaleit M, Metter A, Listing J, Sieper J, Braun J. Inflammatory back pain in ankylosing spondylitis: a reassessment of the clinical history for application as classification and diagnostic criteria. Arthritis Rheum. 2006;54(2):569–78.
11. Wu Q, Inman RD, Davis KD. Neuropathic pain in ankylosing spondylitis: a psychophysics and brain imaging study. Arthritis Rheum. 2013;65(6):1494–503.
12. Salaffi F, De Angelis R, Carotti M, Gutierrez M, Sarzi-Puttini F, Atzeni F. Fibromyalgia in patients with axial spondyloarthritis: epidemiological profile and effect on measures of disease activity. Rheumatol Int. 2014;34(8):1103–10.
13. Latremoliere A, Woolf CJ. Central sensitization: a generator of pain hypersensitivity by central neural plasticity. J Pain. 2009;10(9):895–926.
14. Brionez TF, Assassi S, Reveille JD, Green C, Learch T, Diekman L, et al. Psychological correlates of self-reported disease activity in ankylosing spondylitis. J Rheumatol. 2010;37(4):829–34.
15. Almodovar R, Carmona L, Zarco P, Collantes E, Gonzalez C, Mulero J, et al. Fibromyalgia in patients with ankylosing spondylitis: prevalence and utility of the measures of activity, function and radiological damage. Clin Exp Rheumatol. 2010;28(6 Suppl 63):S33–9.
16. Azevedo VF, Paiva Edos S, Felippe LR, Moreira RA. Occurrence of fibromyalgia in patients with ankylosing spondylitis. Rev Bras Reumatol. 2010;50(6):646–50.
17. Webers C, Essers I, Ramiro S, Stolwijk C, Landewé R, van der Heijde D, et al. Gender-attributable differences in outcome of ankylosing spondylitis: long-term results from the Outcome in Ankylosing Spondylitis International Study. Rheumatology (Oxford). 2016;55(3):419–28.
18. Ramiro S, van Tubergen A, Stolwijk C, van der Heijde D, Royston P, Landewé R. Reference intervals of spinal mobility measures in normal individuals: the MOBILITY study. Ann Rheum Dis. 2015;74(6):1218–24.
19. Sieper J, van der Heijde D, Landewé R, Brandt J, Burgos-Vagas R, Collantes-Estevez E, et al. New criteria for inflammatory back pain in patients with chronic back pain: a real patient exercise by experts from the Assessment of SpondyloArthritis international Society (ASAS). Ann Rheum Dis. 2009;68(6):784–8.
20. Calin A, Garrett S, Whitelock H, Kennedy LG, O'Hea J, Mallorie P, et al. A new approach to defining functional ability in ankylosing spondylitis: the development of the Bath Ankylosing Spondylitis Functional Index. J Rheumatol. 1994;21(12):2281–5.
21. Castro MP, Stebbings SM, Milosavljevic S, Bussey MD. Construct validity of clinical spinal mobility tests in ankylosing spondylitis: a systematic review and meta-analysis. Clin Rheumatol. 2016;35(7):1777–87.
22. Jenkinson TR, Mallorie PA, Whitelock HC, Kennedy LG, Garrett SL, Calin A. Defining spinal mobility in ankylosing spondylitis (AS): the Bath AS Metrology Index. Index J Rheumatol. 1994;21(9):1694–8.
23. Roelofs J, van Breukelen G, Sluiter J, Frings-Dresen MH, Goossens M, Thibault P, et al. Norming of the Tampa Scale for Kinesiophobia across pain diagnoses and various countries. Pain. 2011;152(5):1090–5.
24. Swinnen TW, Vlaeyen JWS, Dankaerts W, Westhovens R, de Vlam K. Activity limitations in patients with axial spondyloarthritis: a role for fear of movement and (re)injury beliefs. J Rheumatol. 2018;45(3):357–66.
25. Chan CY, Tsang HHL, Lau CS, Chung HY. Prevalence of depressive and anxiety disorders and validation of the Hospital Anxiety and Depression Scale as a screening tool in axial spondyloarthritis patients. Int J Rheum Dis. 2017;20(3):317–25.
26. Mease PJ, Goffe BS, Metz J, VanderStoep A, Finck B, Burge DJ. Etanercept in the treatment of psoriatic arthritis and psoriasis: a randomised trial. Lancet. 2000;356(9227):385–90.
27. Wolfe F, Clauw DJ, Fitzcharles MA, Goldenberg DL, Katz RS, Mease P, et al. The American College of Rheumatology preliminary diagnostic criteria for fibromyalgia and measurement of symptom severity. Arthritis Care Res (Hoboken). 2010;62(5):600–10.
28. International Association for the Study of Pain (IASP). Classification of Chronic Pain, Second Edition (Revised). http://www.iasp-pain.org/PublicationsNews/Content.aspx?ItemNumber=1673&navItemNumber=677. Accessed 4 Oct 2017.
29. Slipman CW, Jackson HB, Lipetz JS, Chan KT, Lenrow D, Vresilovic EJ. Sacroiliac joint pain referral zones. Arch Phys Med Rehabil. 2000;81(3):334–8.
30. Landis JR, Koch GG. The measurement of observer agreement for categorical data. Biometrics. 1977;33(1):159–74.
31. Dougados M, Etcheto A, Molto A, Alonso S, Bouvet S, Daures JP, et al. Clinical presentation of patients suffering from recent onset chronic inflammatory back pain suggestive of spondyloarthritis: the DESIR cohort. Joint Bone Spine. 2015;82(5):345–51.
32. Lee W, Reveille JD, Davis JC Jr, Learch TJ, Ward MM, Weisman MH. Are there gender differences in severity of ankylosing spondylitis? Results from the PSOAS cohort. Ann Rheum Dis. 2007;66(5):633–8.
33. Baraliakos X, Landewé R, Hermann KG, Listing J, Golder W, Brandt J, et al. Inflammation in ankylosing spondylitis: a systematic description of the extent and frequency of acute spinal changes using magnetic resonance imaging. Ann Rheum Dis. 2005;64(5):730–4.
34. Blachier M, Coutanceau B, Dougados M, Saraux A, Bastuji-Garin S, Ferkal S, et al. Does the site of magnetic resonance imaging abnormalities match the site of recent-onset inflammatory back pain? The DESIR cohort. Ann Rheum Dis. 2013;72(6):979–85.
35. Szadek KM, Hoogland PV, Zuurmond WW, de Lange JJ, Perez RS. Nociceptive nerve fibers in the sacroiliac joint in humans. Reg Anesth Pain Med. 2008;33(1):36–43.
36. Ford KR, Myer GD, Hewett TE. Valgus knee motion during landing in high school female and male basketball players. Med Sci Sports Exerc. 2003;35(10):1745–50.
37. Jacques P, Lambrecht S, Verheugen E, Pauwels E, Kollias G, Armaka M, et al. Proof of concept: enthesitis and new bone formation in spondyloarthritis are driven by mechanical strain and stromal cells. Ann Rheum Dis. 2014;73(2):437–45.
38. Tournadre A, Pereira B, Lhoste A, Dubost JJ, Ristori JM, Claudepierre P, et al. Differences between women and men with recent-onset axial spondyloarthritis: results from a prospective multicenter French cohort. Arthritis Care Res (Hoboken). 2013;65(9):1482–9.
39. Ramonda R, Lorenzin M, Lo Nigro A, Vio S, Zucchetta P, Frallonardo P, et al. Anterior chest wall involvement in early stages of spondyloarthritis: advanced diagnostic tools. J Rheumatol. 2012;39(9):1844–9.

40. Wendling D, Prati C, Demattei C, Loeuille D, Richette P, Dougados M. Anterior chest wall pain in recent inflammatory back pain suggestive of spondyloarthritis: data from the DESIR cohort. J Rheumatol. 2013;40(7):1148–52.

41. Bogduk N. The innervation of the lumbar spine. Spine (Phila Pa 1976). 1983; 8(3):286–93.

42. Fillingim RB, King CD, Ribeiro-Dasilva MC, Rahim-Williams B, Riley JL 3rd. Sex, gender, and pain: a review of recent clinical and experimental findings. J Pain. 2009;10(5):447–85.

43. Incel NA, Erdem HR, Ozgocmen S, Catal SA, Yorgancioglu ZR. Pain pressure threshold values in ankylosing spondylitis. Rheumatol Int. 2002;22(4):148–50.

44. Wu Q, Inman RD, Davis KD. Tumor necrosis factor inhibitor therapy in ankylosing spondylitis: differential effects on pain and fatigue and brain correlates. Pain. 2015;156(2):297–304.

45. Gerecz-Simon EM, Tunks ER, Heale JA, Kean WF, Buchanan WW. Measurement of pain threshold in patients with rheumatoid arthritis, osteoarthritis, ankylosing spondylitis and healthy controls. Clin Rheumatol. 1989;8(4):467–74.

46. Bagnato G, De Andres I, Sorbara S, Verduci E, Corallo G, Ferrera A, et al. Pain threshold and intensity in rheumatic patients: correlations with the Hamilton Depression Rating Scale. Clin Rheumatol. 2015;34(3):555–61.

47. Kaya A, Ozgocmen S, Kamanli A, Aydogan R, Yildirim A, Ardicoglu O. Evaluation of a quantitative scoring of enthesitis in ankylosing spondylitis. J Clin Rheumatol. 2007;13(6):303–6.

48. Bönisch A, Ehlebracht-König I. The BASDAI-D – an instrument to defining disease status in ankylosing spondylitis and related diseases [in German]. Z Rheumatol. 2003;62(3):251–63.

49. Kilic E, Kilic G, Akgul O, Ozgocmen S. Discriminant validity of the Ankylosing Spondylitis Disease Activity Score (ASDAS) in patients with non-radiographic axial spondyloarthritis and ankylosing spondylitis: a cohort study. Rheumatol Int. 2015;35(6):981–9.

50. van der Horst-Bruinsma IE, Zack DJ, Szumski A, Koenig AS. Female patients with ankylosing spondylitis: analysis of the impact of gender across treatment studies. Ann Rheum Dis. 2013;72(7):1221–4.

51. Fernandez-Espartero C, de Miguel E, Loza E, Tomero E, Gobbo M, Descalzo MA, et al. Validity of the ankylosing spondylitis disease activity score (ASDAS) in patients with early spondyloarthritis from the Esperanza programme. Ann Rheum Dis. 2014;73(7):1350–5.

2

Comparative effectiveness of allopurinol versus febuxostat for preventing incident dementia in older adults: a propensity-matched analysis

Jasvinder A. Singh[1,2,3,4]* (iD) and John D. Cleveland[2]

Abstract

Background: The purpose of this study was to assess the comparative effectiveness of allopurinol versus febuxostat for preventing incident dementia in older adults.

Methods: In a retrospective cohort study using Medicare claims data, we included patients newly treated with allopurinol or febuxostat (baseline period of 365 days without either medication). We used 5:1 propensity-matched Cox regression analyses to compare the hazard ratio (HR) of incident dementia with allopurinol versus febuxostat use and with allopurinol/febuxostat dose and duration.

Results: Crude rates of incident dementia per 100,000 person-days were lower with higher daily dose: allopurinol less than 200, 200 to 299, and at least 300 mg/day with 12, 9, and 8 and febuxostat 40 and 80 mg/day with 9 and 8, respectively. In propensity-matched analyses, compared with allopurinol use, febuxostat use was not significantly different, and the HR of incident dementia was 0.79 (95% confidence interval (CI) 0.61, 1.03). Compared with allopurinol less than 200 mg/day, higher allopurinol doses (200 to 299 and at least 300 mg/day) and the febuxostat 40 mg/day dose were each associated with lower HRs of dementia: 0.80 (95% CI 0.64, 0.98), 0.59 (95% CI 0.50, 0.71), and 0.64 (95% CI 0.47, 0.86), respectively. Compared with allopurinol use for 1 to 180 days, longer allopurinol or febuxostat use durations were not significantly associated with differences in HR of dementia (range of 0.76 to 1.14).

Conclusions: A dose-related reduction in the risk of dementia in older adults was noted with higher allopurinol dose and with febuxostat 40 mg daily dose. Future studies need to examine the mechanism of this benefit.

Keywords: Allopurinol, Febuxostat, Dementia, Older adults, Elderly, Medicare

Background

The association of uric acid levels and dementia is an emerging area of interest. An important unanswered question is whether urate-lowering therapy (ULT) use affects the risk of dementia. We recently showed that, compared with non-use, use allopurinol or febuxostat (the most commonly used ULTs) was not associated with any increase in the risk of dementia in older adults [1]. Important study limitations were that dose and duration

were not examined and that allopurinol and febuxostat were not compared with each other. Allopurinol is a purine analog that non-selectively inhibits the xanthine oxido-reductase (XOR) system and other enzymes in purine and pyrimidine pathways, whereas febuxostat is a non-purine analog that selectively inhibits XOR [2]. XOR exists as xanthine oxidase (XO) or xanthine dehydrogenase (XDH) [3]. The XOR system catalyzes the two terminal reactions of purine metabolism in humans, the conversion of hypoxanthine into xanthine and xanthine into uric acid. The conversion of hypoxanthine into uric acid by XOR leads to the formation of super-oxide species that increases oxidative stress. Additionally, uric acid has both a pro-oxidant action [4, 5] and

* Correspondence: jassingh@uab.edu
[1]Medicine Service, VA Medical Center, 510, 20th Street South, FOT 805B, Birmingham, AL 35233, USA
[2]Department of Medicine at School of Medicine, University of Alabama at Birmingham, 20th Street South, FOT 805B, Birmingham, AL 35294-0022, USA
Full list of author information is available at the end of the article

an anti-oxidant action [6, 7] and is potentially neuroprotective based on its anti-oxidant effect. Thus, hyperuricemia may be associated with oxidative stress, which is implicated in the pathogenesis of dementia [8–10]. Allopurinol or febuxostat potentially reduces the risk of dementia by inhibiting XOR and reducing uric acid production; given its non-selective inhibition of other purine and pyrimidine pathways, allopurinol may differ in effect from febuxostat [2].

Dementia, characterized by progressive deterioration of cognitive ability and function, is a common disease of older adults and for the first time has replaced ischemic heart disease as the leading cause of death in England and Wales [11]. An estimated 36 million people worldwide had dementia in 2010, and the number is expected to double to 66 million by 2030 and quadruple to 115 million by 2050 [12]. Worldwide, the total estimated costs of dementia were USD $604 billion in 2010 [13] and were likely much higher recently [14]. Dementia is associated with the loss of independence and increased morbidity and mortality [15, 16]. Therefore, dementia is a significant public health problem of increasing impact.

A few studies showed that hyperuricemia was associated with a better cognition and a lower risk of dementia [17–19], whereas other studies showed an opposite effect [20–25]; that is, hyperuricemia was a risk factor for dementia. The 2016 European League Against Rheumatism (EULAR) treatment guideline for gout [26] cautioned against long-term lowering of serum urate of less than 3 mg/dL because of a potential risk of adverse neurologic outcome. This was based on low-quality evidence, mainly from studies in neurological conditions other than dementia. In contrast, a large French population-based study showed that hyperuricemia was associated with a higher risk of dementia in older adults [27]. Thus, robust studies are needed for a better understanding of this relationship. One way to examine the potential relationship or hyperuricemia with the risk of dementia, is to examine whether the use of ULT, or ULT dose or duration of use are associated with a reduced risk of dementia in older adults.

We hypothesized that in older adults (65 years or older; population at risk), ULT type, dose, and duration would be associated with the risk of dementia. Specifically, we assessed the hypotheses of whether (1) febuxostat is more effective than allopurinol in preventing dementia and (2) higher doses and longer duration of allopurinol or febuxostat use are associated with a greater risk reduction of dementia than lower doses or shorter use duration.

Methods
Study cohort
This is a retrospective cohort study of Medicare beneficiaries from 2006 to 2012. We examined the 5% random Medicare sample that contains all insurance claims for each beneficiary and has been widely used for epidemiological research. We obtained the data from the Centers for Medicare and Medicaid Services (CMS) Chronic Condition Data Warehouse. We abstracted data from the following files for each beneficiary: (1) a beneficiary summary file: demographics, including birthdate, death date, sex, and race, and monthly entitlement indicators (A/B/C/D); (2) part D file: prescription claims, dose, supply, and drug name; and (3) inpatient and outpatient claim files: diagnosis codes for each claim and claim dates. The Medicare beneficiaries were eligible for this study if they (1) were enrolled in Medicare fee-for-service with pharmacy coverage (parts A, B, and D) and not enrolled in a Medicare Advantage Plan, (2) resided in the US from 2006 to 2012, and (3) received new treatment with allopurinol or febuxostat, defined as any new filled prescription of allopurinol (or febuxostat) with a clean baseline period of 365 days without any allopurinol (or febuxostat) filled prescription (details in a section below). The institutional review board of the University of Alabama at Birmingham approved the study and waived the requirement for informed consent for this database study. Methods and results are being reported as recommended in the STROBE (Strengthening of Reporting in Observational studies in Epidemiology) statement.

Exposure of interest: new treatment with allopurinol or febuxostat
A beneficiary began a new allopurinol (or febuxostat) treatment episode by filling an allopurinol prescription provided that they had not filled an allopurinol (or febuxostat) prescription in the previous 365 days. We assigned days of exposure for each allopurinol (or febuxostat) treatment episode, calculated on the basis of the days' supply variable provided in the Medicare Part D file and included a 30-day residual period. Continuous allopurinol (or febuxostat) episode ended after 30 days of the end of allopurinol (or febuxostat) exposure. If there were more than 30 days between prescription fills, a new allopurinol (or febuxostat) exposure started. If a patient had prescriptions for both drugs, then they were considered exposed to the one that was prescribed second; for example, if a patient was taking allopurinol and got a new prescription of febuxostat, then he or she was considered to be on febuxostat only as of the febuxostat fill date.

If a patient received a 90-day supply of allopurinol (or febuxostat), then we considered them exposed for 120 days: 90 days of supply plus 30 days of residual period. We included a 30-day residual period to capture imperfect medication adherence and to account for any residual protective biological effects related to the medication itself. If the patient switched medications (allopurinol to febuxostat or vice versa), the 30-day latency did not apply and they were immediately classified as exposed to the new medication only. This was done since the ULTs achieve significant blood and tissue concentrations soon after initiation.

The main predictor of interest was febuxostat use, and allopurinol use was the reference category. We assessed all allopurinol doses (200 to 299 and at least 300 mg/day) and febuxostat dose (40 and 80 mg/day), and allopurinol less than 200 mg/day was the reference category. We calculated the daily allopurinol (or febuxostat) dose as the mean daily use for each continuous allopurinol (or febuxostat) episode. For each allopurinol (or febuxostat) treatment episode, we categorized the duration of use as 1 to 180 days, 181 to 365 days, and more than 1 year. Subjects contributed to the "none" category during periods in which they were not in an allopurinol or febuxostat treatment episode.

Study outcome

The outcome of interest for our study was incident dementia, identified by the occurrence of a new diagnostic code for dementia with an absence of any prior diagnostic code in a 183-day baseline period before allopurinol or febuxostat initiation. We used the International Classification of Diseases, ninth revision, common modification (ICD-9-CM) code, 290.xx, 294.1x, or 331.2, for assessing dementia, as in the Quan-Charlson index [28], a validated and commonly used comorbidity index. These ICD-9-CM codes were shown to have high accuracy in the Medicare claims data [29], are valid for identifying patients with dementia with positive and negative predictive values of 96% and 98% (respectively) and specificity of 100% [30], and have been used in other studies to identify cohorts of dementia [31].

Covariates

We assessed several important covariates, including patient demographics, medical comorbidity, and the use of medications for cardiovascular diseases for the baseline period for each episode, obtained from the Medicare denominator and other claims files. Biological variables such as age, sex, and race/ethnicity were included, as were cardiovascular medications and the Charlson-Romano comorbidity index score, a validated comorbidity index developed for claims data analysis [32]. The Charlson-Romano comorbidity index is an adaptation of the Charlson index, the most commonly used comorbidity index in research studies. It is a weighted index that includes comorbidities such as diabetes, myocardial infarction, congestive heart failure, cerebrovascular disease, liver disease, pulmonary disease, peripheral vascular disease, and rheumatic disease. We included statins, beta-blockers, diuretics, and angiotensin-converting enzyme (ACE) inhibitors since these cardiovascular medications (as markers of active cardiovascular disease or by an independent effect), coronary artery disease (CAD), and risk factors for CAD (tobacco use disorder, hyperlipidemia, and hypertension) might impact the risk of dementia.

Statistical analyses

We compared baseline characteristics of episodes with versus without incident dementia and calculated crude incidence rates of incident dementia for new allopurinol (or febuxostat) episodes. For comparative efficacy of allopurinol versus febuxostat, we performed propensity score–matched (matched 5:1 on propensity score) Cox proportional hazard regression analyses to control for differences between patients exposed to allopurinol versus febuxostat. Propensity matching included age, sex, race, Charlson-Romano comorbidity score, region, each Charlson-Romano comorbidity, risk factors for CAD, and the use of medications for cardiovascular diseases (statins, beta-blockers, diuretics, and ACE inhibitors). The analyses for allopurinol and febuxostat daily dose used allopurinol less than 200 mg daily dose as the reference category, and the analyses for allopurinol and febuxostat use duration considered allopurinol use of 1 to 180 days as the reference category.

We used multivariable-adjusted Cox proportional hazard regression models and Huber-White "Sandwich" variance estimator to account for correlations between observations from the same patient [33] and calculated the hazard ratio (HR) of incident dementia for febuxostat use versus allopurinol use (reference category). We conducted additional sensitivity analyses to test the robustness of findings by repeating the propensity-matched analyses only in patients with gout.

Results

Patient characteristics and crude rates in patients receiving allopurinol or febuxostat

We found 42,704 new allopurinol or febuxostat treatment episodes in 35,030 patients, and 2591 of these episodes ended in incident dementia (Fig. 1). Compared with patients with no dementia, patients with a new diagnosis of dementia were older, more likely to be female, White, and living in the South and had a higher Charlson-Romano comorbidity index (Table 1). The crude incidence of dementia in people with allopurinol use, or febuxostat use was 10 and 9 per 100,000 person-days, respectively (Table 2). The crude incidence of dementia by daily ULT dose was as follows: allopurinol less than 200 mg, 200 to 299 mg, and at least 300 mg daily: 12, 9, and 8 per 100,000 person-days; and febuxostat 40 and 80 mg daily, 9 and 8 per 100,000 person-days (Table 2). The mean study follow-up time was 922.5 days, and 86.1% of the people receiving the allopurinol or febuxostat prescription (36,760 out of 42,704) had gout.

Propensity-matched analysis of allopurinol or febuxostat use: risk of dementia

Most of the significant differences noted between allopurinol and febuxostat users before propensity matching (Additional file 1) were eliminated and reduced to

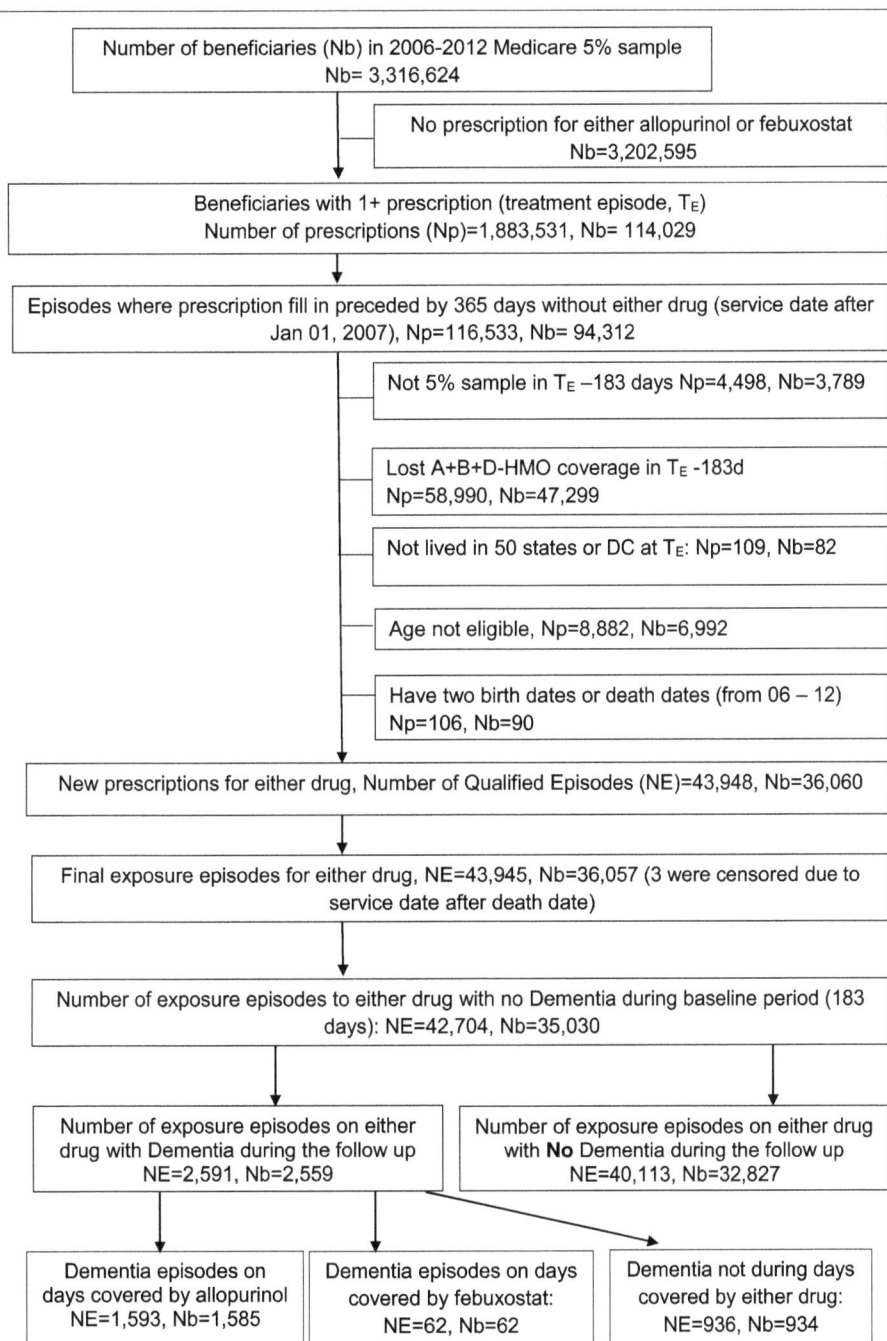

Fig. 1 Patient selection flow chart. The flow chart shows the selection of new allopurinol exposure episodes after applying all the eligibility criteria, including the absence of any allopurinol or febuxostat filled prescription in the baseline period of 365 days (new user design) and an absence of dementia. We found 42,704 new allopurinol or febuxostat exposure episodes in 35,030 patients. Of these, 2591 ended in incident dementia and 40,113 ended without incident dementia. *We followed each eligible patient with a new filled allopurinol or febuxostat prescription until the patient lost full Medicare coverage, had dementia (the outcome of interest), died, or reached the each of the study period on December 31, 2012, whichever came first. For some of these patients, dementia occurred on days covered by allopurinol exposure ($n = 1593$) or febuxostat exposure ($n = 62$), yet other patients had periods of no allopurinol or febuxostat use after an initial qualifying prescription during which dementia occurred ($n = 936$ exposure episodes). Abbreviations: *Nb* number of beneficiaries; *NE* number of qualified episodes of new allopurinol or febuxostat prescriptions, *Np* number of allopurinol or febuxostat prescriptions; T_E treatment episodes

Table 1 Demographic and clinical characteristics of all new episodes* of allopurinol or febuxostat use

| | All episodes | Incident dementia* during the follow-up | | P value |
		Yes	No	
Total, N (episodes)	42,704	2591	40,113	
Age in years, mean (SD)	76.0 (7.38)	80.8 (7.36)	75.7 (7.27)	< 0.0001
Sex, N (%)				< 0.0001
Male	22,125 (51.8%)	1099 (42.4%)	21,026 (52.4%)	
Female	20,579 (48.2%)	1492 (57.6%)	19,087 (47.6%)	
Race/Ethnicity, N (%)				< 0.0001
White	33,409 (78.2%)	1975 (76.2%)	31,434 (78.4%)	
Black	5317 (12.5%)	391 (15.1%)	4926 (12.3%)	
Hispanic	898 (2.1%)	65 (2.5%)	833 (2.1%)	
Asian	2073 (4.9%)	118 (4.6%)	1955 (4.9%)	
Native American	129 (0.3%)	10 (0.4%)	119 (0.3%)	
Other/unknown	878 (1.3%)	32 (1.2%)	846 (2.1%)	
Region, N (%)				< 0.0001
Midwest	10,488 (24.6%)	582 (22.5%)	9906 (24.7%)	
Northeast	6901 (16.2%)	526 (20.3%)	6375 (15.9%)	
South	17,351 (40.6%)	1081 (41.7%)	16,270 (40.6%)	
West	7964 (18.6%)	402 (15.5%)	7562 (18.9%)	
Charlson-Romano comorbidity score, mean (SD)	1.77 (2.09)	2.31 (2.26)	1.74 (2.08)	< 0.0001

Abbreviation: *SD* standard deviation
*Baseline period of 365 days without allopurinol or febuxostat use and without dementia

Table 2 Crude incidence rate of dementia with allopurinol versus febuxostat exposure

	Person-days of follow-up	Number of cases of incident dementia	Dementia incidence rate per 100,000 person-days
Allopurinol	16,999,091	1593	10
Febuxostat	774,291	62	9
Allopurinol duration			
1–180 days	7,775,101	834	11
181–365 days	3,311,650	286	9
>1 year	5,912,340	473	9
Febuxostat duration			
1–180 days	435,872	35	9
181–365 days	167,335	14	9
>1 year	171,084	13	8
Allopurinol dose			
< 200 mg/day	7,701,139	899	12
200–299 mg/day	3,091,767	251	9
≥300 mg/day	6,206,185	443	8
Febuxostat dose			
40 mg/day	634,925	51	9
80 mg/day	139,366	11	8

*Drug exposure considered up to 30 days after last day of medication fill/refill (except when switched to the other ULT, i.e., switched from allopurinol to febuxostat or vice versa); baseline period was 365 days, that is, each new exposure was defined as no previous exposure (allopurinol or febuxostat) in the baseline period

non-significant differences in 5:1 propensity-matched cohorts (Additional file 1). In propensity-matched analyses with 12,135 episodes of exposure to allopurinol and 2427 episodes of febuxostat exposure (5:1 matching), compared with allopurinol use (all doses), febuxostat use (all doses) was not significantly different regarding the risk of incident dementia, and the HR was 0.79 (95% confidence interval (CI) 0.61, 1.03) (Table 3). Compared with allopurinol less than 200 mg/day, higher allopurinol doses (200 to 299 mg/day and at least 300 mg/day) and febuxostat 40 mg/day dose were each associated with significantly lower HRs of dementia: 0.80 (95% CI 0.64, 0.98), 0.59 (95% CI 0.50, 0.71), and 0.64 (95% CI 0.47, 0.86), respectively (Table 3); febuxostat 80 mg/day was not significantly different, and the HR was 0.66 (95% CI 0.36, 1.19). Compared with allopurinol use of 1 to 180 days, longer febuxostat or allopurinol use durations were not significantly associated with differences in HR of dementia, which ranged from 0.76 to 1.14 (Table 3). Sensitivity analyses limited to patients with gout confirmed all the findings above, and there was minimal attenuation of HRs and no change in statistical significance (Additional file 2).

Discussion

In this study of Americans who were at least 65 years old, higher doses of allopurinol and febuxostat 40 mg/

Table 3 Propensity-score adjusted association of allopurinol or febuxostat with the hazard of incident dementia in patients who received allopurinol or febuxostat with a clean baseline period of 365 days*

	Hazard ratio (95% CI)	P value
Allopurinol	Ref	
Febuxostat	0.79 (0.61, 1.03)	0.09
Urate-lowering therapy (ULT) dose		
Allopurinol <200 mg/day	Ref	
Allopurinol 200–299 mg/day	**0.80 (0.64, 0.98)**	**0.03**
Allopurinol ≥300 mg/day	**0.59 (0.50, 0.71)**	**<0.0001**
Febuxostat 40 mg/day	**0.64 (0.47, 0.86)**	**0.003**
Febuxostat 80 mg/day	0.66 (0.36, 1.19)	0.17
ULT duration		
Allopurinol, 1–180 days	Ref	
Allopurinol, 181–365 days	1.14 (0.86, 1.53)	0.36
Allopurinol, >1 year	1.12 (0.84, 1.49)	0.46
Febuxostat, 1–180 days	0.76 (0.53, 1.08)	0.13
Febuxostat, 181–365 days	1.09 (0.61, 1.94)	0.77
Febuxostat, >1 year	0.82 (0.44, 1.53)	0.54

Abbreviations: *CI* confidence interval, *Ref* referent category.
*Baseline period of 365 days without allopurinol or febuxostat use and without any diagnosis of dementia; A bold font indicates associations that are statistically significant with a p-value <0.05

day, compared with low-dose allopurinol (<200 mg/day), were associated with a lower hazard of incident dementia. Compared with allopurinol use duration of 1 to 180 days, longer durations of allopurinol or febuxostat use were not associated with significant reductions of hazard of dementia. Overall, febuxostat did not differ from allopurinol in reducing the risk of dementia. All of our findings were reproduced in propensity-matched analyses limited to people with gout, and there was minimal attenuation of HRs and no change in significance. Since we were inherently interested in examining comparative effectiveness of allopurinol versus febuxostat in people with gout, we did not include gout in propensity matching. Nevertheless, sensitivity analyses performed in people with gout to address this issue essentially reproduced the main findings, as expected. These findings indirectly support and extend the findings of studies that have shown that hyperuricemia is associated with a higher risk of dementia [20–25], including a recent large population-based study [27], although some studies do not agree [17–19]. The existing controversy related to hyperuricemia and the risk of dementia [34] and the lack of studies of ULT led us to assess the comparative efficacy of allopurinol and febuxostat for preventing dementia. Several findings from our study merit further discussion.

Only one previous Taiwanese study reported that, compared with patients without gout, patients with gout receiving ULT had much lower odds of dementia, 0.71 (95% CI 0.65, 0.78), while untreated gout patients did not differ, 0.97 (95% CI 0.87, 1.09) [17]. This indicated a potential beneficial effect related to ULT use, but the evidence was indirect at best. We found that, compared with allopurinol less than 200 mg/day, allopurinol 200 to 299 and at least 300 mg/day were associated with 20% and 41% reductions (respectively) in the hazard of dementia. High-dose allopurinol reduces vascular oxidative stress significantly more than the conventional doses [35, 36], which supports this finding. Allopurinol inactivates XOR and, at high concentrations, can scavenge hydroxyl radicals [37]. Febuxostat, the new XOR inhibitor, also has oxidative stress reduction properties [38, 39]. Evidence has linked oxidative stress and mitochondrial dysfunction [8–10] to neurodegenerative processes in dementia. Oxidative damage to mitochondrial DNA demonstrates an age-dependent increase in human brain [40]. Animal studies also showed that associated oxidative damage in brain [41] and upregulation of genes relating to mitochondrial metabolism and apoptosis in neurons [42] precede Aβ-amyloid deposition and neuronal injury. Thus, inhibition of oxidative stress with febuxostat and higher doses of allopurinol might explain the associated reduced risk of dementia, compared with lower allopurinol doses. It is possible that other indirect urate-related mechanisms (for example, decreased cardiovascular burden) underlie the neuroprotective effect observed with higher doses of ULT in this study.

We noted a biologic gradient with increasing allopurinol dose that satisfied one of Bradford-Hill's criteria for causation versus association [43]. Interestingly, of the three studies that found gout to be protective of dementia, two did not adjust for ULT use [18, 19]. One study that separated patients with gout by treatment found that, compared with matched controls, only patients with ULT-treated gout had a lower hazard of dementia (HR 0.69, 95% CI 0.64, 0.75) but not untreated patients (HR 0.963, 95% CI 0.84, 1.03) [17]. These findings again indicated to us that ULT use might explain these associations of hyperuricemia to lower risk of dementia, which were contrary to other studies that found hyperuricemia to be a risk factor for dementia.

Dementia is a slow process, and a relatively short treatment duration might not be sufficient to counteract the detrimental effect of many years of hyperuricemia with regard to the increased risk of dementia. This may lead to underestimations of the neuroprotective effect of ULT and also may explain the lack of effect of ULT duration on the risk of dementia. Studies of longer duration are needed to further address the questions related to the duration of ULT use and potential reduction of the risk of dementia.

Our finding related to allopurinol dose is interesting and has important clinical implications. Allopurinol, ranging from 100 to 300 mg/day with a mean dose of 230 mg/day, is commonly used in suboptimal doses in patients with gout [44]; less than 50% of those treated at these allopurinol doses achieve the target serum urate of less than 6 mg/dL [45], an important goal associated with lower flare rate [46]. Therefore, higher allopurinol doses are needed in a significant proportion of patients with gout for an appropriate treatment of hyperuricemia and can be given safely [47]. Evidence from studies such as this and others [48] should provide a strong motivation for clinicians to use appropriate (that is, higher) doses of allopurinol to achieve maximum benefits for patients. Additional non-arthritic benefits, such as these, can be considered in decision-making regarding ULT and its dose.

Our study failed to confirm our hypothesis that febuxostat is significantly more effective than allopurinol for the reduction of risk of dementia, which was based on previously observed greater oxidative stress reduction with febuxostat compared with allopurinol [49]. This may be due to either a true lack of difference in mechanism of action between allopurinol and febuxostat related to dementia risk or few events in those exposed to febuxostat. In our study, the majority of febuxostat use was 40 mg/day (82%), while the allopurinol use was split between doses: less than 200 mg/day (45%), 200 to 299 mg/day (18%), and at least 300 mg/day (37%). The lowest marketed dose of febuxostat (40 mg/day) is as efficacious as the allopurinol 300 mg/day dose [50]. Thus, non-significant differences between allopurinol and febuxostat can be explained by the differences in commonly used doses of allopurinol versus febuxostat.

Our study has several limitations that must be considered while interpreting the findings. We examined only older Americans, who were Medicare beneficiaries. Therefore, these findings can be generalized only to Americans 65 years or older; however, this patient population is at high risk of dementia. We examined the most commonly used ULTs: allopurinol and febuxostat. Because few patients received doses higher than 300 mg/day (real-world practice), we were unable to examine the association with higher allopurinol doses (that is, 600 mg/day). We conducted propensity-matched analyses to avoid channeling bias, and most variables matched very closely in propensity-matched cohorts. We included several potential confounders to reduce the risk of confounding bias; however, residual confounding is still possible. Misclassification bias is possible for dementia; however, we used validated codes for dementia [31] shown to have high accuracy [30]. These codes have been used in studies using Medicare claims data [29] and are used in the Quan-Charlson index [28], a very commonly used comorbidity index in research studies. Sensitivity analyses performed by limiting ourselves to one specific code for dementia (290.xx), as in the Charlson-Deyo index, confirmed the findings in the main analysis. Our study was not designed to answer the following questions, which need to be answered by future studies: (1) can allopurinol or febuxostat reduce the progression of cognitive decline in patients with early dementia, (2) does the comparative effectiveness of allopurinol versus febuxostat differ by the type of dementia (that is, Alzheimer's versus vascular dementia), and (3) does the extent of lowering of serum urate correlate with the prevention of dementia and differ for the types of dementia?

Our study has several strengths. We used a new (allopurinol/febuxostat) user design and required all patients to be free of dementia at baseline for a rigorous study design. We examined a representative national sample of the older adults in the US, adjusted for important confounders and covariates, and conducted sensitivity analyses to make sure our results were robust.

Conclusions

We found that, compared with lower allopurinol dose (<200 mg/day), higher allopurinol doses and febuxostat 40 mg/day were associated with a lower risk of a new diagnosis of dementia. This association does not imply causation. This finding provides a rationale for the use of therapeutic allopurinol doses for treatment of conditions such as gout, with an added potential benefit of lower risk of dementia. Mechanistic studies are now needed to better understand how and why this ULT dose-related benefit of reduction of risk of dementia occurs.

Abbreviations
ACE: Angiotensin-converting enzyme; CAD: Coronary artery disease; CI: Confidence interval; HR: Hazard ratio; ICD-9-CM: International Classification of Diseases, ninth revision, common modification; ULT: Urate-lowering therapy; XOR: Xanthine oxido-reductase system

Acknowledgments
We thank Jeffrey Curtis, of the University of Alabama at Birmingham (UAB) Division of Rheumatology, who permitted us to re-use the 5% Medicare data.

Funding
This material is the result of work supported by research funds from the Division of Rheumatology at the UAB and the resources and use of facilities at the Birmingham VA Medical Center (Birmingham, AL, USA). The funding body did not play any role in design; in the collection, analysis, and interpretation of data; in the writing of the manuscript; or in the decision to submit the manuscript for publication.

Authors' contributions
JAS designed the study, developed study protocol, reviewed analyses, and wrote the first draft of the manuscript. JDC performed the data abstraction and data analyses. Both authors made revisions to the manuscript and read and approved the final manuscript.

Consent for publication
Not required.

Competing interests
JAS has received research grants from Takeda and Savient and consultant fees from Savient, Takeda, Regeneron, Merz, Iroko, Bioiberica, Crealta/Horizon and Allergan, WebMD, UBM LLC, and the American College of Rheumatology (ACR). JAS serves as the principal investigator for an investigator-initiated study funded by Horizon through a grant to Dinora, Inc., a 501 (c)(3) entity. JAS is a member of the executive board of OMERACT, an organization that develops outcome measures in rheumatology and receives arms-length funding from 36 companies; a member of the ACR Annual Meeting Planning Committee; chair of the ACR Meet-the-Professor, Workshop and Study Group Subcommittee; and a member of the Veterans Affairs Rheumatology Field Advisory Committee. JAS is the editor and director of the UAB Cochrane Musculoskeletal Group Satellite Center on Network Meta-analysis. JDC declares that he has no competing interests. The authors declare that they have no non-financial competing interests.

Author details
[1]Medicine Service, VA Medical Center, 510, 20th Street South, FOT 805B, Birmingham, AL 35233, USA. [2]Department of Medicine at School of Medicine, University of Alabama at Birmingham, 20th Street South, FOT 805B, Birmingham, AL 35294-0022, USA. [3]Division of Epidemiology at School of Public Health, University of Alabama at Birmingham, 1720 Second Avenue South, Birmingham, AL 35294-0022, USA. [4]University of Alabama, Faculty Office Tower 805B, 510 20th Street South, Birmingham, AL 35294-0022, USA.

References
1. Singh JA, Cleveland JD. Use of urate-lowering therapies is not associated with an increase in the risk of incident dementia in older adults. Ann Rheum Dis. 2018;77(8):1243–5.
2. Grewal HK, Martinez JR, Espinoza LR. Febuxostat: drug review and update. Expert Opin Drug Metab Toxicol. 2014;10(5):747–58.
3. Harrison R. Structure and function of xanthine oxidoreductase: where are we now? Free Radic Biol Med. 2002;33(6):774–97.
4. Bagnati M, Perugini C, Cau C, Bordone R, Albano E, Bellomo G. When and why a water-soluble antioxidant becomes pro-oxidant during copper-induced low-density lipoprotein oxidation: a study using uric acid. Biochem J. 1999;340(Pt 1):143–52.
5. Kanellis J, Kang DH. Uric acid as a mediator of endothelial dysfunction, inflammation, and vascular disease. Semin Nephrol. 2005;25(1):39–42.
6. Squadrito GL, Cueto R, Splenser AE, Valavanidis A, Zhang H, Uppu RM, et al. Reaction of uric acid with peroxynitrite and implications for the mechanism of neuroprotection by uric acid. Arch Biochem Biophys. 2000;376(2):333–7.
7. Yu ZF, Bruce-Keller AJ, Goodman Y, Mattson MP. Uric acid protects neurons against excitotoxic and metabolic insults in cell culture, and against focal ischemic brain injury in vivo. J Neurosci Res. 1998;53(5):613–25.
8. Lin MT, Beal MF. Mitochondrial dysfunction and oxidative stress in neurodegenerative diseases. Nature. 2006;443(7113):787–95.
9. Coyle JT, Puttfarcken P. Oxidative stress, glutamate, and neurodegenerative disorders. Science. 1993;262(5134):689–95.
10. Barnham KJ, Masters CL, Bush AI. Neurodegenerative diseases and oxidative stress. Nat Rev Drug Discov. 2004;3(3):205–14.
11. Dementia and Alzheimer's leading cause of death in England and Wales. https://www.theguardian.com/society/2016/nov/14/dementia-and-alzheimers-leading-cause-of-death-england-and-wales. Accessed 21 July 2018.
12. Prince M, Bryce R, Albanese E, Wimo A, Ribeiro W, Ferri CP. The global prevalence of dementia: a systematic review and metaanalysis. Alzheimers Dement. 2013;9(1):63–75. e62
13. Wimo A, Jönsson L, Bond J, Prince M, Winblad B, Alzheimer Disease International. The worldwide economic impact of dementia 2010. Alzheimers Dement. 2013;9(1):1–11. e13
14. 2016 Alzheimer's disease facts and figures. http://www.alz.org/facts/. Accessed 21 July 2018.
15. Bunn F, Burn AM, Goodman C, Rait G, Norton S, Robinson L, et al. Comorbidity and dementia: a scoping review of the literature. BMC Med. 2014;12:192.
16. Johnson NB, Hayes LD, Brown K, Hoo EC, Ethier KA, Centers for disease C, prevention. CDC National Health Report: leading causes of morbidity and mortality and associated behavioral risk and protective factors--United States, 2005-2013. MMWR Suppl. 2014;63(4):3–27.
17. Hong JY, Lan TY, Tang GJ, Tang CH, Chen TJ, Lin HY. Gout and the risk of dementia: a nationwide population-based cohort study. Arthritis Res Ther. 2015;17:139.
18. Lu N, Dubreuil M, Zhang Y, Neogi T, Rai SK, Ascherio A, et al. Gout and the risk of Alzheimer's disease: a population-based, BMI-matched cohort study. Ann Rheum Dis. 2016;75(3):547–51.
19. Euser SM, Hofman A, Westendorp RG, Breteler MM. Serum uric acid and cognitive function and dementia. Brain. 2009;132(Pt 2):377–82.
20. Afsar B, Elsurer R, Covic A, Johnson RJ, Kanbay M. Relationship between uric acid and subtle cognitive dysfunction in chronic kidney disease. Am J Nephrol. 2011;34(1):49–54.
21. Cicero AF, Desideri G, Grossi G, Urso R, Rosticci M, D'Addato S, et al. Serum uric acid and impaired cognitive function in a cohort of healthy young elderly: data from the Brisighella study. Intern Emerg Med. 2015;10(1):25–31.
22. Perna L, Mons U, Schottker B, Brenner H. Association of cognitive function and serum uric acid: are cardiovascular diseases a mediator among women? Exp Gerontol. 2016;81:37–41.
23. Verhaaren BF, Vernooij MW, Dehghan A, Vrooman HA, de Boer R, Hofman A, et al. The relation of uric acid to brain atrophy and cognition: the Rotterdam scan study. Neuroepidemiology. 2013;41(1):29–34.
24. Beydoun MA, Canas JA, Dore GA, Beydoun HA, Rostant OS, Fanelli-Kuczmarski MT, et al. Serum uric acid and its association with longitudinal cognitive change among urban adults. J Alzheimers Dis. 2016;52(4):1415–30.
25. Ruggiero C, Cherubini A, Lauretani F, Bandinelli S, Maggio M, Di Iorio A, et al. Uric acid and dementia in community-dwelling older persons. Dement Geriatr Cogn Disord. 2009;27(4):382–9.
26. Richette P, Doherty M, Pascual E, Barskova V, Becce F, Castaneda-Sanabria J, et al. 2016 updated EULAR evidence-based recommendations for the management of gout. Ann Rheum Dis. 2017;76(1):29–42.
27. Latourte A, Soumare A, Bardin T, Perez-Ruiz F, Debette S, Richette P. Uric acid and incident dementia over 12 years of follow-up: a population-based cohort study. Ann Rheum Dis. 2018;77(3):328–35.

28. Quan H, Sundararajan V, Halfon P, Fong A, Burnand B, Luthi JC, et al. Coding algorithms for defining comorbidities in ICD-9-CM and ICD-10 administrative data. Med Care. 2005;43(11):1130–9.

29. Taylor DH Jr, Ostbye T, Langa KM, Weir D, Plassman BL. The accuracy of Medicare claims as an epidemiological tool: the case of dementia revisited. J Alzheimers Dis. 2009;17(4):807–15.

30. Quan H, Li B, Saunders LD, Parsons GA, Nilsson CI, Alibhai A, et al. Assessing validity of ICD-9-CM and ICD-10 administrative data in recording clinical conditions in a unique dually coded database. Health Serv Res. 2008;43(4):1424–41.

31. Green AR, Leff B, Wang Y, Spatz ES, Masoudi FA, Peterson PN, et al. Geriatric conditions in patients undergoing defibrillator implantation for prevention of sudden cardiac death: prevalence and impact on mortality. Circ Cardiovasc Qual Outcomes. 2016;9(1):23–30.

32. Romano PS, Roos LL, Jollis JG. Adapting a clinical comorbidity index for use with ICD-9-CM administrative data: differing perspectives. J Clin Epidemiol. 1993;46(10):1075–9. discussion 1081–90

33. Lin DY, Wei LJ. The robust inference for the cox proportional hazards model. J Am Stat Assoc. 1989;84:1074–8.

34. Chen X, Guo X, Huang R, Chen Y, Zheng Z, Shang H. Serum uric acid levels in patients with Alzheimer's disease: a meta-analysis. PLoS One. 2014;9(4):e94084.

35. George J, Carr E, Davies J, Belch JJ, Struthers A. High-dose allopurinol improves endothelial function by profoundly reducing vascular oxidative stress and not by lowering uric acid. Circulation. 2006;114(23):2508–16.

36. Graham S, Day RO, Wong H, McLachlan AJ, Bergendal L, Miners JO, et al. Pharmacodynamics of oxypurinol after administration of allopurinol to healthy subjects. Br J Clin Pharmacol. 1996;41(4):299–304.

37. Moorhouse PC, Grootveld M, Halliwell B, Quinlan JG, Gutteridge JM. Allopurinol and oxypurinol are hydroxyl radical scavengers. FEBS Lett. 1987; 213(1):23–8.

38. Fukui T, Maruyama M, Yamauchi K, Yoshitaka S, Yasuda T, Abe Y. Effects of Febuxostat on oxidative stress. Clin Ther. 2015;37(7):1396–401.

39. Tsuda H, Kawada N, Kaimori JY, Kitamura H, Moriyama T, Rakugi H, et al. Febuxostat suppressed renal ischemia-reperfusion injury via reduced oxidative stress. Biochem Biophys Res Commun. 2012;427(2):266–72.

40. Mecocci P, MacGarvey U, Kaufman AE, Koontz D, Shoffner JM, Wallace DC, et al. Oxidative damage to mitochondrial DNA shows marked age-dependent increases in human brain. Ann Neurol. 1993;34(4):609–16.

41. Pratico D, Uryu K, Leight S, Trojanoswki JQ, Lee VM. Increased lipid peroxidation precedes amyloid plaque formation in an animal model of Alzheimer amyloidosis. J Neurosci. 2001;21(12):4183–7.

42. Reddy PH, McWeeney S, Park BS, Manczak M, Gutala RV, Partovi D, et al. Gene expression profiles of transcripts in amyloid precursor protein transgenic mice: up-regulation of mitochondrial metabolism and apoptotic genes is an early cellular change in Alzheimer's disease. Hum Mol Genet. 2004;13(12):1225–40.

43. Hill AB. The environment and disease: association or causation? Proc R Soc Med. 1965;58:295–300.

44. Sarawate CA, Brewer KK, Yang W, Patel PA, Schumacher HR, Saag KG, et al. Gout medication treatment patterns and adherence to standards of care from a managed care perspective. Mayo Clin Proc. 2006;81(7):925–34.

45. Singh JA, Hodges JS, Asch SM. Opportunities for improving medication use and monitoring in gout. Ann Rheum Dis. 2009;68(8):1265–70.

46. Shoji A, Yamanaka H, Kamatani N. A retrospective study of the relationship between serum urate level and recurrent attacks of gouty arthritis: evidence for reduction of recurrent gouty arthritis with antihyperuricemic therapy. Arthritis Rheum. 2004;51(3):321–5.

47. Stamp LK, O'Donnell JL, Zhang M, James J, Frampton C, Barclay ML, et al. Using allopurinol above the dose based on creatinine clearance is effective and safe in patients with chronic gout, including those with renal impairment. Arthritis Rheum. 2011;63(2):412–21.

48. Noman A, Ang DS, Ogston S, Lang CC, Struthers AD. Effect of high-dose allopurinol on exercise in patients with chronic stable angina: a randomised, placebo controlled crossover trial. Lancet. 2010;375(9732):2161–7.

49. Tausche AK, Christoph M, Forkmann M, Richter U, Kopprasch S, Bielitz C, et al. As compared to allopurinol, urate-lowering therapy with febuxostat has superior effects on oxidative stress and pulse wave velocity in patients with severe chronic tophaceous gout. Rheumatol Int. 2014;34(1):101–9.

50. Becker MA, Schumacher HR, Espinoza LR, Wells AF, MacDonald P, Lloyd E, et al. The urate-lowering efficacy and safety of febuxostat in the treatment of the hyperuricemia of gout: the CONFIRMS trial. Arthritis Res Ther. 2010;12(2):R63.

3

Radiographs in screening for sacroiliitis in children: what is the value?

Pamela F. Weiss[1,3,4,8*] (iD), Rui Xiao[4], Timothy G. Brandon[1,3], David M. Biko[2], Walter P. Maksymowych[5,7], Robert G. Lambert[6,7], Jacob L. Jaremko[6] and Nancy A. Chauvin[2]

Abstract

Background: We aimed to evaluate the diagnostic utility of pelvic radiographs versus magnetic resonance imaging (MRI) of the sacroiliac joints in children with suspected sacroiliitis.

Methods: This was a retrospective cross-sectional study of children with suspected or confirmed spondyloarthritis who underwent pelvic radiograph and MRI within 6 months of one another. Images were scored independently by five raters. Interrater reliability was calculated using Fleiss's kappa coefficient (κ). Test properties of radiographs for depiction of sacroiliitis were calculated using MRI global sacroiliitis impression as the reference standard.

Results: The interrater agreement for global impression was κ = 0.34 (95% CI 0.19–0.52) for radiographs and κ = 0.72 (95% CI 0.52–0.86) for MRI. Across raters, the sensitivity of radiographs ranged from 25 to 77.8% and specificity ranged from 60.8 to 92.2%. Positive and negative predictive values ranged from 25.9 to 52% and from 82.7 to 93.9%, respectively. The misclassification rate ranged from 6 to 17% for negative radiographs/positive MRI scans and from 48 to 74% for positive radiographs/negative MRI scans. When the reference standard was changed to structural lesions consistent with sacroiliitis on MRI, the misclassification rate was higher for negative radiographs/positive MRI scans (9–23%) and marginally improved for positive radiographs/negative MRI scans (33–52%).

Conclusion: Interrater reliability of MRI was superior to radiographs for global sacroiliitis impression. Misclassification for both negative and positive radiographs was high across raters. Radiographs have limited utility in screening for sacroiliitis in children and result in a significant proportion of both false negative and positive findings versus MRI findings.

Keywords: Radiograph, Magnetic resonance imaging, Sacroiliitis, Juvenile spondyloarthritis, Misclassification

Background

Juvenile spondyloarthritis (SpA) is a term that encompasses a group of conditions characterized by inflammatory arthritis, enthesitis, HLA-B27 positivity, acute anterior uveitis, inflammatory bowel disease, and psoriasis. The arthritis of juvenile SpA (JSpA) can be peripheral or axial (sacroiliac joints or spine). While the diagnosis of peripheral arthritis can typically be made by clinical examination, confirmation of sacroiliitis often requires imaging. Prior studies have shown that tenderness to palpation and physical examination maneuvers such as the flexion

abduction external rotation (FABER) hip test have low sensitivity and specificity for sacroiliitis using magnetic resonance imaging (MRI) as the reference standard [1]. For historical reasons, radiographs are currently the gold standard for making the diagnosis of ankylosing spondylitis and are frequently a prerequisite for obtaining an MRI study under many insurance plans in the United States. Radiographs, however, only show bony damage and are not sensitive enough to detect early disease or incremental changes over short periods of time [2]. Given the relatively short disease duration and rare occurrence of ankylosis in children [1, 3, 4], the value of radiographs at the time of diagnosis or in evaluation of suspected early inflammatory sacroiliitis in children is unclear. The practice of routinely obtaining radiographs may cause unnecessary radiation exposure and result in early cases of sacroiliitis going

* Correspondence: weisspa@email.chop.edu
[1]Department of Pediatrics, Division of Rheumatology, Children's Hospital of Philadelphia, Philadelphia, PA, USA
[3]Center for Pediatric Clinical Effectiveness (CPCE), Children's Hospital of Philadelphia, Philadelphia, PA, USA
Full list of author information is available at the end of the article

undetected and untreated if MRI is not subsequently performed [1]. Misdiagnosis may also result in inappropriate therapy.

MRI has become increasingly utilized to detect inflammation in the sacroiliac joints (SIJs) before changes are apparent on radiographs. The Assessment of SpondyloArthritis International Society (ASAS) classification criteria for axial spondyloarthritis specifically include MRI evidence of inflammation in the sacroiliac joints in the criteria for adult SpA [5]. Several studies have shown the value of MRI in evaluation of JSpA [1, 6–8], but only one small study has directly evaluated the diagnostic utility of radiography versus MRI for children with SpA [7]. Concordant with other studies which show unequivocal superiority of MRI over radiographs for detection of active disease [9–11], the positive likelihood ratio (LR+) for a clinical diagnosis of SpA was much higher for MRI findings than radiographic findings in that small study, especially for erosions (LR+ = 6.7 vs 3.5) and global impression (LR+ = 9.4 vs 4.4) [7]. However, that study had a small sample size and a high frequency of abnormalities reported in controls; 55% and 20% had sclerosis and erosions by radiograph, respectively. This may have been due to use of oversensitive criteria for these radiographic findings [12].

The objective of this project was to more fully evaluate the accuracy of radiographs to detect sacroiliitis in children using global impression of the MRI study as the reference standard. Our working hypotheses were that radiographs do not add incremental value to the MRI examination of the sacroiliac joint and that the test properties of radiographs are sufficiently low that follow-up MRI is needed in most cases.

Methods
Human subject protection
The protocol for the conduct of this study was reviewed and approved by the Children's Hospital of Philadelphia Committee for the Protection of Human Subjects (IRB 16-013013).

Study population
This was a retrospective cross-sectional study of all children with suspected or confirmed JSpA who underwent both pelvic radiograph and MRI separated by no more than 6 months between January 2012 and May 2016. Eligible children were ages 6–18 years at the time of clinical care and had the following imaging protocols performed at our institution: anterioposterior (AP) view of the pelvis or dedicated radiographs and MRI of the sacroiliac joints that included coronal oblique T1 and STIR sequences performed at either 1.5 or 3 Tesla. All MRI assessments were made using noncontrast sequences. Demographic characteristics and indications for imaging were abstracted from the electronic medical record and the imaging studies were obtained from the picture archiving and communication system (PACS).

Evaluation of imaging studies
All scoring exercises were completed within a web-based environment (CaREArthritis.com) or Research Electronic Data Capture (REDCap) [13]. REDCap is a secure, web-based application designed to support data capture for research studies. Four raters were musculoskeletal radiologists (DMB, RGL, JLJ, NAC) and one rater was an adult rheumatologist with SIJ imaging expertise (WPM). All images were reviewed in random order and blinded to clinical details. All raters have had extensive training in the interpretation of pelvic radiographs and MRI.

Each radiograph was assessed for erosions, sclerosis, joint space narrowing, joint space widening, and ankylosis. Each rater indicated whether the radiograph was globally representative of sacroiliitis (yes or no) and rated confidence in global impression (ordinal scale – 4 to 4 with anchors of "definitely no" and "definitely yes"). Erosion was defined as a cortical irregularity along the articular surface of the bone. Sclerosis was defined as increased subchondral bone density compared to the subchondral bone density in the hips/spine. Ankylosis was defined as complete obliteration of the joint space with contiguous bone between the sacrum and ilium. Joint space narrowing and widening were determined subjectively as decreased or increased width of the joint space. The presence of each lesion was recorded as occurring in the left or right joint, with an additional specification of quadrant location being made for erosion and sclerosis.

Each MRI study was evaluated for active inflammatory lesions (bone marrow edema, capsulitis, SIJ effusion, enthesitis outside of the SIJ) and structural lesions (erosion, sclerosis, fat metaplasia, backfill, ankylosis). Inflammation was assessed using the CareArthritis platform and the Spondyloarthritis Research Consortium of Canada (SPARCC) SIJ Inflammation Score (SIS) scoring module. Reliability of the SPARCC SIS has been demonstrated in the pediatric population [14, 15]. Details about the platform and scoring have been published previously [16]. All raters previously completed calibration exercises for the SPARCC SIS and SSS with acceptable reliability (intraclass correlation (ICC) ≥ 0.8) [14, 15]. The presence or absence of marrow edema was scored for each joint quadrant (total score per slice 0–8). Marrow edema was deemed present if the intensity was the same or greater than the presacral veins and depth ≥ 1 cm, and was scored dichotomously for each sacroiliac joint. Positive bone marrow edema findings were defined in accordance with the ASAS criteria (bone marrow edema in two or more locations on a single MRI slice or bone marrow edema on two consecutive MRI slices). The ASAS MRImagine consensus-based eCRF for recording MRI data was used to capture the following: rater global impression of acute/active inflammatory lesions compatible with sacroiliitis (yes/no), rater global impression of structural lesions typical of axial SpA, confidence in that assessment (ordinal scale – 4 to 4 with anchors of "definitely no" and "definitely yes"), capsulitis (yes/no), SIJ effusion (yes/no), and enthesitis outside of the SIJ (yes/no) [17, 18].

Structural lesions on MRI (erosion, sclerosis, fat metaplasia, backfill, ankyloses) were assessed using the CareArthritis platform and the SPARCC SIJ structural score (SSS) scoring module. Reliability of the SPARCC SSS has been demonstrated in the pediatric population [19].

Statistical analysis

Subject demographic characteristics and raters' assessments of lesions were summarized by frequencies and percentages or medians and interquartile ranges (IQR). In order to compare radiograph and MRI assessment for lesions, all MRI scoring was dichotomized. Interrater agreement was assessed using Fleiss's kappa statistic with bootstrap confidence intervals [20], with agreement interpreted as poor ≤ 0.40, fair 0.41–0.59, good 0.60–0.74, and excellent ≥ 0.75 [21]. Sensitivity, specificity, positive predictive value, and negative predictive value were calculated to assess the performance of radiographs in identifying sacroiliitis (global impression "yes") using MRI global impression of active sacroiliitis ("yes") as the reference standard. We also conducted two analogous analyses in which the reference standard was altered: to assess performance of radiographs in identifying sacroiliitis using MRI global impression of structural lesions consistent with sacroiliitis (global impression "yes") as the reference standard; and to assess performance of radiographs in identifying sacroiliitis using MRI global impression of active sacroiliitis (global impression "yes") or structural lesions consistent with sacroiliitis (global impression "yes") as the reference standard. All analyses were performed using Stata 14.2 (2015, Stata Statistical Software Release 14; StataCorp. LP, College Station, TX, USA).

Results

Subjects

A total of 228 children had both a radiograph and an MRI ordered during the study window; 60 pairs of images met our inclusion criteria (Fig. 1). The median time between studies was 0 days (IQR 0–10 days). In 41 (68.3%) cases, radiograph and MRI occurred on the same day, 16 (26.7%) cases had a radiograph that preceded the MRI, and the remaining three (5.0%) cases had an MRI prior to the radiograph. The primary indication for imaging in our study population was inclusion in a prior study evaluating the prevalence of sacroiliitis in patients newly diagnosed with

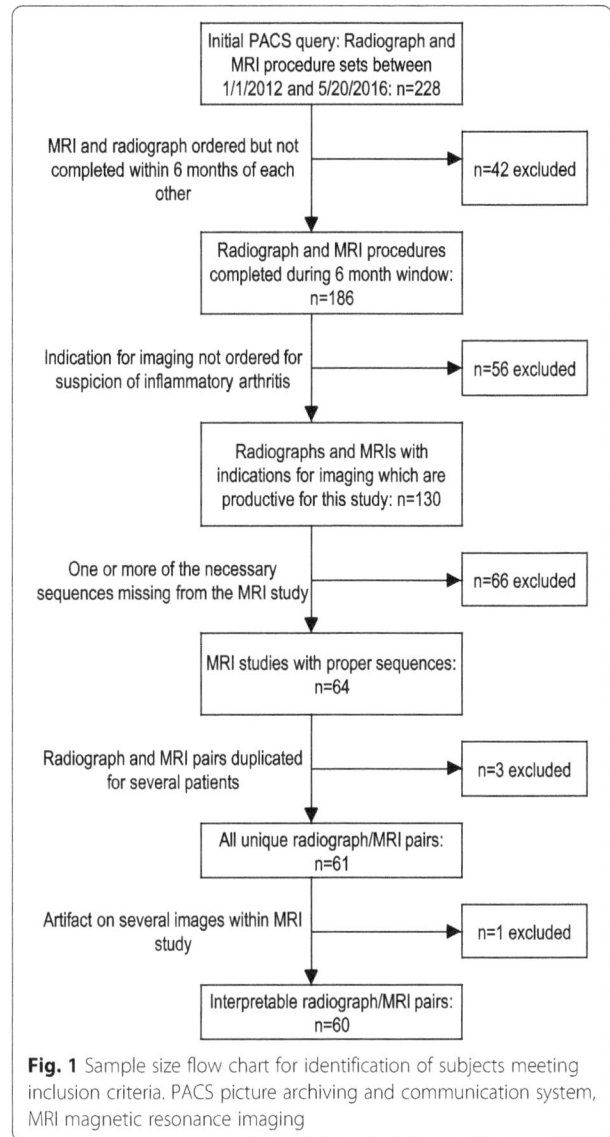

Fig. 1 Sample size flow chart for identification of subjects meeting inclusion criteria. PACS picture archiving and communication system, MRI magnetic resonance imaging

JSpA [1] (n = 38, 63.3%). The remaining subjects were imaged for complaints of back (23.3%) or hip (3.3%) pain, limited range of motion (1.7%), or as follow-up for a previous sacroiliitis diagnosis (8.3%). Demographics are presented in Table 1. Half of the subjects were male and the median age at time of radiograph was 14.4 years (IQR 11.9–16.6 years). Eighty percent of subjects were Caucasian and 12% were African American.

Radiographs

Fifty-four (90%) subjects had a single AP pelvic radiograph, three subjects had AP and frogleg sacroiliac radiographs, and three subjects had AP and bilateral oblique dedicated sacroiliac radiographs performed. Fourteen (23.3%) radiographs were read as abnormal by three or more raters. Of those radiographs with at least three raters reporting abnormal findings, all raters called the study abnormal in five

Table 1 Subject characteristics

	Frequency (%)/median (IQR) (n = 60)
Age at radiograph (years)	14.4 (11.9–16.6)
Age at MRI (years)	14.6 (11.9–16.7)
Time between studies (months)	0 (0–0.3)
Sex, male	30 (50%)
Race	
White/Caucasian	48 (80%)
Black/African American	7 (12%)
Asian	1 (2%)
Other	4 (7%)

IQR interquartile range, MRI magnetic resonance imaging

(35.7%) cases. The most common radiographic findings across 300 reads completed by the five raters were sclerosis (29%), erosion (22%), and joint space widening (14%). The interrater agreement for global impression and all lesions assessed by radiograph are presented in Table 2. The interrater agreement for global impression of active sacroiliitis was poor (κ = 0.34, 95% CI 0.19–0.52). The interrater agreement for each radiographic lesion was either poor or fair. The

interrater reliability could not be determined for ankylosis due to low prevalence. One hundred and seventy three of 300 (57.7%) assessments of active arthritis had a confidence level of "definitely yes" or "definitely no".

Magnetic resonance imaging
Ten (16.7%) pelvic MRI scans were considered indicative of active sacroiliitis by at least three of the raters. Of these MRI studies with at least three raters reporting active sacroiliitis, all raters called the study abnormal in eight (80%) cases. Across all studies, periarticular bone marrow edema was noted in 19%. The most commonly detected structural MRI lesions across all studies were sclerosis (21%) and erosion (18%). The interrater agreement for global impression and all lesions assessed by MRI are presented in Table 2. The kappa value for global MRI impression of active sacroiliitis was good (κ = 0.72, 95% CI 0.52–0.86). The interrater agreement for bone marrow edema, the key lesion for classification according to the ASAS criteria, was excellent (κ = 0.78, 95% CI 0.58–0.9) [22]. The kappa values for other lesions consistent with active sacroiliitis (capsulitis, enthesitis, SIJ effusion) were low (κ ≤ 0.25). The interrater agreement for global impression of structural lesions consistent

Table 2 Radiologist findings and agreement for radiograph and MRI

	Frequency (%)					
	Rater 1	Rater 2	Rater 3	Rater 4	Rater 5	Kappa (95% CI)
Radiograph						
Global impression of sacroiliitis	8 (1)	8 (13)	27 (45)	17 (28)	25 (42)	0.34 (0.19–0.52)
Erosion	7 (12)	6 (10)	25 (42)	12 (20)	15 (26)	0.42 (0.22–0.6)
Sclerosis	8 (13)	8 (13)	21 (35)	19 (32)	32 (53)	0.35 (0.19–0.52)
Ankylosis	0 (0)	0 (0)	2 (3)	3 (5)	4 (7)	–
JSN	1 (2)	1 (2)	10 (17)	18 (30)	8 (13)	0.11 (0.03–0.2)
JSW	7 (12)	5 (8)	13 (22)	10 (17)	8 (13)	0.4 (0.23–0.57)
MRI						
Global impression of acute/active sacroiliitis[a]	12 (20)	9 (15)	9 (15)	10 (17)	17 (28)	0.72 (0.52–0.86)
BME	10 (17)	9 (15)	12 (20)	10 (17)	16 (27)	0.78 (0.58–0.9)
Capsulitis	6 (10)	2 (3)	0 (0)	1 (2)	7 (12)	0.21 (−0.02–0.46)
Enthesitis outside of SIJ	6 (10)	3 (5)	1 (2)	0 (0)	4 (7)	0.25 (− 0.01–0.52)
SIJ effusion	1 (2)	3 (5)	7 (12)	11 (18)	17 (28)	0.19 (0.05–0.34)
Global impression of structural chronic[b] lesions consistent with sacroiliitis	16 (27)	9 (15)	12 (20)	13 (22)	19 (32)	0.58 (0.39–0.74)
Erosion	14 (23)	9 (15)	9 (15)	13 (22)	9 (15)	0.64 (0.48–0.81)
Sclerosis	4 (7)	4 (7)	6 (10)	12 (20)	36 (60)	0.15 (0.01–0.31)
Backfill	11 (18)	4 (7)	6 (10)	4 (7)	6 (10)	0.59 (0.24–0.81)
Fat metaplasia	3 (5)	1 (2)	2 (3)	1 (2)	5 (8)	0.52 (−0.02–0.93)
Ankylosis	0 (0)	1 (2)	0 (0)	1 (2)	1 (2)	–

BME bone marrow edema, CI confidence interval, JSN joint space narrowing, JSW joint space widening, MRI magnetic resonance imaging, SIJ sacroiliac joint
[a]Acute/active inflammatory lesions meeting the Assessment of Spondyloarthritis International Society definition of a positive MRI scan of the sacroiliac joints
[b]Structural chronic lesions refer to the clear presence of typical findings such as sclerosis, erosion, fatty lesions, bone bridges, and ankyloses

with sacroiliitis was fair (κ = 0.58, 95% CI 0.39–0.74). The interrater agreement for each of the structural lesions assessed on MRI were fair to good with the exception of sclerosis (κ = 0.15) and ankylosis, which again could not be assessed secondary to the low prevalence of lesions. Two hundred and thirty of 300 (76.6%) assessments had a confidence level of "definitely yes or definitely no".

Radiograph versus MRI

Table 3 presents the performance of radiographs in identifying sacroiliitis (global impression "yes") using MRI global impression of active sacroiliitis ("yes") as the reference standard. The sensitivity of radiographs for sacroiliitis on MRI ranged from 25 to 77.8% and specificity ranged from 60.8 to 92.2% across raters. Positive and negative predictive values ranged from 25.9 to 52% and from 82.7 to 93.9%, respectively. Across raters, the misclassification rate ranged from 6 to 17% for negative radiographs/positive MRI scans and from 48 to 74% for positive radiographs/negative MRI scans. Examples of agreement from 5/5 raters on positive radiograph/negative MRI and negative radiograph/positive MRI are shown in Fig. 2. Of the 51 cases across raters where positive radiographs were paired with negative MRI scans, 12 (23.5%) of the MRI scans showed structural lesions in the absence of findings consistent with active inflammatory sacroiliitis. The reported structural abnormalities were erosion (n = 6), sclerosis (n = 7), backfill (n = 1), and fat metaplasia (n = 1). Of the five cases where all raters' impression on radiograph was congruent with sacroiliitis, two of those cases were found to be normal on MRI by all raters. Eight cases had

total agreement on global impression of sacroiliitis "yes" among raters on MRI, five of which were paired with a sacroiliitis impression "yes" from three or more raters on the corresponding radiographs.

Table 4 presents the performance of radiographs in identifying sacroiliitis (global impression "yes") when the reference standard was changed to MRI global impression of structural lesions consistent with sacroiliitis ("yes"). Across raters, the sensitivity of radiographs for structural lesions consistent with sacroiliitis on MRI ranged from 25 to 75% and specificity ranged from 70.7 to 90.9%. Positive and negative predictive values ranged from 37.5 to 52% and from 76.9 to 90.9%, respectively. Across raters, the misclassification rate ranged from 9.1 to 23.1% for negative radiographs/positive MRI scans and from 48.0 to 66.7% for positive radiographs/negative MRI scans. When the reference standard was changed to MRI global impression of active *or* structural lesions consistent with sacroiliitis on MRI, the test properties and misclassification rate were similar (Table 5).

In order to examine whether the test properties of radiographs for the detection of inflammatory sacroiliitis were robust to whether the child was acutely symptomatic or not, we performed a sensitivity analysis by excluding those children who were imaged as part of a prior study and were asymptomatic. In the restricted sample of 42 children, the sensitivity of radiographs ranged from 20 to 77.8% and the specificity ranged 69.7 to 90.6%.

Discussion

This is a systematic analysis to compare the utility of radiographs to MRI in the evaluation of suspected sacroiliitis.

Table 3 Test properties of radiograph for detection of active inflammatory sacroiliitis on MRI

	Rater 1	Rater 2	Rater 3	Rater 4	Rater 5
Percentage (95% CI)					
Sensitivity	25.0 (5.5–57.2)	44.4 (13.7–78.8)	77.8 (40.0–97.2)	70.0 (34.8–93.3)	76.5 (50.1–93.2)
Specificity	89.6 (77.3–96.5)	92.2 (81.1–97.8)	60.8 (46.1–74.2)	80.0 (66.3–90.0)	72.1 (56.3–84.7)
PPV	37.5 (8.5–75.5)	50.0 (15.7–84.3)	25.9 (11.1–46.3)	41.2 (18.4–67.1)	52.0 (31.3–72.2)
NPV	82.7 (69.7–91.8)	90.4 (79.0–96.8)	93.9 (79.8–99.3)	93.0 (80.9–98.5)	88.6 (73.3–96.8)
Frequency (%)					
Radiograph–[a]					
Radiograph–/MRI–	43 (83)	47 (90)	31 (94)	40 (93)	31 (89)
Radiograph–/MRI+	9 (17)	5 (10)	2 (6)	3 (7)	4 (11)
Radiograph+ [a]					
Radiograph+/MRI–	5 (63)	4 (50)	20 (74)	10 (59)	12 (48)
Radiograph+/MRI+	3 (37)	4 (50)	7 (26)	7 (41)	13 (52)

Kappa value interpretations: ≤ 0.40 poor agreement, 0.41–0.59 fair agreement, 0.60–0.74 good agreement, and ≥ 0.75 excellent agreement [21]. For sensitivity, specificity, PPV, and NPV calculations, positive radiograph defined as global impression of sacroiliitis (yes) and reference standard was MRI global impression of active sacroiliitis (yes)

CI confidence interval, *MRI* magnetic resonance imaging, *NPV* negative predictive value, *PPV* positive predictive value

[a]MRI and radiograph + or – defined as global impression of sacroiliitis (yes/no)

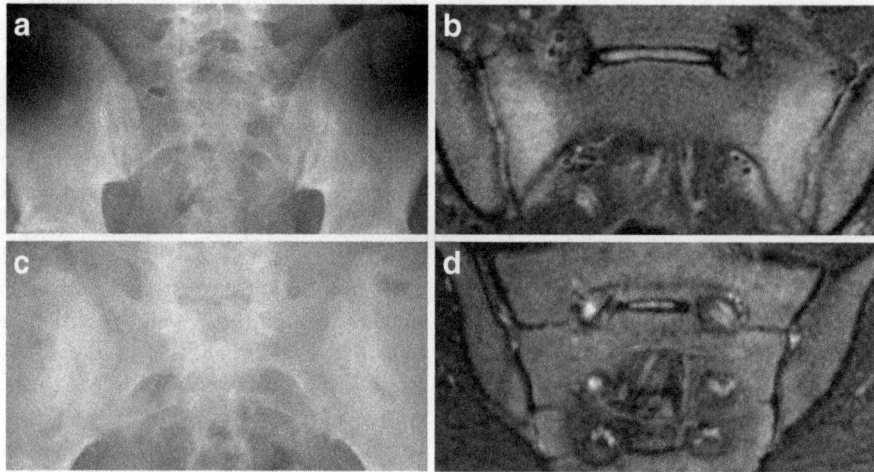

Fig. 2 Samples of discordant radiograph and MRI overall impressions of presence/absence of sacroiliitis. **a** and **b**) 16-year-old HLA-B27+ male with 2 months of hamstring, gluteal, and low back pain. (**a**) Radiograph – normal (no sacroiliitis) by 5/5 raters; two raters noted sclerosis. (**b**) MRI STIR – abnormal (sacroiliitis present) rated by 5/5 raters; bilateral sacral subchondral bone marrow edema is clearly present. Two raters reported a positive erosion finding and 3 raters reported a positive sclerosis finding. (**c** and **d**) 13-year-old HLA-B27 negative female with lower and mid-back pain with accompanying morning stiffness, acute uveitis, and multiple tender entheses. (**c**) Radiograph – rated abnormal (sacroiliitis present) by 5/5 raters; two raters reported a positive finding for erosion, two reported a finding of joint space narrowing, and all five raters reported sclerosis. (**d**) MRI STIR – rated as normal (no sacroiliitis) by 5/5 raters; no abnormalities (erosion, sclerosis, fat metaplasia, ankylosis, or backfill) were reported on MRI. Radiologist raters were blinded to patient clinical details and are included here to provide the reader with relevant medical history

Interrater reliability and confidence of MRI were superior to radiographs for global impression of sacroiliitis. The rates of misclassification were high, with false positive radiographs occurring more frequently than false negative radiographs. Radiographs do remain indispensable for identification of lesions that may be on the differential of pediatric lower back pain including osteomyelitis, septic arthritis, chronic recurrent multifocal osteomyelitis, tumor, and fracture. Our results, however, indicate that radiographs have limited utility in screening for inflammatory or structural lesions consistent with sacroiliitis in children and result in a significant proportion of both false negative and positive findings.

Several limitations should be considered while interpreting our findings. First, our sample size was limited to 60 sets of radiographs and MRI scans. The number of children who had imaging performed at our institution during the study timeframe was much larger, but many

Table 4 Test properties of radiograph for detection of structural lesions consistent with sacroiliitis on MRI

	Rater 1	Rater 2	Rater 3	Rater 4	Rater 5
Percent (95% CI)					
Sensitivity	25.0 (7.3–52.4)	33.3 (7.5–70.1)	75.0 (42.8–94.5)	53.8 (25.1–80.8)	68.4 (43.4–87.4)
Specificity	90.9 (78.3–97.5)	90.2 (78.6–96.7)	62.5 (47.4–76.0)	78.7 (64.3–89.3)	70.7 (54.5–83.9)
PPV	50.0 (15.7–84.3)	37.5 (8.5–75.5)	33.3 (16.5–54.0)	41.2 (18.4–67.1)	52.0 (31.3–72.2)
NPV	76.9 (63.2–87.5)	88.5 (76.6–95.6)	90.9 (75.7–98.1)	86.0 (72.1–94.7)	82.9 (66.4–93.4)
Frequency (%)					
Radiograph–[a]					
Radiograph–/MRI–	40 (76.9)	46 (88.5)	30 (90.9)	37 (86)	29 (82.9)
Radiograph–/MRI+	12 (23.1)	6 (11.5)	3 (9.1)	6 (14)	6 (17.1)
Radiograph+[a]					
Radiograph+/MRI–	4 (50)	5 (62.5)	18 (66.7)	10 (58.8)	12 (48)
Radiograph+/MRI+	4 (50)	3 (37.5)	9 (33.3)	7 (41.2)	13 (52)

Kappa value interpretations: ≤ 0.40 poor agreement, 0.41–0.59 fair agreement, 0.60–0.74 good agreement, and ≥ 0.75 excellent agreement [21]. For sensitivity, specificity, PPV, and NPV calculations, positive radiograph defined as global impression of sacroiliitis (yes) and reference standard was MRI global impression of structural lesions consistent with sacroiliitis (yes)
CI confidence interval, MRI magnetic resonance imaging, NPV negative predictive value, PPV positive predictive value
[a]MRI and radiograph + or – defined as global impression of sacroiliitis (yes/no)

Table 5 Test properties of radiograph for detection of active *or* structural lesions typical of sacroiliitis on MRI

	Rater 1	Rater 2	Rater 3	Rater 4	Rater 5
Percent (95% CI)					
Sensitivity	22.2 (6.4–47.6)	33.3 (9.9–65.1)	75.0 (42.8–94.5)	57.1 (28.9–82.3)	64.0 (42.5–82.0)
Specificity	90.5 (77.4–97.3)	91.7 (80.0–97.7)	62.5 (47.4–76.0)	80.4 (66.1–90.6)	74.3 (56.7–87.5)
PPV	50.0 (15.7–84.3)	50.0 (15.7–84.3)	33.3 (16.5–54.0)	47.1 (23.0–72.2)	64.0 (42.5–82.0)
NPV	73.1 (59.0–84.4)	84.6 (71.9–93.1)	90.9 (75.7–98.1)	86.0 (72.1–94.7)	74.3 (56.7–87.5)
Frequency (%)					
Radiograph–[a]					
Radiograph–/MRI–	38 (73.1)	44 (84.6)	30 (90.9)	37 (86)	26 (74.3)
Radiograph–/MRI+	14 (26.9)	8 (15.4)	3 (9.1)	6 (14)	9 (25.7)
Radiograph +					
Radiograph+/MRI–	4 (50)	4 (50)	18 (66.7)	9 (52.9)	9 (36)
Radiograph+/MRI+	4 (50)	4 (50)	9 (33.3)	8 (47.1)	16 (64)

Kappa value interpretations: ≤ 0.40 poor agreement, 0.41–0.59 fair agreement, 0.60–0.74 good agreement, and ≥ 0.75 excellent agreement [21]. For sensitivity, specificity, PPV, and NPV calculations, positive radiograph defined as global impression of sacroiliitis (yes) and reference standard was MRI global impression of active inflammatory (yes) *or* structural lesions consistent with sacroiliitis (yes)
CI confidence interval, *MRI* magnetic resonance imaging, *NPV* negative predictive value, *PPV* positive predictive value
[a]MRI and radiograph + or – defined as global impression of sacroiliitis (yes/no)

did not have both radiograph and MRI performed within 6 months of each other. Further, MRI at our institution prior to 2012 did not routinely include coronal oblique sacral sequences, which we consider vital for adequate assessment of the sacroiliac joints. Nevertheless, even with our limited sample size we were able to identify significant shortcomings in the use of radiographs in children. Second, this was a retrospective study using sets of images that could have been obtained at any point in the child's disease course. Perhaps the utility of radiographs is higher with longer disease duration or older age and more closely matches the utility seen in adults in these cases of prolonged disease exposure. The vast majority of children, however, have relatively short duration of symptoms and disease at the time imaging is ordered. We think our data reflect the typical use of radiographs for routine practice in the evaluation of the sacroiliac joints in children with both suspected and established JSpA. Third, some of the subjects had imaging performed shortly after spondyloarthritis diagnosis as part of a prior study. Our sensitivity analysis investigating this limitation using a sample restricted to those patients imaged specifically because of pain (no prior research subjects) demonstrated that our range of estimates of the radiograph test properties did not vary between the full and restricted samples. Fourth, since this was not a prospective study, there was no imaging protocol and there were differences in imaging sequences obtained. All children had at least a single AP view radiograph performed, by study design, but some children had dedicated films with multiple views. It is possible that the sensitivity and specificity of a single view radiograph is inferior to multiple views. However, in a study of adults with seronegative spondyloarthritis, there was excellent agreement (greater than 86% for both left and right joints) between AP views and AP plus oblique projections [23]. All MRI sequences, by study design, included coronal oblique views on both T1 and T2 sequences to ensure adequate visualization of the sacroiliac joints. There are no strict measurements for depiction of sacroiliac joint effusions on MRI in children. The presence or absence of abnormality is, therefore, a subjective call which is likely the reason why these lesions had low agreement between the raters. Until there are sufficient normative data in children, definitive characterization of abnormal amounts of fluid for the sacroiliac joints will remain difficult. Fifth, our study results are not applicable to parts of the world in which a MRI scan is difficult to obtain. In these areas, radiographs remain the only option for screening. Sixth, unlike the other prior study [7], this imaging-only study uses MRI findings as the gold standard for sacroiliitis, without direct use of an external reference standard. Pathologic confirmation of sacroiliitis, for example by biopsy, is rarely feasible, and clinical diagnosis of spondyloarthropathy is complex; determining the relation between MRI findings of sacroiliitis and a clinical diagnosis of spondyloarthritis or juvenile idiopathic arthritis is beyond the scope of this work.

A few findings from this study warrant additional consideration. First, the specificity of radiographs for detection of sacroiliitis using MRI as the reference standard was relatively high (60.8–92.2) with slightly higher negative predictive values (82.7–93.9). However, when we looked at the children who actually had sacroiliitis, the majority had normal radiographs. The positive and negative predictive values and rates of misclassification were very similar when the reference standard was changed to structural lesions on MRI. This means that if radiographs remain the gold standard for screening, then almost all cases of sacroiliitis, even if symptoms prompted the imaging, would be missed. If we apply the concept of an early treatment window, as has been shown in rheumatoid arthritis [24], waiting to declare sacroiliitis as a disease manifestation until changes appear on radiographs is a missed opportunity to maximally improve long-term clinical, functional, and radiographic outcomes. Further, radiographs are not without consequences to children and their parents, including anxiety (from extra imaging procedures or false positive results), radiation exposure, and costs. Procedural costs for a single AP pelvic radiograph at our institution is approximately $97.00 for one or two views and $132.00 for dedicated sacroiliac joint views; additional fees are charged for professional interpretation.

Second, imaging studies always need to be clinically correlated, considering both the pretest probability and suspicion for disease. All of the children included in the study had suspected inflammatory sacroiliitis either because of underlying diagnosis or symptoms. The majority of positive MRI studies had normal radiographs but, given clinical suspicion, MRI studies were ordered anyway. At least half of the radiographs considered indicative of sacroiliitis by all raters were accompanied by a normal MRI scan. Further, even when we think the radiograph is truly depicting evidence of joint damage and not a false positive result, the findings do not indicate whether the disease remains active and requires treatment or whether the disease has already burnt out. Therefore, abnormal radiographs are almost always followed by an MRI study. If the pretest suspicion of sacroiliitis is high enough that we are going to order the MRI scan regardless of the radiograph findings, why not save the patient and family from anxiety, radiation exposure, and healthcare dollars and jump straight to the MRI?

Conclusions

This is a systematic comparison of the utility of radiographs and MRI in children with suspected inflammatory sacroiliitis. Our results demonstrate very limited utility of radiographs for the detection of sacroiliitis. In parts of the world where MRI is readily available, obtaining or requiring radiographs prior to MRI is an antiquated practice.

Abbreviations

AP: Anterioposterior; ASAS: Assessment of Spondyloarthritis International Society; FABER: Flexion abduction external rotation; IQR: Interquartile range; JSpA: Juvenile spondyloarthritis; MRI: Magnetic resonance imaging; PACS: Picture archiving and communication system; REDCap: Research Electronic Data Capture; SIJ: Sacroiliac joint; SIS: Sacroiliac joint inflammation score; SPARCC: Spondyloarthritis Research Consortium of Canada; SSS: Sacroiliac joint structural score

Acknowledgements
The authors would like to acknowledge Joe Paschke for his assistance with the development and management of the data collection within the CaRE Arthritis platform.

Funding
PFW's work was supported by the Rheumatology Research Foundation.JLJ is supported by the Capital Health Chair in Diagnostic Imaging.

Authors' contributions
All authors made substantial contributions to conception and design, acquisition of data, or analysis and interpretation of data; were involved in drafting of the manuscript or revising it critically for important intellectual content; gave final approval of the version to be published; and agreed to be accountable for all aspects of the work in ensuring that questions related to the accuracy or integrity of any part of the work are appropriately investigated and resolved.

Competing interests
The authors declare that they have no competing interests.

Author details
[1]Department of Pediatrics, Division of Rheumatology, Children's Hospital of Philadelphia, Philadelphia, PA, USA. [2]Department of Radiology, Children's Hospital of Philadelphia, Philadelphia, PA, USA. [3]Center for Pediatric Clinical Effectiveness (CPCE), Children's Hospital of Philadelphia, Philadelphia, PA, USA. [4]Center for Clinical Epidemiology and Biostatistics, Perelman School of Medicine at the University of Pennsylvania, Philadelphia, PA, USA. [5]Department of Medicine, University of Alberta, Edmonton, AB, Canada. [6]Department of Radiology and Diagnostic Imaging, University of Alberta, Edmonton, AB, Canada. [7]Canadian Research and Education (CaRE) Arthritis Organization, Edmonton, AB, Canada. [8]The Children's Hospital of Philadelphia, Roberts Center for Pediatric Research, 2716 South Street, Room 11121, Philadelphia, PA 19146, USA.

References
1.   Weiss PF, Xiao R, Biko DM, Chauvin NA. Sacroiliitis at diagnosis of juvenile spondyloarthritis assessed by radiography, magnetic resonance imaging, and clinical examination. Arthritis Care Res. 2015;68(2):187–94.
2.   Baraliakos X, Maksymowych WP. Imaging in the diagnosis and management of axial spondyloarthritis. Best Pract Res Clin Rheumatol. 2016;30(4):608–23.
3.   Herregods N, Dehoorne J, Joos R, Jaremko JL, Baraliakos X, Leus A, Van den Bosch F, Verstraete K, Jans L. Diagnostic value of MRI features of sacroiliitis in juvenile spondyloarthritis. Clin Radiol. 2015;70(12):1428–38.
4.   Weiss PF, Xiao R, Biko DM, Johnson AM, Chauvin NA. Detection of inflammatory sacroiliitis in children with magnetic resonance imaging: is gadolinium contrast enhancement necessary? Arthritis Rheumatol. 2015; 67(8):2250–6.
5.   Sieper J, Rudwaleit M, Baraliakos X, Brandt J, Braun J, Burgos-Vargas R, Dougados M, Hermann KG, Landewe R, Maksymowych W, et al. The assessment of SpondyloArthritis International Society (ASAS) handbook: a guide to assess spondyloarthritis. Ann Rheum Dis. 2009;68(Suppl 2):ii1–ii44.
6.   Lin C, MacKenzie JD, Courtier JL, Gu JT, Milojevic D. Magnetic resonance imaging findings in juvenile spondyloarthropathy and effects of treatment observed on subsequent imaging. Ped Rheumatol Online J. 2014;12:25.
7.   Jaremko JL, Liu L, Winn NJ, Ellsworth JE, Lambert RG. Diagnostic utility of magnetic resonance imaging and radiography in juvenile spondyloarthritis: evaluation of the sacroiliac joints in controls and affected subjects. J Rheumatol. 2014;41(5):963–70.
8.   Pagnini I, Savelli S, Matucci-Cerinic M, Fonda C, Cimaz R, Simonini G. Early predictors of juvenile sacroiliitis in enthesitis-related arthritis. J Rheumatol. 2010;37(11):2395–401.
9.   Puhakka KB, Jurik AG, Egund N, Schiottz-Christensen B, Stengaard-Pedersen K, van Overeem Hansen G, Christiansen JV. Imaging of sacroiliitis in early seronegative spondylarthropathy. Assessment of abnormalities by MR in comparison with radiography and CT. Acta Radiol. 2003;44(2):218–29.

10. Blum U, Buitrago-Tellez C, Mundinger A, Krause T, Laubenberger J, Vaith P, Peter HH, Langer M. Magnetic resonance imaging (MRI) for detection of active sacroiliitis—a prospective study comparing conventional radiography, scintigraphy, and contrast enhanced MRI. J Rheumatol. 1996;23(12):2107–15.

11. Oostveen J, Prevo R, den Boer J, van de Laar M. Early detection of sacroiliitis on magnetic resonance imaging and subsequent development of sacroiliitis on plain radiography. A prospective, longitudinal study. J Rheumatol. 1999; 26(9):1953–8.

12. Weiss PF, Colbert RA. Radiography versus magnetic resonance imaging (MRI) in juvenile spondyloarthritis: is the MR image everything? J Rheumatol. 2014;41(5):832–3.

13. Harris PA, Taylor R, Thielke R, Payne J, Gonzalez N, Conde JG. Research Electronic Data Capture (REDCap)—a metadata-driven methodology and workflow process for providing translational research informatics support. J Biomed Inform. 2009;42(2):377–81.

14. Weiss PF, Maksymowych W, Lambert RG, Jaremko JL, Biko DM, Paschke J, Brandon T, Chauvin NA. Feasibility and reliability of the Spondyloarthritis Research Consortium of Canada sacroiliac joint structural score for children with spondyloarthritis. J Rheumatol. 2018; https://doi.org/10.3899/jrheum.171329.

15. Weiss PF, Maksymowych W, Lambert RG, Jaremko JL, Biko DM, Paschke J, Brandon T, Chauvin NA. Feasibility and reliability of the Spondyloarthritis Research Consortium of Canada sacroiliac joint inflammation score for children with spondyloarthritis. Arthritis Res Ther. 2018;20(1):56. https://doi.org/10.1097/PEC.0000000001460.

16. Maksymowych WP, Lambert RG, Brown LS, Pangan AL. Defining the minimally important change for the SpondyloArthritis Research Consortium of Canada spine and sacroiliac joint magnetic resonance imaging indices for ankylosing spondylitis. J Rheumatol. 2012;39(8):1666–74.

17. Maksymowych W, Lambert RG, Ostergaard M, de Hooge M, Pedersen SJ, Bennett AN, Burgos-Vagas R, Eshed I, Landewé R, Machado P, et al. MRI lesion definitions in axial spondyloarthritis: a consensus reappraisal from the assessments in SpondyloArthritis International Society (ASAS) [abstract]. Ann Rheum Dis. 2018;77(Suppl 2):356–57.

18. Maksymowych W, Ostergaard M, Lambert RG, Weber U, Pedersen SJ, Sieper J, Poddubnyy D, Wichuk S, Machado P, Baraliakos X. The contribution of structural MRI lesions to detection of sacroiliitis in patients in the assessments in SpondyloArthritis International Society (ASAS) classification cohort [abstract]. Ann Rheum Dis. 2018;77(Supll2):173–74.

19. Chauvin N, Maksymowych W, Lambert R, Jaremko J, Biko D, Brandon T, Paschke J, Weiss P. Feasibility and reliability of the Spondyloarthritis Research Consortium of Canada Sacroiliac joint structural score for children with spondyloarthritis [abstract]. Arthritis Rheumatol. 2016;68(suppl 10). https://acrabstracts.org/abstract/feasibility-and-reliability-of-the-spondyloarthritis-research-consortium-ofcanada-sacroiliac-joint-inflammation-score-for-children-with-spondyloarthritis/.

20. Fleiss JL. Measuring nominal scale agreement among many raters. Psychol Bull. 1971;76:378–82.

21. Landis JR, Koch GG. The measurement of observer agreement for categorical data. Biometrics. 1977;33:159–74.

22. Rudwaleit M, Jurik AG, Hermann K-GA, Landewé R, van der Heijde D, Baraliakos X, Marzo-Ortega H, Østergaard M, Braun J, Sieper J. Defining active sacroiliitis on magnetic resonance imaging (MRI) for classification of axial spondyloarthritis: a consensual approach by the ASAS/OMERACT MRI group. Ann Rheum Dis. 2009;68(10):1520–7.

23. Battistone MJ, Manaster BJ, Reda DJ, Clegg DO. Radiographic diagnosis of sacroiliitis—are sacroiliac views really better? J Rheumatol. 1998;25(12):2395–401.

24. Monti S, Montecucco C, Bugatti S, Caporali R. Rheumatoid arthritis treatment: the earlier the better to prevent joint damage. RMD Open. 2015; 1(Suppl 1):e000057.

4

Resolution of synovitis and arrest of catabolic and anabolic bone changes in patients with psoriatic arthritis by IL-17A blockade with secukinumab: results from the prospective PSARTROS study

Eleni Kampylafka[1], Isabelle d'Oliveira[1], Christina Linz[1], Veronika Lerchen[1], Fabian Stemmler[1], David Simon[1], Matthias Englbrecht[1], Michael Sticherling[2], Jürgen Rech[1], Arnd Kleyer[1], Georg Schett[1] and Axel J. Hueber[1]*

Abstract

Background: Although the effects of interleukin-17A (IL-17A) inhibition on the signs and symptoms of psoriatic arthritis (PsA) are well defined, little is known about its impact of local inflammatory and structural changes in the joints. The PSARTROS study was designed to elucidate the effects of IL-17A inhibition on inflammation and bone changes in joints affected by PsA.

Methods: This was a prospective open-label study in 20 patients with active PsA receiving 24 weeks of treatment with the IL-17A inhibitor secukinumab. Magnetic resonance imaging (MRI), power Doppler ultrasound (PDUS), and high-resolution peripheral quantitative computer tomography (HR-pQCT) of the hands were performed at baseline and after 24 weeks to assess synovitis, periarticular inflammation, bone erosion, enthesiophyte formation, and bone structure. Demographic and clinical measures of joint disease (DAPSA and DAS28-ESR), skin disease (PASI and BSA), and composite measures (minimal disease activity, or MDA) were also recorded.

Results: Treatment with secukinumab led to significant improvement of signs and symptoms of PsA; 46% reached MDA and 52% DAPSA low disease activity. MRI synovitis ($P = 0.034$) and signal in PDUS ($P = 0.030$) significantly decreased after 24 weeks of treatment. Bone erosions in MRI and HR-pQCT and enthesiophytes in the HR-pQCT did not show any progression, and structural integrity and functional bone strength remained stable.

Conclusions: IL-17 inhibition by secukinumab over 24 weeks led to a significant decrease of synovial inflammation and no progression of catabolic and anabolic bone changes in the joints of patients with PsA.

Keywords: Psoriatic arthritis, Bone, Erosions, Enthesiophytes, Synovitis, bDMARDs

* Correspondence: axel.hueber@uk-erlangen.de
[1]Department of Internal Medicine 3 – Rheumatology and Immunology, Friedrich-Alexander-Universität Erlangen-Nürnberg (FAU) and Universitätsklinikum Erlangen, Ulmenweg 18, 91054 Erlangen, Germany
Full list of author information is available at the end of the article

Background

Psoriatic arthritis (PsA) is a chronic inflammatory disease affecting the joints and the entheses and leads to bone damage [1]. In the joints, the inflammatory process in PsA afflicts the synovium and the periosteal insertions of tendons and ligaments. Chronic inflammation at these synovial and entheseal sites leads to bone erosions and enthesiophytes, respectively, and a link to the intestinal microbiome has been suggested [1, 2]. Cytokines are considered to trigger both the inflammatory and structural changes in patients with PsA and to provide the essential link between inflammation and damage [3, 4]. Aside from tumor necrosis factor (TNF), interleukin-17A (IL-17A) has been identified as a key cytokine in psoriatic skin and joint disease [5]. Inhibition of IL-17A by neutralizing antibodies has been shown to improve the signs and symptoms of joint disease in patients with PsA [6–8].

Despite unequivocal evidence that IL-17 inhibition works on the signs and symptoms of PsA, its local effects on the joint are inadequately characterized. Radiographic studies suggest that IL-17A inhibition retards the progression of bone erosion; however, the overall progression rate in conventional radiographs is low in PsA [9]. Although the reduction of the burden of synovitis seems to be crucial for achieving protection from bone erosion, it is not fully clear whether these targets are indeed achieved by IL-17A inhibition. On the other hand, no data are available on whether IL-17A inhibition retards or arrests the progression of enthesiophyte formation in PsA. In this context, reduction of enthesitis appears to be important [10].

Preclinical data have suggested that Il-17 is a cytokine that modulates bone structure during inflammation. Thus, IL-17 increases osteoclast differentiation and mediates bone erosion in experimental arthritis by upregulating receptor activator of nuclear factor-kappa B ligand (RANKL) and IL-1 [11, 12]. Furthermore, IL-17–producing TH17 cells induce osteoclast differentiation [13, 14]. These observations provide a rationale for the protection from bone erosion by IL-17 inhibition in PsA. Additional data suggest that the IL-23–IL-17 pathway is involved in enthesial inflammation, which is linked to new bone formation in PsA and axial spondyloarthritis [10, 15–18]. Finally, IL-17 has been shown to be a key mediator for bone loss in psoriatic disease both in mice and in humans [19]. PsA has been shown to be associated with increased fracture risk, which is likely triggered by the prolonged effect of inflammatory cytokines such as IL-17 [20]. Hence, the ideal protection from structural bone damage in PsA would mean an arrest of bone erosion, retardation of enthesiophyte formation, and maintenance of bone architecture and strength.

In this work, we performed a meticulous assessment of joints and bones of patients with PsA treated with secukinumab, a fully human monoclonal antibody selective for IL-17A, for 24 weeks. Patients with active PsA were enrolled in the prospective observational PSARTROS imaging study. Assessments were carried out by a combination of magnetic resonance imaging (MRI), power Doppler ultrasound (PDUS), and high-resolution peripheral quantitative computed tomography (HR-pQCT) to assess synovitis, periarticular inflammation, bone erosions, enthesiophytes, and bone architecture and strength at baseline and 24 weeks of secukinumab treatment. In addition, the clinical effects of secukinumab on the signs and symptoms of PsA were recorded.

Methods

Study design and patients

The PSARTROS study (ClinicalTrials.gov Identifier: NCT02483234) is a single-arm prospective exploratory open-label study to assess the effects of secukinumab treatment on the inflammatory and structural changes in the joints of patients with PsA. All patients received subcutaneous treatment with 300 mg secukinumab once weekly for the first five applications and then once monthly for a total of 24 weeks. Eligible patients were above 18 years of age and had been diagnosed with PsA according to the Classification Criteria for Psoriatic Arthritis (CASPAR) for at least 6 months prior to their inclusion in the study and had active joint disease with at least three tender and three swollen joints out of a 78/76-joint count. Corticosteroid treatment was allowed at stable doses of not more than 10 mg/day prednisone for at least 2 weeks before baseline and had to remain on a stable dose until the end of the study. Concomitant non-biologic treatment was allowed if on a stable dose for at least 4 weeks before randomization and throughout the study. Previous TNF inhibitor therapy was allowed after appropriate washout periods. Patients who had previously used drugs targeting IL-17 or IL-23p40, had received any recent live vaccines, had a history of tuberculosis, were pregnant, were using opioid analgesics, had a history of alcohol or drug abuse within the last 6 months, or had any uncontrolled medical condition were not eligible. All patients provided written informed consent, and institutional review boards/ethics committees approved the protocol.

Magnetic resonance imaging

MRI was used to assess inflammatory and structural changes in the joints. MRI scans of the dominant hand were performed at baseline and after 24 weeks of secukinumab treatment by using a 1.5 T Magneton Avanto system (Siemens, Erlangen, Germany) as described before [21]. T1-weighted images with and without contrast agent as well as T2-weighted coronal fat saturated turbo inversion recovery magnitude (TIRM) sequences were assessed for synovitis, periarticular inflammation, tenosynovitis, bone erosions, and bone proliferations as well as osteitis. T1-weighted coronal images without contrast were used to assess erosions and bone proliferation. T1-weighted axial images after intravenous gadolinium injection were used to assess synovitis and tenosynovitis. The same T1-weighted images were assessed to evaluate periarticular inflammation. TIRM sequences were used to assess osteitis. Images were evaluated by two independent assessors (IO and CL) blinded to the identity of the patients and the sequence of the images using standardized Psoriatic Arthritis Magnetic Resonance Imaging Score–OMERACT (PsAMRIS-OMERACT) scoring [22].

Power Doppler ultrasound

PDUS was used to assess the inflammatory changes in the joints. PDUS was performed at baseline and after 24 weeks of secukinumab treatment by using a Mylab twice ultrasound machine (Esaote Biomedica, Genova, Italy) with a 6- to 18-MHz probe (LA435). In 28 joints, comprising the metacarpophalangeal (MCP) 2–5, proximal interphalangeal (PIP) 2–5, wrist, knee and

metatarsophalangeal (MTP) 2–5 joints of both sides, synovial hypertrophy and power Doppler signals were scored in accordance with the Global OMERACT EULAR Ultrasound Synovitis Score (GLOESS) [23, 24]. In this score, synovial hypertrophy and power Doppler signals are graded as absent (0), mild (1), moderate (2), or severe (3). In addition, the presence of effusion was assessed. Scans were performed and evaluated by an experienced sonographer (AK).

High-resolution peripheral quantitative computed tomography

HR-pQCT was used to assess the structural changes in the joints and the bone composition and function. HR-pQCT of the dominant hand was performed at baseline and after 24 weeks of secukinumab treatment by using an XtremeCT I scanner (Scanco Medical, Brüttisellen, Switzerland). Scans were performed at MCP joints 2 and 3, PIP joints 2 and 3, and the distal radius. MCPs and PIPs were evaluated for erosions (numbers and volume) by using HR-pQCT Software [25] and enthesiophytes in accordance with the following grading: grade 1: maximum height ≤ 4 mm; grade 2: maximum height >

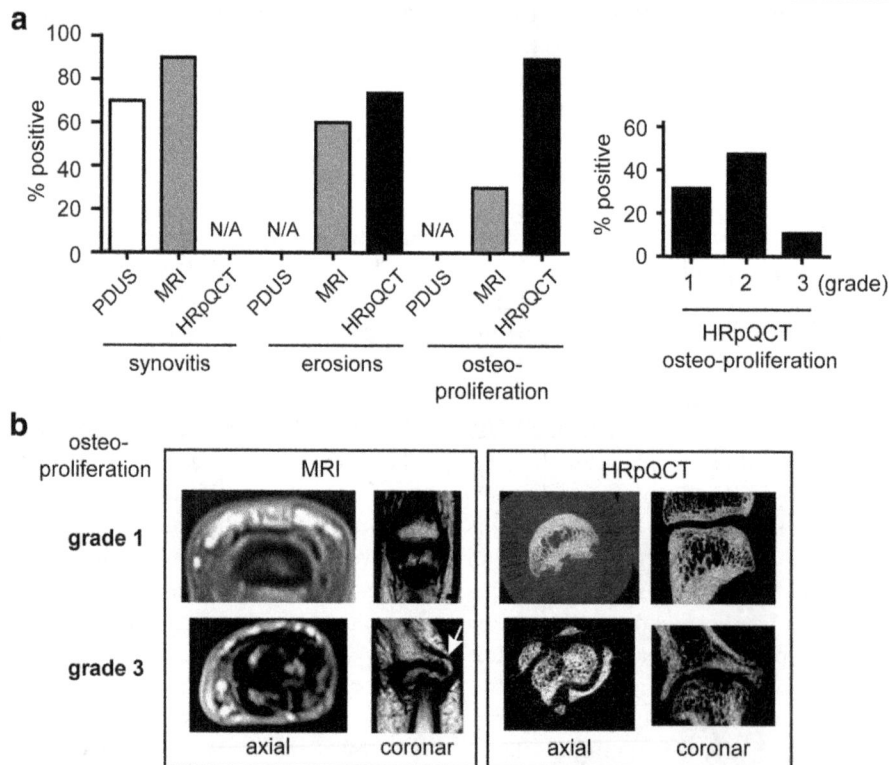

Fig. 1 Prevalence of inflammatory and structural changes in the joints of patients with psoriatic arthritis. **a** On left, baseline imaging analysis and comparative presentation of the prevalence of synovitis, bone erosions, and enthesiophytes in power Doppler ultrasound (PDUS), magnetic resonance imaging (MRI), and high-resolution peripheral quantitative computed tomography (HR-pQCT); on right, prevalence of enthesiophytes according to size using HR-pQCT (grade 1: height < 4 mm, grade 2: height ≥ 4 mm, grade 3: diffuse proliferation). **b** Coronal and axial images of the same enthesiophytes (upper panel: grade 1, lower panel: grade 3) in MRI and HR-pQCT. Arrow indicates the lesion. Abbreviation: *N/A* not applicable

4 mm; and grade 3: diffuse osteoproliferation [26]. The MCP 2 and MCP 3 joints were additionally evaluated for the volume of erosions present by using the HR-pQCT Software [25]. The distal radius was evaluated for bone structural and microstructural parameters as described previously [20]. In addition, biomechanical properties of bone (stiffness and failure load) were assessed through micro-finite element analysis of the radius (FAIM software, version 8.0, Numerics88 Solutions Ltd., Calgary, AB, Canada) [27].

Clinical assessments

Clinical evaluation at baseline and 24 weeks included tender joint counts (TJCs) 78, swollen joint counts (SJCs) 76, and visual analogue scales for patients and physicians global disease activity and patients pain. Activity of skin disease was assessed by psoriasis area severity index (PASI) and body surface area (BSA). Activity of PsA and response in signs and symptoms of PsA was assessed by Disease Activity in PSA (DAPSA) [28], Disease Activity Score (DAS) 28, Minimal Disease Activity (MDA) [29], and Psoriatic Arthritis Response Criteria (PsARC) as well as by American Colleague of Rheumatology (ACR) 20, 50, and 70 responses.

Statistical analysis

The hypothesis of the study was that secukinumab treatment (a) leads to significant improvement of synovitis and periarticular inflammation and (b) arrests progression of both erosions and enthesiophytes in the joints of PsA patients after 24 weeks. The Wilcoxon signed-rank test was used for paired comparisons between baseline and week 24. Cross-sectional analyses were performed by using the Mann–Whitney U test for differences and Spearman correlation for relations. Statistical significance was set at $P \leq 0.05$, and data were presented as median and quartiles. All analyses were performed in a two-tailed manner by using IBM SPSS version 21 (IBM, Armonk, NY, USA).

Results

Patient characteristics

In total, 20 patients with PsA were prospectively included in the study, and 60% of them were females. The median age was 50.5 years (interquartile range (IQR) 44–59), and median disease duration was 5.5 (1.25–11.75) years. Patients had moderate-to-high PsA activity according to Disease Activity Score 28-joint count–erythrocyte sedimentation rate (DAS28-ESR) (median 4.94; IQR 4.31–5.8) and DAPSA (median 27.55; IQR 22.53–38.35) with a median TJC of 10 (6.25–20) and SJC of 4 (3–5.75). Both oligo- and poly-articular PsA patients were included, and all patients showed clinical and imaging involvement of the hands (Additional file 1: Table S1). Skin involvement

was low; PASI was 0.4 (0.2–1.9) and BSA was 0.4 (0.2–1.5); 55% of the patients were biological disease-modifying antirheumatic drug (bDMARD)–naïve entering secukinumab treatment, while 45% had previously experienced TNF inhibitor. Forty percent had concomitant conventional DMARD (cDMARD) treatment, which was kept stable during the treatment phase. Three patients dropped out during the 24-week study period: one due to recurrent pharyngitis, one due to lack of efficacy, and one due to consent withdrawal. Treatment with secukinumab showed an overall good safety profile, and no serious adverse events, including infection requiring hospitalization, were reported; neither deaths nor major lab abnormalities or injection site reactions occurred. The longitudinal imaging

Table 1 Baseline imaging characteristics

Magnetic resonance imaging	
Synovitis %	90%
PSAMRIS Synovitis (median, IQR)	2.5 (1.25, 6)
Osteitis %	20%
PSAMRIS Osteitis (median, IQR)	0 (0, 0)†
PSAMRIS Osteitis (mean ± SD)	1 ± 2.8
Erosion %	60%
PSAMRIS Erosion (median, IQR)	1 (0, 2.75)
Proliferation %	30%
PSAMRIS Proliferation (median, IQR)	0 (0, 1)†
PSAMRIS Proliferation (mean ± SD)†	1.1 ± 2.4
Periarticular %	25%
PSAMRIS Periarticular (median, IQR)	0 (0, 1.5)†
PSAMRIS Periarticular (mean ± SD)†	0.8 ± 1.6
Tenosynovitis %	35%
PSAMRIS Tenosynovitis (median, IQR)	0 (0, 1.75)†
PSAMRIS Tenosynovitis (mean ± SD)†	1.6 ± 2.9
Total PSAMRIS (median, IQR)	5.5 (3, 19.5)
PDUS	
Synovitis %	70%
OMERACT Hypertrophy (median, IQR)	5.5. (2.25, 10.75)
OMERACT Effusion (median, IQR)	4.5 (1, 8.5)
OMERACT Power Doppler (median, IQR)	2 (1.25, 5.75)
OMERACT Global (median, IQR)	5 (3, 11)
HR-pQCT	
Erosions (%)	73.7%
Enthesiophytes (%)	89.5%

HR-pQCT high-resolution peripheral quantitative computed tomography, *IQR* interquartile range, *OMERACT* outcome measures in rheumatoid arthritis clinical trials, *PDUS* power Doppler ultrasound, *PSAMRIS* psoriatic arthritis magnetic resonance imaging scoring system. †Additionally reported as mean and standard deviation (mean ± standard deviation) because median was equal to zero. Data are based on all 20 psoriatic arthritis patients recruited into the study evaluation was performed in the 17 patients completing the study.

Baseline imaging features and comparison of imaging modalities

Baseline MRI investigation revealed synovitis in the vast majority (90%) of patients. Synovitis was also found in the majority of patients (70%) when using PDUS (Fig. 1a, Table 1). The median total PSAMRIS score was 5.5 (IQR 3–19.5), the median global OMERACT score was 8.5 (IQR 4.25–12.75), and MRI showed other forms of inflammation such as tenosynovitis, periarticular inflammation, and osteitis in a substantial number of patients (Table 1). The majority of patients with PsA had erosions in the MRI at baseline (60%) and this number was even higher when assessing the joints by HR-pQCT (73.7%). Enthesiophytes were found in only 30% of the patients when MRI was used, but these bone lesions were much more detectable by HR-pQCT, where most patients with PsA (89%) showed enthesiophytes. The majority of enthesiophytes were graded as mild (grade 1) or moderate (grade 2) and only few were severe (grade 3), which were then also detected by MRI (Fig. 1b).

Effects of secukinumab on joint inflammation

Sequential assessment of joint inflammation by MRI showed a significant decrease in global PsAMRIS ($P = 0.039$) and PsAMRIS synovitis score ($P = 0.034$) (Fig. 2a and b; Table 2; Additional file 1: Figure S1 and 2A; Additional file 1: Table S5) after 24 weeks of secukinumab treatment. Furthermore, periarticular inflammation completely disappeared (Table 2). With respect to PDUS assessment, global OMERACT EULAR ultrasound score ($P = 0.005$), synovial hypertrophy ($P = 0.009$), and power Doppler activity ($P = 0.030$) significantly improved after 24 weeks of secukinumab treatment (Table 2, Fig. 2c, Additional file 1: Figure S2B), confirming the data

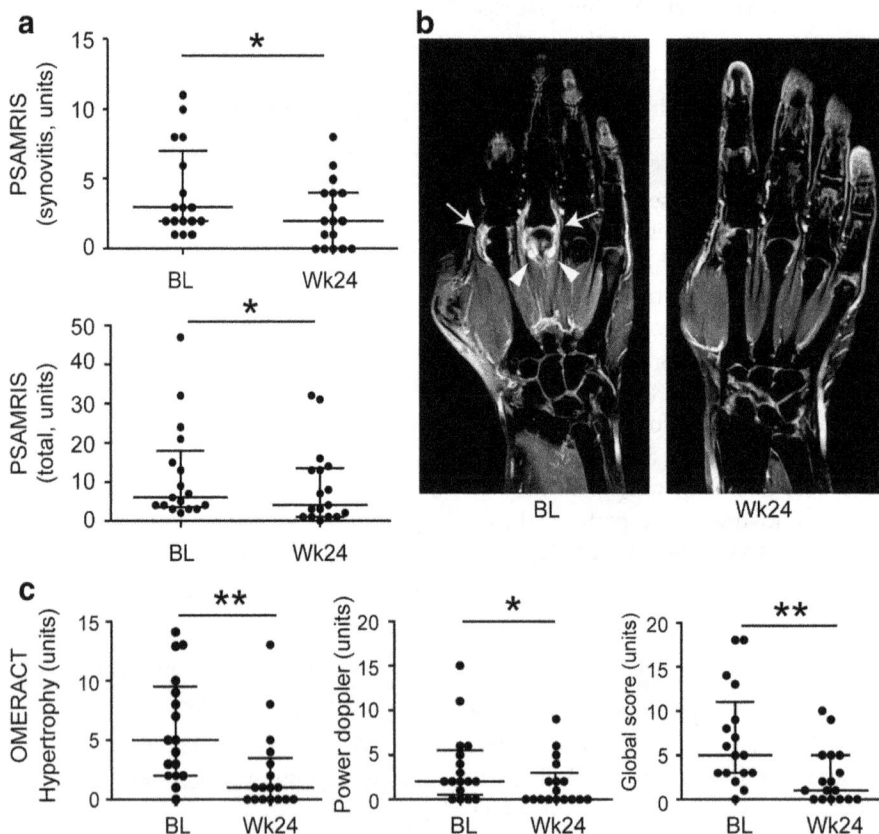

Fig. 2 Effects of secukinumab treatment on the inflammatory changes in the joints of patients with psoriatic arthritis. **a** Comparison of inflammatory changes in the joints of psoriatic arthritis (PsA) patients using magnetic resonance imaging (MRI) at baseline (BL) and after 24 weeks (Wk24) of secukinumab treatment. Psoriatic arthritis MRI scores (PsAMRIS) for synovitis and total PsAMRIS scores are shown. **b** Representative coronal T1-weighted fat-suppressed post-gadolinium MRI images of the hand of the same patient with PsA at baseline and after 24 weeks are depicted. Baseline image shows synovitis (arrows) and periarticular inflammation at enthesial sites (arrowheads), which resolved after 24 weeks of secukinumab treatment. **c** Comparison of inflammatory changes in the joints of PsA patients using power Doppler ultrasound (PDUS) at baseline (BL) and after 24 weeks (Wk24) of secukinumab treatment. OMERACT ultrasound scores for synovial hypertrophy and power Doppler activity as well as global OMERACT ultrasound scores are shown. Data are presented as median and interquartile ranges. *$P \leq 0.05$; **$P \leq 0.01$

Table 2 Changes of the inflammatory and structural parameters between baseline and week 24

Characteristic	Baseline	Week 24	P value
MRI			
PSAMRIS Synovitis (median,IQR)	3 (2, 7)	2 (0, 4)	0.034*
PSAMRIS Osteitis (median,IQR), (mean ± SD)†	0 (0, 5)†, 1.2 ± 3.1	0 (0, 0)†, 0.5 ± 1.3	0.180
PSAMRIS Periarticular (median,IQR) (mean ± SD)†	0 (0, 1)†, 0.7 ± 1.6	0 (0, 0)†, 0 ± 0	0.059
PSAMRIS Tenossynovitis (median,IQR) (mean ± SD)†	0 (0, 1.5)†, 1.2 ± 2.2	0 (0, 0)†, 0.7 ± 1.7	0.400
PSAMRIS Erosions (median, IQR)	1 (0, 3)	1 (0, 4)	0.167
PSAMRIS Proliferation (median,IQR) (mean ± SD)†	0 (0, 1)†, 1.2 ± 2.6	0 (0, 1)†, 1.2 ± 2.6	0.655
Total PSAMRIS (median, IQR)	6 (3.5, 18)	4 (1, 13.5)	0.039*
PDUS			
OMERACT Hypertrophy (median, IQR)	5 (2, 9.5)	1 (0, 3.5)	0.009**
OMERACT Effusion (median, IQR) (mean ± SD)†	4 (0.5, 6.5)†, 4.1 ± 3.9	0 (0, 4)†, 2.3 ± 3.2	0.084
OMERACT Power Doppler (median, IQR) (mean ± SD)†	2 (0.5, 5.5)†, 3.6 ± 4.1	0 (0, 3)†, 1.8 ± 2.7	0.030**
Global OMERACT (median, IQR)	5 (3, 11)	1 (0, 5)	0.003**
HR-pQCT			
Erosion Number (median, IQR)	2 (0.5, 4.5)	2 (1, 4)	0.059
Erosion Volume (median, IQR)	3.29 (0.40, 14.68)	3.87 (0.41, 16.7)	0.859
Proliferation Grade (median, IQR)	2 (1,2)	2 (1.5, 2)	0.083

HR-pQCT high-resolution peripheral quantitative computed tomography, *IQR* interquartile range, *MRI* magnetic resonance imaging, *OMERACT* outcome measures in rheumatoid arthritis clinical trials, *PDUS* power Doppler ultrasound, *PSAMRIS* psoriatic arthritis magnetic resonance imaging scoring system. †Additionally reported as mean and standard deviation (mean ± standard deviation) because median was equal to zero. Data are based on 17 psoriatic arthritis patients with complete baseline and 24 week data. Wilcoxon signed-rank test. *P ≤0.05, **P ≤0.01

obtained by MRI. The effects of secukinumab on the reduction of synovitis in MRI and PDUS were not different between patients naïve or experienced to TNF inhibitors (Additional file 1: Table S2). When comparing previous or concomitant cDMARD treatment also no difference in response was detected (Additional file 1: Table S3 and S4).

Effects of secukinumab on bone erosions
We next examined whether secukinumab therapy arrests the progression of bone erosions in patients with PsA. Bone erosions were assessed at baseline and after 24 weeks of secukinumab treatment by using MRI and HR-pQCT. In MRI, PSAMRIS bone erosion score remained stable over the 24 weeks of treatment with no signs of progression (Table 2; Fig. 3a). In HR-pQCT, erosion numbers and erosion volume did not show any significant progression either (Table 2; Fig. 3a).

Effects of secukinumab on enthesiophyte progression
Since enthesiophytes are a hallmark of structural damage in PsA, we were interested in whether the progression of these lesions is inhibited by secukinumab. In MRI, where osteoproliferation is also scored, no progression was found (Table 2; Fig. 3b). In HR-pQCT, which is more sensitive for enthesiophytes, no progression was detected (Table 2,

Fig. 3b), suggesting that secukinumab also leads to an arrest of progression of anabolic bone changes in PsA.

Effects of secukinumab on bone structure and functional properties
We next investigated bone structure and bone functional properties at the distal radius. Cortical and trabecular bone structure remained stable over 24 weeks of secukinumab treatment (Fig. 3c). Furthermore, cortical thickness, as the key microstructural parameter of cortical bone, and trabecular number, as the key microstructural parameter of trabecular bone, did not change between baseline and week 24 (Fig. 3c). Finally, functional bone parameters such as failure load and stiffness resembling bone strength according to micro-finite element analysis remained stable (Fig. 3d).

Effects of secukinumab on clinical outcomes
DAS28-ESR declined from a median of 4.93 units at baseline to 2.93 units ($P = 0.001$) after 24 weeks, resembling low disease activity (Table 3). DAPSA declined from a median of 27.5 units at baseline to 5.7 units ($P < 0.001$) after 24 weeks, also resembling low disease activity. Effects of DAPSA responses were similar between patients naïve or experienced to TNF inhibitors, while DAS28-ESR responses were better ($P = 0.01$; Mann–Whitney U test) in TNF inhibitor–naïve (2.4; 2.1–3.5) than experienced (1.5; 1.2–2.1) patients.

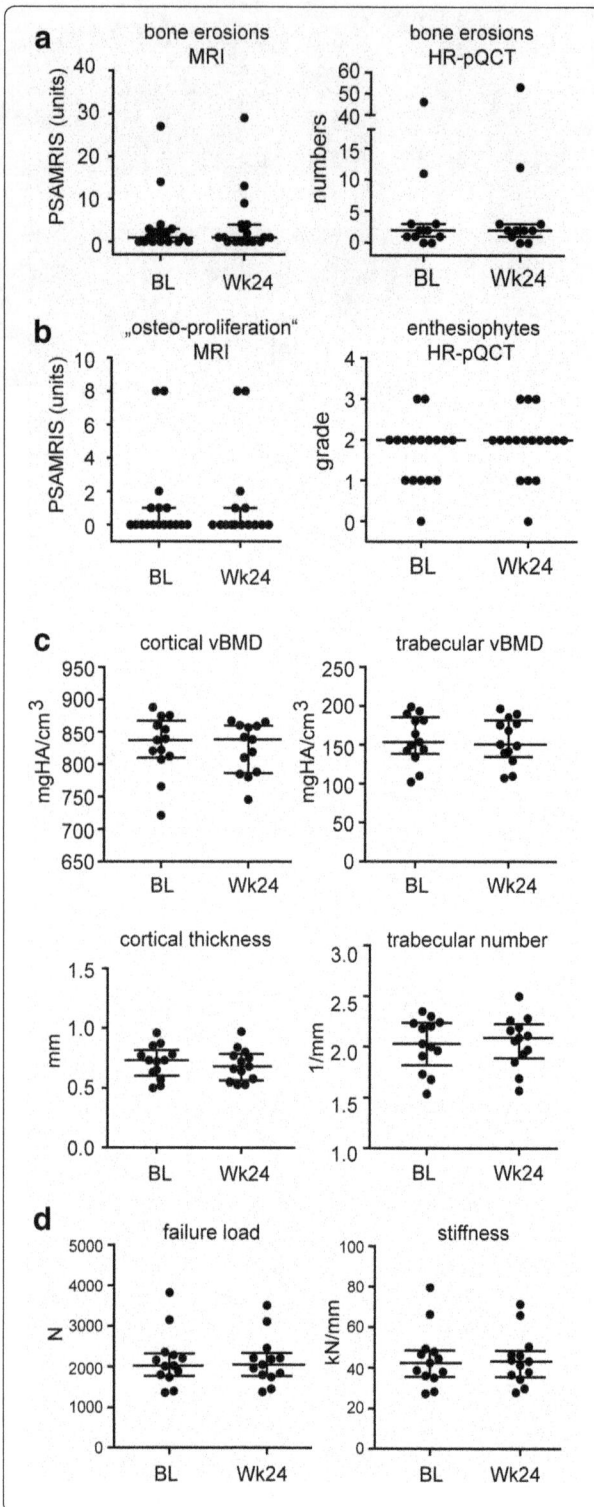

Fig. 3 Effects of secukinumab treatment on the articular and extra-articular structural bone changes in patients with psoriatic arthritis. **a** Comparison of bone erosions in the joints of psoriatic arthritis (PsA) patients using magnetic resonance imaging (MRI, left) and high-resolution peripheral quantitative computed tomography (HR-pQCT, right) at baseline (BL) and after 24 weeks (Wk24) of secukinumab treatment. MRI data represent Psoriatic arthritis MRI scores (PsAMRIS) for erosions, and HR-pQCT data represent erosion volumes. **b** Comparison of enthesiophytes in the joints of PsA patients using MRI (left) and HR-pQCT (right) at baseline (BL) and after 24 weeks (Wk24) of secukinumab treatment. MRI data represent Psoriatic arthritis MRI scores (PsAMRIS) for proliferations, and HR-pQCT data represent enthesiophyte grades according to size. **c** Comparison of bone micro-structural data of the distal radius of PsA patients using HR-pQCT at baseline (BL) and after 24 weeks (Wk24) of secukinumab treatment. Cortical and trabecular volumetric bone density (vBMD), cortical thickness, and trabecular numbers are shown. **d** Comparison of biomechanical properties of radial bones of PsA patients using HR-pQCT measurements at baseline (BL) and after 24 weeks (Wk24) of secukinumab treatment. Data show failure load and bone stiffness based on micro-finite element analysis. Data are presented as median and interquartile ranges. Abbreviations: *kN* kiloNewton, *mgHA/cm³* milligram of hydroxyapatite per cube centimeter, *N* Newton

ACR 20, 50, and 70 were achieved in 82.4%, 52.9%, and 35.3% of patients, respectively. MDA was achieved in 46.2% of the patients after 24 weeks (Table 3). Patients reaching MDA had significantly better response in PDUS parameters of inflammation (OMERACT synovium hypertrophy and GLOESS, $P < 0.05$) than those not reaching MDA.

Discussion

The data from the PSARTROS study show that inhibition of IL-17A by secukinumab improves the local inflammatory changes in the joints of patients with PsA and also arrests the progression of structural changes. These data add knowledge to the existing clinical trial data on the effects of IL-17A inhibition on the signs and symptoms of PsA. Importantly, both MRI and PDUS analysis of the joints showed a consistent improvement of synovitis in PsA patients and no sign of structural progression, even with high-quality imaging such as MRI and HR-pQCT.

Clinical studies to date have shown compelling evidence that secukinumab improves pain, swelling, function, and quality of life. These data have led to the approval of secukinumab for the treatment of PsA. The effects of IL-17A inhibition by secukinumab on the local inflammatory and structural pathologies in the joints of patients with PsA are less well defined. Analysis of the joints by conventional radiography showed that secukinumab was associated with significant retardation of radiographic progression after 24 weeks [9]. This finding essentially supports the function of secukinumab as DMARD in PsA. However, overall radiographic

Table 3 Changes in signs and symptoms of psoriatic arthritis between baseline and week 24

Characteristic	Baseline	Week 24	P value
TJC 78 (median, IQR)	10 (6, 16.5)	1 (0, 3.5)	< 0.001**
SJC 76 (median, IQR), (mean ± SD)	4 (3, 7), 5.1 ± 2.5	0 (0, 0)†, 0.2 ± 0.4	< 0.001**
DAS28-ESR (median, IQR)	4.93 (4.08, 5.74)	2.93 (2.01, 3.70)	0.001**
DAPSA (median, IQR)	27.55 (22.53, 38.35)	5.73 (3.63, 3.70)	< 0.001**
PASI (median, IQR)	0.4 (0.2, 2.3)	0.1 (0, 1.3)	0.062
BSA% (median, IQR)	0.3 (0.2, 1.5)	0.2 (0, 1.9)	0.325
ACR20	-	82.4%	-
ACR50	-	52.9%	-
ACR70	-	35.3%	-
EULAR moderate	-	68.8%	-
EULAR good	-	25.0%	-
PSARC	-	88.2%	-
DAPSA minor#	-	11.8%	-
DAPSA moderate#	-	29.4%	-
DAPSA good#	-	35.3%	-
DAPSA high##	-	0%	-
DAPSA moderate##	-	17.6%	-
DAPSA low##	-	52.9%	-
DAPSA remission##	-	29.4%	-
MDA	-	46.2%	-

ACR American College of Rheumatology, *BSA%* percent body surface area, *DAPSA* disease activity in psoriatic arthritis score, *DAS28-ESR* disease activity score 28 based on erythrocyte sedimentation rate, *EULAR* European League Against Rheumatism, *IQR* interquartile range, *MDA* minimal disease activity, *PASI* psoriasis area and severity index, *PsARC* psoriatic arthritis response criteria, *SJC* swollen joint count, *TJC* tender joint count. #Minor (change ≥50%), moderate (≥75%), good (≥85%). ##Remission (DAPSA ≤4), low (>4 and ≤14), moderate (>14 and ≤28), high (>28). †Additionally reported as mean and standard deviation (mean ± standar deviation) because median was equal to zero. Data are based on 17 psoriatic arthritis patients with complete baseline and 24 week data. Wilcoxon signed-rank test. *P ≤0.05, **P ≤0.01

progression rate is low, raising the question of whether conventional radiography may miss substantial aspects of structural pathology in PsA. Limitations associated with conventional radiography are (i) its resolution, (ii) the fact that anabolic features of bone damage are not analyzed, and (iii) the fact that no information on the inflammatory pathologies in the joints of patients with PsA is obtained.

MRI und PDUS are the techniques of choice to analyze inflammatory changes in patients with PsA, especially since instruments such as PSAMRIS and OMERACT ultrasound scores for grading have been developed [22, 23]. Unfortunately, these instruments have not been consistently implemented in evaluating the therapeutic responses of cytokine inhibitors in PsA. Herein, we show that it is feasible to find significant therapeutic responses by MRI und PDUS in even small numbers of patients with PsA. Hence, the burden of synovitis was consistently reduced by secukinumab irrespectively of whether MRI or PDUS was used to quantify inflammation. Furthermore, periarticular inflammation in the MRI, which, in part, resembles enthesitis, completely resolved upon secukinumab treatment. These

data suggest that IL-17A inhibition allows full or at least partial resolution of inflammatory lesions in the joints. Given that clinical and imaging signs of inflammation are often not well aligned [30], these findings are particularly valuable, indicating that it is possible to clear inflammation from PsA joints by neutralizing IL-17A.

With respect to bone erosions, the observation that even highly sensitive techniques, such as MRI and particularly HR-pQCT, did not show any signs of progression provides solid evidence that the aforementioned reduction of synovitis by secukinumab is followed by protection from progression of structural damage. Direct effects of IL-17A inhibition on osteoclast differentiation may add to the observed protection from erosion in PsA. Even more importantly, PSARTROS provides the first evidence that enthesiophyte formation can be arrested in PsA. Hence, HR-pQCT assessment of this central structural change in patients with PsA [31] showed no signs of progression of bony spurs. In contrast, previous longitudinal data on enthesiophytes suggested progression of these anabolic bone lesions in both methotrexate- and TNF inhibitor-treated PsA patients [32]. Hence, these data provide the first evidence that enthesiophyte growth can be stopped in patients with PsA. These findings also support the increasingly recognized role of IL-17 in enthesitis [10].

IL-17 is a cytokine which negatively influences bone homeostasis by upregulating bone resorption [11–14] and inhibiting bone formation [19, 33]. Patients with PsA are characterized by bone loss and increased fracture risk [20]. We therefore took the opportunity to assess the effects of secukinumab on bone structure and strength. In this detailed analysis of bone mass, microstructure, and strength, no significant decline of bone parameters could be observed over a period of 24 weeks. These data represent the first longitudinal data on bone microstructure and strength during the treatment of arthritis and provide strong evidence that IL-17A targeting maintains the structural and functional properties of bone in patients with PsA.

Although this study provides the first comprehensive and in-depth imaging analysis of the joints of PsA patients during bDMARD therapy, several limitations have to be discussed. First, there is no placebo control arm, which does not completely rule out the possibility that in placebo-treated patients no structural progression would have occurred. However, inclusion of a placebo arm over 24 weeks would have been ethically challenging given that active PsA patients failing on methotrexate or biologic therapy were included. Furthermore, it seems unlikely that placebo treatment would have led to significant responses on synovitis. Second, this is an exploratory study with a small sample size using high-end imaging. Hence, generalizability of the data needs to be regarded with caution, and it cannot be excluded that, in larger samples, some patients progress despite secukinumab treatment. Nonetheless, in this study, significant effects on the inflammatory changes by MRI and PDUS were detected. Finally, long-term effects of secukinumab treatment on bone structure are not assessed by this study, which lasted for 24 weeks. Hence, especially the effects on bone structure may take more time than only 24 weeks and could have been missed.

Conclusions

In summary, the PSARTROS study shows that targeting IL-17 by secukinumab effectively controls synovitis and leads to an arrest of catabolic as well as anabolic structural bone changes in patients with PsA. These data underline a causative role of IL-17 in triggering joint disease in the context of psoriasis.

Abbreviations

ACR: American Colleague of Rheumatology; bDMARD: Biological disease-modifying antirheumatic drug; BSA: Body surface area; DAPSA: Disease Activity in psoriatic arthritis; DAS: Disease Activity Score; DMARD: Disease-modifying antirheumatic drug; ESR: Erythrocyte sedimentation rate; EULAR: European League Against Rheumatism; GLOESS: Global OMERACT EULAR Ultrasound Synovitis Score; HR-pQCT: High-resolution peripheral quantitative computer tomography; IL-17: Interleukin-17; IQR: Interquartile range; MCP: Metacarpophalangeal; MDA: Minimal disease activity; MRI: Magnetic resonance imaging; OMERACT: Outcome Measures in Rheumatoid Arthritis Clinical Trials; PASI: Psoriasis area severity index; PDUS: Power Doppler ultrasound; PIP: Proximal interphalangeal; PsA: Psoriatic arthritis; SJC: Swollen joint count; TJC: Tender joint count; TNF: Tumor necrosis factor

Acknowledgments
We thank Catherina Kühl for her support in conducting this study.

Funding
This work was supported by a research grant from the FOREUM Foundation for Research in Rheumatology and by a research grant from Novartis. We acknowledge support by Deutsche Forschungsgemeinschaft and Friedrich-

Authors' contributions
EK, DS, JR, AK, and AJH collected the data. EK, IS, CL, VL, FS, DS, ME, MS, JR, AK, and AJH analyzed and interpreted the data. EK, GS, and AJH prepared and revised the manuscript. GS and AJH designed the study. All authors read and approved the final manuscript.

Consent for publication
Not applicable.

Competing interests
The authors declare that they have no competing interests.

Author details
[1]Department of Internal Medicine 3 – Rheumatology and Immunology, Friedrich-Alexander-Universität Erlangen-Nürnberg (FAU) and Universitätsklinikum Erlangen, Ulmenweg 18, 91054 Erlangen, Germany. [2]Department of Dermatology, Friedrich-Alexander-Universität Erlangen-Nürnberg (FAU) and Universitätsklinikum Erlangen, Ulmenweg 18, 91054 Erlangen, Germany.

References
1. Ritchlin CT, Colbert RA, Gladman DD. Psoriatic arthritis. N Engl J Med. 2017; 376(21):2095–6.
2. Scher JU, Ubeda C, Artacho A, Attur M, Isaac S, Reddy SM, et al. Decreased bacterial diversity characterizes the altered gut microbiota in patients with psoriatic arthritis, resembling dysbiosis in inflammatory bowel disease. Arthritis Rheumatol. 2015;67(1):128–39.
3. Mease P. New pathways of treatment for psoriatic arthritis. Lancet (London, England). 2017;389(10086):2268–70.
4. Veale DJ. Psoriatic arthritis: recent progress in pathophysiology and drug development. Arthritis Res Ther. 2013;15(6):224.
5. Schett G, Elewaut D, McInnes IB, Dayer JM, Neurath MF. How cytokine networks fuel inflammation: toward a cytokine-based disease taxonomy. Nat Med. 2013;19(7):822–4.
6. McInnes IB, Mease PJ, Kirkham B, Kavanaugh A, Ritchlin CT, Rahman P, et al. Secukinumab, a human anti-interleukin-17A monoclonal antibody, in patients with psoriatic arthritis (FUTURE 2): a randomised, double-blind, placebo-controlled, phase 3 trial. Lancet (London, England). 2015;386(9999):1137–46.
7. Mease PJ, van der Heijde D, Ritchlin CT, Okada M, Cuchacovich RS, Shuler CL, et al. Ixekizumab, an interleukin-17A specific monoclonal antibody, for the treatment of biologic-naive patients with active psoriatic arthritis: results from the 24-week randomised, double-blind, placebo-controlled and active (adalimumab)-controlled period of the phase III trial SPIRIT-P1. Ann Rheum Dis. 2017;76(1):79–87.
8. Mease PJ, McInnes IB, Kirkham B, Kavanaugh A, Rahman P, van der Heijde D, et al. Secukinumab inhibition of interleukin-17A in patients with psoriatic arthritis. N Engl J Med. 2015;373(14):1329–39.
9. van der Heijde D, Landewe RB, Mease PJ, McInnes IB, Conaghan PG, Pricop L, et al. Brief report: Secukinumab provides significant and sustained inhibition of joint structural damage in a phase III study of active psoriatic arthritis. Arthritis Rheumatol. 2016;68(8):1914–21.
10. Schett G, Lories RJ, D'Agostino MA, Elewaut D, Kirkham B, Soriano ER, et al. Enthesitis: from pathophysiology to treatment. Nat Rev Rheumatol. 2017; 13(12):731–41.

11. Koenders MI, Lubberts E, Oppers-Walgreen B, van den Bersselaar L, Helsen MM, Di Padova FE, et al. Blocking of interleukin-17 during reactivation of experimental arthritis prevents joint inflammation and bone erosion by decreasing RANKL and interleukin-1. Am J Pathol. 2005;167(1):141–9.

12. Adamopoulos IE, Chao CC, Geissler R, Laface D, Blumenschein W, Iwakura Y, et al. Interleukin-17A upregulates receptor activator of NF-kappaB on osteoclast precursors. Arthritis Res Ther. 2010;12(1):R29.

13. Sato K, Suematsu A, Okamoto K, Yamaguchi A, Morishita Y, Kadono Y, et al. Th17 functions as an osteoclastogenic helper T cell subset that links T cell activation and bone destruction. J Exp Med. 2006;203(12):2673–82.

14. Kotake S, Udagawa N, Takahashi N, Matsuzaki K, Itoh K, Ishiyama S, et al. IL-17 in synovial fluids from patients with rheumatoid arthritis is a potent stimulator of osteoclastogenesis. J Clin Invest. 1999;103(9):1345–52.

15. Sherlock JP, Joyce-Shaikh B, Turner SP, Chao CC, Sathe M, Grein J, et al. IL-23 induces spondyloarthropathy by acting on ROR-gammat+ CD3+CD4-CD8- entheseal resident T cells. Nat Med. 2012;18(7):1069–76.

16. Lories RJ, McInnes IB. Primed for inflammation: enthesis-resident T cells. Nat Med. 2012;18(7):1018–9.

17. Reinhardt A, Yevsa T, Worbs T, Lienenklaus S, Sandrock I, Oberdorfer L, et al. Interleukin-23-dependent gamma/delta T cells produce Interleukin-17 and accumulate in the Enthesis, aortic valve, and Ciliary body in mice. Arthritis Rheumatol. 2016;68(10):2476–86.

18. Cuthbert RJ, Fragkakis EM, Dunsmuir R, Li Z, Coles M, Marzo-Ortega H, et al. Brief report: group 3 innate lymphoid cells in human Enthesis. Arthritis Rheumatol. 2017;69(9):1816–22.

19. Uluckan O, Jimenez M, Karbach S, Jeschke A, Grana O, Keller J, et al. Chronic skin inflammation leads to bone loss by IL-17-mediated inhibition of Wnt signaling in osteoblasts. Sci Transl Med. 2016;8(330):330ra337.

20. Kocijan R, Englbrecht M, Haschka J, Simon D, Kleyer A, Finzel S, et al. Quantitative and qualitative changes of bone in psoriasis and psoriatic arthritis patients. J Bone Miner Res. 2015;30(10):1775–83.

21. Faustini F, Simon D, Oliveira I, Kleyer A, Haschka J, Englbrecht M, et al. Subclinical joint inflammation in patients with psoriasis without concomitant psoriatic arthritis: a cross-sectional and longitudinal analysis. Ann Rheum Dis. 2016;75(12):2068–74.

22. Ostergaard M, McQueen F, Wiell C, Bird P, Boyesen P, Ejbjerg B, et al. The OMERACT psoriatic arthritis magnetic resonance imaging scoring system (PsAMRIS): definitions of key pathologies, suggested MRI sequences, and preliminary scoring system for PsA hands. J Rheumatol. 2009;36(8):1816–24.

23. Bruyn GA, Naredo E, Iagnocco A, Balint PV, Backhaus M, Gandjbakhch F, et al. The OMERACT ultrasound working group 10 years on: update at OMERACT 12. J Rheumatol. 2015;42(11):2172–6.

24. D'Agostino MA, Boers M, Wakefield RJ, Berner Hammer H, Vittecoq O, Filippou G, et al. Exploring a new ultrasound score as a clinical predictive tool in patients with rheumatoid arthritis starting abatacept: results from the APPRAISE study. RMD Open. 2016;2(1):e000237.

25. Figueiredo CP, Kleyer A, Simon D, Stemmler F, d'Oliveira I, Weissenfels A, et al. Methods for segmentation of rheumatoid arthritis bone erosions in high-resolution peripheral quantitative computed tomography (HR-pQCT). Semin Arthritis Rheum. 2018;47(5):611–8.

26. Finzel S, Sahinbegovic E, Kocijan R, Engelke K, Englbrecht M, Schett G. Inflammatory bone spur formation in psoriatic arthritis is different from bone spur formation in hand osteoarthritis. Arthritis Rheumatol. 2014;66(11): 2968–75.

27. Macneil JA, Boyd SK. Bone strength at the distal radius can be estimated from high-resolution peripheral quantitative computed tomography and the finite element method. Bone. 2008;42(6):1203–13.

28. Smolen JS, Schoels M, Aletaha D. Disease activity and response assessment in psoriatic arthritis using the disease activity index for PSoriatic arthritis (DAPSA). A brief review. Clin Exp Rheumatol. 2015;33(5 Suppl 93):S48–50.

29. Coates LC, Fransen J, Helliwell PS. Defining minimal disease activity in psoriatic arthritis: a proposed objective target for treatment. Ann Rheum Dis. 2010;69(1):48–53.

30. Lackner A, Duftner C, Ficjan A, Gretler J, Hermann J, Husic R, et al. The association of clinical parameters and ultrasound verified inflammation with patients' and physicians' global assessments in psoriatic arthritis. Semin Arthritis Rheum. 2016;46(2):183–9.

31. Finzel S, Englbrecht M, Engelke K, Stach C, Schett G. A comparative study of periarticular bone lesions in rheumatoid arthritis and psoriatic arthritis. Ann Rheum Dis. 2011;70(1):122–7.

32. Finzel S, Kraus S, Schmidt S, Hueber A, Rech J, Engelke K, et al. Bone anabolic changes progress in psoriatic arthritis patients despite treatment with methotrexate or tumour necrosis factor inhibitors. Ann Rheum Dis. 2013;72(7):1176–81.

33. Shaw AT, Maeda Y, Gravallese EM. IL-17A deficiency promotes periosteal bone formation in a model of inflammatory arthritis. Arthritis Res Ther. 2016; 18(1):104.

5

Ten years of follow-up data in psoriatic arthritis: results based on standardized monitoring of patients in an ordinary outpatient clinic in southern Norway

Glenn Haugeberg[1,2]*, Brigitte Michelsen[1], Stig Tengesdal[1], Inger Johanne Widding Hansen[1], Andreas Diamantopoulos[3] and Arthur Kavanaugh[4]

Abstract

Background: Over the last decade, a treat-to-target (T2T) strategy has been recommended for psoriatic arthritis (PsA) and new treatment options have become available. There is a lack of data on PsA regarding any changes that may have occurred over these past years. Thus, the main aim of this study was to look for changes in clinical disease status and treatment in a PsA outpatient clinic population monitored over the period 2008 to 2017.

Methods: Annual data collection included demographic data, laboratory (erythrocyte sedimentation rate (ESR) and C-reactive protein (CRP)) and clinic measures of disease activity (e.g., 28 and 32 joint count Disease Activity Score (DAS28), Clinical Disease Activity Index (CDAI), and modified Disease Activity index for Psoriatic arthritis (DAPSA)), evaluator's global assessment, and patient-reported outcomes (PROs), including for example measures of physical function, pain, and patient global assessment. Disease-modifying antirheumatic drug (DMARD) use was also registered.

Results: In the PsA outpatient clinic population over the 10-year period (annual mean number of patients, 331) the mean (standard deviation) age was 58.4 (12.4) years, disease duration was 9.6 (7.9) years, 49.4% were female, and 17.6% were current smokers. From 2008 to 2017, no statistically significant increase in remission rates was seen for DAPSA (13.5% and 22.0%) or Boolean remission (6.6% and 8.9%), whereas a statistically significant increase was seen for DAS28-ESR (36.8% and 50.6%) and CDAI (20.0% and 29.6%), but not for the last 5 years (DAS28-ESR, 42.3% and 50.6%; CDAI, 27.9% and 29.6%). Furthermore, over the 10-year period no significant improvement for PROs and no significant change in the use of synthetic (annual mean 53.0%) and biologic DMARDs (annual mean 29.9%) was found.

Conclusion: Our data suggest that even in the biologic treatment era there is an unmet need for treating PsA patients to target remission. New treatment options and the development of more feasible and valid outcome measures for use in a T2T strategy in ordinary clinical practice may in the future to further improve clinical outcomes in PsA.

Keywords: Psoriatic arthritis, Clinical outcome, Disease activity, Patient-reported outcome measures, Treat to target, Real life registries

* Correspondence: glenn.haugeberg@sshf.no
[1]Division of Rheumatology, Department of Medicine, Hospital of Southern Norway Trust, Servicebox 416, 4604 Kristiansand, Norway
[2]Department of Neuroscience, Division of Rheumatology, Norwegian University of Science and Technology, Trondheim, Norway
Full list of author information is available at the end of the article

Background

In the new millennium, new treatment strategies (early intervention and treat-to-target (T2T)) have become the new standard of clinical follow-up for patients with chronic inflammatory joint disorders [1]. The T2T strategy was first recommended for use in rheumatoid arthritis (RA) where its significant impact on improved clinical outcome has been convincingly documented [2, 3]. Encouraged by the evidence in RA, an international task force in 2012 recommended the T2T strategy also be used in spondyloarthritis (SpA), including psoriatic arthritis (PsA). The recommendations, however, were mainly based on expert opinion [4]. With new data available strengthening these recommendations, a revised updated version was published in 2018 [5].

In the new millennium, new treatment options with a broad range of targeted modes of action have become available for treatment of chronic inflammatory joint disorders, including PsA [6].

Most data available in the literature are based on selected patient groups included in, for example, registries or clinical studies. Data reflecting unselected outpatient clinic cohorts with data obtained from patients monitored using clinical outcome measures are rare.

We have previously published data on 10-year change in disease status and treatment for RA based on standardized monitoring in an ordinary outpatient clinic in southern Norway [7]. In that study, we documented the dramatic improvement in clinical outcomes and prognosis for RA that took place in a Norwegian outpatient clinic in the period from 2004 to 2013 [7]. To our knowledge, no longitudinal observational study data exist on changes in clinical outcomes and treatment for PsA outpatients reflecting an entire PsA outpatient clinic cohort monitored with standardized outcome measures as part of ordinary clinical practice.

Thus, the aim of this study was to explore the long-term changes in clinical disease status and treatment in Norwegian PsA outpatients, monitored as part of standard clinical care in the era of biologic treatment.

Methods

Patients and data collection

The outpatient rheumatology clinic serves a population of approximately 290,000 inhabitants living in the two most southern counties in Norway. In the same geographic era there are also two private practicing rheumatologists.

At the outpatient clinic, the standard for monitoring patients with recommended outcome measures was first introduced in 2003 for RA patients. In 2005, the computer software program GoTreatIT® Rheuma (www.diagraphit.com) was implemented at the outpatient clinic, facilitating patient monitoring with selected outcome measures. During 2007, regularly monitoring of not only

RA but also PsA patients was implemented as part of standard clinical care. For RA patients, no specific protocol for tight control or any specific treatment protocol was used [7]. Treatment and follow-up visits were based on the treating doctor's judgment performed in accordance with national recommendations and, after 2007, also in accordance with the Norwegian tender system for prescription of biologic disease-modifying antirheumatic drugs (bDMARDs).

The same standard outcome measures used for monitoring RA patients at the outpatient clinic were also applied to monitor the PsA patients. Patient-reported outcome (PRO) measures included the Modified Health Assessment Questionnaire (MHAQ) assessing physical function [8], visual analog scales (VAS; 0–100 mm) used to report pain, joint pain, fatigue, and patient global assessment (PGA). Morning stiffness was reported in 15-min units. Standard assessment did not include assessment of skin, nails, entheses, or dactylitis.

Standardized 28 and 32 swollen and tender joint counts were performed by rheumatologists or by trained nurses. The 32-joint count included the 28-joint count plus standardized joint count of ankles and metatarsophalangeal joints (MTP) joints, both scored from 0–2 (the MTP joints were scored as one joint). Laboratory markers of inflammation included C-reactive protein (CRP; mg/L) and erythrocyte sedimentation rate (ESR; mm/h). The 28-joint composite Disease Activity Score (DAS) with ESR (DAS28-ESR) [9], the Clinical Disease Activity Index (CDAI) [10], and a modified version of the Disease Activity index for Psoriatic arthritis (DAPSA) including a 32-joint count instead of the original 66/68-joint count was calculated [11]. The evaluator's (trained nurse or rheumatologist) global assessment (EGA) of disease activity was reported on a VAS (0–100 mm). Data on rheumatoid factor (RF) were also recorded.

We used the cut-offs for DAS28-ESR, CDAI, and DAPSA to define remission, low disease activity, moderate disease activity, and high disease activity [10, 12, 13]. We also applied the suggested DAS28-ESR cut-off from Salaffi et al. of 2.4 instead of 2.6 for defining remission in PsA [14]. Furthermore, the Boolean remission criteria in accordance with the new American College of Rheumatology/European League Against Rheumatism (ACR/EULAR) guidelines for remission were tested [15].

Previous and current treatment use was systematically registered and updated at all visits, including use of prednisolone, synthetic DMARDs (sDMARDs), and bDMARDs. Demographic data collected included gender, age, weight, height, body mass index (BMI), smoking status, disease duration, and work status. From 2010 onwards, self-reported height and weight, smoking status, years of education, and work status were included as part of the standard routine with the use of the computer program. In the analysis we only included PsA patients who fulfilled the Classification for Psoriatic Arthritis criteria (CASPAR) and who were 18 years or older [16]. Data retrieved from the computer were based on data from the last annual patient visit for each year.

Statistical analysis
Continuous variables are presented as mean and standard deviation (SD). Categorical variables are presented as numbers and percentages. To look for a change in variables and associations over the 10-year period and the last 5 years of this period we used linear regression for continuous variables and the Chi-square test for categorical variables. A p value of < 0.05 was taken to be statistically significant.

Results
The number of PsA patients with at least one annual visit during the follow-up period ranged from 106 patients in 2008 to a maximum of 412 in 2014, with a mean annual number of 331 patients. From 2008 to 2010, the number of PsA patients increased from 106 to 318 and thereafter stabilized at a mean annual number of 367 patients in the subsequent years.

Data for gender, age, BMI, years of education, full time job status, smoking status, disease duration, and RF status are shown in Table 1. Apart from age and disease duration, no statistically significant differences during follow-up were seen, as shown in Table 1. Over the 10-year period, mean annual proportions were: females 49.4%; patients with a full-time job (age < 65 years) 35.8%; current smokers 17.6%; and RF-positive patients 4.8%. Mean (SD) annual values for the period were: age, 58.4 (12.4) years; BMI 27.6 (4.7) kg/m^2; education 12.5 (3.6) years; and disease duration 9.6 (7.9) years.

Table 2 shows the measures of disease activity displayed for each year in the 10-year period. A statistically significant improvement in all disease activity measures was seen for the 10-year period; however, for the last 5 years of follow-up (2013–2017) a statistically significant improvement was only seen for ESR and for DAS28-ESR, but not for CRP, joint count, CDAI, modified DAPSA, or EGA.

Comparing the two joint counts, the swollen/tender 32-joint count was a mean of 0.1/0.3 higher than the 28-joint count (annual detailed data for 32-joint counts are not shown).

As shown in Fig. 1, the proportion of patients in remission was dependent on the composite measures used. The lowest remission rates were found when applying the ACR/EULAR Boolean criteria (range 3.6% to 9.5%) and the modified DAPSA criteria (range 12.2% to 23.0%). The highest remission rates were shown for the

DAS28-ESR criteria (range 42.1% to 63.1%) and CDAI criteria (range 13.5% to 30.2%), both developed and validated for use in RA. When using the DAS28-ESR cut off ≤ 2.4, as recommended by Salaffi et al. to be applied when used in PsA [14], the remission rates were lower (range 32.4% to 50.6%); however, these were still significantly higher than for DAPSA and the ACR/EULAR Boolean remission criteria. A significant increase over the 10-year period was only seen for DAS28-ESR and CDAI remission and not for Boolean and DAPSA remission. For the last 5 years of follow-up, no significant change in remission rates occurred for any of the remission criteria.

As shown in Table 3, no significant improvement was seen for either the 10-year period or the last 5 years of follow-up for PRO measures. In contrast, in the last 5 years of follow-up, a small but statistically significant deterioration was seen for MHAQ, pain, joint pain, and morning stiffness, but not for fatigue or PGA.

In Table 4 the proportions of PsA patients treated with prednisolone, sDMARD, and bDMARD monotherapy or combination therapy are shown. The proportion of patients on no treatment declined significantly over the 10-year period from approximately 30% in 2008 to approximately 20% in 2017. The proportion of PsA patients using prednisolone (annual mean 14.9%, range 12.6% to 22.6%), sDMARDs (annual mean 53.0%, range 50.7% to 56.3%), and bDMARDs (annual mean 29.9%, range 23.5% to 32.8%) remained stable overall over the 10-year period. The use of sDMARDs was dominated by the use of methotrexate, and bDMARDs by the use of tumor necrosis factor (TNF) inhibitors. The annual mean percentage of PsA patients using the different sDMARDs was 38.5% for methotrexate, 11.2% for leflunomide, 2.4% for sulfasalazine, and 0.9% for other sDMARDs. Only a few PsA patients were treated with bDMARDs with modes of action other than TNF inhibitors: ustekinumab and sekukinumab. However, the use of sekukinumab, which was introduced in Norway in 2016, for PsA-treated patients increased from 0.6% in 2016 to 2.6% in 2017.

The use of a combination of sDMARDs and bDMARDs was also stable over the years (annual mean 15.9%, range 13.4% to 18.9%). Detailed information on use of specific sDMARDs and bDMARDs is shown in Table 4.

Over the 10-year period, significantly more PsA patients had been ever-users of bDMARDs, ranging from 27.6% in 2009 to 46.0% in 2017; however, for the last 5 years no significant increase for ever-use of bDMARDs was found.

Discussion
In our PsA outpatient clinic population for the 2008 to 2017 period, a statistically significant improvement in

Table 1 Clinical and demographic data for our study sample

Year (patients)	Females, n (%)	Age (years)	BMI (kg/m²)	Education (years)	Full-time job if aged < 65 years, n (%)	Current smoker, n (%)	Disease duration (years)	RF-positive, n (%)
2008 (n = 106)	52 (49.1%) [100%]	59.5 (13.5) [100%]	NA	NA	NA	NA	7.3 (8.0) [100%]	4 (7.1%) [52.8%]
2009 (n = 268)	140 (52.2%) [100%]	60.3 (11.8) [100%]	NA	NA	NA	NA	8.2 (7.4) [100%]	10 (6.7%) 150 [56.0%]
2010 (n = 318)	158 (49.7%) [100%]	60.5 (12.1) [100%]	27.4 (4.8) [91.8%]	12.3 (3.5) [94.0%]	73 (39.2%) 194a [95.9%]	59 (19.6%) [94.7%]	8.3 (7.2) [100%]	14 (6.8%) [64.5%]
2011 (n = 365)	181 (49.6%) [100%]	59.4 (12.5) [100%]	27.6 (4.8) [97.3%]	12.3 (3.7) [88.5%]	84 (40.2%) 233a [89.7%]	71 (21.8%) [89.3%]	8.9 (7.4) [100%]	15 (5.6%) [73.4%]
2012 (n = 377)	179 (47.5%) [100%]	58.6 (12.3) [100%]	27.4 (4.8) [96.6%]	12.3 (3.7) [97.3%]	86 (35.5%) 250a [96.8%]	70 (19.1%) [97.1%]	9.2 (7.4) [100%]	17 (5.8%) [78.2%]
2013 (n = 397)	197 (49.6%) [100%]	58.8 (12.3) [100%]	27.6 (4.4) [98.0%]	12.4 (3.6) [98.2%]	93 (35.6%) 264a [98.9%]	69 (17.6%) [98.5%]	9.7 (7.9) [100%]	17 (5.1%) 335 [84.4%]
2014 (n = 412)	208 (50.5%) [100%]	58.3 (12.3) [100%]	27.7 (4.6) [96.8%]	12.6 (3.4) [97.1%]	107 (39.1%) 282a [97.2%]	71 (17.7%) [97.3%]	9.8 (7.9) [100%]	13 (3.9%) [81.1%]
2015 (n = 384)	197 (51.3%) [100%]	56.8 (12.6) [100%]	27.7 (4.7) [98.2%]	12.5 (3.6) [97.7%]	90 (32.8%) 280a [97.9%]	60 (15.9%) [98.2%]	10.3 (8.1) [100%]	10 (3.3%) [79.9%]
2016 (n = 340)	165 (48.5%) [100%]	57.1 (12.6) [100%]	27.7 (5.0) [97.4%]	12.6 (3.5) [96.8%]	68 (29.2%) 239a [97.5%]	51 (15.4%) [97.6%]	10.6 (8.3) [100%]	9 (3.2%) [82.4%]
2017 (n = 341)	158 (46.3%) [100%]	56.0 (12.3) [100%]	28.0 (4.8) [97.9%]	12.9 (3.4) [97.1%]	87 (36.0%) 249a [97.2%]	47 (14.1%) [97.7%]	11.3 (8.5) [100%]	10 (3.6%) [80.6%]
Mean for the period	49.4%	58.4 (12.4)	27.6 (4.7)	12.5 (3.6)	35.8%	17.6%	9.6 (7.9)	4.8%
P value b 2008–2017	0.94	< 0.001	NA	NA	NA	NA	< 0.001	0.41
P value b 2013–2017	0.71	0.001	0.38	0.11	0.34	0.64	0.003	0.74

Values are shown as mean (standard deviation) unless otherwise indicated

Percentages within square brackets represent patients with available data

BMI body mass index, RF rheumatoid factor, NA not available

aNumbers of patients aged > 65 years

bχ² test for categorical and linear regression for continuous variables was used to test for differences during follow-up

Table 2 Measures of disease activity for each year from 2008 to 2017 for patients with psoriatic arthritis monitored with outcome measures in an ordinary outpatient clinic

Year (patients)	ESR (mm/h)	CRP (mg/L)	28 tender joint count	28 swollen joint count	DAS28-ESR	CDAI	DAPSA	EGA (VAS, mm)
2008 (n = 106)	15.8 (13.1) [80.2%]	7.6 (10.2) [86.8%]	3.3 (5.6) [92.5%]	1.5 (2.0) [92.5%]	3.32 (1.49) [53.8%]	10.09 (8.98) [51.9%]	13.0 (9.9) [49.1%]	14.5 (14.5) [84.9%]
2009 (n = 268)	15.3 (14.0) [71.3%]	5.8 (9.2) [79.9%]	2.5 (4.6) [96.6%]	1.2 (2.2) [96.6%]	3.05 (1.29) [64.6%]	9.25 (7.97) [80.2%]	12.4 (8.6) [67.5%]	13.2 (12.6) [90.3%]
2010 (n = 318)	15.8 (14.5) [77.7%]	5.4 (8.9) [83.3%]	1.7 (3.5) [96.9%]	0.8 (1.7) [96.9%]	2.79 (1.13) [74.2%]	7.35 (6.34) [89.9%]	11.1 (7.9) [78.6%]	11.6 (11.2) [93.7%]
2011 (n = 365)	14.1 (12.4) [77.8%]	4.9 (11.1) [82.2%]	1.6 (3.6) [93.4%]	0.6 (1.6) [93.4%]	2.64 (1.06) [75.9%]	6.94 (6.30) [87.9%]	10.6 (8.0) [77.5%]	11.6 (11.8) [90.4%]
2012 (n = 377)	12.6 (9.9) [71.4%]	4.2 (6.8) [78.0%]	1.3 (3.2) [93.9%]	0.5 (1.3) [93.9%]	2.52 (1.08) [66.3%]	6.45 (5.90) [87.8%]	9.9 (7.3) [71.6%]	9.7 (11.2) [92.0%]
2013 (n = 397)	14.2 (13.1) [77.6%]	4.5 (9.0) [82.9%]	1.5 (3.3) [94.0%]	0.4 (1.1) [94.0%]	2.66 (1.07) [75.1%]	6.60 (5.54) [87.7%]	10.3 (7.1) [78.3%]	10.0 (10.8) [91.9%]
2014 (n = 412)	14.6 (13.5) [78.6%]	4.7 (6.9) [83.3%]	1.3 (3.1) [96.6%]	0.4 (1.3) [96.6%]	2.56 (1.08) [74.0%]	6.27 (5.58) [90.0%]	9.8 (7.2) [76.0%]	8.4 (9.4) [95.4%]
2015 (n = 384)	14.0 (13.8) [78.9%]	4.5 (9.8) [86.7%]	1.4 (3.3) [97.4%]	0.4 (1.4) [97.4%]	2.59 (1.12) [74.2%]	6.66 (6.11) [91.1%]	10.4 (7.9) [78.9%]	9.0 (9.5) [96.4%]
2016 (n = 340)	13.2 (12.8) [77.9%]	5.2 (9.4) [87.1%]	1.3 (3.0) [93.8%]	0.4 (1.0) [93.8%]	2.46 (1.03) [68.5%]	6.39 (5.17) [82.6%]	10.0 (6.8) [74.1%]	9.2 (9.9) [91.5%]
2017 (n = 341)	10.9 (11.2) [59.8%]	4.1 (7.4) [69.2%]	1.6 (3.6) [78.9%]	0.6 (1.5) [78.9%]	2.46 (1.12) [49.3%]	6.76 (6.08) [68.3%]	10.4 (7.6) [54.5%]	8.6 (11.4) [80.1%]
Mean for the period	14.0 (12.9)	4.9 (8.9)	1.6 (3.6)	0.6 (1.5)	2.64 (1.13)	6.93 (6.19)	10.5 (7.7)	10.2 (11.0)
P value[a] 2008–2017	< 0.001	0.01	< 0.001	< 0.001	< 0.001	< 0.001	0.001	< 0.001
P value[a] 2013–2017	0.004	0.92	0.94	0.28	0.03	0.71	0.48	0.32

Values are shown as mean (standard deviation)

The percentages within square brackets represent patients with available data

CDAI Clinical Disease Activity Index, CRP C-reactive protein, DAPSA Disease Activity index for Psoriatic arthritis, DAS Disease Activity Score, EGA evaluator's global assessment, ESR erythrocyte sedimentation rate, VAS visual analog scale

[a]Linear regression was used to test for differences during follow-up

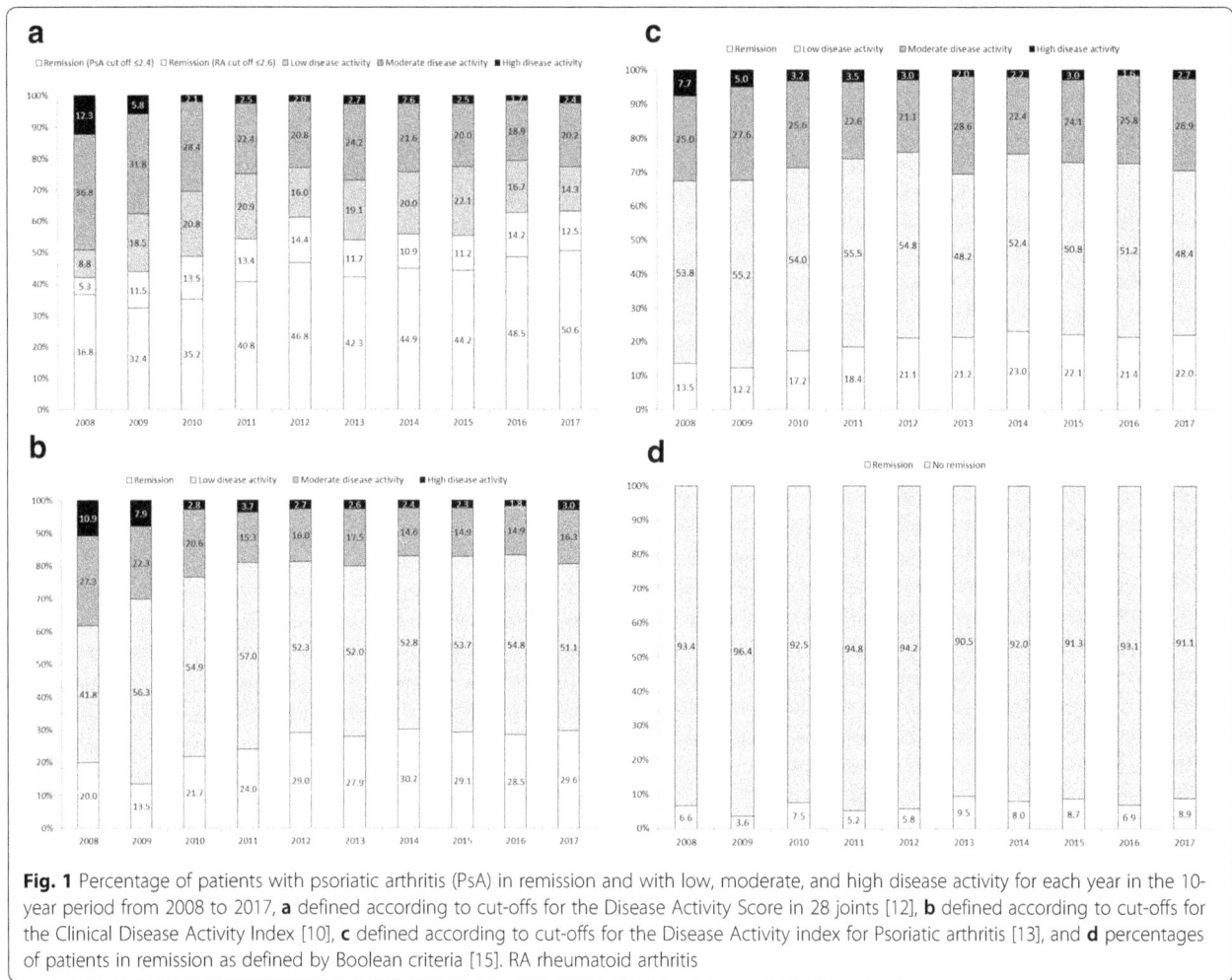

Fig. 1 Percentage of patients with psoriatic arthritis (PsA) in remission and with low, moderate, and high disease activity for each year in the 10-year period from 2008 to 2017, **a** defined according to cut-offs for the Disease Activity Score in 28 joints [12], **b** defined according to cut-offs for the Clinical Disease Activity Index [10], **c** defined according to cut-offs for the Disease Activity index for Psoriatic arthritis [13], and **d** percentages of patients in remission as defined by Boolean criteria [15]. RA rheumatoid arthritis

measures reflecting disease activity was observed. However, for the last 5 years of follow-up, a statistically significant improvement was only seen for ESR and DAS28-ESR and not for CRP, 28-joint count, CDAI, EGA, or DAPSA. Furthermore, no significant improvement in physical functioning or patient perception of, for example, fatigue, pain, and morning stiffness was found. A statistically significant increase in remission rates was only found for the entire period for DAS28-ESR (range 32.4% to 50.6%) and CDAI (range 13.5% to 30.2%), but not for ACR/EULAR Boolean (range 3.6% to 9.5%) and DAPSA (range 12.2% to 23.0%) remission or for DAS28-ESR (range 42.3 to 50.6%) and CDAI (range 27.9 to 30.2%) remission for the last 5 years of follow-up.

The remission rates observed in our PsA cohort seems to be lower than that found in our RA outpatient clinic population for the period 2004 to 2013, where remission rates increased significantly not only for DAS28-ESR but also for ACR/EULAR Boolean remission [7]. For comparison with the period 2008 to 2013, the remission rates in the reported RA patients increased from 24.7%

to 55.5% for DAS28-ESR and from 6.8% to 17.7% for Boolean remission, whereas the remission rates in our PsA patients increased from 32.4% to 46.8% for DAS28-ESR and from 3.5% to 9.5% for the ACR/EULAR Boolean. However, this comparison should be interpreted with caution. Our data confirm the results from others that DAS28-ESR and CDAI (developed for use in RA) overestimates the remission rates in PsA compared with DAPSA [17], and this occurs even when using the recommended DAS28-ESR remission cut-off ≤ 2.4 from Salaffi et al. to define remission in PsA [14]. When aiming for a less stringent T2T goal, including low disease activity, the differences between DAS28-ESR, CDAI, and DAPSA was less striking, as shown in Fig. 1.

The reduced access over the last years to modern treatment options with different modes of action other than TNF inhibitors in PsA compared with RA patients may partly explain the impression of a less significant improvement in clinical outcomes seen in our study. This is illustrated by 13.5% of RA patients from our outpatient clinic using non-TNF inhibitor bDMARDs in 2013, whereas the figures for our PsA patients were 1.3%

Table 3 Patient-reported outcome measures for each year from 2008 to 2017 for patients with psoriatic arthritis monitored in an ordinary outpatient clinic

Year (patients)	MHAQ (0–3)	Pain (VAS, mm)	Joint pain (VAS, mm)	Fatigue (VAS, mm)	Morning stiffness (h)	PGA (VAS, mm)
2008 (n = 106)	0.59 (0.53) 59.4%]	37.5 (24.6) [56.6%]	41.1 (25.2) 36 [34.0%]	44.5 (32.4) [58.5%]	1.24 (1.48) [58.5%]	41.3 (26.0) [58.5%]
2009 (n = 268)	0.46 (0.44) [85.8%]	37.5 (22.1) [84.3%]	38.1 (23.0) [84.3%]	47.0 (30.2) [84.7%]	0.93 (1.05) [85.1%]	40.3 (24.4) [87.3%]
2010 (n = 318)	0.45 (0.43) [93.4%]	37.4 (23.4) [93.1%]	36.2 (23.5) [91.8%]	43.2 (31.1) [92.1%]	0.90 (1.15) [92.8%]	37.6 (23.3) [93.7%]
2011 (n = 365)	0.44 (0.42) [89.9%]	36.1 (24.2) [89.6%]	35.4 (24.1) [89.3%]	44.9 (30.6) [89.3%]	0.90 (1.21) [90.4%]	37.1 (23.9) [91.5%]
2012 (n = 377)	0.44 (0.43) [89.7%]	36.2 (24.5) [89.7%]	35.6 (24.7) [89.7%]	42.9 (30.2) [89.7%]	0.93 (1.27) [89.1%]	37.6 (25.6) [91.0%]
2013 (n = 397)	0.42 (0.40) [90.1%]	33.9 (25.5) [90.2%]	33.8 (23.7) [90.7%]	42.6 (31.0) [90.4%]	0.87 (1.15) [90.7%]	37.4 (26.2) [90.9%]
2014 (n = 412)	0.45 (0.44) [90.0%]	35.8 (24.7) [89.1%]	35.0 (24.7) [87.1%]	42.7 (31.3) [87.1%]	0.89 (1.14) [86.7%]	37.9 (26.5) [91.3%]
2015 (n = 384)	0.47 (0.43) [91.4%]	38.4 (26.5) [91.1%]	36.2 (26.6) [90.1%]	45.5 (32.6) [90.4%]	0.97 (1.27) [89.8%]	40.1 (28.2) [93.0%]
2016 (n = 340)	0.51 (0.46) [87.6%]	38.8 (26.8) [86.2%]	38.3 (26.5) [87.4%]	45.2 (32.2) [87.6%]	1.06 (1.36) [86.8%]	40.6 (27.8) [87.9%]
2017 (n = 341)	0.51 (0.45) [89.4%]	39.8 (26.4) [89.4%]	38.7 (26.3) [89.4%]	45.1 (32.7) [89.1%]	1.03 (1.27) [89.7%]	40.6 (27.9) [90.6%]
Mean for the period	0.46 (0.44)	37.0 (24.8)	36.3 (24.9)	44.2 (31.3)	0.95 (1.22)	38.8 (26.0)
P value[a] 2008–2017	0.11	0.10	0.44	0.90	0.26	0.18
P value[a] 2013–2017	0.002	0.001	0.003	0.16	0.025	0.06

Values are shown as mean (standard deviation)

The percentages within square brackets represent patients with available data

MHAQ Modified Health Assessment Questionnaire, PGA patient's global assessment, VAS visual analog scale

[a] Linear regression was used to test for differences during follow-up

Table 4 Treatment is displayed for each year in the 10-year period from 2008 to 2017 for patients with psoriatic arthritis monitored with outcome measures in an ordinary outpatient clinic

Treatment	2008 (n = 106)	2009 (n = 268)	2010 (n = 318)	2011 (n = 365)	2012 (n = 377)	2013 (n = 397)	2014 (n = 412)	2015 (n = 384)	2016 (n = 340)	2017 (n = 341)	Annual mean	P value[a] 2008–17 and 2013–17
No treatment[b] (%)	29 (27.4)	92 (34.3)	96 (30.2)	115 (31.5)	115 (30.5)	112 (28.2)	113 (27.4)	102 (26.6)	72 (21.2)	65 (19.1)	27.5%	<0.001 0.011
bDMARD (%)	32 (30.2)	63 (23.5)	88 (27.7)	99 (27.1)	113 (30.0)	120 (30.2)	129 (31.3)	125 (32.6)	107 (31.5)	112 (32.8)	29.9%	0.29 0.94
TNF inhibitor (%)	31 (29.2)	59 (22.0)	83 (26.1)	94 (25.8)	110 (29.2)	115 (29.0)	121 (29.4)	118 (30.7)	99 (29.1)	100 (29.3)	28.1%	0.43 0.99
Non-TNF inhibitors (%)	1 (0.9)	4 (1.5)	5 (1.6)	5 (1.4)	3 (0.8)	5 (1.3)	8 (1.9)	7 (1.8)	8 (2.4)	12 (3.5)	1.8%	0.32 0.30
sDMARD (%)	59 (55.7)	136 (50.7)	168 (52.8)	188 (51.5)	192 (50.9)	208 (52.4)	215 (52.2)	206 (53.6)	188 (55.3)	192 (56.3)	53.0%	0.89 0.75
One sDMARD (%)	59 (55.7)	136 (50.7)	168 (52.8)	188 (51.5)	191 (50.7)	208 (52.4)	214 (51.9)	205 (53.4)	188 (55.3)	191 (56.0)	52.8%	0.96 0.87
Two sDMARDs (%)	0 (0)	0 (0)	0 (0)	0 (0)	1 (0.3)	0 (0)	1 (0.2)	1 (0.3)	0 (0)	1 (0.3)	0.1%	–
bDMARD and sDMARD (%)	20 (18.9)	36 (13.4)	51 (16.0)	52 (14.2)	61 (16.2)	66 (16.6)	68 (16.5)	68 (17.7)	52 (15.3)	53 (15.5)	15.9%	0.91 0.91
TNF inhibitor and sDMARD (%)	20 (18.9)	35 (13.1)	50 (15.7)	52 (14.2)	61 (16.2)	64 (16.1)	65 (15.8)	64 (16.7)	49 (14.4)	47 (13.8)	15.3%	0.89 0.81
Prednisolone (%)	24 (22.6)	39 (14.6)	49 (15.4)	52 (14.2)	49 (13.0)	56 (14.1)	52 (12.6)	54 (14.1)	59 (17.4)	60 (17.6)	14.9%	0.22 0.23
Prednisolone and sDMARD (%)	16 (15.1)	23 (8.6)	29 (9.1)	32 (8.8)	26 (6.9)	28 (7.1)	25 (6.1)	28 (7.3)	31 (9.1)	31 (9.1)	8.1%	0.19 0.44
Prednisolone, sDMARD, and bDMARD (%)	4 (3.8)	8 (3.0)	9 (2.8)	7 (1.9)	5 (1.3)	9 (2.3)	5 (1.2)	5 (1.3)	5 (1.5)	5 (1.5)	1.9%	0.47 0.77
Biologic DMARDs												
Adalimumab (%)	11 (10.4)	31 (11.6)	41 (12.9)	44 (12.1)	46 (12.2)	48 (12.1)	44 (10.7)	41 (10.7)	25 (7.4)	28 (8.2)	10.9%	0.33 0.18
Certolizumab (%)	0 (0)	0 (0)	0 (0)	1 (0.3)	1 (0.3)	1 (0.3)	12 (2.9)	16 (4.2)	18 (5.3)	15 (4.4)	1.9%	<0.001 0.001
Etanercept (%)[c]	8 (7.5)	20 (7.5)	26 (8.2)	37 (10.1)	44 (11.7)	33 (8.3)	34 (8.3)	31 (8.1)	30 (8.8)	34 (10.0)	9.0%	0.69 0.90
Golimumab (%)	0 (0)	0 (0)	9 (2.8)	5 (1.4)	7 (1.9)	23 (5.8)	19 (4.6)	12 (3.1)	11 (3.2)	8 (2.3)	2.8%	<0.001 0.11
Infliximab (%)[d]	12 (11.3)	8 (3.0)	7 (2.2)	7 (1.9)	12 (3.2)	10 (2.5)	12 (2.9)	19 (4.9)	15 (4.4)	15 (4.4)	3.5%	0.001 0.31
Abatacept (%)	1 (0.9)	4 (1.5)	4 (1.3)	2 (0.5)	2 (0.5)	4 (1.0)	2 (0.5)	2 (0.5)	1 (0.3)	1 (0.3)	0.7%	0.65 0.66
Ustekinumab (%)	0 (0)	0 (0)	0 (0)	1 (0.3)	0 (0)	1 (0.3)	6 (1.5)	4 (1.0)	5 (1.5)	2 (0.6)	0.6%	0.022 0.33
Sekukinumab (%)	0 (0)	0 (0)	0 (0)	0 (0)	0 (0)	0 (0)	0 (0)	0 (0)	2 (0.6)	9 (2.6)	0.3%	<0.001 <0.001
Other biologics (%)	0 (0)	0 (0)	1 (0.3)	2 (0.5)	1 (0.3)	0 (0)	0 (0)	1 (0.3)	0 (0)	0 (0)	0.2%	0.55 0.42
Synthetic DMARDs (%)												
Leflunomide	6 (5.7)	19 (7.1)	27 (8.5)	37 (10.1)	48 (12.7)	53 (13.4)	58 (14.1)	49 (12.8)	36 (10.6)	37 (10.9)	11.2%	0.037 0.52
Methotrexate	48 (45.3)	106 (39.6)	124 (39.0)	134 (36.7)	130 (34.5)	144 (36.3)	151 (36.7)	147 (38.3)	141 (41.5)	149 (43.7)	38.5%	0.22 0.18
Sulfasalazine	4 (3.8)	8 (3.0)	13 (4.1)	13 (3.6)	11 (2.9)	7 (1.8)	4 (1.0)	8 (2.1)	8 (2.4)	5 (1.5)	2.4%	0.16 0.62
Other synthetic DMARDs[e]	1 (0.9)	3 (1.1)	4 (1.3)	4 (1.1)	4 (1.1)	4 (1.0)	3 (0.7)	3 (0.8)	3 (0.9)	2 (0.6)	0.9%	1.00 0.98

Table 4 Treatment is displayed for each year in the 10-year period from 2008 to 2017 for patients with psoriatic arthritis monitored with outcome measures in an ordinary outpatient clinic (*Continued*)

Treatment	2008 (n = 106)	2009 (n = 268)	2010 (n = 318)	2011 (n = 365)	2012 (n = 377)	2013 (n = 397)	2014 (n = 412)	2015 (n = 384)	2016 (n = 340)	2017 (n = 341)	Annual mean	P value[a] 2008–17 and 2013–17
Ever users												
Biologic DMARDs (%)	41 (38.7)	74 (27.6)	106 (33.3)	123 (33.7)	138 (36.6)	152 (38.3)	165 (40.0)	171 (44.5)	150 (44.1)	157 (46.0)	38.6%	< 0.001 0.16
TNF inhibitor (%)	41 (38.7)	74 (27.6)	105 (33.0)	122 (33.4)	137 (36.3)	150 (37.8)	164 (39.8)	168 (43.8)	147 (43.2)	156 (45.7)	38.2%	< 0.001 0.17
Non-TNF inhibitors (%)	2 (1.9)	5 (1.9)	8 (2.5)	7 (1.9)	7 (1.9)	11 (2.8)	16 (3.9)	17 (4.4)	21 (6.2)	20 (5.9)	3.4%	0.004 0.15

Data are presented as n (%)

bDMARD biologic disease-modifying antirheumatic drug, *sDMARD* synthetic disease-modifying antirheumatic drug, *TNF* tumor necrosis factor

[a]χ^2 test used to test for differences during follow-up for the period 2008–2017 and 2013–2017

[b]No prednisolone, bDMARD or sDMARD

[c]Includes the originator and SB4

[d]Includes the originator and the biosimilar CT-P13

[e]Includes hydroxychloroquine, auranofin, azathioprine

in 2013 and 3.5% in 2017 [7]. The new drugs with mode of actions other than TNF inhibition used in our study included interleukin (IL)-12/23 inhibition (ustekinumab) and IL-17A inhibition (sekukinumab). The Janus kinase inhibitor tofacitinib has also been shown to be effective in treating PsA and is expected to soon reach the Norwegian market [18]. The number of PsA patients receiving no treatment (neither prednisolone nor DMARDs) in our study was in the range 20–30%. These figures are high compared with those we reported in RA, where approximately 10% of RA patients received no prednisolone or DMARD treatment [7]. One reason for this may be that a large proportion of PsA patients present as mono- or oligoarthritis. For example, in a Norwegian PsA study, 5.8% had mono- and 22.9% had oligoarthritis [19]. These patients may be less likely than the polyarthritis PsA patients to be treated with DMARDs and this may partly explain the rather high proportion of PsA patients receiving no treatment in our study.

According to EULAR recommendations, it is recommended that RA patients in need of bDMARDs (especially TNF inhibitors) be treated in combination with sDMARDs because of the superior efficacy compared with monotherapy using either sDMARDs or bDMARDs [20]. In PsA there is no such strong evidence for combination treatment, as is also reflected in the EULAR recommendations for the management of PsA [21]. In our study, approximately 50% of the TNF inhibitor-treated PsA patients were also on sDMARDs. In comparison, approximately 75% of the TNF inhibitor-treated RA patients in 2013 were treated in combination with sDMARDs [7]. The rather high rate of bDMARD-treated PsA patients on concomitant sDMARDs may not only be explained by the physician's belief of a better effect using the combination, but could also be explained by a physician's concern about immunogenicity using bDMARD monotherapy without combination with, for example, methotrexate [22].

Challenges related to the heterogeneity of the PsA disease are reflected in the use of outcome measures in our study but are also shown by the different recommendations on use of outcome measures; some favor the use of unidimensional composite scores (e.g., DAPSA) focusing on articular inflammation [23], and some favor the use of multidimensional scores [24] including the different disease domains [5]. This heterogeneity of the PsA disease is therefore a major challenge when assessing the burden of disease both in the clinic and in research. Despite all these challenges, the concept of remission as a treatment goal in PsA is gaining more and more acceptance among rheumatologists. Higher scores for PROs (e.g., pain and fatigue) have been reported in PsA compared with RA, in spite of lower swollen joint counts [25]. The higher scores for pain reported in PsA patients seen in the literature may be explained by the inflammatory involvement of entheses and the presence of dactylitis which were not assessed in our study.

Despite recommendations for treating PsA patients to target, and agreement among rheumatologist favoring this approach, there is a discrepancy with what occurs in real life. This issue was explored in the study by Gvozdenovic and colleagues [26]. In their study, 83% agreed that composite measures should be recorded regularly in RA patients; however, the real-life data revealed that in only 54% of the patients were composite scores actually recorded at ≥ 50% of the patient visits. There is reason to believe that this is also the case for PsA and, due to the heterogeneity of the PsA disease, the figures may be even worse in PsA than in RA. One strategy to improve the use of outcome measures in clinical practice could be the use of dedicated and trained nurse practitioners and physician assistants [27]. Further systematic education in outpatient clinics, for example implementing a learning collaborative, may also improve the adherence to a T2T strategy [28]. Another strategy could be developing patient self-assessment tools. For example, for the psoriasis area and severity index (PASI), a validated patient self-administered psoriasis score has been developed called the self-administered psoriasis area and severity index (SAPASI) [29, 30]. The implementation of outcome measures in daily clinical practice can also be facilitated by the use of computer technology as, for example, in our study and in DANBIO [31, 32].

Our study has several limitations, including the use of outcome measures developed and validated for use in RA, no examination of the skin, nails, entheses or dactylitis, and the use of the 32-joint count and not the 66/68-swollen and tender joint count in the calculation of DAPSA [11]. This most likely has underestimated the DAPSA score in our PsA outpatients since the use of a reduced joint count has been shown to miss a significant number of PsA patients with active disease [33]. However, the mean difference between 28- and 32-joint count was minor in our study (mean 0.1 for swollen and 0.3 for tender joints). We also emphasize that the composite scores of DAS28 and CDAI with their cut-offs to define disease status and the Boolean remission criteria have not been validated for use in PsA. It is, however, a paradox that even recent approval of novel therapies for PsA have been based on clinical trials using primary endpoints derived from RA.

Other limitations of our study include assessment bias through examination by various physicians at various time points, and missing data, which may affect the internal validity of the results. The generalizability of the results may also have been affected by patient recruitment being only from one center. However, there is no obvious reason to believe that the examined PsA out-patient clinic cohort is different from other outpatient clinic cohorts in Norway. Despite all the limitations in this study, the long-term monitoring of PsA patients reflecting an entire PsA outpatient clinic population is in itself rather unique, and our data may thus be of interest both for clinicians and researchers in contributing to an increased understanding of the disease burden in PsA in our time.

Conclusions

The overall interpretation of our results is that there is still an unmet need in treating PsA patients to target, even in the era of biologic treatment. There is also an urgent need to develop, validate, and agree on feasible outcome measures to be used in ordinary clinical care, capturing the heterogenic expression of the PsA disease. However, in the meantime, our study should encourage clinicians to implement the use of available and feasible outcome measures in ordinary clinical care, for example DAPSA, to improve patient outcome.

Abbreviations

ACR/EULAR: American College of Rheumatology/European League Against Rheumatism; bDMARD: Biologic disease-modifying antirheumatic drug; BMI: Body mass index; CDAI: Clinical Disease Activity Index; CRP: C-reactive protein; DAPSA: Disease Activity index for Psoriatic arthritis; DAS: Disease Activity Score; DMARD: Disease-modifying antirheumatic drug; EGA: Evaluator's global assessment; ESR: Erythrocyte sedimentation rate; MHAQ: Modified Health Assessment Questionnaire; MTP: Metatarsophalangeal; PGA: Patient global assessment; PRO: Patient-reported outcome; PsA: Psoriatic arthritis; RA: Rheumatoid arthritis; RF: Rheumatoid factor; SD: Standard deviation; sDMARD: Synthetic disease-modifying antirheumatic drug; T2T: Treat-to-target; TNF: Tumor necrosis factor; VAS: Visual analog scale

Acknowledgements

We thank all secretaries, nurses, and doctors at the Division of Rheumatology, Department of Internal Medicine, Hospital of Southern Norway Trust who contributed to implementation of the strategy of monitoring PsA patients at the outpatient clinic.

Funding

This study was supported by an unrestricted grant from Pfizer Norway.

Authors' contributions

GH contributed to study conception and design, statistical analysis, and interpretation of results and was mainly responsible for drafting the manuscript. BM contributed to data collection, study conception, and interpretation of results. ST contributed to data collection, study conception, and interpretation of results. IJWH contributed to data collection, study conception, and interpretation of results. AD contributed to data collection, study conception, and interpretation of results. AK contributed to study design, interpreting statistical analysis, and interpretation of results. All authors were involved in drafting and revising the manuscript and approved the final version.

Consent for publication

Not applicable.

Competing interests

GH is a founder and shareholder for DiaGraphIT AS, manufacturing the GoTreatIT® Rheuma software. The remaining authors declare that they have no competing interests.

Author details

[1]Division of Rheumatology, Department of Medicine, Hospital of Southern Norway Trust, Servicebox 416, 4604 Kristiansand, Norway. [2]Department of Neuroscience, Division of Rheumatology, Norwegian University of Science and Technology, Trondheim, Norway. [3]Department of Rheumatology, Martina Hansens Hospital, Bærum, Norway. [4]Division of Rheumatology, Allergy, and Immunology, School of Medicine, University of California, San Diego, USA.

References

1. Smolen JS. Treat-to-target as an approach in inflammatory arthritis. Curr Opin Rheumatol. 2016;28:297–302.
2. Smolen JS, Aletaha D, Bijlsma JW, Breedveld FC, Boumpas D, Burmester G, et al. Treating rheumatoid arthritis to target: recommendations of an international task force. Ann Rheum Dis. 2010;69:631–7.
3. Smolen JS, Breedveld FC, Burmester GR, Bykerk V, Dougados M, Emery P, et al. Treating rheumatoid arthritis to target: 2014 update of the recommendations of an international task force. Ann Rheum Dis. 2016;75:3–15.
4. Smolen JS, Braun J, Dougados M, Emery P, Fitzgerald O, Helliwell P, et al. Treating spondyloarthritis, including ankylosing spondylitis and psoriatic arthritis, to target: recommendations of an international task force. Ann Rheum Dis. 2014;73:6–16.
5. Smolen JS, Schols M, Braun J, Dougados M, FitzGerald O, Gladman DD, et al. Treating axial spondyloarthritis and peripheral spondyloarthritis, especially psoriatic arthritis, to target: 2017 update of recommendations by an international task force. Ann Rheum Dis. 2018;77:3–17.
6. Ramiro S, Smolen JS, Landewe R, van der Heijde D, Dougados M, Emery P, et al. Pharmacological treatment of psoriatic arthritis: a systematic literature review for the 2015 update of the EULAR recommendations for the management of psoriatic arthritis. Ann Rheum Dis. 2016;75:490–8.
7. Haugeberg G, Hansen IJ, Soldal DM, Sokka T. Ten years of change in clinical disease status and treatment in rheumatoid arthritis: results based on standardized monitoring of patients in an ordinary outpatient clinic in southern Norway. Arthritis Res Ther. 2015;17:219.
8. Pincus T, Summey JA, Soraci SA Jr, Wallston KA, Hummon NP. Assessment of patient satisfaction in activities of daily living using a modified Stanford health assessment questionnaire. Arthritis Rheum. 1983;26:1346–53.
9. Prevoo ML, van 't Hof MA, Kuper HH, van Leeuwen MA, van de Putte LB, van Riel PL. Modified disease activity scores that include twenty-eight-joint counts. Development and validation in a prospective longitudinal study of patients with rheumatoid arthritis. Arthritis Rheum. 1995;38:44–8.
10. Aletaha D, Smolen JS. The simplified disease activity index (SDAI) and clinical disease activity index (CDAI) to monitor patients in standard clinical care. Best Pract Res Clin Rheumatol. 2007;21:663–75.
11. Schoels M, Aletaha D, Funovits J, Kavanaugh A, Baker D, Smolen JS. Application of the DAREA/DAPSA score for assessment of disease activity in psoriatic arthritis. Ann Rheum Dis. 2010;69:1441–7.
12. van Gestel AM, Haagsma CJ, van Riel PL. Validation of rheumatoid arthritis improvement criteria that include simplified joint counts. Arthritis Rheum. 1998;41:1845–50.
13. Schoels MM, Aletaha D, Alasti F, Smolen JS. Disease activity in psoriatic arthritis (PsA): defining remission and treatment success using the DAPSA score. Ann Rheum Dis. 2016;75:811–8.
14. Salaffi F, Ciapetti A, Carotti M, Gasparini S, Gutierrez M. Disease activity in psoriatic arthritis: comparison of the discriminative capacity and construct validity of six composite indices in a real world. Biomed Res Int. 2014;2014:528105.

15. Felson DT, Smolen JS, Wells G, Zhang B, van Tuyl LH, Funovits J, et al. American College of Rheumatology/European League Against Rheumatism provisional definition of remission in rheumatoid arthritis for clinical trials. Arthritis Rheum. 2011;63:573–86.

16. Taylor W, Gladman D, Helliwell P, Marchesoni A, Mease P, Mielants H. Classification criteria for psoriatic arthritis: development of new criteria from a large international study. Arthritis Rheum. 2006;54(8):2665–73.

17. Michelsen B, Diamantopoulos AP, Hoiberg HK, Soldal DM, Kavanaugh A, Haugeberg G. Need for improvement in current treatment of psoriatic arthritis: study of an outpatient clinic population. J Rheumatol. 2017;44:431–6.

18. Mease P, Hall S, FitzGerald O, van der Heijde D, Merola JF, Avila-Zapata F, et al. Tofacitinib or adalimumab versus placebo for psoriatic arthritis. N Engl J Med. 2017;377:1537–50.

19. Madland TM, Apalset EM, Johannessen AE, Rossebo B, Brun JG. Prevalence, disease manifestations, and treatment of psoriatic arthritis in western Norway. J Rheumatol. 2005;32:1918–22.

20. Smolen JS, Landewe R, Bijlsma J, Burmester G, Chatzidionysiou K, Dougados M, et al. EULAR recommendations for the management of rheumatoid arthritis with synthetic and biological disease-modifying antirheumatic drugs: 2016 update. Ann Rheum Dis. 2017;76:960–77.

21. Gossec L, Smolen JS, Ramiro S, de Wit M, Cutolo M, Dougados M, et al. European League Against Rheumatism (EULAR) recommendations for the management of psoriatic arthritis with pharmacological therapies: 2015 update. Ann Rheum Dis. 2016;75:499–510.

22. Garces S, Demengeot J, Benito-Garcia E. The immunogenicity of anti-TNF therapy in immune-mediated inflammatory diseases: a systematic review of the literature with a meta-analysis. Ann Rheum Dis. 2013;72:1947–55.

23. Smolen JS, Schoels M, Aletaha D. Disease activity and response assessment in psoriatic arthritis using the disease activity index for psoriatic arthritis (DAPSA). A brief review. Clin Exp Rheumatol. 2015;33(5 Suppl 93):S48–50.

24. Mease PJ, Coates LC. Considerations for the definition of remission criteria in psoriatic arthritis. Seminar Arthritis Rheum. 2018 Epub ahead; https://doi.org/10.1016/j.semarthrit.2017.10.021.

25. Michelsen B, Fiane R, Diamantopoulos AP, Soldal DM, Hansen IJ, Sokka T, et al. A comparison of disease burden in rheumatoid arthritis, psoriatic arthritis and axial spondyloarthritis. PLoS One. 2015;10:e0123582.

26. Gvozdenovic E, Allaart CF, van der Heijde D, Ferraccioli G, Smolen JS, Huizinga TW, et al. When rheumatologists report that they agree with a guideline, does this mean that they practise the guideline in clinical practice? Results of the international recommendation implementation study (IRIS). RMD open. 2016;2:e000221.

27. Smith BJ, Bolster MB, Slusher B, Stamatos C, Scott JR, Benham H, et al. Core curriculum to facilitate the expansion of a rheumatology practice to include nurse practitioners and physician assistants. Arthritis Care Res. 2018;70:672–8.

28. Solomon DH, Losina E, Lu B, Zak A, Corrigan C, Lee SB, et al. Implementation of treat-to-target in rheumatoid arthritis through a learning collaborative: results of a randomized controlled trial. Arthritis Rheumatol. 2017;69:1374–80.

29. Fleischer AB Jr, Rapp SR, Reboussin DM, Vanarthos JC, Feldman SR. Patient measurement of psoriasis disease severity with a structured instrument. J Invest Dermatol. 1994;102:967–9.

30. Feldman SR, Fleischer AB Jr, Reboussin DM, Rapp SR, Exum ML, Clark AR, et al. The self-administered psoriasis area and severity index is valid and reliable. J Invest Dermatol. 1996;106:183–6.

31. Hetland ML. DANBIO—powerful research database and electronic patient record. Rheumatology. 2011;50:69–77.

32. Sokka T, Haugeberg G, Pincus T. Assessment of quality of rheumatoid arthritis care requires joint count and/or patient questionnaire data not found in a usual medical record: examples from studies of premature mortality, changes in clinical status between 1985 and 2000, and a QUEST-RA global perspective. Clin Exp Rheumatol. 2007;25(6 Suppl 47):86–97.

33. Coates LC, FitzGerald O, Gladman DD, McHugh N, Mease P, Strand V, et al. Reduced joint counts misclassify patients with oligoarticular psoriatic arthritis and miss significant numbers of patients with active disease. Arthritis Rheum. 2013;65:1504–9.

6

Methods for high-dimensional analysis of cells dissociated from cryopreserved synovial tissue

Laura T. Donlin[1,2†], Deepak A. Rao[3†], Kevin Wei[3], Kamil Slowikowski[3,4], Mandy J. McGeachy[5], Jason D. Turner[6], Nida Meednu[7], Fumitaka Mizoguchi[3], Maria Gutierrez-Arcelus[3,4], David J. Lieb[4], Joshua Keegan[3], Kaylin Muskat[8], Joshua Hillman[8], Cristina Rozo[1], Edd Ricker[1,2], Thomas M. Eisenhaure[4], Shuqiang Li[4], Edward P. Browne[4], Adam Chicoine[3], Danielle Sutherby[4], Akiko Noma[4], Accelerating Medicines Partnership RA/SLE Network, Chad Nusbaum[4], Stephen Kelly[9], Alessandra B. Pernis[1,2], Lionel B. Ivashkiv[1,2], Susan M. Goodman[1,2], William H. Robinson[10], Paul J. Utz[10], James A. Lederer[3], Ellen M. Gravallese[11], Brendan F. Boyce[7], Nir Hacohen[4,12], Costantino Pitzalis[13], Peter K. Gregersen[14], Gary S. Firestein[8], Soumya Raychaudhuri[3], Larry W. Moreland[5], V. Michael Holers[15], Vivian P. Bykerk[1,2], Andrew Filer[6], David L. Boyle[8], Michael B. Brenner[3] and Jennifer H. Anolik[7*]

Abstract

Background: Detailed molecular analyses of cells from rheumatoid arthritis (RA) synovium hold promise in identifying cellular phenotypes that drive tissue pathology and joint damage. The Accelerating Medicines Partnership RA/SLE Network aims to deconstruct autoimmune pathology by examining cells within target tissues through multiple high-dimensional assays. Robust standardized protocols need to be developed before cellular phenotypes at a single cell level can be effectively compared across patient samples.

Methods: Multiple clinical sites collected cryopreserved synovial tissue fragments from arthroplasty and synovial biopsy in a 10% DMSO solution. Mechanical and enzymatic dissociation parameters were optimized for viable cell extraction and surface protein preservation for cell sorting and mass cytometry, as well as for reproducibility in RNA sequencing (RNA-seq). Cryopreserved synovial samples were collectively analyzed at a central processing site by a custom-designed and validated 35-marker mass cytometry panel. In parallel, each sample was flow sorted into fibroblast, T-cell, B-cell, and macrophage suspensions for bulk population RNA-seq and plate-based single-cell CEL-Seq2 RNA-seq.

Results: Upon dissociation, cryopreserved synovial tissue fragments yielded a high frequency of viable cells, comparable to samples undergoing immediate processing. Optimization of synovial tissue dissociation across six clinical collection sites with ~ 30 arthroplasty and ~ 20 biopsy samples yielded a consensus digestion protocol using 100 μg/ml of Liberase™ TL enzyme preparation. This protocol yielded immune and stromal cell lineages with preserved surface markers and minimized variability across replicate RNA-seq transcriptomes. Mass cytometry analysis of cells from cryopreserved synovium distinguished diverse fibroblast phenotypes, distinct populations of memory B cells and antibody-secreting cells, and multiple CD4[+] and CD8[+] T-cell activation states. Bulk RNA-seq of sorted cell populations demonstrated robust separation of synovial lymphocytes, fibroblasts, and macrophages. Single-cell RNA-seq produced transcriptomes of over 1000 genes/cell, including transcripts encoding characteristic lineage markers identified.

(Continued on next page)

* Correspondence: jennifer_anolik@urmc.rochester.edu
†Laura T. Donlin and Deepak A. Rao contributed equally to this work.
David L. Boyle, Michael B. Brenner and Jennifer H. Anolik are joint co-authors.
[7]University of Rochester Medical Center, Rochester, NY 14642, USA
Full list of author information is available at the end of the article

(Continued from previous page)

Conclusions: We have established a robust protocol to acquire viable cells from cryopreserved synovial tissue with intact transcriptomes and cell surface phenotypes. A centralized pipeline to generate multiple high-dimensional analyses of synovial tissue samples collected across a collaborative network was developed. Integrated analysis of such datasets from large patient cohorts may help define molecular heterogeneity within RA pathology and identify new therapeutic targets and biomarkers.

Keywords: Rheumatoid arthritis, Synovial tissue, Accelerating Medicines Partnership, RNA sequencing, CyTOF, Mass cytometry, Arthroplasty, Synovial biopsy,

Background

The destructive inflammatory environment in rheumatoid arthritis (RA) synovium results from the activity of various cell types, including synovial fibroblasts, macrophages, lymphocytes, osteoclasts, and vascular endothelial cells [1–5]. Multiple pathways can be targeted to treat RA, including inhibition of tumor necrosis factor (TNF) or interleukin-6 (IL-6) signaling, blockade of T-cell costimulation, depletion of B cells, and inhibition of the JAK/STAT pathway [6]. However, despite the advent of biologic therapies, up to ~ 2/3 of RA patients do not achieve sustained disease remission [7], and there are no reliable biomarkers that serve to guide selection of specific therapeutic options for the individual patient. A more comprehensive interrogation of cells present in rheumatoid synovium may identify additional pathologic pathways targetable by therapeutics and aid in stratifying patients into disease subsets and treatment response categories based on informative biomarkers [8, 9]. Such studies have previously been limited by the lack of methods to simultaneously recover and assay the diversity of cell types in the synovium and by the challenge of applying high-dimensional single cell analytics to sufficient numbers of patient samples. In addition, comparisons of identical cell lineages isolated from targeted tissues in patients with RA and other diseases such as systemic lupus erythematosus (SLE) have not been performed.

In recognition of these needs, the NIH Accelerating Medicines Partnership (AMP) RA/SLE Network was assembled with the goal of generating detailed analyses of synovial tissue samples from a large number of RA patients. The RA Working Group of the AMP RA/SLE Network (or AMP RA network) has developed a pipeline to study RA synovial tissue samples through parallel high-dimensional analyses including mass cytometry, bulk RNA-seq of selected cell populations, and single cell RNA-seq. Mass cytometry can define the cellular landscape of tissues, while RNA-seq delves deeper into the gene expression profile for each cell type. When performed at scale on a large patient cohort, these assays have the potential to aid in developing personalized therapeutic approaches for RA.

To amass an RA cohort of sufficient size, numerous clinical collection sites contributed synovial tissue samples. The network set out to develop a pipeline for uniform and reproducible sample handling involving cryopreservation of intact synovial tissue samples. The frozen tissue fragments were then shipped to a central processing site capable of performing multiple high-dimensional analyses in parallel for each sample. The protocol was optimized for two sources of tissue: synovial biopsy obtained for research and clinically indicated excision during arthroplasty.

Here, we report the AMP RA network protocol for dissociation and analysis of immune and stromal cells from cryopreserved synovial tissue by multiple high-dimensional technologies. We describe a consensus protocol for synovial tissue disaggregation that results in high yields of viable cells with preserved surface marker expression—for both larger arthroplasty and millimeter-sized biopsy samples. We also describe an experimental pipeline to analyze each sample in parallel using single-cell RNA-seq and low-input bulk RNA-seq on selected populations, as well as mass cytometry with defined markers for synovial cells. This pipeline allows for cytometric identification and quantification of numerous immune and stromal cell populations, as well as robust transcriptomic analyses of small populations of cells from pathologic synovial samples. These methods are adaptable for use in multiple sites and have been adopted and utilized by the AMP RA network.

Methods
Human patient samples

Patients with RA fulfilled the ACR 2010 Rheumatoid Arthritis classification criteria or were identified by the participating site rheumatologist as having clinical RA [6]. A diagnosis of osteoarthritis (OA) was defined by the treating surgeon and confirmed by chart review. Synovial tissue samples were acquired by two different methods: arthroplasty and ultrasound-guided synovial biopsy. Arthroplasty samples were acquired after removal as part of standard of care at four US institutions (Hospital for Special Surgery, NY; University California San Diego, CA; University of Pittsburgh, PA; and University of Rochester, NY). All synovial biopsy samples were acquired from clinically inflamed joints under research protocols at the University of Birmingham, UK and Barts & the London School of Medicine and Dentistry, UK. The study received institutional review board approval at each site.

Arthroplasty synovial tissue collection

Synovial tissue excised as standard of care during arthroplasty was transported from the operating room to a laboratory in ice-cold PBS. The tissue was identified as synovium by characteristic features: a fibrous or elastic tissue, pink or reddish in appearance. Small fragments (~ 1–2 mm^3) were generated by dissecting with forceps or surgical scissors. Six fragments (~ 150 mg total) across the tissue were randomly combined to make individual aliquots [10, 11].

Synovial biopsy procedures

Synovial biopsy samples were obtained under ultrasound guidance by an experienced interventionist using either a needle biopsy or portal and forceps. For needle biopsy procedures, a 14G or 16G spring-loaded Cook Quick-Core® Biopsy needle was used to obtain multiple fragments [12, 13]. For the portal-based approach, a portal (Merit Medical Prelude 7F) was initially inserted into the synovial cavity with multiple samples and then retrieved using flexible 2.0–2.2 mm forceps [14, 15]. Six biopsy fragments were randomly allocated per aliquot.

Synovial tissue cryopreservation and thawing

Synovial tissues were either (1) disaggregated immediately followed by cryopreservation of dissociated cells or (2) cut into fragments that were cryopreserved for subsequent disaggregation at a central processing site. Dissociated synovial cells were resuspended in CryoStor® CS10 (Bio-Life Solutions) at ~ 2 million cells/ml to viably freeze them. Intact synovial tissue samples were divided into fragments as already described and transferred to a cryovial (1.5 ml; Nalgene) containing 1 ml of CryoStor® CS10 for viable freezing. Cryovials were then placed in an insulated container with isopropanol in the bottom chamber for slow freezing (Mr. Frosty; Nalgene), which comprised incubation at 4 °C for 10 min followed by 1 day at – 80 °C. The samples were then either shipped on dry ice or transferred into liquid nitrogen for long-term storage.

Synovial fragments were thawed by rapidly warming the cryovial in a 37 °C water bath. The preservation media was filtered out through a 70-μm strainer. The tissue was then rinsed through a series of incubations in a six-well culture plate: 10 min in 10% FBS/RPMI at room temperature with intermittent swirling, a quick rinse in 10% FBS/RPMI, and a final rinse in serum-free RPMI. Frozen synovial cells were thawed rapidly in a 37 °C water bath and transferred into 20 ml of 10% FBS/RPMI, centrifuged to pellet cells, and then resuspended in media for downstream analyses.

Dissociation of synovial tissue

Both arthroplasty and synovial biopsy samples were dissociated by a combination of enzymatic digestion and mechanical disruption with various test conditions described in Results. The final consensus AMP RA network enzyme digestion uses RPMI media with Liberase™ TL enzyme preparations (100 μg/ml; Roche) and DNase I (100 μg/ml; Roche).

Arthroplasty tissue

To achieve consistent mechanical disruption and proteolytic enzyme exposure across a fragment of tissue, large synovial specimens (> 150 mg) were cut into small fragments (~ 2 mm^3) using surgical scissors. Mechanical disruption of arthroplasty samples (six tissue fragments totaling ≥ 500 mg) was carried out by a gentleMACS dissociator system (Miltenyi) with the m_Spleen 04.01 setting, which involves churning and shredding in a sterile disposable tube. Enzymatic digestion was performed in RPMI medium at 37 °C for 30 min. A large volume of 5% FBS/RPMI was then added to terminate the enzymatic reaction. The tissue was ground through a 70-μm filter using the flat plastic end of a 3-ml syringe plunger to disperse the remaining intact tissue and dispense dissociated cells.

Synovial biopsy tissue

For the samples obtained by synovial biopsy, tissue fragments were minced into small fragments (~ 1 mm^3) using a scalpel. Samples were then subjected to enzymatic digestion at 37 °C while being exposed to continuous stirring in a U-bottom polystyrene tube (12×75 mm^2) with a magnetic stir bar for 30 min. Halfway through the enzymatic digestion, samples were passed gently through a 16G syringe needle 10 times for additional mechanical disruption.

RNA extraction from whole synovial tissue fragments

For samples used in the aforementioned dissociation protocol, synovial tissue fragments were also preserved for whole tissue RNA extraction. Three whole tissue replicates were collected for each sample, with six fragments placed into a cryovial containing 1 ml of RNALater (Qiagen) and inverted three times. The cryovials were incubated overnight at 4 °C. The next day, the cryovials were spun at $\sim 1000 \times g$ for 30 s and most of the RNALater was removed, leaving only enough RNALater to cover the tissue. The cryovials were then placed in storage at – 70 °C. For RNA extraction, samples were thawed and fragments transferred into RLT lysis buffer (Qiagen) + 1% β-mercaptoethanol (Sigma) and homogenized using a TissueLyser II (Qiagen) before RNA isolation using RNeasy columns.

Flow cytometry cell sorting

Synovial cell suspensions were stained with an 11-color flow cytometry panel designed to identify synovial stromal and leukocyte populations. Antibodies included anti-CD 45-FITC (HI30), anti-CD90-PE(5E10), anti-podoplanin-PerCP/eFluor710 (NZ1.3), anti-CD3-PECy7 (UCHT1), anti-CD19-BV421 (HIB19), anti-CD14-BV510 (M5E2), anti-CD34-BV605 (4H11), anti-CD4-BV650 (RPA-T4), anti-CD8-BV711 (SK1), anti-CD31-AlexaFluor700 (WM59), anti-CD27-APC (M-T271), anti-CD235a-APC/AF750, TruStain FcX, and propidium iodide. Cells were stained in HEPES-buffered saline (20 mM HEPES, 137 mM NaCl, 3 mM KCl, 1 mM $CaCl_2$) with 1% bovine serum albumin (BSA) for 30 min, then washed once, resuspended in the same buffer with propidium iodide added, vortexed briefly, and passed through a 100-μm filter.

Cells were sorted on a three-laser BD FACSAria Fusion cell sorter. Intact cells were gated according to FSC-A and SSC-A. Doublets were excluded by serial FSC-H/FSC-W and SSC-H/SSC-W gates. Nonviable cells were excluded based on propidium iodide uptake. Cells were sorted through a 100-μm nozzle at 20 psi.

A serial sorting strategy was used to sequentially capture cells for bulk RNA-seq and then single-cell RNA-seq if sufficient numbers of cells were present. First, 1000 cells of the targeted cell type were sorted for low-input RNA-seq into a 1.7-ml Eppendorf tube containing 350 μl of RLT lysis buffer (Qiagen) + 1% β-mercaptoethanol. Once 1000 cells of a particular cell type were collected, the sort was stopped and the tube was exchanged for a second tube containing FACS buffer. Sorting was then resumed and the rest of the cells of that type were collected into the second tube as viable cells. This process was carried out for four targeted populations. Live cells of each population that were sorted into FACS buffer were then resorted as single cells into wells of 384-well plates containing 1 μl of 1% NP-40, targeting up to 144 cells of each type per sample.

RNA sequencing on low-input bulk populations
RNA from sorted bulk cell populations was isolated using RNeasy columns (Qiagen). RNA from up to 1000 cells was treated with DNase I (New England Biolabs), and then concentrated using Agencourt RNAClean XP beads (Beckman Coulter). Full-length cDNA and sequencing libraries were prepared using the Smart-Seq2 protocol as described previously [16]. Libraries were sequenced on a MiSeq (Illumina) to generate 25-base-pair, paired-end reads totaling a fragment length of 50 base pairs.

Single-cell RNA sequencing
Single cell RNAseq (scRNA-Seq) was performed using the CEL-Seq2 method [17] with the following modifications. Single cells were sorted into 384-well plates containing 0.6 μl of 1% NP-40 buffer in each well. Then, 0.6 μl dNTPs (10 mM each; NEB) and 5 nl of barcoded reverse transcription primer (1 μg/μl) were added to each well

along with 20 nl of ERCC spike-in (diluted 1:800,000). Reactions were incubated at 65 °C for 5 min, and then moved immediately to ice. Reverse transcription reactions were carried out as described previously [17] and cDNA was purified using 0.8× volumes of AMPure XP beads (Beckman Coulter). In-vitro transcription reactions (IVT) were performed as described followed by EXO-SAP treatment. Amplified RNA (aRNA) was fragmented at 80 °C for 3 min and purified using RNAClean XP beads (Beckman Coulter). The purified aRNA was converted to cDNA using an anchored random primer and Illumina adaptor sequences were added by PCR. The final cDNA library was purified using AMPure XP beads (Beckman Coulter). Libraries were sequenced on a Hiseq 2500 (Illumina) in Rapid Run Mode to generate paired-end reads. Forward reads (35 nt) were mapped to human reference genome hg19 using STAR v2.5 [18], while reverse reads (15 nt) included cellular and molecular barcodes (6 nt each). Basic analyses of single-cell RNA-seq data, including quantification of genes detected per cell, filtering of cells with less than 1000 detected genes, and principal components analyses, were performed using RSEM [19].

Differential expression
To examine differential gene expression profiles between RA and OA synovial tissues processed through the consensus disaggregation protocol, tissue samples were collected from 10 RA patients and 10 OA patients. From these 20 patients, 2–8 replicates were generated per donor for a total of 87 samples. We performed differential expression analysis by fitting a linear mixed model to each gene, in which we controlled for unwanted technical variation with donor and site as random effects.

Gene Ontology term enrichment analysis
We tested Gene Ontology (GO) enrichment with differentially expressed genes. We used Ensembl gene IDs downloaded in April 2016, including 9797 GO terms and 15,693 genes. The minimal hypergeometric test was used to test for significance [20].

Mass cytometry
Synovial cells were resuspended in PBS/1%BSA with primary antibody cocktails at 1:100 dilution for 30 min (Additional file 1: Table S1). All antibodies were obtained from the Longwood Medical Area CyTOF Antibody Resource Core (Boston, MA, USA). Cisplatin was added at 1:400 dilution for the last 5 min of the stain to assess viability. Cells were then washed and fixed in 1.6% paraformaldehyde for 10 min at room temperature. Cells were then washed and incubated with Ebioscience Transcription Factor Fix/Perm Buffer for 30 min, washed in Ebioscience perm buffer, and stained for intracellular markers at 1:100 for 30 min. Cells were refixed in 1.6%

paraformaldehyde for 10 min and stored overnight in PBS/1%BSA. The following day, cells were incubated with MaxPar Intercalator-Ir 500 µM 1:4000 in PBS for 20 min, and then washed twice with MilliQ water, filtered, and analyzed on a Helios instrument (Fluidigm). Mass cytometry data were normalized using EQ™ Four Element Calibration Beads (Fluidigm) as described previously [21]. viSNE analysis was performed using the Barnes-Hut SNE implementation on Cytobank (www.cytobank.org). Gated live cells (DNA-positive, cisplatin-negative) were analyzed using all available protein markers. Biaxial gating was performed using FlowJo 10.0.7.

Results

Synovial tissue dissociation: optimizing cell yield and surface marker preservation

Laboratories within the AMP RA network (Fig. 1a) initially set out to collectively establish a standard operating procedure for isolating cells of differing lineages from synovial tissue. This protocol required balancing rigorous dissociation of stromal cells that adhere tightly to the tissue matrix, while minimizing perturbations and maintaining viability, RNA stability, and key surface proteins required for downstream isolation and assays. In addition, methods were needed to handle both large arthroplasty samples and small synovial biopsy samples (Fig. 1b).

Selection of methods for mechanical disruption

Pilot experiments across several sites suggested that various forms of mechanical disruption could be used, including manual inversion of the tube or incubation in a Stomacher® 400 circulator. Dissociation using the gentleMACS was selected for arthroplasty as this method provided an automated and standardized protocol that could be implemented across laboratories (Fig. 1c). However, dissociation of small synovial biopsy fragments (~ 0.5–1 mm^3) using the gentleMACS system generated variable and insufficient yields, possibly due to cell retention in the dissociation container. Therefore, synovial biopsy samples were subjected to mechanical disruption by continuous magnetic stirring, combined with trituration through a syringe needle.

Enzymatic dissociation combined with mechanical disruption generates high cell yields

To test the impact of combining enzymatic treatment with mechanical dissociation, proteolytic enzymes were added to the media during mechanical dissociation. For the majority of tissue samples, higher cell yields were obtained when synovial fragments were incubated with enzyme in addition to mechanical disruption (Fig. 2a). Importantly for highly adherent stromal (PDPN$^+$CD45$^-$) lineages, the proportion recovered increased with enzymatic digestion (Fig. 2b, c).

Proteolytic enzyme preparations differ in surface marker preservation

Focusing on highly purified enzyme formulations designed for standardized protocols, the consortium tested Liberase™ mixtures containing thermolysin (T) or dispase (D) in combination with collagenase. As proteolytic enzymes can cleave cell surface proteins [22, 23], we tested the enzyme panel to identify a formulation that preserved important cell surface proteins such as CD3 and CD4. Certain formulations compromised the detection of cell surface proteins. For example, on CD3$^+$ T cells isolated from synovium, a decline in CD4 surface detection was observed with Liberase™ Dispase-High (DH), Thermolysin-Medium (TM), and Thermolysin-High (TH) compared to no enzyme treatment or Thermolysin-Low (TL) and Dispase-Low (DL) (Fig. 2d). As peripheral blood mononuclear cell preparations with equal numbers of circulating T cells resulted in a similar pattern of loss in CD4 detection when treated with the enzymes, the decline in CD4 levels in the synovial preparations is likely due to direct degradation of the cell surface protein by proteases rather than a selective reduction in extracting CD4$^+$ T subsets (Additional file 1: Figure S1a). As Liberase™ TL versus TM mixtures proved equally efficient at dissociating out both stromal and hematopoietic cells (Additional file 1: Figure S1b), Liberase™ TL was chosen for both high cell yields and preservation of cell surface markers for downstream analyses, including mass cytometry.

Optimization of proteolytic enzyme concentrations

To determine the optimal concentration of proteolytic enzyme for consistent cell recovery and reproducibility of downstream assays, four network sites processed arthroplasty samples using three different Liberase™ TL concentrations, with three technical replicates for each concentration. In comparison to the 25 and 50 µg/ml concentrations, the 100 µg/ml concentration yielded the highest amount of intact RNA after tissue dissociation (Fig. 2e). In addition, synovial samples processed with 100 µg/ml enzyme concentration demonstrated the lowest variance in RNA-seq gene expression across replicate samples, visually depicted in the principal component analysis (PCA) plots where distance between replicates is minimized with the 100 µg/ml concentration (Fig. 2f). Next, we computed the sum of squares within (SSW) to quantify replicate similarities within each of the three enzyme concentrations. Here, we also observed that replicates processed with 100 µg/ml had the least variation (Fig. 2g).

To gain insight into the source of gene expression variation across synovial samples, we applied analysis of variance (ANOVA) to each principal component to assess the contribution of the following sources: site, donor, and the potential impact of the dissociation process (Additional file 1: Figure S1c). The majority of gene expression

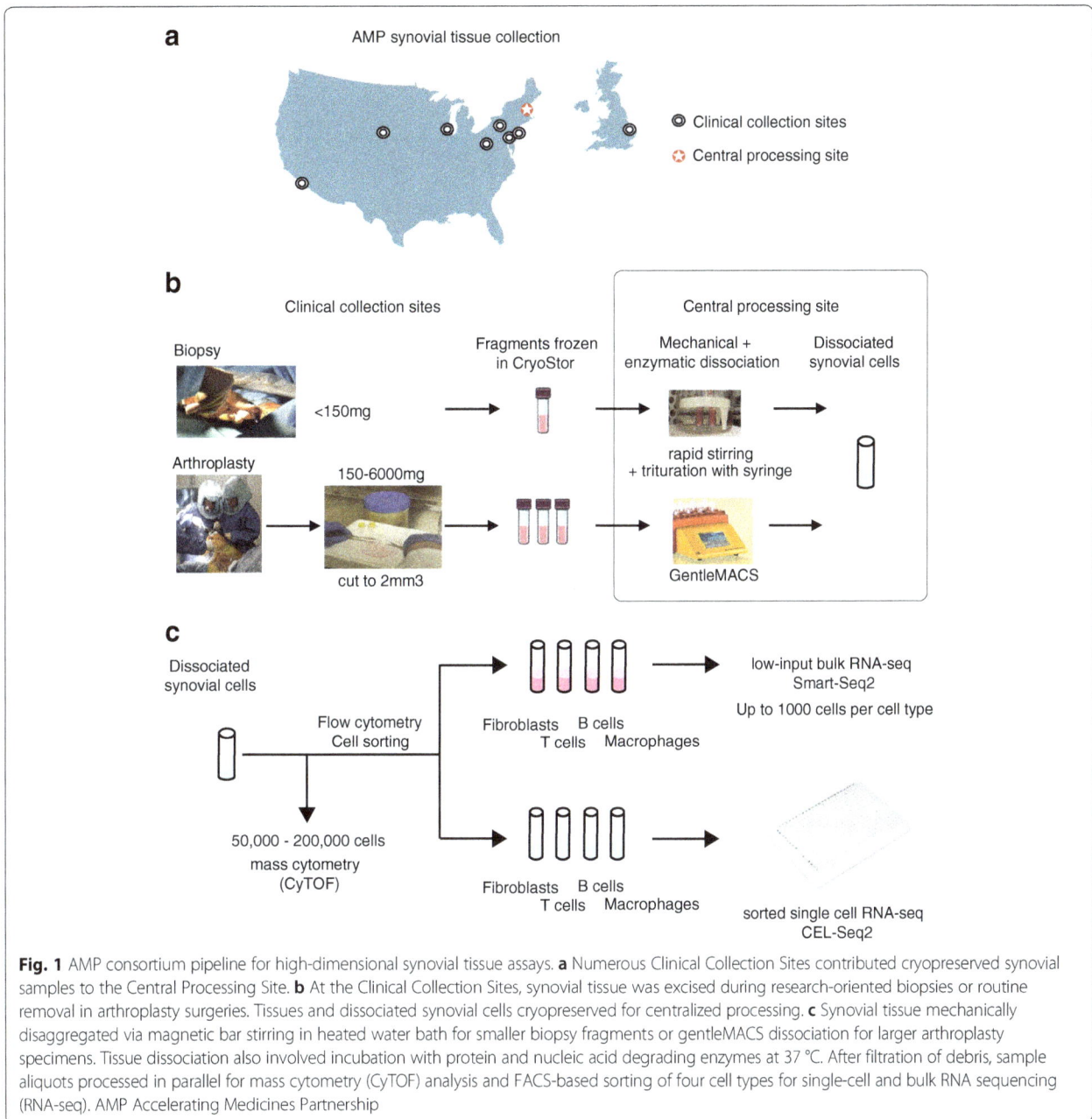

Fig. 1 AMP consortium pipeline for high-dimensional synovial tissue assays. **a** Numerous Clinical Collection Sites contributed cryopreserved synovial samples to the Central Processing Site. **b** At the Clinical Collection Sites, synovial tissue was excised during research-oriented biopsies or routine removal in arthroplasty surgeries. Tissues and dissociated synovial cells cryopreserved for centralized processing. **c** Synovial tissue mechanically disaggregated via magnetic bar stirring in heated water bath for smaller biopsy fragments or gentleMACS dissociation for larger arthroplasty specimens. Tissue dissociation also involved incubation with protein and nucleic acid degrading enzymes at 37 °C. After filtration of debris, sample aliquots processed in parallel for mass cytometry (CyTOF) analysis and FACS-based sorting of four cell types for single-cell and bulk RNA sequencing (RNA-seq). AMP Accelerating Medicines Partnership

variation associated with donor differences (PC1 and PC2), which encompasses biological differences such as disease state. Site-specific collection and/or processing differences also contributed variation (PC1). Of note, the AMP Network has designated a central processing site to eliminate site-specific dissociation effects.

Sample variability in PC3 and PC6 also related to gene expression differences that were identified in a separate RNAseq analysis comparing whole versus dissociated synovial preparations (Additional file 1: Figure S1c–e). The analysis comparing dissociated versus whole tissue RNAseq was intended to identify dissociation-induced effects, but involved mixtures of various cell types and,

correspondingly, much of the gene expression differences indicated cell composition differences. These differences likely relate to differences in the preparation protocols; for example, adipocytes escape during spinning and aspiration steps in the dissociation protocol, while red blood cells may inadvertently be removed in whole tissue preparations during a salt solution incubation and subsequent aspiration. Nonetheless, outside of cell type-specific genes, there was an increase in stress response genes in dissociated cell preparations, similar to a previous report on dissociation-induced effects in single cells [24]. This included an upregulation in heat shock protein genes (*HSP1A1*, *HSP6A*, *HSP90AA*) and early response genes

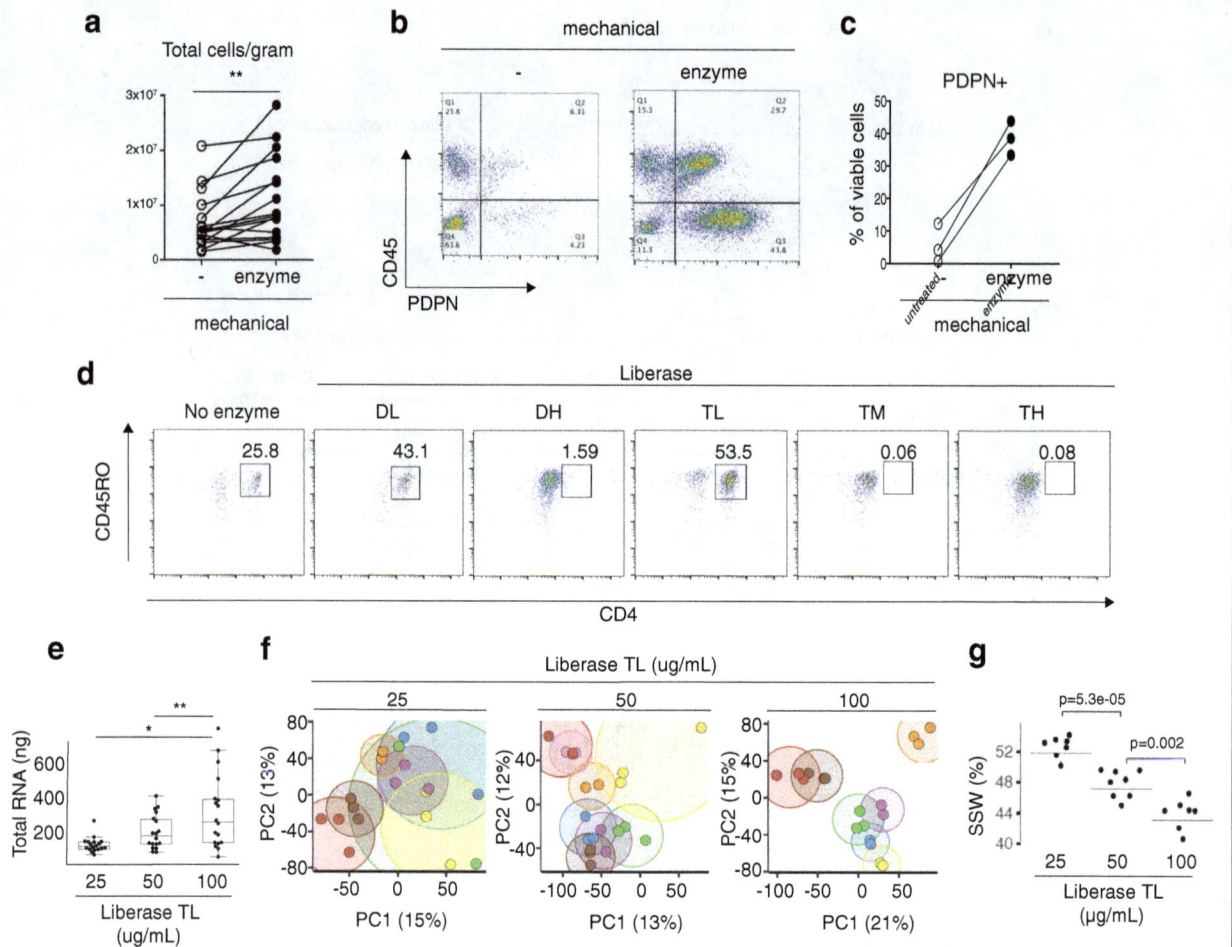

Fig. 2 High synovial cell yield, preserved surface markers, and reproducible transcriptomic results with mechanical and enzymatic disaggregation protocol. **a** Total cell counts per gram from synovial tissue mechanically disaggregated with or without Liberase™ TL proteolytic enzyme treatment. $n = 16$, paired t test. **b, c** Flow cytometry detection and quantification of stromal cells (CD45⁻PDPN⁺) upon mechanical disaggregation with or without Liberase™ TL proteolytic enzyme treatment. **d** Flow cytometry of dissociated synovial cells treated with panel of proteolytic Liberase™ TL formulations. Cells gated for viability and CD3 T-cell receptor subunit. Plots representative of $n = 4$ biologic replicates. **e** Total RNA yield from synovial tissue dissociated with three concentrations of Liberase™ TL. Two or three technical replicates from nine tissues used for each enzyme concentration. ANOVA with Tukey's comparison, *$p<0.05$ and **$p<0.01$. **f** Principal component analyses on RNA-seq gene expression results for samples from (**e**), whereby each technical replicate of same sample is represented by a dot of same color while variation between replicates is indicated by size of encircling cloud of same color. **g** Sum of squares within (SSW) replicates from same donor divided by total sum of squares, using gene expression profiles from (**e**) and (**f**). Horizontal lines indicate SSW values using all replicates. Individual dots are SSW values computed after leave-one-out strategy where replicates from one donor are left out and SSW is computed with remaining samples. Student's t test used to test whether bootstrapped SSW values differ significantly. DH Dispase-High, DL Dispase-Low, PC principal component, PDPN podoplanin, TH Thermolysin-High, TL Thermolysin-Low, TM Thermolysin-Medium

(*FOS, JUN, ATF3*) (Additional file 1: Figure S1d, e). Thus, synovial cells demonstrating specific upregulation in this signature could indicate a dissociation-induced gene expression pattern rather than a cell subset-specific program. For subsequent single-cell RNAseq studies, individual synovial cells with high levels of this stress response could either be removed from the analyses or the signature could be adjusted for computationally.

Overall, these results suggest that dissociation with 100 µg/ml Liberase™ TL produces consistent and robust

recovery of diverse synovial stromal and immune cell populations with the largest source of variation in the samples due to donor biological differences.

Development of cryopreservation methods

Having established synovial dissociation methods, we then focused on establishing a strategy to analyze samples acquired at distant sites through a uniform high-dimensional analysis pipeline. We first evaluated the feasibility of studying synovial cells cryopreserved after tissue dissociation.

From three different arthroplasty samples analyzed either immediately after dissociation (fresh) or after freezing the cells in a cryopreservation solution for at least 1 day, comparable cell frequencies were extracted for synovial fibroblasts, monocytes, T cells, and B cells (Fig. 3a). This result, although based on only three samples, suggested that synovial cells generally survive cryopreservation well, consistent with prior studies [5, 25, 26].

In addition to cryopreserving dissociated synovial cells, we next evaluated the feasibility of cryopreserving intact synovial tissue fragments prior to dissociation. Notably, three synovial biopsy tissues processed after cryopreservation yielded cells with comparable viability to paired tissue analyzed immediately after isolation (Fig. 3b). In addition, flow cytometric analysis of cells from cryopreserved synovial tissue showed robust detection of stromal and hematopoietic cell populations, similar to fresh synovial tissue (Fig. 3c). These results indicate that intact synovial tissue can be cryopreserved for subsequent cellular analyses.

We next examined whether application of the protocol implementing 100 μg/ml of Liberase™ TL, mechanical disaggregation, and viable freezing could detect robust expression pattern differences between dissociated synovial cells from tissues from patients with RA and osteoarthritis (OA). Importantly, an RNA-seq analysis of disaggregated total synovial cells demonstrated an upregulation in RA of genes involved in immune processes, such as immunoglobulin binding, cellular response to molecules of bacterial origin, leukocyte chemotaxis and migration, cytokine production, and antigen processing and presentation by MHC class II (Fig. 3d).

High-dimensional assays of synovial cells

A goal of the AMP Network is to generate both mass cytometry and RNA-seq analyses of cells from cryopreserved synovial samples dissociated by the protocol described earlier. Acquisition of data for both of these technologies from the same synovial sample allows the coupling of detailed quantification of cell populations with genome-wide transcriptomic analyses. These combined analyses enable interrogation of correlations between cell populations and transcriptomic signatures with unprecedented resolution for a human autoimmune disease tissue target. Because synovial samples vary widely in both cell yield and composition, we developed an algorithm to allocate cells for different analyses in a step-wise fashion without prior knowledge of the cell composition (Fig. 1c). Preliminary experiments indicated that reproducible mass cytometry analyses could be obtained from 100,000 synovial cells; therefore, for samples that yielded over 200,000 synovial cells, approximately half of the cells were allocated to mass cytometry, with the rest were used for sequential low-input and

single-cell RNA-seq analyses. When less than 200,000 synovial cells were obtained, mass cytometric analysis was omitted and only RNA-seq analyses were performed.

Mass cytometry of synovial cells

A 35-parameter mass cytometry panel was developed to identify stromal, vascular, and immune cells within synovial samples (Fig. 4a). Visualization of the mass cytometry data obtained from a cryopreserved synovial biopsy sample using the dimensional reduction tool viSNE [27] revealed clear discrimination of synovial fibroblasts (cadherin-11$^+$), endothelial cells (VE-cadherin$^+$), and immune cell subsets from cryopreserved RA synovial tissue (Fig. 4b). viSNE visualization highlighted the heterogeneity within immune cell populations, which was confirmed by biaxial gating. For example, two populations of B cells were easily resolved, including one CD19$^+$CD20$^+$ population and a distinct CD19$^+$CD20$^-$CD38^{hi} population comprised of antibody-secreting cells (Fig. 4b, c) [28, 29]. Marked heterogeneity within the CD3$^+$ T-cell population was also evident, with multiple lobes of T cells visualized, including a subset of PD-1^{hi}ICOS$^+$CD4$^+$ T cells (Fig. 4b, c) [5]. This visualization also demonstrated heterogeneity among the podoplanin$^+$ synovial fibroblasts, including fibroblast subpopulations that express CD90 and/or CD34 [25, 26]. These results indicate that high-resolution mass cytometry data can be obtained from synovial cells collected from cryopreserved intact synovial tissue that is subsequently thawed and dissociated.

RNA-seq transcriptomics of synovial cell populations and single cells

In addition to mass cytometry analyses, a major goal of the AMP Network is to define molecular signatures and pathways of disease by transcriptome analysis. Low-input RNA-seq provided robust gene expression values for a large number of protein coding genes averaged across approximately 1000 cells. The complementary single-cell RNA-seq approach provided a high-resolution view of the heterogeneity of expression profiles between individual cells. We designed a cell sorting workflow that prioritized collecting cells for low-input RNA-seq, with a goal of collecting 1000 cells from each of the four targeted cell types. If more than 1000 cells of a targeted cell type were available, the remaining cells were sorted into a second collection tube for subsequent single-cell RNA-seq analysis (Fig. 1c). This sorting scheme enabled capture of virtually all of the cells for each of the four target populations for low-input and single-cell RNA-seq.

Synovial cells were stained with a multidimensional flow cytometry panel that could identify diverse cell populations including fibroblasts (CD45$^-$podoplanin$^+$CD31$^-$), endothelial cells (CD45$^-$podoplanin$^-$CD31$^+$), macrophages (CD45$^+$CD14$^+$CD3$^-$), and T cells (CD45$^+$CD14$^-$CD3$^+$)

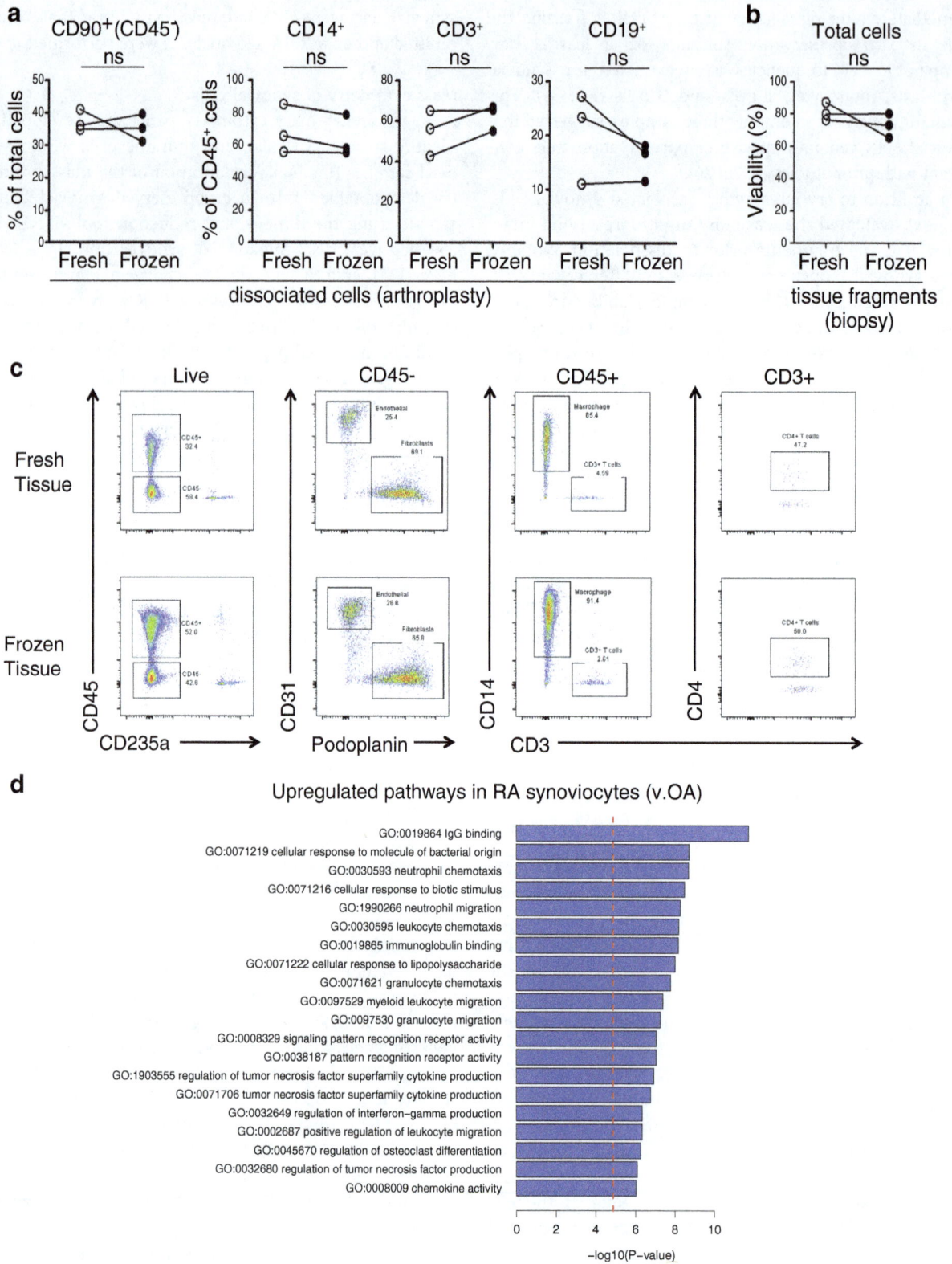

Fig. 3 (See legend on next page.)

Fig. 3 Cryopreservation of synovial fragments retains stromal and hematopoietic cell viability and RA synovial gene expression patterns. **a** Frequency of synovial cell subpopulations from arthroplasty samples dissociated from freshly isolated or cryopreserved aliquots. **b** Cell viability frequency assayed by flow cytometry for synovial biopsy samples dissociated from fresh or cryopreserved tissue fragments. **c** Flow cytometry analysis of cells dissociated from synovial tissue either immediately or after cryopreservation. **d** Top 20 GO terms enriched for genes upregulated in RA patient disaggregated synovial cells in comparison to patients with OA. $N = 10$ RA and 10 OA samples with 2–8 replicates per donor. ns no significant difference, OA osteoarthritis, RA rheumatoid arthritis

(Fig. 5a). Low-input RNA-seq analysis of fibroblasts, macrophages, endothelial cells, and T cells sorted from three cryopreserved RA synovial biopsy samples yielded transcriptomes with 8000–13,000 genes detected from cell inputs ranging from 1000 cells down to 83 cells (Fig. 5a, b). Principal components analysis robustly distinguished the different cell types at the global transcriptomic level (Fig. 5c). These results indicate that cells obtained from cryopreserved biopsies yield transcriptomes that reflect the expected cell identity.

Transcriptomes of single cells sorted from cryopreserved RA synovium were obtained by RNA-seq through the CEL-Seq2 platform. High-quality transcriptomes from both single-cell fibroblasts and leukocytes from RA synovium were generated, with fibroblasts generally yielding higher gene counts (Fig. 6a). Principal components analysis of single cells from an RA synovial sample separated the fibroblasts from the immune cells along PC1, and mostly separated macrophages from T and B lymphocytes along PC2 (Fig. 6b). Importantly, single cells from each sorted cell population expressed markers expected for that cell type. For example, the *podoplanin* transcript was expressed primarily in fibroblasts, consistent with flow cytometry and mass cytometry data, while the *CD14* transcript was identified in sorted macrophages, an expected finding since the cells were flow sorted by CD14 protein expression (Fig. 6c). Similarly, the *CD3E* transcript was uniquely detected in sorted T cells, while *CD79A* expression was unique to sorted B cells. These results indicate that high-quality transcriptomes can be generated from bulk populations and single cells obtained from cryopreserved RA synovial tissue samples.

Discussion

Here we describe the development of an experimental pipeline to analyze synovial tissue with multiple high-dimensional technologies, aimed at deconstructing the cellular and molecular features of RA. This standardized and validated strategy enables single-cell analytics on large sample numbers collected from numerous clinical sites.

The integration of contemporary high-dimensional assays provides the opportunity to dissect the properties of tissues affected by rheumatic disease with a resolution not previously possible. Histologic and immunohistochemical assessments of synovium have revealed marked

heterogeneity in RA synovial pathology [13, 30]. Gene expression analyses of synovium by microarray have added gene expression signatures to these histologic patterns [31–34]. However, broad analyses of gene expression in synovium have thus far been limited mainly to assessments of whole tissue, which cannot distinguish which cell types express the relevant genes [31, 35–38]. The analysis pipeline described here enables simultaneous quantification of a wide range of stromal and leukocyte subpopulations by mass cytometry, paired with genome-wide transcriptional analyses, both of targeted cell populations and of single cells. Mass cytometry alone provides a powerful, broad assessment of the cell types and phenotypes within the tissue on a relatively large number of cells [5]. Transcriptomic analyses of sorted subpopulations can identify the cell types contributing specific gene expression signatures derived in the synovium, including signatures specific to RA synovium. Single-cell transcriptomics allow a high-powered characterization of the heterogeneity of cells across a tissue [39] and within cell subsets that were previously classified as the same cell type [25, 26, 40]. We propose that integrating the multiple high-dimensional datasets acquired with this pipeline will reveal how distinct cell types relate to specific aspects of RA pathology. Applied to a large patient cohort, these analyses have the potential to reveal functional pathologic markers that distinguish patients with distinct clinical trajectories and therapeutic responses [5].

Implementing these technologies requires robust tissue processing protocols. The validation studies described here, which were carried out by a collaboration among laboratories with expertise in synovial tissue and RA, provide a widely applicable, reproducible method for obtaining single cells from RA synovium that performs well in cytometric and transcriptomic analyses. Classically, synovial tissue has been disaggregated by crude collagenase preparations, which often cleave cell surface proteins and may contain bacterial products that stimulate immune cells. Here, varied concentrations of highly purified proteolytic enzyme preparations were assessed for preservation of vulnerable cell surface proteins required for downstream assays, as well as cell viability, RNA integrity, and applicability to next-generation sequencing. Combining limited enzyme incubation time with mechanical disaggregation yielded viable cell populations from disparate lineages that performed well in downstream assays. It is

a

CyTOF Panel	
CD45	VE-Cadherin
CD66b	VCAM-1
CD14	Podoplanin
CD64	Cadherin-11
CD16	FAP
CD11c	CD146
CCR2	CD90
CD3	CD34
CD4	CD19
CD8	CD20
CD69	CD38
CD45RO	CD138
CXCR5	IgD
PD-1	IgM
ICOS	IgA
HLA-DR	FcRL4
TCRgd	RANKL
FoxP3	Live/dead

b

c

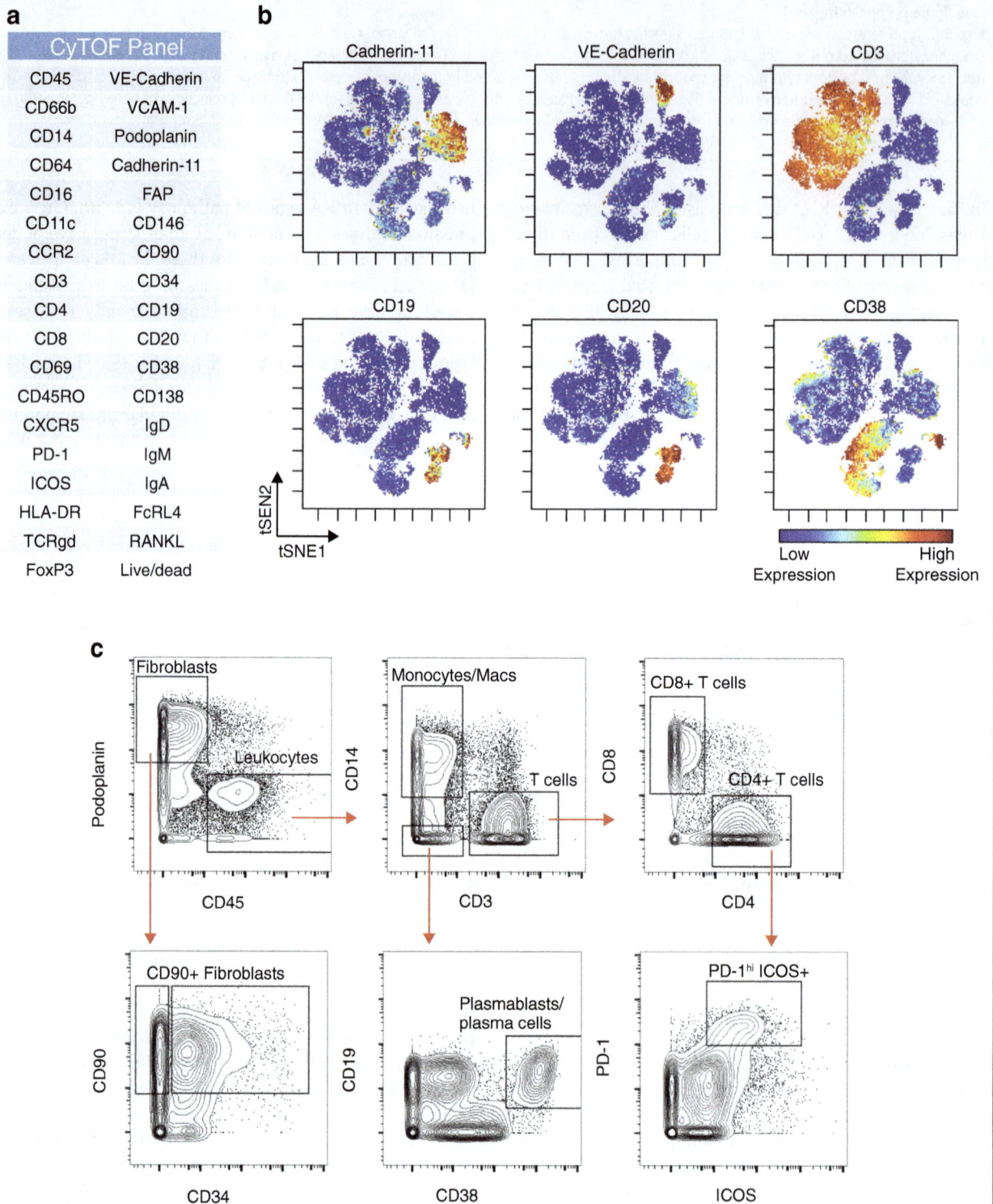

Fig. 4 Mass cytometry analysis of dissociated synovial tissue reveals synovial cell heterogeneity via surface marker detection. **a** Antibody marker panel for synovial cell mass cytometry analysis. **b** viSNE visualization of synovial cells analyzed by mass cytometry from cryopreserved synovial biopsy sample obtained from knee of an RA patient. Each dot is a cell. Color reflects level of expression of marker indicated at top of plot. **c** Biaxial contour plots of same mass cytometry data shown in (**b**), showing serial gating of cell subpopulations. Representative of at least six synovial samples

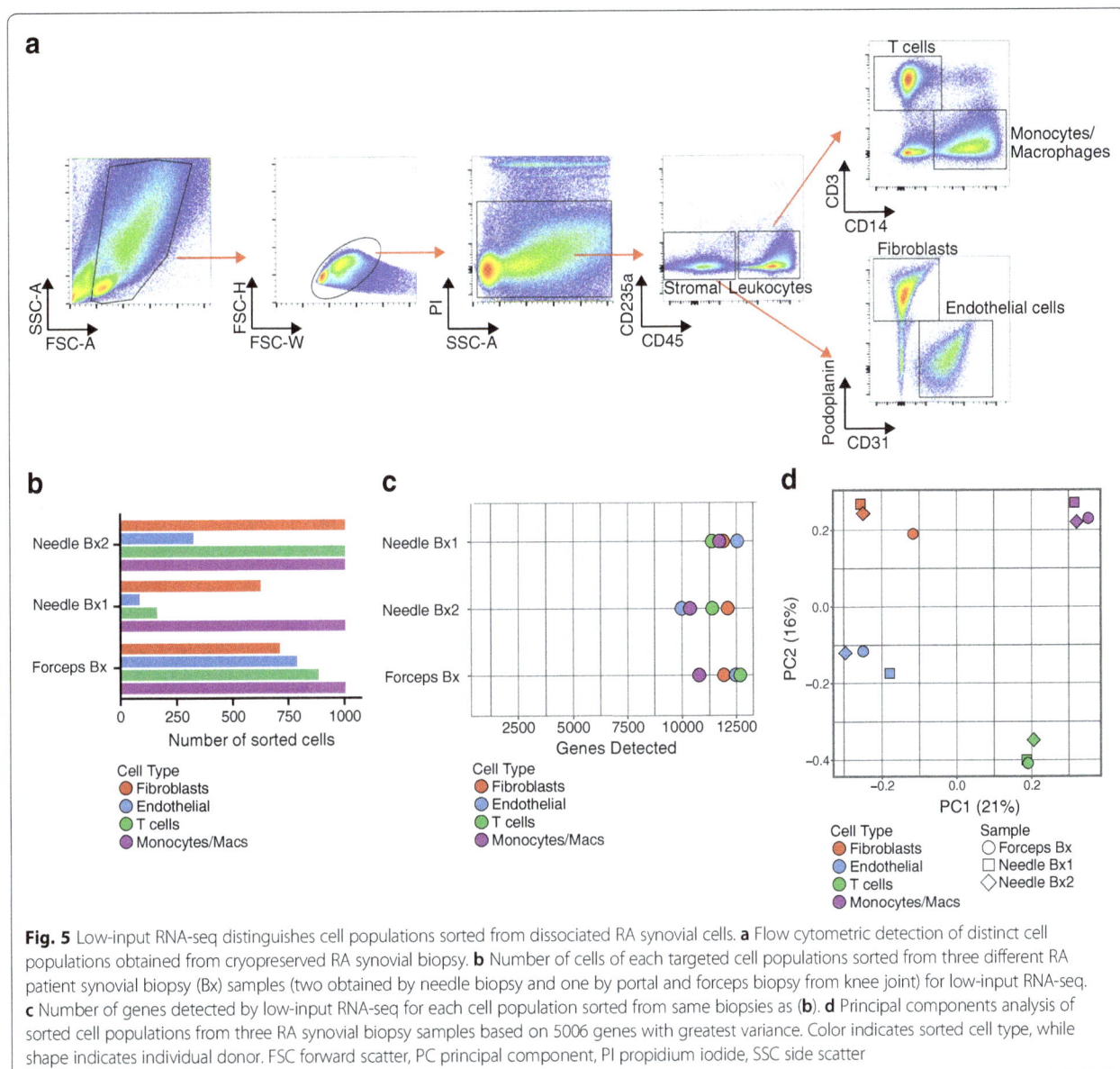

Fig. 5 Low-input RNA-seq distinguishes cell populations sorted from dissociated RA synovial cells. **a** Flow cytometric detection of distinct cell populations obtained from cryopreserved RA synovial biopsy. **b** Number of cells of each targeted cell populations sorted from three different RA patient synovial biopsy (Bx) samples (two obtained by needle biopsy and one by portal and forceps biopsy from knee joint) for low-input RNA-seq. **c** Number of genes detected by low-input RNA-seq for each cell population sorted from same biopsies as (**b**). **d** Principal components analysis of sorted cell populations from three RA synovial biopsy samples based on 5006 genes with greatest variance. Color indicates sorted cell type, while shape indicates individual donor. FSC forward scatter, PC principal component, PI propidium iodide, SSC side scatter

important to recognize that dissociating tissues into cell suspensions may introduce processing signatures [24]. However, differences in transcriptome between intact and dissociated tissue may arise from a number of sources. These may include better representation of genes from cells difficult to extract in the intact tissue samples, in addition to potentially adverse consequences such as a cellular response to tissue manipulation. Importantly, with the synovial tissue disaggregation protocols developed here, mass cytometry of the single cells obtained clearly identified multiple expected cell populations in striking detail. RNA-seq transcriptomic analyses also robustly distinguished cells of different types at both the low-input and single-cell level. Further, transcriptomic analysis of synovial cells identified RA-specific gene signatures even in the relatively small sample set presented with the

largest source of variation in the transcriptome due to donor biological differences. While dissociation-induced gene signatures are identifiable, they can be adjusted for computationally if necessary. Taken together, these observations strongly argue for the potential of this approach to discover new aspects of RA cellular pathology, which can be further validated in intact tissues.

The ability to effectively cryopreserve synovial tissue marks a major technical advance for synovial research. The viability and flow cytometric phenotypes of cells from cryopreserved synovial tissue samples were comparable to those from freshly processed tissues. Cells obtained from cryopreserved tissue samples were largely viable and readily used for all of the mass cytometric and RNA-seq analyses presented in this report. Cryopreservation of intact synovial tissue provides a simple, rapid technique to

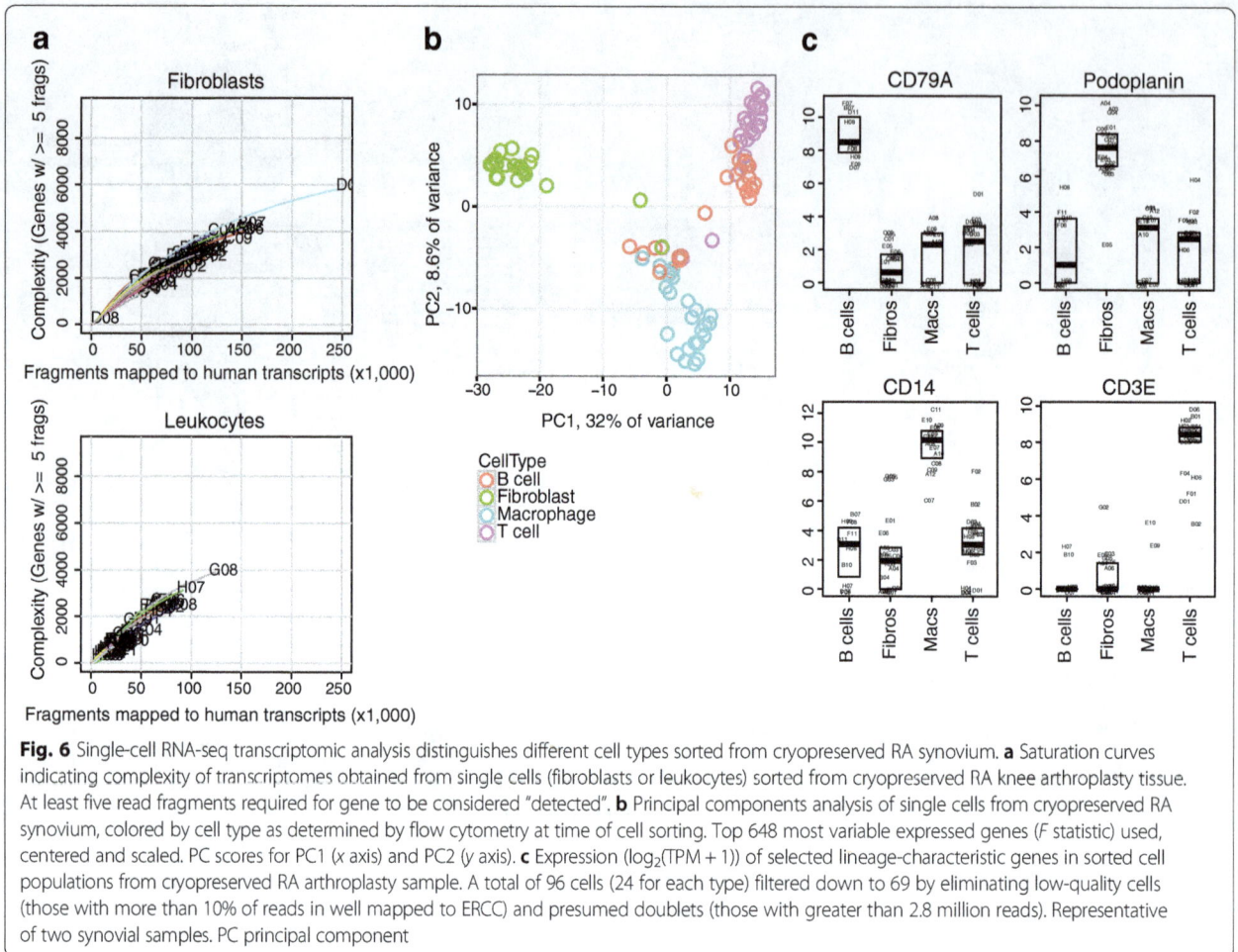

Fig. 6 Single-cell RNA-seq transcriptomic analysis distinguishes different cell types sorted from cryopreserved RA synovium. **a** Saturation curves indicating complexity of transcriptomes obtained from single cells (fibroblasts or leukocytes) sorted from cryopreserved RA knee arthroplasty tissue. At least five read fragments required for gene to be considered "detected". **b** Principal components analysis of single cells from cryopreserved RA synovium, colored by cell type as determined by flow cytometry at time of cell sorting. Top 648 most variable expressed genes (F statistic) used, centered and scaled. PC scores for PC1 (x axis) and PC2 (y axis). **c** Expression (log2(TPM + 1)) of selected lineage-characteristic genes in sorted cell populations from cryopreserved RA arthroplasty sample. A total of 96 cells (24 for each type) filtered down to 69 by eliminating low-quality cells (those with more than 10% of reads in well mapped to ERCC) and presumed doublets (those with greater than 2.8 million reads). Representative of two synovial samples. PC principal component

preserve and transport affected tissues for cellular studies in a multisite consortium. Tissue fragment cryopreservation enables sample collection from numerous clinical sites, including those lacking the resources for tissue dissociation. This approach also eliminates site-specific processing effects, allowing samples to be processed at a central site that possesses multiple high-dimensional technologies, and to utilize batch processing of samples to minimize technical variation and confounding effects. While it remains to be determined how long cryopreserved synovial tissue can be stored, samples have been routinely stored in liquid nitrogen for several months, and a small number of samples have been analyzed over 1 year after freezing without obvious decreases in cell yield.

In an ongoing phase I study, the AMP RA Network has implemented this synovial tissue pipeline to study cryopreserved synovial samples from a pilot cohort of over 40 RA and OA patients with the goal of defining RA disease-specific cellular populations and pathways. Greater than half of the synovial samples processed yielded sufficient cells for both mass cytometry and RNA-seq analyses,

with cell viabilities comparable to those reported here. Analysis of cells from these phase I samples is in progress.

The phase I pilot study will be followed by a phase II study involving a much larger cohort of RA patients, including those with early disease, with a focus on identifying RA tissue biomarkers and novel tissue drug targets. A similar strategy of tissue cryopreservation has been adopted by the AMP for single-cell transcriptomic analyses of kidney biopsy samples from patients with lupus nephritis, including development of a dissociation protocol optimized for human kidney tissue [41]. Although different tissues and cellular subsets may respond to cryopreservation differently, the strategy of analyzing cells from cryopreserved tissue appears readily adaptable to multicenter studies of tissues in other inflammatory diseases.

Conclusions

These studies demonstrate the feasibility and potential of analyzing viable cells from cryopreserved synovial tissue samples by multiple, complementary high-dimensional analyses. Using an optimized dissociation protocol that provides high yields of viable cells with preserved cell surface and transcriptomic features, synovial tissue samples acquired across a multisite network can be analyzed in a uniform way in order to identify dominant cell types and pathways, as well as to characterize previously unidentified cellular heterogeneity. Such approaches applied to large numbers of patients offer new opportunities to discover rheumatic disease biomarkers, targets for drug development, and molecular stratification of synovial pathology.

Abbreviations

AMP RA network: RA Working Group of the AMP RA/SLE Network; AMP: Accelerating Medicines Partnership; ANOVA: Analysis of variance; DH: Dispase-High; DL: Dispase-Low; GO: Gene Ontology; IL-6: Interleukin-6; OA: Osteoarthritis; PCA: Principal component analysis; RA: Rheumatoid arthritis; RNA-seq: RNA sequencing; SLE: Systemic lupus erythematosus; SSW: Sum of squares within; TH: Thermolysin-High; TL: Thermolysin-Low; TM: Thermolysin-Medium; TNF: Tumor necrosis factor

Acknowledgements

The authors acknowledge the many clinical coordinators and patients who helped to provide samples for analysis in this study. They appreciate the many efforts of Mina Pichavant, Clinical Research Project Manager for the AMP, and Bill Apruzzese, Associate Director of Operations and Management for the AMP. Dr. Anolik gratefully acknowledges the UR Flow Cytometry Core and the Genomics Research Center. The following additional AMP members have contributed to the consortium through a variety of efforts: Jane Buckner, Derrick Todd, Michael Weisman,
Ami Ben Artzi, Lindsy Forbess, Joan Bathon, John Carrino, Oganna Nwawka, Eric Matteson, Robert Darnell, Dana Orange, Rahul Satija, Diane Horowitz, Harris Perlman, Art Mandelin, Louis Bridges, Laura B. Hughes, Arnold Ceponis, Peter Lowry, Paul Emery, Ahmed Zayat, Amir Aslaam, Karen Salomon-Escoto, David Fox, Robert Ike, Andy Cordle, Aaron Wise, John Ashton, Javier Rangel-Moreno, Christopher Ritchlin, Darren Tabechian, Ralf Thiele, Deborah Parks, John Akinson, Chiam Putterman, Evan Der, Elena Massarotti, Michael Weisman, David Hildeman, Richard Furie, Betty Diamond, Michelle Petri, Diane Kamen, Melissa Cunningham, Jill Buyon, Iris Lee, Hasan Salameh, Maureen McMahon, Ken Kalunian, Maria Dall'Era, David Wofsy, Mattias Kretzler, Celine Berthier, William McCune, Ruba Kado, Wiliam Pendergraft, Dia Waguespack, Yanyan Liu, Gerald Watts, Arnon Arazi, Rohit Gupta, Holden Maecker, Patrick Dunn, Rong Mao, Mina Pichavant, Quan Chen, John Peyman, Ellen Goldmuntz, Justine Buschman, Jennifer Chi, Su-Yau Mao, Susana Serrate-Sztein, Yan Wang, Thomas Tuschl, Yvonne Lee, Chamith Fonseka, Fan Zhang, Ilya Korsunskiy, Judith A. James, and Joel Guthridge.

Funding

This work was supported by the Accelerating Medicines Partnership (AMP) in Rheumatoid Arthritis and Lupus Network (AMP RA/SLE Network). The AMP is a public–private partnership (AbbVie Inc., Arthritis Foundation, Bristol-Myers Squibb Company, Lupus Foundation of America, Lupus Research Alliance, Merck Sharp & Dohme Corp., National Institutes of Health, Pfizer Inc., Rheumatology Research Foundation, Sanofi, and Takeda Pharmaceuticals International, Inc.) created to develop new ways of identifying and validating promising biological targets for diagnostics and drug development. Funding was provided through grants from the National Institutes of Health (UH2-AR067676, UH2-AR067677, UH2-AR067679, UH2-AR067681, UH2-AR067685, UH2-AR067688, UH2-AR067689, UH2-AR067690, UH2-AR067691, UH2-AR067694, and UM2-AR067678). This report includes independent research supported by the National Institute for Health Research/Wellcome Trust Clinical Research Facility at University Hospitals Birmingham NHS Foundation Trust. The views expressed in this publication are those of the author(s) and not necessarily those of the NHS, the National Institute for Health Research, or the Department of Health. Funding was also provided by Arthritis Research UK (Fellowship 18547) and the RACE Rheumatoid Arthritis Pathogenesis Centre of Excellence (grant 20298).

Authors' contributions

LTD, MJM, JDT, NM, KM, JH, SK, SMG, CP, EMG, LWM, VPB, AF, DLB, and JHA contributed to tissue collection, acquisition of data, and data interpretation. LTD, DAR, KW, MJM, JDT, NM, FM, JK, KM, JH, CR, ER, AC, SK, ABP, JAL, LBI, CP, GSF, LWM, AF, DLB, and MBB contributed to tissue processing and validation studies, acquisition of data, and data interpretation. LTD, MJM, JDT, NM, FM, KM, JH, AF, DLB, MBB, and JHA contributed to the AMP Tissue Working Group and experimental design. DAR, KW, FM, DJL, JK, TME, SL, EPB, CN, and NH contributed to RNA purification, library prep, and sequencing. KS, MG-A, DJL, TME, SL, EPB, DS, AN, CN, JAL, NH, SR, and MBB contributed to computational data analysis. DAR and JAL contributed to mass cytometry experimental design, data acquisition, and data interpretation. KS, MG-A, DJL, TME, SL, EPB, WHR, NH, SR, and MBB contributed to the AMP Systems Biology Group. LTD, DAR, AF, MBB, and JHA contributed to manuscript drafting. All authors contributed to manuscript review. EMG, PKG, LWM, VPB, DLB, MBB, and JHA contributed to the AMP RA Disease Focus Group and experimental design. MJM, ABP, LBI, WHR, PJU, EMG, BFB, JAL, NH, CP, PKG, GSF, SR, LWM, VMH, VPB, AF, DLB, MBB, and JHA were AMP Principal Investigators. All authors read and approved the final manuscript.

Competing interests

The authors declare that they have no competing interests.

Author details

[1]Hospital for Special Surgery, New York, NY 10021, USA. [2]Weill Cornell Medical College, New York, NY 10065, USA. [3]Brigham and Women's Hospital, Harvard Medical School, Boston, MA 02115, USA. [4]Broad Institute of MIT and Harvard University, Cambridge, MA 02142, USA. [5]University of Pittsburgh School of Medicine, Pittsburgh, PA 15261, USA. [6]University of Birmingham, Queen Elizabeth Hospital, B15 2WB, Birmingham, UK. [7]University of Rochester Medical Center, Rochester, NY 14642, USA. [8]University of California San Diego School of Medicine, La Jolla, CA 92093, USA. [9]Mile End Hospital, Barts Health NHS Trust, E1 1BB, London, UK. [10]Stanford University School of Medicine, Stanford, CA 94305, USA. [11]University of Massachusetts Medical School, Worcester, MA 01605, USA. [12]Massachusetts General Hospital, Harvard Medical School, Boston, MA 02114, USA. [13]Queen Mary University of London, E1 4NS, London, UK. [14]The Feinstein Institute for Medical Research, Manhasset, NY 11030, USA. [15]University of Colorado of Denver School of Medicine, Aurora, CO 80045, USA.

References

1. Gravallese EM, Manning C, Tsay A, Naito A, Pan C, Amento E, Goldring SR. Synovial tissue in rheumatoid arthritis is a source of osteoclast differentiation factor. Arthritis Rheum. 2000;43(2):250–8.
2. Meednu N, Zhang H, Owen T, Sun W, Wang V, Cistrone C, Rangel-Moreno J, Xing L, Anolik JH. Production of RANKL by memory B cells: a link between B cells and bone Erosion in rheumatoid arthritis. Arthritis Rheumatol. 2016;68(4):805–16.
3. McInnes IB, Schett G. The pathogenesis of rheumatoid arthritis. N Engl J Med. 2012;365(23):2205–19.
4. Ai R, Hammaker D, Boyle DL, Morgan R, Walsh AM, Fan S, Firestein GS, Wang W. Joint-specific DNA methylation and transcriptome signatures in rheumatoid arthritis identify distinct pathogenic processes. Nat Commun. 2016;7:11849.
5. Rao DA, Gurish MF, Marshall JL, Slowikowski K, Fonseka CY, Liu Y, Donlin LT, Henderson LA, Wei K, Mizoguchi F, et al. Pathologically expanded peripheral T helper cell subset drives B cells in rheumatoid arthritis. Nature. 2017;542(7639):110–4.

6. Smolen JS, Landewe R, Bijlsma J, Burmester G, Chatzidionysiou K, Dougados M, Nam J, Ramiro S, Voshaar M, van Vollenhoven R, et al. EULAR recommendations for the management of rheumatoid arthritis with synthetic and biological disease-modifying antirheumatic drugs: 2016 update. Ann Rheum Dis. 2017;76(6):960–77.

7. Nagy G, van Vollenhoven RF. Sustained biologic-free and drug-free remission in rheumatoid arthritis, where are we now? Arthritis Res Ther. 2015;17:181.

8. Tak P. A personalized medicine approach to biological treatment of rheumatoid arthritis: a preliminary treatment algorithm. Rheumatol. 2012;17:2012.

9. Orr C, Vieira-Sousa E, Boyle DL, Buch MH, Buckley CD, Canete JD, Catrina AI, Choy EHS, Emery P, Fearon U, et al. Synovial tissue research: a state-of-the-art review. Nat Rev Rheumatol. 2017;13(8):463–75.

10. Dolhain RJ, Ter Haar NT, De Kuiper R, Nieuwenhuis IG, Zwinderman AH, Breedveld FC, Miltenburg AM. Distribution of T cells and signs of T-cell activation in the rheumatoid joint: implications for semiquantitative comparative histology. Br J Rheumatol. 1998;37(3):324–30.

11. Boyle DL, Rosengren S, Bugbee W, Kavanaugh A, Firestein GS. Quantitative biomarker analysis of synovial gene expression by real-time PCR. Arthritis Res Ther. 2003;5(6):R352–60.

12. Kelly S, Humby F, Filer A, Ng N, Di Cicco M, Hands RE, Rocher V, Bombardieri M, D'Agostino MA, McInnes IB, et al. Ultrasound-guided synovial biopsy: a safe, well-tolerated and reliable technique for obtaining high-quality synovial tissue from both large and small joints in early arthritis patients. Ann Rheum Dis. 2015;74(3):611–7.

13. Pitzalis C, Kelly S, Humby F. New learnings on the pathophysiology of RA from synovial biopsies. Curr Opin Rheumatol. 2013;25(3):334–44.

14. Koski JM, Helle M. Ultrasound guided synovial biopsy using portal and forceps. Ann Rheum Dis. 2005;64(6):926–9.

15. Choi IY, Karpus ON, Turner JD, Hardie D, Marshall JL, de Hair MJH, Maijer KI, Tak PP, Raza K, Hamann J, et al. Stromal cell markers are differentially expressed in the synovial tissue of patients with early arthritis. PLoS One. 2017;12(8):e0182751.

16. Picelli S, Faridani OR, Bjorklund AK, Winberg G, Sagasser S, Sandberg R. Full-length RNA-seq from single cells using smart-seq2. Nat Protoc. 2014;9(1):171–81.

17. Hashimshony T, Senderovich N, Avital G, Klochendler A, de Leeuw Y, Anavy L, Gennert D, Li S, Livak KJ, Rozenblatt-Rosen O, et al. CEL-Seq2: sensitive highly-multiplexed single-cell RNA-Seq. Genome Biol. 2016;17:77.

18. Dobin A, Davis CA, Schlesinger F, Drenkow J, Zaleski C, Jha S, Batut P, Chaisson M, Gingeras TR. STAR: ultrafast universal RNA-seq aligner. Bioinformatics. 2013;29(1):15–21.

19. Li B, Dewey CN. RSEM: accurate transcript quantification from RNA-Seq data with or without a reference genome. BMC Bioinformatics. 2011;12:323.

20. Wagner F. The XL-mHG test for gene set enrichment. PeerJ Preprints. 2017; https://doi.org/10.7287/peerj.preprints.1962v3.

21. Finck R, Simonds EF, Jager A, Krishnaswamy S, Sachs K, Fantl W, Pe'er D, Nolan GP, Bendall SC. Normalization of mass cytometry data with bead standards. Cytometry Part A. 2013;83(5):483–94.

22. Van Landuyt KB, Jones EA, McGonagle D, Luyten FP, Lories RJ. Flow cytometric characterization of freshly isolated and culture expanded human synovial cell populations in patients with chronic arthritis. Arthritis Res Ther. 2010;12(1):R15.

23. Cush JJ, Lipsky PE. Phenotypic analysis of synovial tissue and peripheral blood lymphocytes isolated from patients with rheumatoid arthritis. Arthritis Rheum. 1988;31(10):1230–8.

24. van den Brink SC, Sage F, Vertesy A, Spanjaard B, Peterson-Maduro J, Baron CS, Robin C, van Oudenaarden A. Single-cell sequencing reveals dissociation-induced gene expression in tissue subpopulations. Nat Methods. 2017;14(10):935–6.

25. Stephenson W, Donlin LT, Butler A, Rozo C, Bracken B, Rashidfarrokhi A, Goodman SM, Ivashkiv LB, Bykerk VP, Orange DE, et al. Single-cell RNA-seq of rheumatoid arthritis synovial tissue using low-cost microfluidic instrumentation. Nat Commun. 2018;9(1):791.

26. Mizoguchi F, Slowikowski K, Wei K, Marshall JL, Rao DA, Chang SK, Nguyen HN, Noss EH, Turner JD, Earp BE, et al. Functionally distinct disease-associated fibroblast subsets in rheumatoid arthritis. Nat Commun. 2018;9(1):789.

27. Amir el AD, Davis KL, Tadmor MD, Simonds EF, Levine JH, Bendall SC, Shenfeld DK, Krishnaswamy S, Nolan GP, Pe'er D. viSNE enables visualization of high dimensional single-cell data and reveals phenotypic heterogeneity of leukemia. Nat Biotechnol. 2013;31(6):545–52.

28. Anolik J, Barnard J, Cappione A, Pugh-Bernard A, Felgar R, Looney J, Sanz I. Rituximab improves peripheral B cell abnormalities in human systemic lupus erythematosus. Arthritis Rheumatism. 2004;50:3580–90.

29. Tipton CM, Fucile CF, Darce J, Chida A, Ichikawa T, Gregoretti I, Schieferl S, Hom J, Jenks S, Feldman RJ, et al. Diversity, cellular origin and autoreactivity of antibody-secreting cell population expansions in acute systemic lupus erythematosus. Nat Immunol. 2015;16(7):755–65.

30. Slansky E, Li J, Haupl T, Morawietz L, Krenn V, Pessler F. Quantitative determination of the diagnostic accuracy of the synovitis score and its components. Histopathology. 2010;57(3):436–43.

31. Dennis G Jr, Holweg CT, Kummerfeld SK, Choy DF, Setiadi AF, Hackney JA, Haverty PM, Gilbert H, Lin WY, Diehl L, et al. Synovial phenotypes in rheumatoid arthritis correlate with response to biologic therapeutics. Arthritis Res Ther. 2014;16(2):R90.

32. Belasco J, Louie JS, Gulati N, Wei N, Nograles K, Fuentes-Duculan J, Mitsui H, Suarez-Farinas M, Krueger JG. Comparative genomic profiling of synovium versus skin lesions in psoriatic arthritis. Arthritis Rheumatol. 2015;67(4):934–44.

33. van Baarsen LG, Wijbrandts CA, Timmer TC, van der Pouw Kraan TC, Tak PP, Verweij CL. Synovial tissue heterogeneity in rheumatoid arthritis in relation to disease activity and biomarkers in peripheral blood. Arthritis Rheum. 2010;62(6):1602–7.

34. Hogan VE, Holweg CT, Choy DF, Kummerfeld SK, Hackney JA, Teng YK, Townsend MJ, van Laar JM. Pretreatment synovial transcriptional profile is associated with early and late clinical response in rheumatoid arthritis patients treated with rituximab. Ann Rheum Dis. 2012;71(11):1888–94.

35. Badot V, Galant C, Nzeusseu Toukap A, Theate I, Maudoux AL, Van den Eynde BJ, Durez P, Houssiau FA, Lauwerys BR. Gene expression profiling in the synovium identifies a predictive signature of absence of response to adalimumab therapy in rheumatoid arthritis. Arthritis Res Ther. 2009;11(2):R57.

36. Lauwerys BR, Hernandez-Lobato D, Gramme P, Ducreux J, Dessy A, Focant I, Ambroise J, Bearzatto B, Nzeusseu Toukap A, Van den Eynde BJ, et al. Heterogeneity of synovial molecular patterns in patients with arthritis. PLoS One. 2015;10(4):e0122104.

37. Lindberg J, Wijbrandts CA, van Baarsen LG, Nader G, Klareskog L, Catrina A, Thurlings R, Vervoordeldonk M, Lundeberg J, Tak PP. The gene expression profile in the synovium as a predictor of the clinical response to infliximab treatment in rheumatoid arthritis. PLoS One. 2010;5(6):e11310.

38. Orange DE AP, DiCarlo EF, Szymonifka J, McNamara M, Cummings R, Andersen KM, Mirza S, The Accelerating Medicine Partnership: RA/SLE Network, Figgie M, Ivashkiv L, Pernis AB, Jiang C, Frank M, Darnell R, Gravallese E, Bykerk VP, Goodman SM, Donlin LT: Machine Learning integration of rheumatoid arthritis synovial histology and RNAseq data identifies three disease subtypes. Arthritis Rheumatol. 2018;70(5):690–701

39. Der E, Ranabothu S, Suryawanshi H, Akat KM, Clancy R, Morozov P, Kustagi M, Czuppa M, Izmirly P, Belmont HM, et al. Single cell RNA sequencing to dissect the molecular heterogeneity in lupus nephritis. JCI Insight. 2017;2(9)

40. Villani AC, Satija R, Reynolds G, Sarkizova S, Shekhar K, Fletcher J, Griesbeck M, Butler A, Zheng S, Lazo S, et al. Single-cell RNA-seq reveals new types of human blood dendritic cells, monocytes, and progenitors. Science. 356(6335):eaah4573.

41. Rao DA BC, Arazi A, Davidson A, Liu Y, Browne E, Eisenhaure T, Chicoine A, Lieb D, Smilek D, Tosta P, Lederer J, Brenner M, Hildeman D, Woodle ES, Wofsy D, Anolik JH, Kretzler M, Accelerating Medicines Partnership RA/SLE Network, Hacohen N, Diamond B: A protocol for single-cell transcriptomics from cryopreserved renal tissue and urine for the Accelerating Medicines Partnership (AMP) RA/SLE network. bioRxiv. 2017; https://doi.org/10.1101/275859.

7

Cytokine profiling in active and quiescent SLE reveals distinct patient subpopulations

John A. Reynolds[1,2], Eoghan M. McCarthy[2], Sahena Haque[3], Pintip Ngamjanyaporn[1,4], Jamie C. Sergeant[1,5], Elaine Lee[6], Eileen Lee[6], Stephen A. Kilfeather[6], Ben Parker[1,2] and Ian N. Bruce[1,2]*

Abstract

Background: Patients with SLE display marked clinical and immunlogical heterogeneity. The purpose of the study was to investigate patterns of serum cytokines in patients with active and stable systemic lupus erythematosus (SLE) and to determine how they relate to clinical phenotype.

Methods: Serum levels of 10 cytokines were measured retrospectively in a cohort of patients with SLE and in healthy controls using a high-sensitivity multiplex bead array. Disease activity was determined using the Systemic Lupus Erythematosus Disease Activity Index 2000 (SLEDAI-2K) and British Isles Lupus Assessment Group (BILAG-2004) indices. Logistic regression models were used to determine the association between cytokine levels and active SLE. Principal component analysis (PCA) and cluster analysis was then used to identify subgroups of patients on the basis of cytokine levels.

Results: Serum chemokine (C-X-C motif) ligand 10 (CXCL10) and CXCL13 were significantly higher in patients with SLE compared to healthy controls. Two cytokines (pentraxin-related protein (PTX3) and CXCL10) were significantly higher in patients with active disease after adjustment for potential confounding factors. Measurement of four cytokines (CXCL10, IL-10, IL-21 and PTX3) significantly improved the performance of a model to identify patients with clinically active disease. Cluster analysis revealed that the patients formed 3 distinct groups, characterised by higher levels of interferon alpha (IFNα) and B lymphocyte stimulator (BLyS) (group 1), increased CXCL10 and CXCL13 (group 2) or low levels of cytokines (group 3). Group 2 had significantly lower serum complement and higher anti-double-stranded DNA antibodies and increased prevalence of inflammatory arthritis.

Conclusions: Multiplex analysis has identified a serum cytokine signature for active SLE. Within the SLE population distinct cytokine subgroups were identified, with differing clinical and immunological phenotypes that appeared stable over time. Assessment of cytokine profiles may reveal unique insights into disease heterogeneity.

Keywords: Systemic lupus erythematosus, Cytokines, Biomarkers, Disease activity, Cluster analysis

Background

Systemic lupus erythematosus (SLE) is a systemic inflammatory autoimmune disease with a broad clinical and immunological phenotype, and marked variability in response to treatment. The ability to understand this heterogeneity and to develop relevant biomarkers, in order to better direct therapeutic decision-making, is an important unmet need in the care of patients with lupus [1].

The observed clinical heterogeneity likely reflects differences in underlying immunopathological processes. Recently a landmark study by Banchereau et al. used whole blood transcriptional profiling to identify seven transcriptionally distinct groups in a paediatric SLE population [2]. A number of studies have also identified autoantibody clusters in SLE, again reflecting the immunopathological heterogeneity within this patient group [3, 4].

Although a number of genetic, epigenetic and protein biomarkers have been proposed, many of these currently have limited clinical utility [5]. Cytokine levels may be

* Correspondence: ian.bruce@manchester.ac.uk
[1]Arthritis Research UK Centre for Epidemiology, Centre for Musculoskeletal Research, Manchester Academic Health Science Centre, University of Manchester, Manchester M13 9PT, UK
[2]The Kellgren Centre for Rheumatology, NIHR Manchester Biomedical Research Centre, Manchester University Hospitals NHS Foundation Trust, Manchester Academic Health Science Centre, Manchester, UK
Full list of author information is available at the end of the article

influenced by a number of endogenous and exogenous factors including clinical disease activity, circadian variation, the presence of infection and immunosuppressant treatment [6]. Although patients with SLE are reported to have increased levels of many cytokines including interleukin (IL)-10, IL-17 and interferon alpha (IFNα) these are often measured in isolation making it difficult to understand how cytokine networks exist in SLE [7].

A number of cytokines have been implicated in the pathogenesis of SLE (reviewed by Yu et al. 2012 [8]). However there are currently no reliable cytokine biomarkers to differentiate between active and inactive SLE. Biomarkers that can assist in the identification of active disease are desirable as the clinical assessment of patients can be difficult due to the accrual of damage and the presence of other comorbidities (including concurrent infection).

Furthermore, it is possible that some cytokines are more strongly related to a specific disease phenotype rather than disease activity. As an example, IL-17 has been associated with central nervous system disease in patients with SLE independently of disease activity [9]. This suggests that cytokine levels may reveal important additional information about the immunophenotype of patients with SLE. In addition, although it is recognised that cytokines are unlikely to function in isolation from one another, relatively little is known about how individual cytokines relate to each other in the disease state.

To date, the majority of studies have used singleplex plate-based enzyme-linked immunosorbent assays (ELISAs) to detect serum or plasma cytokine levels. These methods may have disadvantages including a narrow dynamic range, ability to measure only a single analyte and in some cases relatively low sensitivity. Initial multiplexing systems have relatively low sensitivity and have been used by many as "screening systems" prior to further exploration of observed trends with singleplex assays. The sensitivity of multiplexing, however, has evolved to match singleplex assays and, in certain areas, surpasses single ELISA assay sensitivity.

The aim of the present study was to use a high-sensitivity multiplex bead-based assay to investigate serum cytokine levels in patients with stable and active SLE. We incorporated the highest-sensitivity assay system available to us in a customised multiplex system to provide simultaneous cytokine measurement, in order to better understand cytokine relationships in SLE. Specifically we aimed to determine how these cytokines related to disease activity and to determine whether individual cytokines or groups of cytokines were associated with specific SLE disease features.

Methods

Patients with SLE (scoring ≥ 4 in the 1997 updated American College of Rheumatology (ACR) classification

criteria [10]) were recruited from Manchester University Hospitals National Health Service (NHS) Foundation Trust between 2007 and 2013. All patients provided informed written consent, and the study was approved by UK Research Ethics Committees. Demographic details including ethnicity and smoking status were recorded, patients' disease activity and concurrent medication was assessed by a physician and fasting blood samples were taken. Clinical features and serological data relevant to the ACR classification criteria were collected retrospectively from hospital records. Serum autoantibodies and complement levels were measured using standard laboratory assays. In a subset of patients with clinically stable SLE, repeat samples were obtained after 3 months.

Measurement of disease activity

SLE disease activity was measured using the Systemic Lupus Disease Activity Index 2000 (SLEDAI-2 K) [11] and the British Isles Lupus Assessment Group 2004 (BILAG-2004) [12]. Active disease was defined as (i) SLEDAI-2 K > 4, and/or (ii) one BILAG-2004 "A" score and/or (iii) two BILAG-2004 "B" scores.

Cytokine measurement

Serum samples were stored at − 80 °C until analysis. We performed a literature review of studies of the immunopathogenesis of SLE and we selected a panel of 10 cytokines to cover the principle pathways deemed to be relevant to the pathogenesis of SLE: IFNα, B lymphocyte stimulator (BLyS), IL-10, IL-17, IL-18, IL-21, C-X-C motif chemokine ligand (CXCL10), CXCL13, monocyte chemotactic protein-1 (MCP-1) and pentraxin related protein 3 (PTX3). These cytokines therefore addressed monocytes/innate cells (IFNα, IL-10, IL-18, CXCL10, MCP-1 and PTX3), B cells (BLyS and CXCL13) and T cells (IL-10, IL-17 and IL-21). Serum cytokine levels were measured using a high-sensitivity bead-based multiplex ELISA (Aeirtec Ltd., UK). Limits of detection (LOD) values in picogram/millilitre determined within the analysis were as follows: BLyS, 0.05; CXCL13, 0.03; IFNα, 0.11; IL-10, 0.18; IL-17, 0.07; IL-18, 0.64; IL-21, 0.06; CXCL10, 0.05; MCP-1, 0.15 and PTX3, 1.43.

Statistical methods

Cytokine levels were compared between groups using non-parametric tests. Logistic regression models were used to compare patients with SLE and healthy controls and patient groups with active and inactive disease. In order to investigate which cytokines were most associated with the presence of active disease, multivariable models were developed (using a modified definition of active disease, which excluded the contribution of low serum complement/high anti-double-stranded (ds)DNA to the SLEDAI score) and adjusted for age, ethnicity, disease duration and serological markers. Non-significant predictors were removed using backwards elimination (probability threshold for removal 0.1). The ability of the model to discriminate between patients with active and inactive disease was measured using the area under the receiver operating characteristic curve (AUC).

To investigate networks, a Spearman correlation matrix was constructed. For the cluster analysis, principal component analysis (PCA) was undertaken using the cytokine data alone to determine the number of groups present. Following this, K-means clustering of the standardised cytokine levels was conducted. The clinical and serological features of patients were then compared among the three cytokine-based groups. Statistical analysis was carried out using GraphPad Prism v7.0

(GraphPad Software, Inc), STATA/MP v13.0 (StataCorp LLC) and R v3.3.2.

Results

A total of 96 patients with SLE and 13 healthy volunteers were recruited, of whom 95/96 (99.0%) and 12/13 (92.3%) were female, with a median (IQR) age of 50.7 (43.5, 58.8) and 40.0 (31.5, 48.5) years, respectively (Table 1). All healthy subjects were Caucasian and the patients with SLE were predominantly Caucasian (74/96, 77%) reflecting the patient population of Greater Manchester. The median disease duration was 11.7 (6.8, 21.3) years. All 10 cytokines were measurable in most patients. With the exception of IL-17, all cytokines were quantifiable in > 80% samples (see Additional file 1). Serum levels of CXCL10 and CXCL13 were significantly higher in patients with SLE compared to control (38.5

Table 1 Characteristics of patients with SLE by disease activity status

	SLE (n = 96)	Healthy subject (n = 13)	p value
Age (years)	50.7 (43.9, 58.8)	40.0 (31.5, 48.5)	0.012
Gender (female)	95 (99.0%)	12 (92.3%)	0.626
Ethnicity			1.000
Caucasian	74 (77.1%)	13 (100%)	
Black Caribbean	6 (6.3%)		
Black African	3 (3.1%)		
Indian	2 (2.1%)		
Pakistani	3 (3.1%)		
Chinese	1 (1.0%)		
Other	3 (3.1%)		
Disease duration (years)	11.7 (6.84, 21.4)	–	–
≥ 4 ACR criteria	82 (85.4%)	–	–
ACR criteria			–
Malar rash	54 (56.3%)		
Discoid rash	16 (16.7%)		
Photosensitivity	60 (62.5%)		
Oral ulcers	54 (56.3%)		
Arthritis	62 (64.6%)		
Serositis	32 (33.3%)		
Renal	26 (27.1%)		
Neurological	10 (10.4%)		
Haematological	57 (59.4%)		
Immunological	48 (50.0%)		
ANA	82 (85.4%)		
Oral prednisolone use	41/93 (44.1%)		
Antimalarial use	66/93 (71.0%)		
Immunosuppressant use	32/92 (34.8%)		

Results show the number (percentage) or median (IQR) values. The Mann-Whitney U test or Fisher's exact test was used to compare values in the active and the inactive groups

SLE systemic lupus erythematosus, ACR American College of Rheumatology, ANA antinuclear antibody

(19.9, 69.6) vs 11.8 (7.28, 16.9) pg/ml, $p < 0.0001$) and (351.6 (231.4, 568.2) vs. 234.7 (185.2, 239.2) pg/ml, $p = 0.002$), respectively (Fig. 1). Healthy subjects were younger, but in logistic regression models including age and gender, CXCL10 and CXCL13 remained significantly associated with the presence of SLE (OR 1.18 (1.06, 1.31), $p = 0.002$ and OR 1.01 (1.00, 1.01), $p = 0.016$). In an exploratory analysis, patients with SLE with arthritis (according to the ACR criteria) had increased levels of both CXCL10 and CXCL13. CXCL10 was also increased in patients with neurological involvement, and lower in patients with serositis (see Additional file 1).

Cytokine profiles and disease activity

In the SLE patient group, 22/96 patients (23%) had active disease as defined above. The active group was younger (42.5 (31.0, 53.0) vs 52.5 (45.7, 60.7) years, $p = 0.0016$) and had a shorter duration of disease (7.16 (3.58, 15.0) vs 12.7 (8.11, 25.1) years, $p = 0.0174$) than patients with inactive SLE. The frequency of steroid prescription (19/22 (86.3%) vs 22/71 (31.0%), $p < 0.0001$) and the median daily dose (12.5 (7.5, 17.5) vs 7 (5, 10) mg, $p = 0.002$) was also greater in patients with active disease. There was no difference in the frequency of anti-malarial or immunosuppressant use between patients with active and inactive disease ($p = 0.594$ and $p = 0.305$, respectively). Serum levels of BLyS, IL-17, IL-18, CXCL10

and PTX3 were all significantly higher in patients with active disease (Fig. 2). In logistic regression models adjusted for age, gender, disease duration, ethnicity and concomitant steroid use, PTX3 and CXCL10 remained significantly associated with the presence of active disease (OR 1.23 (1.05, 1.45) per 1000 pg/ml and 1.02 (1.00, 1.03) per pg/ml) (Table 2). In a sensitivity analysis, addition of immunosuppressant use to the model did not change these associations (data not shown).

Multivariable logistic regression models were used to determine whether measurement of these 10 cytokines could help to better identify patients with active disease, beyond the commonly used markers of low serum complement and raised anti-dsDNA. In a backwards stepwise logistic regression model, CXCL10, IL-10, IL-21 and PTX3 were all retained with $p < 0.1$.

The AUC of a basic multivariable model comprising age, ethnicity, disease duration, low serum complement and raised anti-dsDNA was 0.7445. The addition of the four cytokines (CXCL10, IL-10, IL-21 and PTX3) significantly increased the AUC to 0.9337 ($p = 0.002$) suggesting that measurement of these cytokines significantly improved the ability of the model to differentiate between patients with active and inactive disease (Fig. 2). There was no additional benefit of using all 10 cytokines in the model (data not shown).

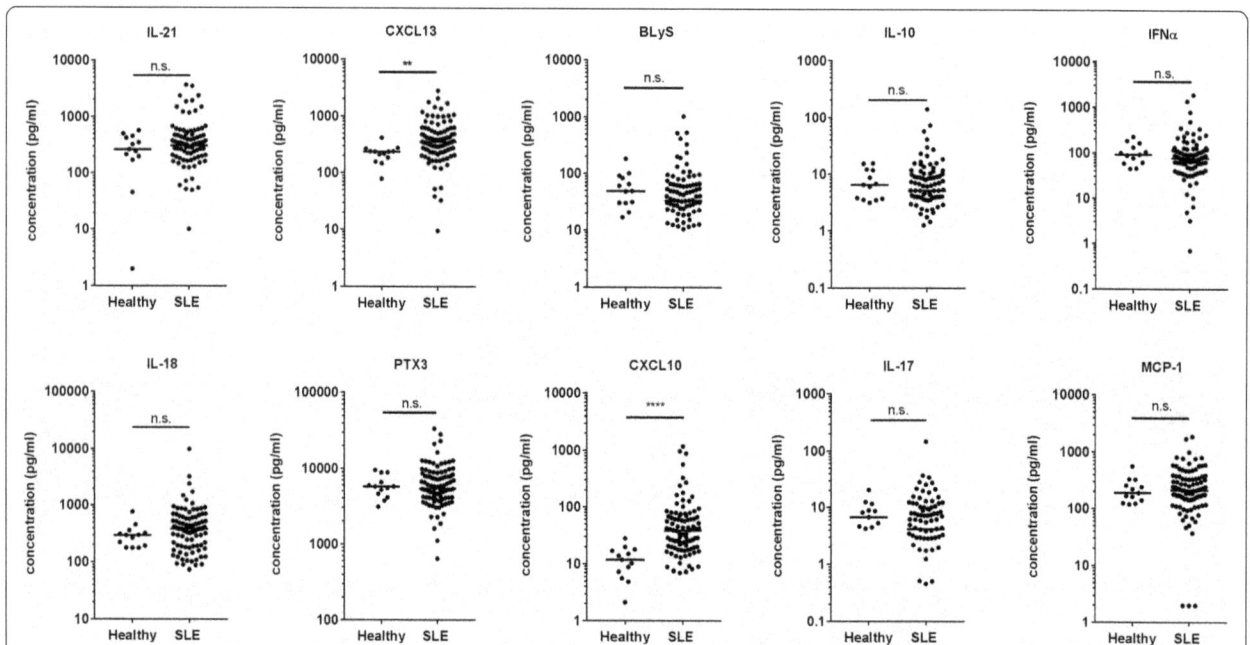

Fig. 1 Differences in cytokine levels between patients with systemic lupus erythematosus (SLE) and healthy subjects. The plots show the serum level (picograms/millilitre) of each of the 10 cytokines in patients with SLE and in healthy controls. The bar represents the median value. Data were compared using the Mann-Whitney test; n.s. = not significant, **$p < 0.01$, ****$p < 0.0001$. Both values remained significant after Bonferroni correction. CXCL, chemokine (C-X-C motif) ligand; BLyS B, lymphocyte stimulator; IFNα, interferon alpha; PTX, pentraxin-related protein; MCP, monocyte chemotactic protein

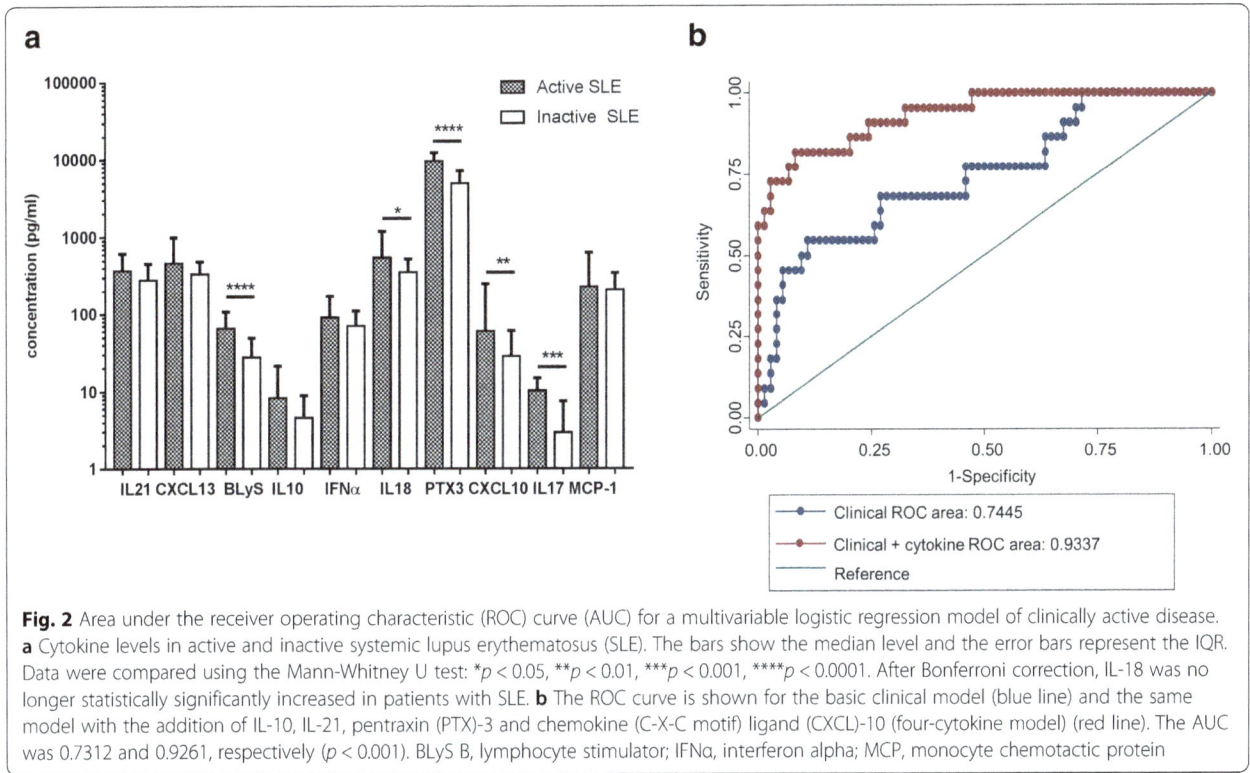

Fig. 2 Area under the receiver operating characteristic (ROC) curve (AUC) for a multivariable logistic regression model of clinically active disease. **a** Cytokine levels in active and inactive systemic lupus erythematosus (SLE). The bars show the median level and the error bars represent the IQR. Data were compared using the Mann-Whitney U test: *$p < 0.05$, **$p < 0.01$, ***$p < 0.001$, ****$p < 0.0001$. After Bonferroni correction, IL-18 was no longer statistically significantly increased in patients with SLE. **b** The ROC curve is shown for the basic clinical model (blue line) and the same model with the addition of IL-10, IL-21, pentraxin (PTX)-3 and chemokine (C-X-C motif) ligand (CXCL)-10 (four-cytokine model) (red line). The AUC was 0.7312 and 0.9261, respectively ($p < 0.001$). BLyS B, lymphocyte stimulator; IFNα, interferon alpha; MCP, monocyte chemotactic protein

Cytokine clustering in patients with SLE

Immune/inflammatory mediators, including cytokines and chemokines, do not necessarily function in isolation from one another and therefore examination of cytokine/chemokine groups may be more informative than individual cytokines. A Spearman correlation matrix demonstrated that with the exception of MCP-1, each cytokine was significantly correlated ($p < 0.05$) with at least one other cytokine (Fig. 3). The strongest correlation was observed between IL-10 and IFNα (Spearman $r = 0.464$, $p < 0.0001$). There was only modest correlation between some cytokines that were increased in patients with active disease, for example for correlation between BLyS and CXCL10, Spearman $r = 0.248$ ($p = 0.015$), suggesting that active disease may be associated with more than one discrete pattern of cytokines.

Principal component analysis (PCA) of the 10 cytokines was performed in the patients with SLE to

Table 2 Association between cytokine expression and presence of active disease in patients with SLE

	Unadjusted		Adjusted for age and gender		Fully adjusted[a]	
	OR (95% CI)	p value	OR (95% CI)	p value	OR (95% CI)	p value
IL-21[b]	1.06 (0.99, 1.13)	0.081	1.08 (0.99, 1.17)	0.077	1.06 (0.95, 1.18)	0.326
CXCL13[b]	1.07 (0.97, 1.18)	0.178	1.08 (0.97, 1.19)	0.177	1.05 (0.94, 1.18)	0.385
BLyS[b]	1.38 (0.96, 1.98)	0.079	1.58 (1.03, 2.42)	0.037	1.20 (0.82, 1.77)	0.350
IL-10	1.07 (1.01, 1.13)	0.013	1.08 (1.02, 1.14)	0.009	1.04 (0.99, 1.10)	0.143
IFNα[b]	1.27 (0.98, 1.64)	0.069	1.30 (0.99, 1.71)	0.056	1.14 (0.88, 1.48)	0.330
IL-18[b]	1.20 (1.05, 1.37)	0.009	1.25 (1.06, 1.47)	0.007	1.18 (0.98, 1.43)	0.075
PTX3[c]	1.33 (1.13, 1.56)	0.001	1.29 (1.11, 1.50)	0.001	1.23 (1.04, 1.46)	0.013
CXCL10	1.00 (1.00, 1.02)	0.022	1.01 (1.00, 1.02)	0.003	1.02 (1.00, 1.03)	0.008
IL-17	1.07 (1.01, 1.13)	0.020	1.06 (1.00, 1.13)	0.062	1.03 (0.98, 1.09)	0.279
MCP-1[b]	1.16 (1.00, 1.36)	0.056	1.20 (0.99, 1.45)	0.070	1.13 (0.90, 1.41)	0.294

Logistic regression models to show the odds of having active disease for every 1 pg/ml increase in the concentration of cytokine

SLE systemic lupus erythematosus, OR odds ratio, 95% CI 95% confidence intervals, CXCL chemokine (C-X-C motif) ligand, BLyS B lymphocyte stimulator, IFNα interferon alpha, PTX pentraxin-related protein, MCP monocyte chemotactic protein

[a]Model adjusted for age, gender, disease duration, ethnicity (Caucasian vs non-Caucasian) and current steroid use

[b]Per 100 pg/ml increase

[c]Per 1000 pg/ml increase

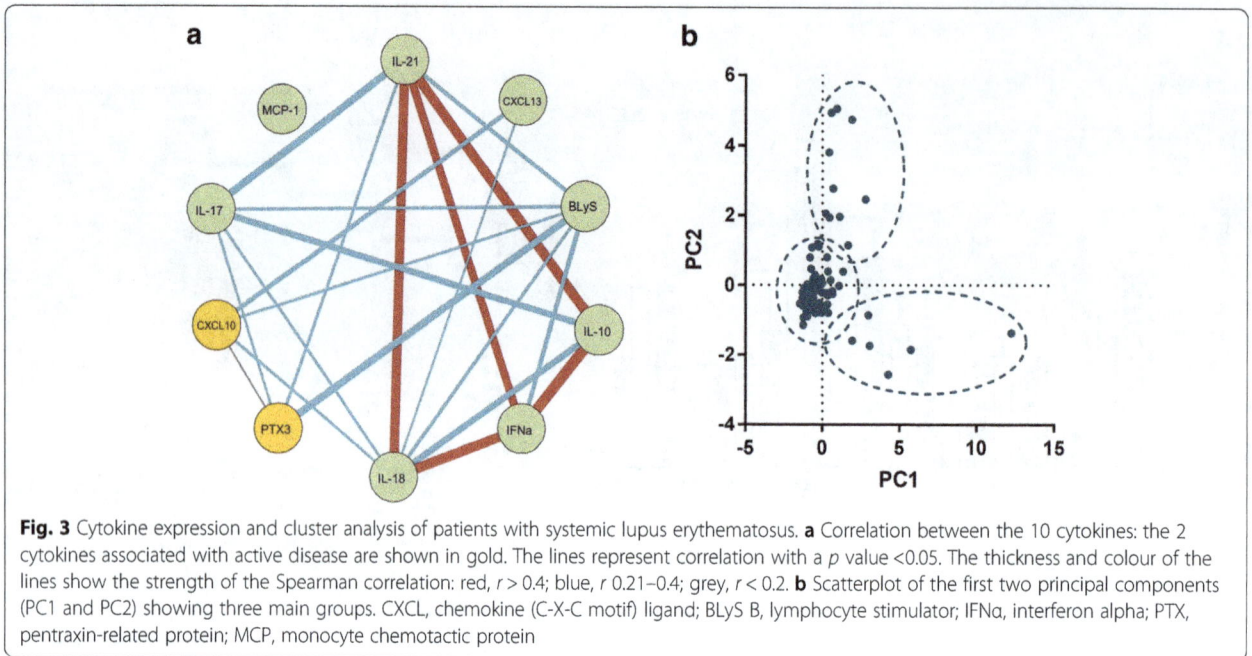

Fig. 3 Cytokine expression and cluster analysis of patients with systemic lupus erythematosus. **a** Correlation between the 10 cytokines: the 2 cytokines associated with active disease are shown in gold. The lines represent correlation with a *p* value <0.05. The thickness and colour of the lines show the strength of the Spearman correlation: red, *r* > 0.4; blue, *r* 0.21–0.4; grey, *r* < 0.2. **b** Scatterplot of the first two principal components (PC1 and PC2) showing three main groups. CXCL, chemokine (C-X-C motif) ligand; BLyS B, lymphocyte stimulator; IFNα, interferon alpha; PTX, pentraxin-related protein; MCP, monocyte chemotactic protein

determine whether any unique groups of cytokines could be identified. Using the Kaiser criterion, three components were retained that had an Eigenvalue > 1. These three components described 57.9% of the variance in cytokine levels in our cohort. A scatterplot of the first two principal components are shown in Fig. 3. K-means clustering of the standardised levels of the 10 cytokines was then performed to cluster patients into k = 3 groups (Fig. 3). The 3 groups comprised 6, 11 and 79 patients, respectively. Groups 1 and 2 were formed principally of patients with active disease (4/6 (67%) and 8/11 (73%), respectively) whilst only 10/79 (12.7%) patients in group 3 had active disease ($p < 0.0001$). In keeping with this, oral corticosteroid use was higher in groups 1 and 2 compared to group 3 ($p = 0.002$), but there were no significant differences in antimalarial or other immunosuppressant use. In a sensitivity analysis including the healthy control samples all healthy subjects were clustered into group 3 (data not shown).

In terms of the cytokines contributing to each cluster, IL-21, BLyS, IL-10, IFNα and IL-17 were increased in group 1 (median fold change between 3.6 and 9.6 compared to group 2). In contrast, CXCL10 and CXCL13 were highly expressed in group 2 (fold change compared to group 1, 4.8 and 7.2, respectively). IL-18 was strongly increased in both groups 1 and 2 and levels of PTX3 were moderately higher in group 2. All 10 cytokines were lower in group 3 than in groups 1 and 2. It was notable that levels of those cytokines that were increased in group 1 were much lower both in groups 2 and 3 (Fig. 4).

Clinical features of clusters

The groups were similar in terms of age, ethnicity and disease duration (not shown). More patients in group 1 (3/6, 50%) were likely to be current smokers compared to groups 2 and 3 (0/11 and 6/79 (8%), respectively) ($p = 0.001$), but there was no difference in the frequency of those who ever smoked ($p = 0.289$). Patients with inflammatory arthritis (according to the updated 1997 ACR classification criteria for SLE) were significantly enriched in group 2 (11/11, 100%) compared to groups 1 (4/6, 67%) and 3 (47/79, 59%) ($p = 0.031$). There were no differences in the frequency of any of the other ACR classification criteria.

The 3 groups also differed in terms of serological markers. At the time of sampling, patients in group 2 were more likely to have a positive anti-dsDNA titre ($p = 0.044$) and lower levels of C3 ($p = 0.003$) and C4 ($p = 0.034$) complement. The cytokine, clinical and serological features of the 3 groups are summarised in Fig. 5.

Stability in cytokine levels over time

Cytokine levels were measured at a second time point in a subgroup of clinically stable patients with SLE. The median (IQR) time between samples was 107 (91, 133) days. The intra-individual differences in cytokine levels between study visits were largest for MCP-1 (14.1%) and smallest for IFNα (− 1.35%). Cytokine levels only differed significantly between the two study visits for MCP-1 (see Additional file 1).

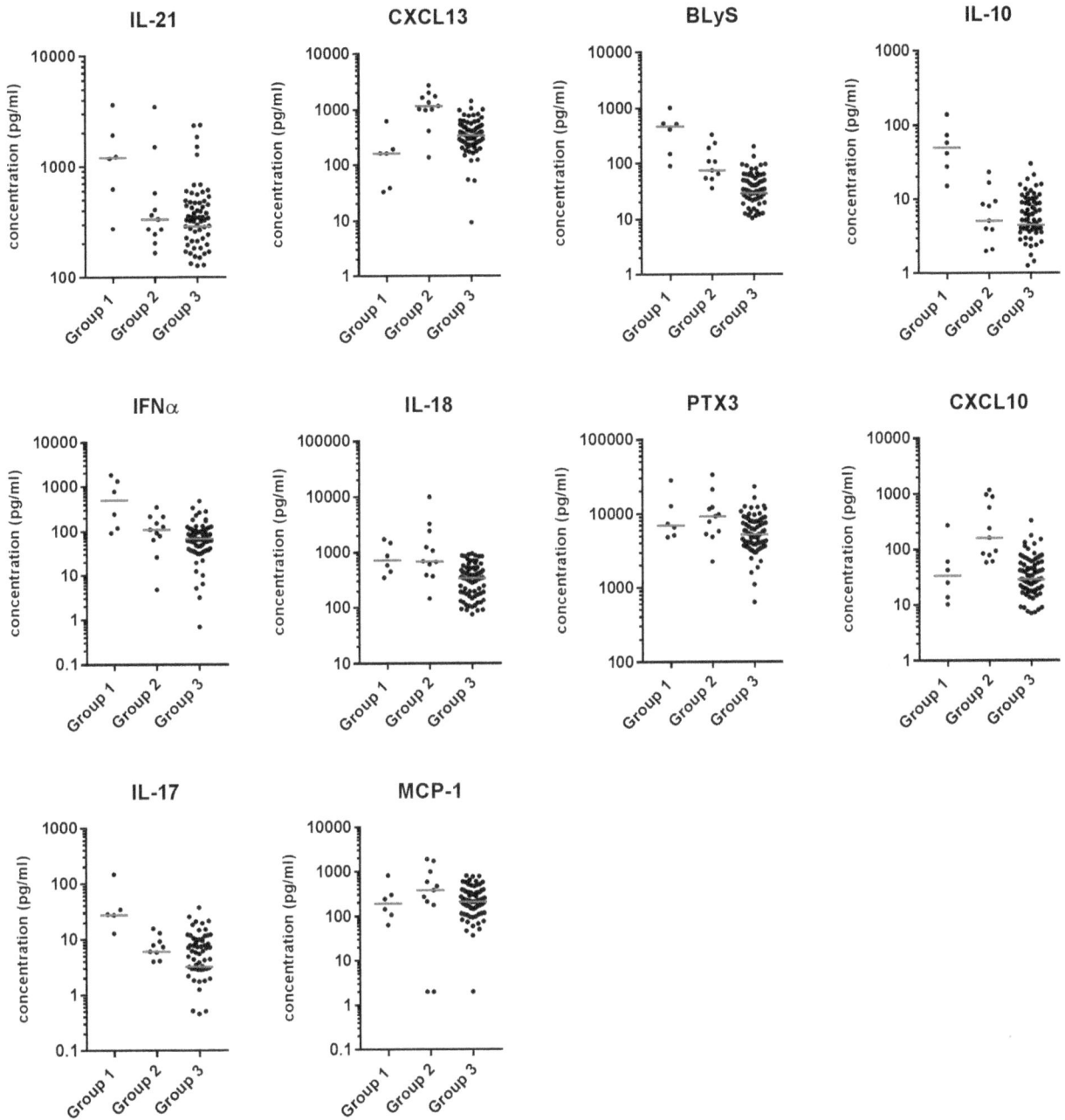

Fig. 4 Cytokine levels in the 3 groups of patients with systemic lupus erythematosus (SLE). The serum levels of the 10 cytokines in the patients with SLE are shown according to the group allocation. Each dot represents a single patient and the bar shows the median value for the group. CXCL, chemokine (C-X-C motif) ligand; BLyS B, lymphocyte stimulator; IFNα, interferon alpha; PTX, pentraxin-related protein; MCP, monocyte chemotactic protein

Discussion

In this study cytokine profiles were identified in patients with SLE that were associated with the presence of active disease and with specific clinical features. The use of high-sensitivity quantification enabled detection of all 10 cytokines in the majority of patient samples, offering advantages over singleplex plate-based ELISA. Only a small number of samples had undetectable levels, which facilitated comparison of the levels of all 10 cytokines across the cohort. Both CXCL10 and CXCL13 were increased in patients with SLE compared to healthy subjects after adjustment for potential confounding factors. In a small case-control study by Bauer et al. (2006) a number of chemokines including CXCL10, CXCL13, CXCL9, MCP-1 (CCL2) and CCL8 were found to be increased in patients with SLE compared to controls [13].

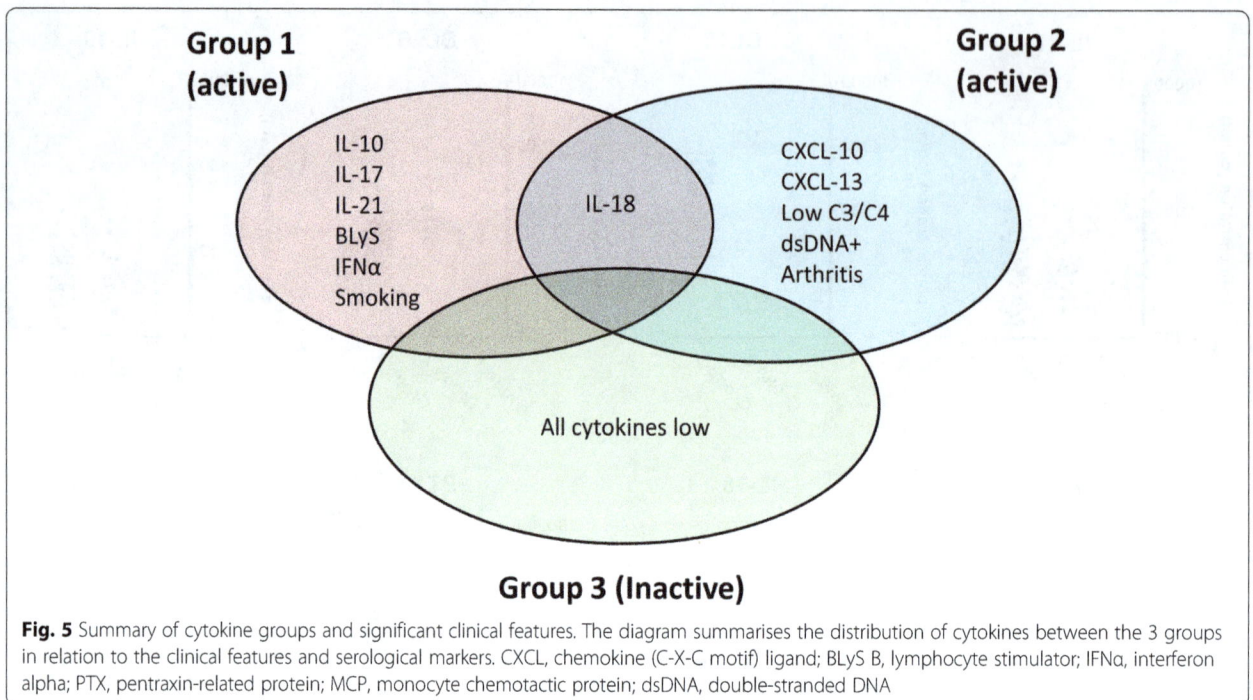

Fig. 5 Summary of cytokine groups and significant clinical features. The diagram summarises the distribution of cytokines between the 3 groups in relation to the clinical features and serological markers. CXCL, chemokine (C-X-C motif) ligand; BLyS B, lymphocyte stimulator; IFNα, interferon alpha; PTX, pentraxin-related protein; MCP, monocyte chemotactic protein; dsDNA, double-stranded DNA

This study compared patients with SLE on the basis of their IFN levels, which may therefore bias the observations towards IFN-related cytokines.

In this SLE cohort approximately 25% of patients had clinically active disease. As expected, those with active disease were younger, with shorter disease duration, and were receiving significantly higher doses of prednisolone whilst awaiting changes to their immunosuppressant therapy. Two cytokines, CXCL10 and PTX3, remained associated with active disease after adjustment for important confounding factors (including steroid use). Of these, CXCL10 had the strongest association with disease activity. The association between CXCL10 and active disease in SLE supports the results of two similar-sized studies [14, 15]. Interestingly, CXCL10/13 levels were not uniformly increased across the SLE cohort but appeared to be restricted to a subset of patients who were more likely to have serologically active disease (high anti-dsDNA and low complement) and inflammatory arthritis. Recently a small study by Ribeiro et al. (2018) identified that patients with SLE with Jaccoud's arthropathy were significantly more likely to be ds-DNA positive and tended to have higher CXCL13 levels, although in this study there was no association between CXCL13 and synovitis or the arthritis component of the SLEDAI score [16]. CXCL13 has also been identified in the serum of patients with rheumatoid arthritis where it is associated with active disease [17].

PTX3 is an acute phase protein predominantly released by the innate immune system. In our study, PTX3 was significantly associated with disease activity both in isolation and as part of the four-cytokine model. Whilst this confirms the work of Assandri et al. [18], others have not found such an association [19].

In a combined model, the addition of four cytokines (IL-21, CXCL13, IL-10 and PTX3) significantly improved the ability of the model to predict the presence of active disease beyond the established markers of raised anti-dsDNA titre and low serum complement. These cytokines in combination were better predictors than any one alone (not shown). These cytokines may therefore have value as novel biomarkers for active SLE, although validation in further cohorts is needed.

The majority of the cytokines measured were significantly correlated with at least one other cytokine. A notable exception was MCP-1, which was not associated with any of the other nine cytokines. The importance of serum MCP-1 levels in SLE remains uncertain, as in a study by Zivkovic et al. (2017) urinary, but not serum levels were associated with the presence of lupus nephritis [20]. Cluster analysis identified three groups of patients, the largest of which had lower levels of all 10 cytokines and contained predominantly clinically inactive patients. The remaining two groups had mostly active disease and, with the exception of IL-18, had distinct cytokine profiles.

Group 1 had high levels of known lupus-related cytokines, including IFNα and BLyS, and pro-inflammatory cytokines including IL-17. Interestingly, group 1 patients were more likely to be smokers and the effect of smoking on the levels of these cytokines warrants further investigation. In contrast, group 2 contained increased levels of

CXCL10 and CXCL13. In a study of 67 patients by Pacheco et al. (2017), using cytokine levels alone four groups were identified: neutral, chemokine, G-colony stimulating factor (G-CSF)-dominant and IFNα/pro-inflammatory [21]. Despite marked differences in the cytokines measures, our larger study also demonstrates "chemokine" and "cytokine" clusters of patients.

The clustering of BLyS in group 1 but low complement/high ds-DNA in group 2 was an unexpected finding. In the clinical trials of the anti-BLyS monoclonal antibody, belimumab, patients with low C3/4 and/or high anti-dsDNA were more likely to respond to BLyS inhibition [22]. The split of BLyS and these serological markers into different groups therefore requires validation and further study.

Limitations of the study
Although this study identifies important associations between cytokines and disease in SLE, it has a number of limitations. First, cytokines were measured at either a single time point or at two time points, which may not adequately capture any fluctuations over time. Further studies are needed to determine how these individual cytokines and groups of cytokines change in response to disease flare/remission in patients with SLE. Second, the number of healthy subjects was relatively small, which may limit the ability to detect differences between healthy controls and patients with SLE, especially as we observed different cytokine patterns within the SLE group. The comparison between active and inactive SLE was also limited by modest numbers. Despite this, however, we identified a number of cytokines that were associated with active disease. Finally, the patients had established disease and some were receiving background treatment, which may affect cytokine levels. It is therefore not possible to comment on whether these findings are relevant to the early disease period.

Conclusions
We have identified novel subsets of patients with active SLE on the basis of cytokine levels using a high-sensitivity bead array. These two groups have different clinical and serological features suggesting differences in pathogenesis. The number of subjects in our study was relatively small and so larger studies are required to confirm these findings and to more accurately classify patients on the basis of their immunophenotype.

Abbreviations
ACR: American College of Rheumatology; BILAG: British Isles Lupus Assessment Group; BLyS: B lymphocyte stimulator; CXCL: Chemokine (C-X-C motif); dsDNA: Double-stranded DNA; ELISA: Enzyme-linked immunosorbent assay; IFN: Interferon; IL: Interleukin; IQR: Interquartile range; MCP: Monocyte chemotactic protein; NHS: National Health Service; NIHR: National Institute for Health Research; PCA: Principal component analysis; PTX: Pentraxin-related protein; SLE: Systemic lupus erythematosus; SLEDAI-2K: Systemic lupus erythematosus disease activity index 2000

Acknowledgements
Dr Bruce is a National Institute for Health Research (NIHR) Senior Investigator and is funded by Arthritis Research UK, the National Institute for Health Research Manchester Biomedical Research Unit and the NIHR/Wellcome Trust Manchester Clinical Research Facility. We acknowledge the support of the NIHR Manchester Clinical Research Facility.

Funding
This research was funded by Manchester University Hospitals Foundation Trust Strategic Investment Scheme and supported by the NIHR Manchester Biomedical Research Centre. The views expressed are those of the author(s) and not necessarily those of the NHS, the NIHR or the Department of Health. We also thank the Arthritis Research UK for their support: Arthritis Research UK Grant number 20380.

Authors' contributions
The research project was conceived by IB, BP, EM, PN, JR and SK. Clinical assessments were performed by JR, BP and SH. Laboratory tests were performed by SK and EL (both). Data analysis was principally performed by JR, JS, PN and SK although all authors contributed. JS contributed expert statistical advice. All authors contributed to the writing of the manuscript. All authors read and approved the final manuscript.

Consent for publication
Not applicable.

Competing interests
The authors declare that they have no competing interests.

Author details
[1]Arthritis Research UK Centre for Epidemiology, Centre for Musculoskeletal Research, Manchester Academic Health Science Centre, University of Manchester, Manchester M13 9PT, UK. [2]The Kellgren Centre for Rheumatology, NIHR Manchester Biomedical Research Centre, Manchester University Hospitals NHS Foundation Trust, Manchester Academic Health Science Centre, Manchester, UK. [3]Rheumatology Department, Wythenshawe Hospital, Manchester University Hospitals NHS Foundation, Manchester, UK. [4]Division of Allergy, Immunology and Rheumatology, Department of Internal Medicine, Faculty of Medicine, Ramathibodi Hospital, Mahidol University, Bangkok, Thailand. [5]Centre for Biostatistics, Manchester Academic Health Science Centre, University of Manchester, Manchester, UK. [6]Aeirtec Ltd, The SmokeHouses Building, Clifford Fort, North Shields, Newcastle upon Tyne, UK.

References
1. Winthrop KL, Strand V, van der Heijde DM, Mease PJ, Crow MK, Weinblatt M, et al. The unmet need in rheumatology: reports from the targeted therapies meeting 2016. Clin Exp Rheumatol. 2016;34:69–76.
2. Banchereau R, Hong S, Cantarel B, Baldwin N, Baisch J, Edens M, et al. Personalized immunomonitoring uncovers molecular networks that stratify lupus patients. Cell. 2016;165:1548–50.
3. Artim-Esen B, Cene E, Sahinkaya Y, Ertan S, Pehlivan O, Kamali S, et al. Cluster analysis of autoantibodies in 852 patients with systemic lupus erythematosus from a single center. J Rheumatol. 2014;41:1304–10.
4. Ching KH, Burbelo PD, Tipton C, Wei C, Petri M, Sanz I, et al. Two major autoantibody clusters in systemic lupus erythematosus. PLoS One. 2012;7:e32001.
5. Wu H, Zeng J, Yin J, Peng Q, Zhao M, Lu Q. Organ-specific biomarkers in lupus. Autoimmun Rev. 2017;16:391–7.
6. Davis LS, Hutcheson J, Mohan C. The role of cytokines in the pathogenesis and treatment of systemic lupus erythematosus. J Interf Cytokine Res. 2011;31:781–9.
7. Lee HM, Sugino H, Nishimoto N. Cytokine networks in systemic lupus erythematosus. J Biomed Biotechnol. 2010;2010:676284.
8. Yu SL, Kuan WP, Wong CK, Li EK, Tam LS. Immunopathological roles of cytokines, chemokines, signalling molecules, and pattern-recognition receptors in systemic lupus erythematosus. Clin Dev Immunol. 2012;2012:715190.
9. Vincent FB, Northcott M, Hoi A, Mackay F, Morand EF. Clinical associations of serum interleukin-17 in systemic lupus erythematosus. Arthritis Res Ther. 2013;15:R97.

10. Hochberg MC. Updating the American college of rheumatology revised criteria for the classification of systemic lupus erythematosus. Arthritis Rheum. 1997;40:1725.

11. Gladman DD, Ibañez D, Urowitz MB. Systemic lupus erythematosus disease activity index 2000. J Rheumatol. 2002;29:288–91.

12. Yee C-S, Farewell V, Isenberg DA, Rahman A, Teh L-S, Griffiths B, et al. British Isles Lupus Assessment Group 2004 index is valid for assessment of disease activity in systemic lupus erythematosus. Arthritis Rheum. 2007;56:4113–9.

13. Bauer JW, Baechler EC, Petri M, Batliwalla FM, Crawford D, Ortmann WA, et al. Elevated serum levels of interferon-regulated chemokines are biomarkers for active human systemic lupus erythematosus. PLoS Med. 2006;3:e491.

14. Rose T, Grutzkau A, Hirseland H, Huscher D, Dahnrich C, Dzionek A, et al. IFN alpha and its response proteins, IP-10 and SIGLEC-1, are biomarkers of disease activity in systemic lupus erythematosus. Ann Rheum Dis. 2013;72:1639–45.

15. Dominguez-Gutierrez PR, Ceribelli A, Satoh M, Sobel ES, Reeves WH, Chan EK. Reduced levels of CCL2 and CXCL10 in systemic lupus erythematosus patients under treatment with prednisone, mycophenolate mofetil, or hydroxychloroquine, except in a high STAT1 subset. Arthritis Res Ther. 2014;16:R23.

16. Ribeiro DS, Lins CF, Galvao V, Santos WGD, Rosa G, Machicado V, et al. Association of CXCL13 serum level and ultrasonographic findings of joints in patients with systemic lupus erythematosus and Jaccoud's arthropathy. Lupus. 2018;27(6):939–46.

17. Greisen SR, Schelde KK, Rasmussen TK, Kragstrup TW, Stengaard-Pedersen K, Hetland ML, et al. CXCL13 predicts disease activity in early rheumatoid arthritis and could be an indicator of the therapeutic 'window of opportunity'. Arthritis Res Ther. 2014;16:434.

18. Assandri R, Monari M, Colombo A, Dossi A, Montanelli A. Pentraxin 3 plasma levels and disease activity in systemic lupus erythematosus. Autoimmune Dis. 2015;2015:354014.

19. Skare TL, Nisihara R, Ramos GP, Utiyama SR, Messias-Reason I. Pentraxin-3 levels in systemic lupus erythematosus: association with cumulative damage but not with disease activity. Joint Bone Spine. 2015;82:466–7.

20. Zivkovic V, Cvetkovic T, Mitic B, Stamenkovic B, Stojanovic S, Radovanovic-Dinic B, et al. Monocyte chemoattractant protein-1 as a marker of systemic lupus erythematosus: an observational study. Rheumatol Int. 2018;38(6):1003-8.

21. Pacheco Y, Barahona-Correa J, Monsalve DM, Acosta-Ampudia Y, Rojas M, Rodriguez Y, et al. Cytokine and autoantibody clusters interaction in systemic lupus erythematosus. J Transl Med. 2017;15:239.

22. van Vollenhoven RF, Petri MA, Cervera R, Roth DA, Ji BN, Kleoudis CS, et al. Belimumab in the treatment of systemic lupus erythematosus: high disease activity predictors of response. Ann Rheum Dis. 2012;71:1343–9.

8

Expansion and activation of monocytic-myeloid-derived suppressor cell via STAT3/arginase-I signaling in patients with ankylosing spondylitis

Yu-feng Liu[1,2], Kun-hai Zhuang[2], Bin Chen[2], Pei-wu Li[2], Xuan Zhou[3], Hua Jiang[4], Li-mei Zhong[3*] and Feng-bin Liu[1,2*]

Abstract

Background: Ankylosing spondylitis (AS) is a chronic inflammatory rheumatic disease. The dysregulated immune system plays an important role in the pathogenesis of AS. Myeloid-derived suppressor cells (MDSCs) play a key immunoregulatory role in autoimmune arthritis. The aim of this study was to clarify the underlying immunoregulatory mechanism of MDSCs in patients with AS.

Methods: Flow cytometry was used to analyze the phenotype of MDSCs among peripheral blood mononuclear cells (PBMCs) from 46 patients with AS and 46 healthy control subjects. The correlation between MDSC frequency and the disease index of patients with AS was evaluated. A T cell proliferation experiment was used to evaluate the immunosuppressive function of MDSCs.

Results: Polymorphonuclear (PMN) and monocytic (M)-MDSCs were significantly elevated in the PBMCs of patients with AS, when compared with levels in healthy controls. Additionally, M-MDSC levels correlated positively with the clinical index of AS, including the Bath ankylosing spondylitis disease activity index (BASDAI) score, erythrocyte sedimentation rate (ESR) and C-reactive protein (CRP) levels. M-MDSCs derived from patients with AS suppressed T cell responses, and this effect was dependent on the induction of arginase-I. Furthermore, AS-derived M-MDSCs showed high levels of phosphorylated STAT3. Stattic, a STAT3-specific inhibitor, and STAT3-targeted siRNA abrogated the immunosuppressive function of M-MDSCs. Inhibition of STAT3 signaling also resulted in decreased arginase-I activity.

Conclusions: STAT3/arginase-I signaling plays an important role in both the expansion and activation of M-MDSCs in patients with AS. This information may be beneficial in developing novel therapeutic strategies for preventing AS.

Keywords: Ankylosing spondylitis, Myeloid-derived suppressor cells, STAT3/arginase-I signaling, T cell suppression

* Correspondence: 854458483@qq.com; liufb163@163.com
[3]Department of Laboratory Medicine, Guangdong Second Provincial General Hospital, Guangzhou 510317, People's Republic of China
[1]Guangzhou University of Chinese Medicine, Guangzhou, People's Republic of China
Full list of author information is available at the end of the article

Key messages

- Expansion of M-MDSCs subset in PBMCs derived patients of AS.
- STAT3/arginase-I pathway mediated the expansion of M-MDSC.

Background

Ankylosing spondylitis (AS) is a chronic inflammatory disease that affects the axial skeleton, causing characteristic inflammatory back pain [1]. The prevalence of different types of spondyloarthritis is 0.5–1.9%, and interaction between a strong genetic component, mainly by specific HLA-B27 subtypes, and bacteria seems to be crucial for the development of the disease [2]. Although there have been significant findings in understanding the pathogenesis of AS, the exact mechanisms have not yet been identified [3, 4]. Clinical therapy and diagnosis are mainly dependent on the radiographic progression of AS [5]. Therefore, understanding the molecular progression of AS would facilitate early diagnosis and treatment during pathogenesis. Immunohistological studies on sacroiliac joint biopsies have shown immune cell infiltrates, including T cells and macrophages, suggesting that both innate and adaptive immune responses could play a role in AS pathogenesis [6]. Further studies determined that gut immunity, T-lymphocyte activation, and peptide processing before HLA class I presentation are involved in the pathogenesis of AS [7]. Studies showing increased frequencies of interleukin (IL)-17-positive CD4$^+$ T cells in peripheral blood mononuclear cells (PBMCs) obtained from patients with AS support the fact that T helper (Th)17 cells are involved in the pathogenesis of inflammatory arthritis [8, 9]. Moreover, imbalances in the T lymphocyte subset ratios, Th1/Th2 and Th17/regulatory T (Treg), were demonstrated in patients with AS [10]. These studies collectively indicate that AS progression may be associated with the degree of immune abnormality.

Myeloid-derived suppressor cells (MDSCs) are a heterogeneous population of cells that consists of myeloid progenitor cells and immature myeloid cells (iMCs). In healthy individuals, iMCs generated in the bone marrow quickly differentiate into mature granulocytes, macrophages, or dendritic cells [11]. In pathological conditions, such as in cancer and some autoimmune diseases, a partial block in the differentiation of iMCs into mature myeloid cells results in the expansion of the MDSC population [12]. MDSCs constitute a unique component of the immune system that regulates immune responses in healthy individuals and in the context of various diseases [13, 14]. MDSCs are classified into two major subsets based on their phenotypic and morphological features: polymorphonuclear (PMN)-MDSCs and monocytic (M)-MDSCs [15]. In mice, MDSCs are defined as cells expressing both Gr-1 and CD11b, and are further classified into two subpopulations based on Ly6G and Ly6C: PMN-MDSC (CD11b$^+$ Ly6G$^+$ Ly6C^{lo}) and M-MDSC (CD11b$^+$ Ly6G$^-$ Ly6C^{hi}) [16]. In human PBMCs, the equivalent subsets to PMN-MDSCs and M-MDSCs are defined as HLA-DR$^{low/-}$ CD11b$^+$CD33$^+$CD14$^-$CD15$^+$ and HLA-DR$^{low/-}$ CD11b$^+$CD33$^+$CD14$^+$CD15$^-$, respectively [17]. MDSCs are characterized by an immunosuppressive phenotype. L-arginine metabolism plays a central role in the immunosuppressive activity of MDSCs. L-arginine can be metabolized by inducible nitric oxide synthase (iNOS or Nos2), generating citrulline and nitric oxide (NO), or can be converted into urea and L-ornithine by arginase [18]. MDSCs expressing arginase-I (ARG1) reduce the availability of L-arginine, which can result in the loss of CD3ζ expression and impaired T cell function [19].

Several recent reports show that MDSCs play crucial roles in the regulation of autoimmune diseases. The MDSC population showed significant expansion in arthritic mice and in patients with rheumatoid arthritis (RA) and produced high levels of inflammatory cytokines [20]. In addition, MDSCs from collagen-induced arthritis (CIA) model mice and patients with RA promoted the polarization of Th17 cells, displaying T cell suppressive ability [21]. Furthermore, the transfer of these CIA mouse-derived MDSCs facilitated disease progression in CIA model mice [22]. These studies collectively show the potential association of MDSCs with autoimmune arthritis disease as well as the therapeutic value of MDSCs. However, the association between MDSCs and AS has not been examined.

In this study, we report that MDSCs showed expansion in patients with AS compared with healthy controls, and the level of M-MDSCs significantly correlated with the AS disease activity index. AS-derived M-MDSCs displayed a T cell suppressive function, which was mediated through the production of arginase-I and activation of STAT3 (signal transducer and activator of transcription 3) signaling. Our study provides novel insights into a valuable role of M-MDSCs in promoting AS pathogenesis and suggests that M-MDSCs represent a potential immune therapeutic target in AS treatment.

Methods
Ethics statement
This research was approved by the ethics review board of Guangdong Second Provincial General Hospital. Written, informed consent was provided by each participant and/or their legal guardian.

Patients
Peripheral blood samples were obtained from 46 AS patients and 46 healthy control subjects. Patients with AS met the modified New York criteria for AS [23]. The

Table 1 Characteristics of the patients with ankylosing spondylitis

Variable	Healthy control	Ankylosing spondylitis
Number of samples (n)	46	46
Age (years)	32.3 ± 1.2	23.6 ± 9.8
Gender, male/female (n)	22/24	25/21
Duration of disease (years)	–	5.6 ± 3.6
BASDAI score	–	2.76 ± 1.07
ESR mm/hour	9.2 ± 3.5	24.1 ± 12.4
CRP, mg/liter	2.5 ± 1.2	28 ± 17.1
HLA-B27, positive member	–	12

BASDAI Bath Ankylosing Spondylitis Disease Activity Index (range 0–10), CRP C-reactive protein, ESR erythrocyte sedimentation rate

Bath Ankylosing Spondylitis Disease Activity Index (BASDAI) score [24] was measured for the majority of patients with AS at the time when the blood samples were obtained. Age, sex, disease duration, erythrocyte sedimentation rate (ESR), and C-reactive protein (CRP) levels were recorded (Table 1).

Reagents and antibodies

RPMI 1640, DMEM, Lipofectamine 2000, FBS, β-ME, penicillin, 5-(and-6)-chloromethyl-2,7-dichlorodihydrofluorescein diacetate, acetyl ester (CM-H2DCFDA), and 5(6)-carboxyfluorescein diacetate succinimidyl ester (CFSE) were obtained from Invitrogen (Grand Island, NY, USA). NW-hydroxy-nor-arginine (NOHA) and L-NG-monomethyl-arginine (L-NMMA) were obtained from Cayman Chemical (Ann Arbor, MI), N-acetylcysteine (NAC) and dimethyl sulfoxide were purchased from Sigma-Aldrich (Merck, Germany). The following anti-human Abs was purchased from Thermo Fisher Scientific (Waltham, MA, USA): CD11b-FITC, CD 33-PE, CD14-PE-Cy7, CD15-eFluor450, HLA-DR-PE-Cy5, CD4-PE, CD8-PE-Cy5, CD3-PE-Cy7, and their corresponding isotype controls.

PBMCs isolation and flow cytometric analysis

PBMC were isolated from whole blood by Ficoll centrifugation and analyzed immediately. The cell phenotype was analyzed by flow cytometer (BD LSR fortessa; BD Biosciences, San Jose, CA, USA), and the data were analyzed with the FlowJo 10.0 software package (TreeStar Inc., Ashland, OR, USA). Data were acquired as the fraction of labeled cells within a live-cell gate set for 50,000 events. A FACS Aria III (BD Biosciences) was used for flow cytometric sorting. The strategy for MDSCs sorting was to gate HLA-DR$^{-/low}$CD11b$^+$CD33$^{int/high}$ cells from PBMC. In some experiment, MDSCs were sorted from PBMC; then, the remaining PBMC were used for the T cell proliferation assay.

T cell proliferation assay

T cell proliferation was evaluated by CFSE dilution. Purified T cells were labeled with CFSE (3 μM; Invitrogen), stimulated with antiCD3/CD28 antibodies (5 μg/ml, Thermo Fisher Scientific), and cultured alone or co-cultured with autologous PMN-MDSCs or M-MDSCs at the indicated ratios. The cells were then stained for surface marker expression with CD4-PE or CD8-PE-Cy5 antibodies, and T cell proliferation was analyzed on a flow cytometer. T cells without stimulation were used as the negative control.

Arginase enzymatic activity assay

Arginase-I activity was measured in PMN-MDSC lysates, as previously described [13] with slight modifications. Briefly, cells were lysed with 0.1% Triton X-100 for 30 min, followed by the addition of 25 mM Tris-HCl and10 mM MnCl$_2$. The enzyme was activated by incubation for 10 min at 56 °C. Arginine hydrolysis was performed by incubating the lysate with 0.5 M l-arginine at 37 °C for 2 h. The urea concentration was measured at 540 nm after the addition of alpha-isonitrosopropiophenone (dissolved in 100% ethanol), followed by heating at 95 °C for 30 min.

Reactive oxygen species (ROS) production

Cells (5×10^5) were incubated at 37 °C in the presence of 1 μM CMH$_2$DCFDA (Thermo Fisher Scientific) for 30 min and were then labeled with fluorescence-conjugated antibodies (Abs) against CD33 and CD11b. The ROS content in PMN-MDSCs was analyzed by flow cytometry.

Enzyme-linked immunosorbent assay (ELISA)

The production of interferon (IFN)-γ in culture supernatants was determined by ELISA, following the manufacturer's instructions (R&D Systems, Minneapolis, MN, USA).

Transwell assays

PMN-MDSCs isolated by flow cytometric sorting were cultured in Transwell inserts (0.4 mm pore size; EMD Millipore, Billerica, MA, USA), and fresh autologous T cells (1×10^6 cells/ml) were cultured in 96-well plates.

Intracellular staining

Intracellular staining of phosphorylated STAT-3 (pSTAT-3, phospho Tyr705) was performed following the manufacturer's protocol (Cell Signaling Technology, Beverly, MA, USA). Cells (5×10^5) were fixed with formaldehyde to stabilize the cell membrane, and permeabilized using BD Fix&Perm Solution (BD Biosciences, Franklin Lakes, NJ, USA). After washing, cells were then stained with Alexa Fluor 488-conjugated pSTAT-3 and analyzed by flow cytometry.

STAT3 inhibition

Stattic, a STAT3-specific small molecule inhibitor (Calbiochem, MilliporeSigma, Burlington, MA, USA) and short interfering (si) RNA targeting *STAT3* (siSTAT3 ID: 116558, Thermo Fisher Scientific) were used to inhibit *STAT3* signaling. Stattic was diluted to 1% in dimethyl sulfoxide (DMSO). PMN-MDSCs were treated with 10 μM Stattic at 37 °C for 24 h. Scrambled and *STAT3*-targeted siRNAs were transduced into PMN-MDSCs cells using lentiviral vectors [25].

Generation of retrovirus

Two hunderd ninety three T cells were transfected with a mixture of DNA containing 2.5 μg VSVG, 2.5 μg Δ8.2, and scrambled or *STAT3*-targeted siRNA vectors using Lipofectamine 2000 according to the manufacturer's instructions. Media containing scrambled or *STAT3* siRNA retroviruses were collected 72 h after transfection and filtered through a 0.45 μm pore-size filter.

Statistics analysis

All data are presented as the mean ± SEM. Clinical and immunological parameters were compared by non-parametric Mann-Whitney U tests. For in vitro experiments, statistical analyses were performed using unpaired or paired t tests. Correlations between different parameters were analyzed using a Spearman rank test. Statistical tests were performed using GraphPad Prism version 5.0a (GraphPad Software, San Diego, CA, USA) and SPSS Statistics 17.0 (SPSS Inc., Chicago, IL, USA). P values of 0.05 or 0.01 were considered significant.

Results

Increased frequency of MDSCs in peripheral blood of patients with AS

To determine whether MDSCs play a role in patients with AS, using flow cytometry, we first compared the MDSC frequencies and absolute cell counts in the peripheral blood of patients with AS ($n = 46$) with those in age-matched healthy donors (n = 46). The HLA-DR$^{-/low}$CD11b^{int}CD33^{int} and HLA-DR$^{-/low}$CD11b^{high}CD33^{high} populations corresponded to the PMN-MDSC and M-MDSC subsets, respectively, further based on the expression of CD14 or CD15 (Fig. 1a). By analyzing the MDSC percentage and absolute numbers of PBMCs, we found significant elevations in the frequency ($0.1697 \pm 0.03879\%$ vs $2.049 \pm 0.1810\%$, $P < 0.001$) and absolute cell counts (1.346 ± 0.1367 vs 28.38 ± 2.516, $P < 0.001$) of M-MDSCs (Fig. 1b–c) and in the frequency ($0.8685 \pm 0.1229\%$ vs $12.13 \pm 0.9299\%$, $P < 0.001$) and absolute cell counts (52.76 ± 8.316 vs 825.3 ± 57.58, $P < 0.001$) of PMN-MDSCs (Fig. 1b, d) in patients with AS compared with healthy controls. We further assessed the MDSC levels in 18 AS patients receive treatment [anti-tumor

necrosis factor (TNF), nonsteroidal anti-inflammatory drugs (NSAIDs) and steroid drugs]. Compared with treatment-naive AS patients, patients who received treatment exhibited lower disease activity (BASDAI, treatment-naive vs treatment: 2.76 ± 1.07 vs 1.091 ± 0.1668) (Additional file 1: Table S1), but still had higher percentages of MDSCs than healthy controls (Additional file 1: Figure S1). Furthermore, we found no significant difference in MDSC levels among the different stages of diseases, including axial disease only and axial plus peripheral disease (Additional file 1: Figure S2). Therefore, we believe that MDSCs may play an important predictive role in early diagnosis of disease. Furthermore, Wright-Giemsa staining showed that the M-MDSCs (Fig. 1e) and PMN-MDSCs (Fig. 1f) from patients with AS exhibited typical immature cellular morphology. These observations collectively demonstrated that the MDSC subset is elevated significantly in the peripheral blood of patients with AS.

Elevated M-MDSCs correlate with disease index in patients with AS

To further investigate the clinical significance of increased MDSCs in patients with AS, we evaluated the correlation between MDSC numbers and AS disease index. The BASDAI score is one of a group of classification criteria for spondyloarthropathies and an important predictor of treatment in patients with AS [24]. We found statistically positive correlations between the frequencies of M-MDSCs and the BASDAI scores ($P = 0.007$). In contrast, there was no correlation between the frequencies of PMN-MDSCs and the BASDAI scores ($P = 0.6304$) (Fig. 2a). In addition to BASDAI, further analysis revealed that the frequency of M-MDSCs, but not PMN-MDSCs, correlated positively with the ESR (Fig. 2b) and CRP levels (Fig. 2c) in patients with AS ($P = 0.001$ and $P = 0.0209$, respectively). A previous study reported that PBMCs from patients with AS showed increased numbers of IL-17-positive CD4$^+$ T cells compared with control subjects, and the numbers were positively correlated with index of disease activity [9]. Interestingly, we also determined that the levels of M-MDSCs in our study were positively correlated with the concentration of IL-17 ($P = 0.0104$) (Fig. 2d). These results suggested that M-MDSC levels were intimately correlated with disease activity index in patients with AS and indicated that M-MDSCs may represent a novel immunological marker of disease progression in AS.

M-MDSCs derived from patients with AS suppress T cell responses

MDSCs are known to suppress T cell immune responses under some pathological conditions [26]. Therefore, we evaluated the effect of AS-derived MDSCs on T cell responses. First, MDSCs were depleted from PBMCs-MDSCs by flow cytometric sorting, after which the PBMCs were stimulated with anti-CD3/CD28 antibodies. The results

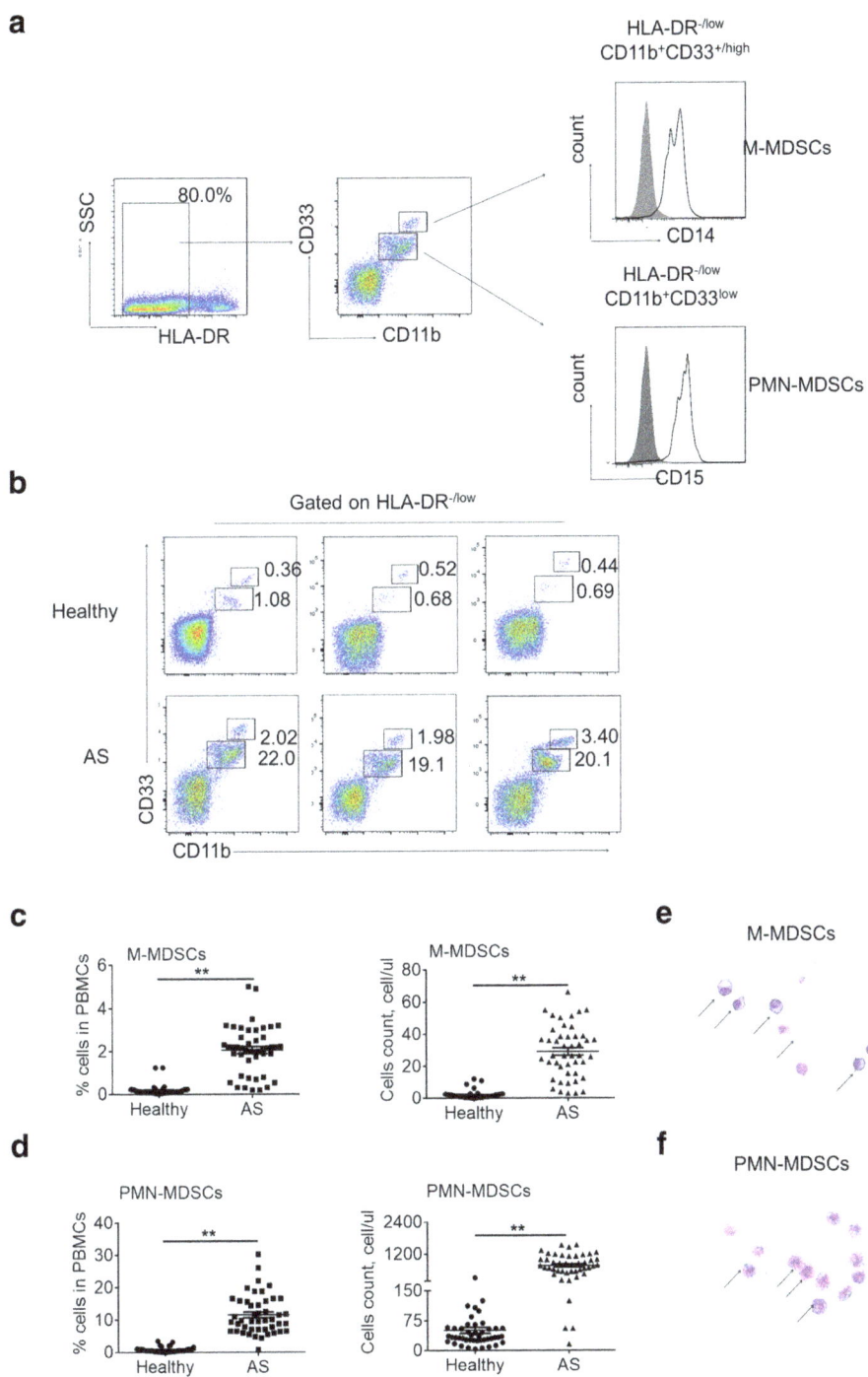

Fig. 1 (See legend on next page.)

(See figure on previous page.)
Fig. 1 Increased frequency of MDSCs in peripheral blood of patients with AS. **a** Gating strategy of MDSCs by flow cytometry analysis. HLA-DR$^{-/low}$ cells were first selected from live PBMCs, the HLA-DR$^{-/low}$CD11b^{int}CD33^{int} and HLA-DR$^{-/low}$CD11b^{high}CD33^{high} populations corresponded to the PMN-MDSCs and M-MDSCs subsets, respectively. The expression of cell surface markers CD14$^+$ (M-MDSCs) and CD15$^+$ (PMN-MDSCs) on this population was subsequently evaluated. *Black*, CD14 or CD15; *gray*, isotype. **b** Representative flow cytometry data for PMN-MDSCs and M-MDSCs from ankylosing spondylitis patients and healthy controls. The *boxed areas* represent the cells percentage in PBMCs, respectively. **c** Statistical analysis of M-MDSCs frequency (*left*) and absolute cell counts (*right*) in the peripheral blood from ankylosing spondylitis patients (n = 46) and healthy controls (n = 46). **P<0.01, unpaired *t* test. **d** Statistical analysis of PMN-MDSCs frequency (*left*) and absolute cell counts (*right*) in the peripheral blood from ankylosing spondylitis patients (n = 46) and healthy controls (n = 46). **P<0.01, unpaired *t* test. **e** Wright-Giemsa staining exhibited that M-MDSCs from patients with ankylosing spondylitis showed typical immature cellular morphology. **f** Wright-Giemsa staining exhibited that PMN-MDSCs from patients with ankylosing spondylitis showed typical immature cellular morphology. *AS* ankylosing spondylitis, *M-MDSCs* monocytic myeloid-derived suppressor cells, *PMN-MDSC* polymorphonuclear myeloid-derived suppressor cells

showed that the proliferation of both CD4 and CD8 T cells was enhanced significantly upon MDSC depletion (Fig. 3a). This suggested that the presence of MDSCs in patients with AS suppressed T cell responses. The suppressive activity of MDSCs was further confirmed by co-culture of M-MDSCs or PMN-MDSCs with T cells. M-MDSCs actively suppressed the autologous T cell responses, including cell proliferation (Fig. 3b) and IFN-γ production (Fig. 3c), in a dose-dependent manner. However, PMN-MDSCs from the PBMCs of patients with AS did not suppress T cell responses (Additional file 1: Figure S3A–B). Secondly, to determine whether M-MDSCs function through direct contact with T cells, M-MDSC/T cell co-culture experiments were performed using Transwells. The separation of M-MDSCs from T cells eliminated their suppressive activity (Fig. 3d), demonstrating that the function of M-MDSCs is cell contact-dependent. Our observations from this series of experiments demonstrated that M-MDSCs present in patients with AS actively suppressed T cells in a cell contact-dependent manner.

AS-derived M-MDSCs suppress T cell responses in an arginase-I-dependent manner

Based on the observation that M-MDSCs derived from patients with AS could suppress T cell responses, we further explored the underlying mechanisms controlling M-MDSC-mediated T cell suppression. Inhibition of l-arginine is believed to mediate the immunosuppressive effect of MDSCs under certain pathological conditions [11]. Therefore, we measured the arginase activity, NO content, and ROS levels in M-MDSCs derived from patients with AS and healthy controls. No significant changes were observed in ROS levels (Fig. 4a) or NO content (Fig. 4b). A significant increase in arginase activity was observed in AS-derived M-MDSCs compared with healthy controls (Fig. 4c). To further test this possibility, M-MDSC/T cell co-culture experiments were performed in the presence of different inhibitors, including L-arginine-metabolizing enzymes (N-hydroxy-nor-l-arginine, NOHA). The results showed that the suppression of T cell proliferation (Fig. 4d) and IFN-γ production

(Fig. 4e) in the presence of M-MDSCs were almost completely recovered after the administration of the arginase inhibitor NOHA, while no similar effects were observed for the NOS inhibitor L-NMMA or the ROS inhibitor N-acetylcysteine (NAC) (Fig. 4d–e). Given the functional significance of STAT3 signaling in myeloid cell [27], we analyzed the intracellular phosphorylated STAT3 (pSTAT3) expression level in AS-derived M-MDSCs. AS-derived M-MDSCs had significantly higher expression of pSTAT3 in comparison with healthy control (Fig. 4f). These results demonstrated that AS-derived M-MDSCs suppress T cells in an arginase-dependent manner.

Inhibition of pSTAT3/arginase-I signaling abrogates the suppressive activity of AS-derived M-MDSCs

Increased levels of pSTAT3 in tumors have been correlated with the increased suppressive activity of tumor-infiltrating MDSCs in patients with cancer [28]. Therefore, we directly investigated the significance of STAT3 signaling in M-MDSCs in patients with AS by inhibiting STAT3 signaling using two independent methods: we used either Stattic, a specific small molecule inhibitor of pSTAT3, or siRNA suppression via lentiviral vector to inhibit STAT3 signaling. Our results showed that both STAT3 signaling inhibition methods appropriately decreased the level of pSTAT3 in M-MDSCs (Fig. 5a–b). Interestingly, both methods of STAT3 signaling inhibition also affected the expression of ARG1 in M-MDSCs (Fig. 5c–d). After treatment with Stattic or siRNA, we found significant decreases in ARG1 activity in AS-derived M-MDSCs (Fig. 5e–f). These data suggest that STAT3 may regulate ARG1 in AS-derived M-MDSCs. Furthermore, both inhibition methods showed that the inhibition of STAT3 signaling abrogated the T cell suppressive function of M-MDSCs derived from patients with AS (Fig. 5g–h). Collectively, these results determined that STAT3 inhibition decreased the ARG1 level and the suppressive activity in AS-derived M-MDSCs.

Discussion

Although MDSCs have been intensively investigated in autoimmune arthritis, recent studies have shown

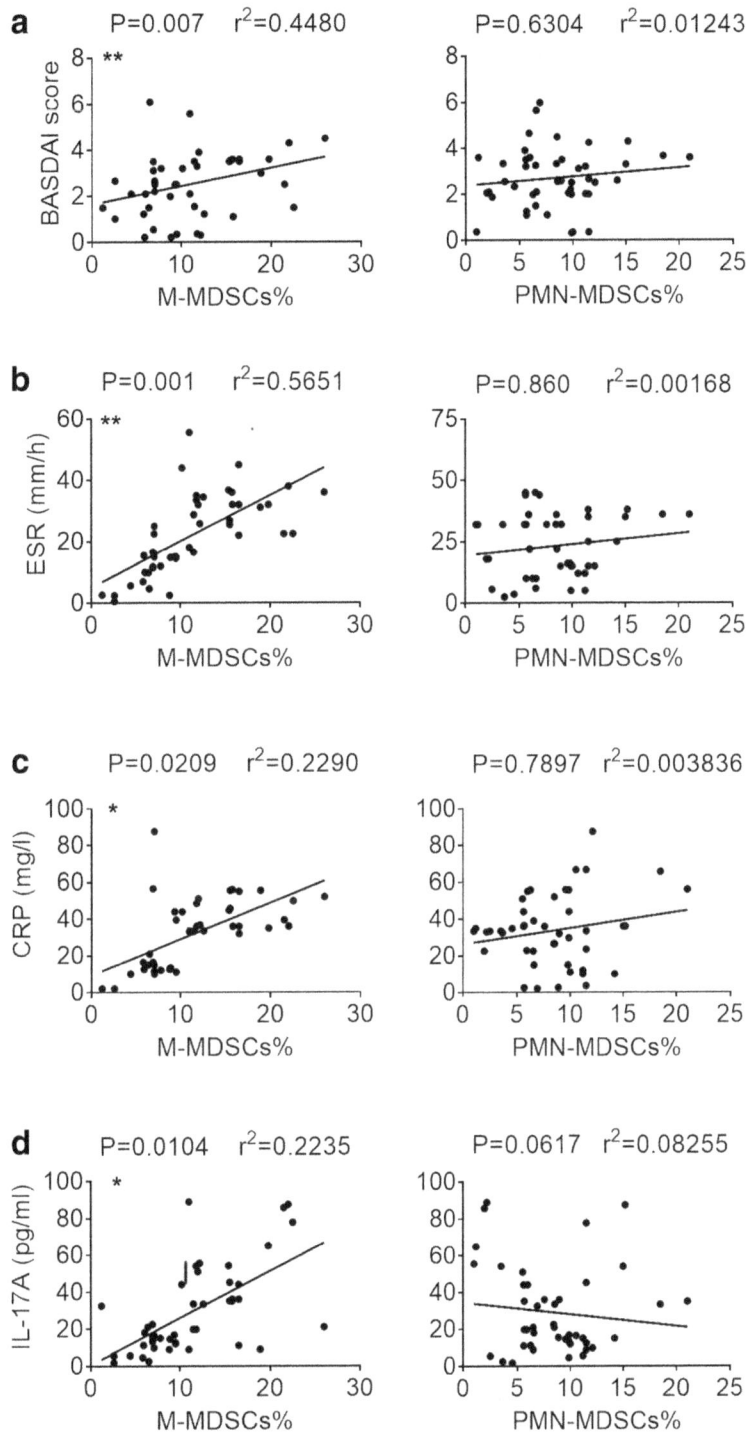

Fig. 2 Elevated M-MDSCs correlate with disease index in patients with AS. Correlation between M-MDSCs (*left*) or PMN-MDSCs (*right*) and disease markers in ankylosing spondylitis patients including BASDAI score (**a**), ESR (**b**), CRP (**c**), and concentration of IL-17 (**d**). *CRP* C-reactive protein, *ESR* erythrocyte sedimentation rate, *IL* interleukin, *M-MDSCs* monocytic myeloid-derived suppressor cells, *PMN-MDSC* polymorphonuclear myeloid-derived suppressor cells

an emerging role for MDSCs in the pathogenesis of RA [20]. However, the mechanisms for the aberrant expansion of MDSCs in AS as well as their immunological and clinical significance remain unclear. Delineating these important issues will advance our understanding of the relationship between MDSCs and AS, which will benefit the development of immunotherapies to treat human AS diseases.

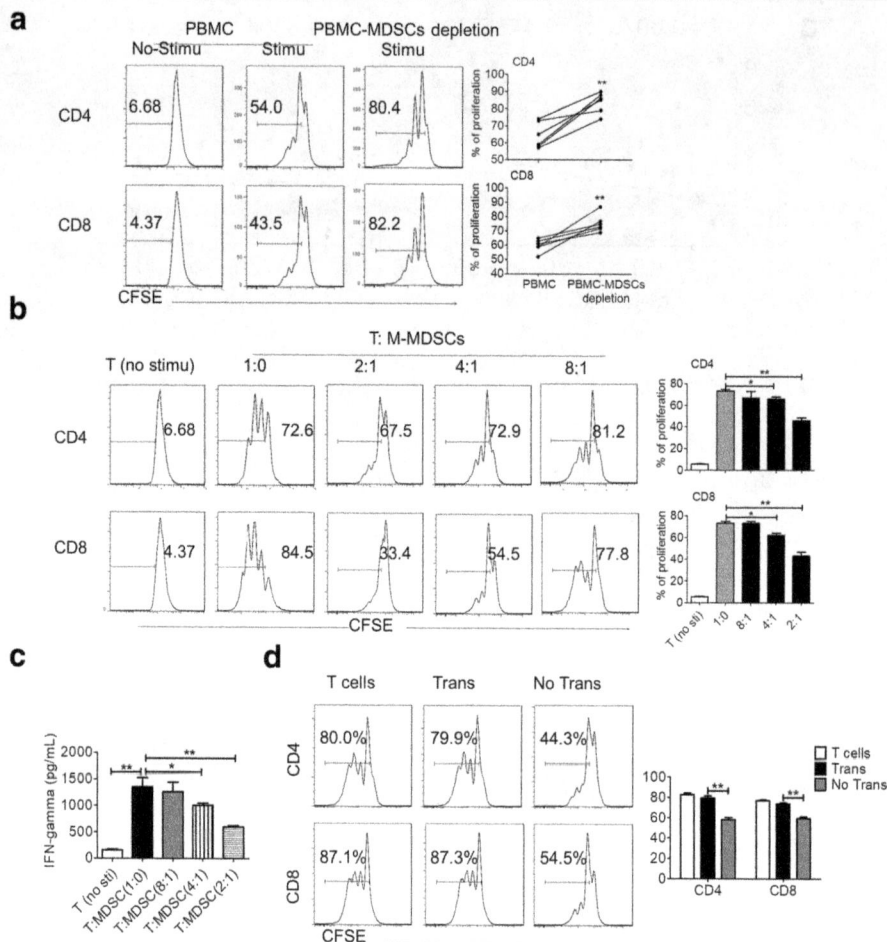

Fig. 3 M-MDSCs derived from patients with AS suppress T cell responses. **a** Depletion of MDSCs enhanced T cell function. PBMCs or PBMCs with MDSC depletion (PBMC-MDSC depletion) from fresh peripheral blood of AS patients were stimulated with CD3/CD28, and proliferation of T cells was examined by CFSE dilution. *Left panels*: representative flow cytometry data from one individual; *right* panel: results of stimulated samples from six individuals. **b** CD3[+] T cell from patients at ankylosing spondylitis patients were stimulated with anti-CD3/CD28, co-cultured with M-MDSCs from the same donors at different ratios for 3d, and T cell proliferation was evaluated by CFSE labeling; unstimulated T cells were used as a negative control. *Left panels*: representative flow cytometry data from one individual; *right panel*: results from five individuals. **c** Production of IFN-γ by T cells in supernatants from panel (**b**) was measured by ELISA. Means and SD are shown; $n = 6$. **d** Co-culture of M-MDSCs-T cell (1:2) experiments as in panel (**b**) were performed, with or without Transwells. $^{*}P < 0.05$; $^{**}P < 0.01$, compared with controls by unpaired t test. *AS* ankylosing spondylitis, *CFSE* carboxyfluorescein succinimidyl ester, *IFN* interferon, *M-MDSCs* monocytic myeloid-derived suppressor cells, *PMN-MDSC* polymorphonuclear myeloid-derived suppressor cells

Here, we report a significant elevation of both subsets of M-MDSCs and PMN-MDSCs in the peripheral blood of patients with AS. Consistent with the CIA mice model and patients with RA, MDSCs significantly expanded in arthritic mice and patients with RA, suggesting that MDSCs play a key role in autoimmune arthritis. However, the mechanism underlying the MDSC expansion in autoimmune arthritis has not yet been determined. In CIA mice, inflammatory cytokines promote myelopoiesis by stimulating the production of myeloid precursors in the bone marrow. Increased levels of TNF-α and/or granulocyte-macrophage colony-stimulating factor (GM-CSF) may promote MDSC accumulation in the PBMC and spleen. In addition, interleukin 6

(IL-6) and transforming growth factor-beta 1 (TGFβ1) genes most likely cause the expansion of MDSCs in inflammatory or cancerous conditions [29]. Similarly, MDSCs from arthritic mice also express higher levels of inflammatory cytokines (e.g. TNF-α, IL-1β) than those from control mice, supporting an inflammatory activation in these cells. These studies suggest that in inflamed tissues, pro-inflammatory cytokines could promote MDSC aggregation, and in turn, MDSCs can releases more pro-inflammatory factors to aggravate inflammatory responses. Moreover, MDSCs from CIA mice and patients with RA promoted the polarization of Th17 cells in vitro [22]. Interestingly, Th17 cells are also involved in the pathogenesis of AS [9]. In our study, we also found that

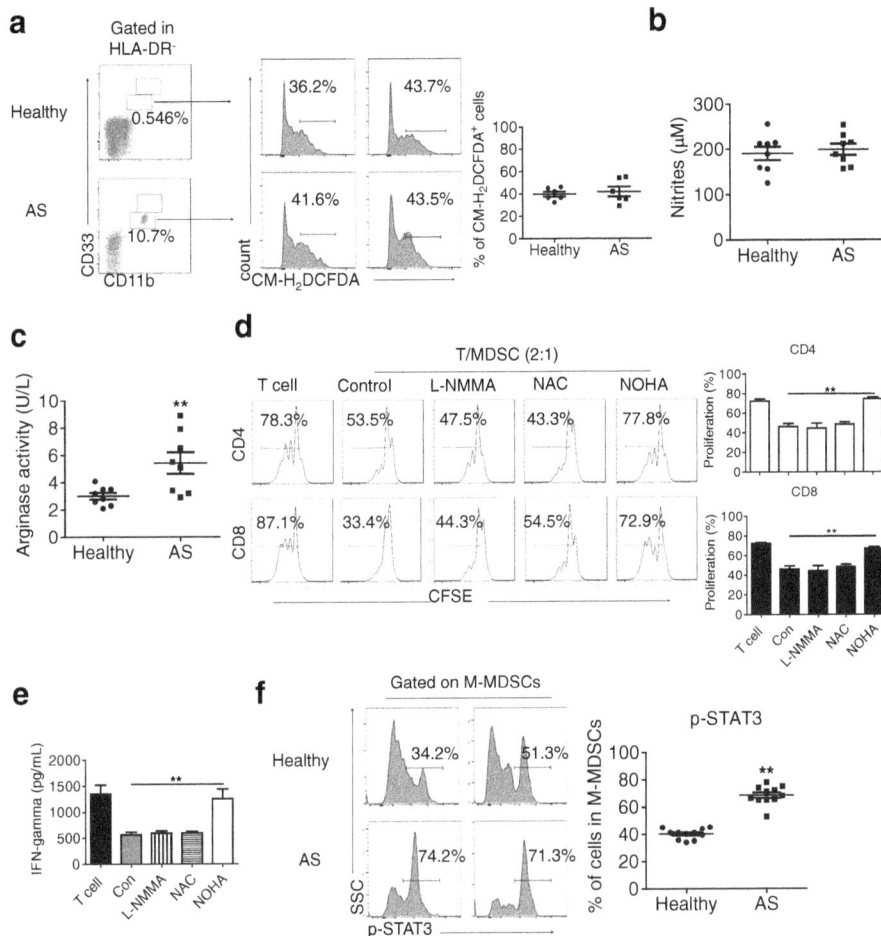

Fig. 4 AS-derived M-MDSCs suppress T cell responses in an arginase-I dependent manner. **a** ROS levels in M-MDSCs from patients with ankylosing spondylitis or healthy controls (n = 6) were measured by flow cytometric analysis (*left*). HLA-DR$^{-/low}$CD11b^{int}CD33^{int} cells were first gated, and the percentage of CM-H$_2$DCFDA$^+$ cells is shown. Both representative results (*left*) and means ± SEM from three independent experiments (*right*) are included. **b** NO content in plasma in sorted M-MDSCs from ankylosing spondylitis patients and healthy controls. **c** Arginase activity in M-MDSCs from healthy controls (n = 6) and from patients at ankylosing spondylitis. **d** Effects of different inhibitors on the suppressive function of M-MDSCs from ankylosing spondylitis patients were evaluated by allogeneic mixed lymphocytes reaction. T cells were labeled with carboxyfluorescein succinimidyl ester (CFSE) and stimulated with anti-CD3/anti-CD28 (5 ng/ml). These cells were then co-cultured with M-MDSCs from the same donor at a 2:1 ratio with treatments as indicated for 3 days, and T cell proliferation was evaluated by a flow cytometry. N-hydroxy-L-arginine (NOHA) (an arginase inhibitor, 100 mM); L-NG-monomethyl-L-arginine [L-NMMA, an inducible nitric oxide synthase (iNOS) inhibitor, 100 mM]; N-acetylcysteine (NAC, a ROS inhibitor, 1 mM). **e** Production of interferon (IFN)-γ by T cell supernatants from (**d**) was measured by enzyme-linked immunosorbent assay (ELISA). **f** p-STAT3 levels in M-MDSCs from ankylosing spondylitis patients (n = 11) and the control population from healthy donors (n = 11) were measured by flow cytometric analysis. *AS* ankylosing spondylitis, *CFSE* carboxyfluorescein succinimidyl ester, *IFN* interferon, *L-NMMA* L-NG-monomethyl-L-arginine, *M-MDSCs* monocytic myeloid-derived suppressor cells, *NAC* N-acetylcysteine, *NOHA* N-hydroxy-nor-L-arginine

there is a positive correlation between the percentages of M-MDSCs and IL-17 levels in patients with AS. In addition to IL-17, circulating M-MDSCs are elevated significantly in patients with AS with positive correlations to elevated disease activity index, including BASDAI, ESR, and CRP. These data suggest that MDSCs play crucial roles in the regulation of AS.

MDSC-mediated suppression of T cell responses could be beneficial in pathological conditions characterized by the unopposed activation of the immune system such as

autoimmune diseases [11]. However, the therapeutic potential of MDSCs in autoimmune arthritis is contradictory. One study showed that the transfer of MDSCs derived from CIA mice and patients with RA facilitated disease progression [30]. In contrast, another study found that the adoptive transfer of CIA-derived MDSCs could reduce the severity of CIA, and the number of Th17 cells also decreased [31]. These inconsistent outcomes may arise from the heterogeneity of MDSCs, factors within the autoimmune inflammatory environment,

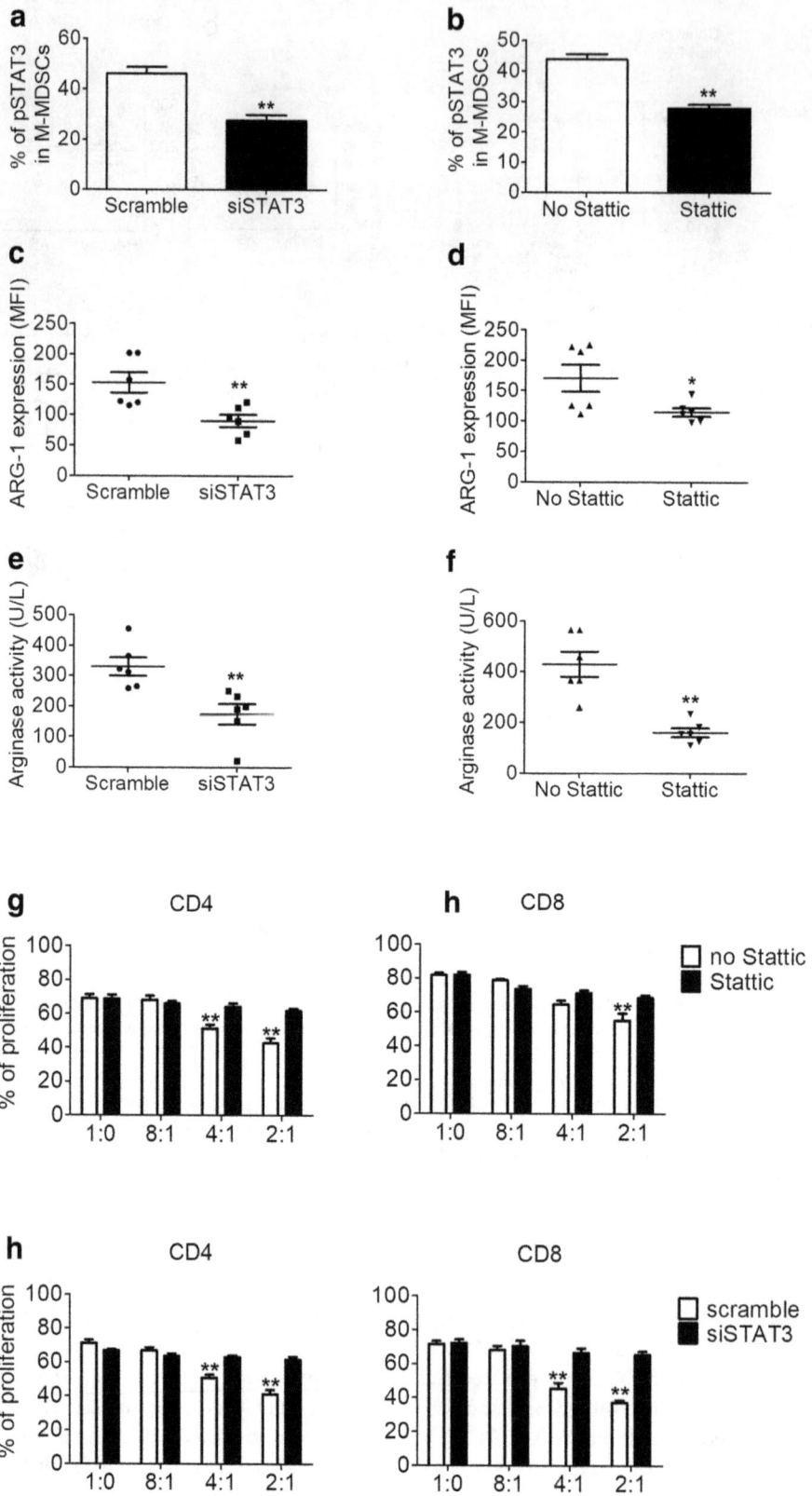

Fig. 5 (See legend on next page.)

(See figure on previous page.)
Fig. 5 Inhibition of pSTAT3- arginase-I signaling abrogates the suppressive activity of AS-derived M-MDSCs. **a** Inhibition of siSTAT3 signaling on M-MDSCs by scramble or siSTAT3 appropriately decreased the level of pSTAT3 (*$P < 0.05$). **b** Inhibition of STAT3 signaling on M-MDSCs by Stattic (10 μM) appropriately decreased the level of pSTAT3. Intracellular level of ARG1 is decreased with two independent methods of STAT3 signaling inhibition, including siSTAT3 (**c**) and Stattic (**d**). *y* axis shows MFI (*$P < 0.05$). ARG1 activity of ankylosing spondylitis patients derived M-MDSCs after pSTAT3 inhibition with siSTAT3 (**e**) and Stattic (**f**). Inhibition of STAT3 signaling ablates the suppressive activity of M-MDSCs from ankylosing spondylitis patients. Both pSTAT3 small molecule inhibitor (Stattic) (**g**), and STAT3 siRNA (**h**) were able to block the functional suppressive capability of ankylosing spondylitis patients derived M-MDSCs. *$P < 0.05$; **$P < 0.01$, compared with controls by unpaired *t* test *ARG1* arginase-I, *M-MDSCs* monocytic myeloid-derived suppressor cells, *pSTAT* phosphorylated signal transducer and activator of transcription 3

and different states of the disease. Further investigations are required to study the therapeutic effect of MDSCs in an AS model through AS-derived-M-MDSC transfer, which will be beneficial in understanding the pathological mechanism of AS and provide key insights for developing MDSC-based therapies to treat AS.

MDSCs are primarily defined by their suppressive function [32], however, the functions of MDSCs in patients with AS remain unclear. The T cell suppressive effect of MDSCs in malignant tumors is due to M-MDSCs rather than PMN-MDSCs [33]. However, PMN-MDSCs have been reported to show suppressive functions in autoimmune disease models [34]. It is possible that the phenotypes of MDSCs responsible for suppressing T cell functions differ between tumors and autoimmune diseases. In our study, we found that the T cell suppressive effect of MDSCs in patients with AS is due to M-MDSCs rather than PMN-MDSCs. We examined regulatory factors in M-MDSCs that could control its suppressive function. A critical pathway in tumors and periphery is mediated by STAT3 signaling in the M-MDSC population [35]. In murine models, pSTAT3 regulates the expansion of MDSCs; however, STAT3 has not been reported to directly regulate the T cell suppressive function of MDSCs [11]. In contrast, the immunosuppressive activity of human MDSCs derived from patients with cancer was found to be STAT3-dependent [36]. In this study, we demonstrated that STAT3 signaling plays a functional role in M-MDSCs derived from patients with AS by mediating their ability to suppress autologous T cell proliferation. STAT3 inhibition decreased the level of arginase-I and the T cell suppressive activity in AS-derived M-MDSCs. We also demonstrated that both siRNA suppression and pSTAT3 inhibition using a STAT3-specific inhibitor could abrogate the T cell suppressive function of AS-derived M-MDSCs as well as decrease the level and activity of arginase-I. These results demonstrate that STAT3 signaling is upstream of the arginase-I activity that mediates the suppression of T cell proliferation in patients with AS.

Several STAT3-dependent genes have been reported to play critical roles in M-MDSC function, indicating that there may be multiple pathways of STAT3-dependent immunosuppression. For instance, STAT3-dependent C/EBPβ transcription factor is critical in regulating immunosuppression [37]. HIF1α, another STAT3-dependent gene, mediates the differentiation into tumor-infiltrating macrophages [38]. Further investigations will be beneficial in testing some of these STAT3-dependent pathways in M-MDSCs.

Conclusions

We report that M-MDSCs were significantly elevated in patients with AS. M-MDSC numbers positively correlated with the AS disease index. The STAT3/arginase-I signaling pathway drove the expansion of M-MDSCs, and mediated the activation of the T cell suppressive function in AS-derived M-MDSCs. Our results collectively suggest that M-MDSCs play an important immunoregulatory role in patients with AS, and therapeutic approaches directed against M-MDSCs may lead to the alleviation of this disease.

Abbreviations
ARG1: Arginase-I; AS: Ankylosing spondylitis; BASDAI: Bath Ankylosing Spondylitis Disease Activity Index; CFSE: Carboxyfluorescein succinimidyl ester; CIA: Collagen-induced arthritis; CRP: C-reactive protein; ELISA: Enzyme-linked immunosorbent assay; ESR: Erythrocyte sedimentation rate; IL: Interleukin; iMCs: Immature myeloid cells; INF: Interferon; L-NMMA: L-NG-monomethyl-L-arginine; M-MDSCs: Monocytic myeloid-derived suppressor cells; NAC: N-acetylcysteine; NOHA: N-hydroxy-nor-L-arginine; PBMCs: Peripheral blood mononuclear cells; PMN-MDSC: Polymorphonuclear myeloid-derived suppressor cells; RA: Rheumatoid arthritis; ROS: Reactive oxygen species; STAT3: Signal transducer and activator of transcription 3; Th: T helper; Tregs: Regulatory T cells

Acknowledgements
We thank Shao-hua Song from the Department of Laboratory Medicine, Guangdong Second Provincial General Hospital, for kindly providing assistance in the clinical sample collection.

Funding
This work was supported by the National Natural Science Foundation of China (81700512) to YL; Natural Science Foundation of Guangdong Province (2016A030310252) to YL; Guandong Second Provincial General Hospital Youth Fund (YQ2016-007) to ZL.

Authors' contributions

All authors were involved in drafting the article or revising it critically for important intellectual content, and all authors approved the final version to be published. FL and LZ had full access to all of the data in the study and takes responsibility for the integrity of the data and the accuracy of the data analysis. YL, LZ, and FL contributed to study conception and design. YL, KZ, HJ, XZ, BC, and PL contributed to acquisition of data. YL, LZ, and FL contributed to analysis and interpretation of data:.

Consent for publication

Not applicable.

Competing interests

The authors declare that they have no competing interests.

Author details

[1]Guangzhou University of Chinese Medicine, Guangzhou, People's Republic of China. [2]The First Affiliated Hospital of Guangzhou University of Chinese Medicine, The Lingnan Medicine Research Center, Guangzhou 510405, People's Republic of China. [3]Department of Laboratory Medicine, Guangdong Second Provincial General Hospital, Guangzhou 510317, People's Republic of China. [4]Department of Hematology Oncology, Guangzhou Medical University, Guangzhou Women and Children's Medical Center, Guangzhou 510623, People's Republic of China.

References

1. Braun J, Sieper J. Ankylosing spondylitis. Lancet. 2007;369(9570):1379–90.
2. Braun J, Brandt J, Listing J, Zink A, Alten R, Golder W, Gromnica-Ihle E, Kellner H, Krause A, Schneider M, et al. Treatment of active ankylosing spondylitis with infliximab: a randomised controlled multicentre trial. Lancet. 2002;359(9313):1187–93.
3. Smith JA. Update on ankylosing spondylitis: current concepts in pathogenesis. Curr Allergy Asthma Rep. 2015;15(1):489.
4. Dakwar E, Reddy J, Vale FL, Uribe JS. A review of the pathogenesis of ankylosing spondylitis. Neurosurg Focus. 2008;24(1):E2.
5. Calin A. Comment on article by van der Linden et al. Evaluation of diagnostic criteria for ankylosing spondylitis: a proposal for modification of the New York criteria. Arthritis Rheum. 1985;28(3):357–9.
6. Appel H, Kuhne M, Spiekermann S, Ebhardt H, Grozdanovic Z, Kohler D, Dreimann M, Hempfing A, Rudwaleit M, Stein H, et al. Immunohistologic analysis of zygapophyseal joints in patients with ankylosing spondylitis. Arthritis Rheum. 2006;54(9):2845–51.
7. Cortes A, Hadler J, Pointon JP, Robinson PC, Karaderi T, Leo P, Cremin K, Pryce K, Harris J, Lee S, et al. Identification of multiple risk variants for ankylosing spondylitis through high-density genotyping of immune-related loci. Nat Genet. 2013;45(7):730–8.
8. Arroyo-Villa I, Bautista-Caro MB, Balsa A, Aguado-Acin P, Nuno L, Bonilla-Hernan MG, Puig-Kroger A, Martin-Mola E, Miranda-Carus ME. Frequency of Th17 CD4+ T cells in early rheumatoid arthritis: a marker of anti-CCP seropositivity. PLoS One. 2012;7(8):e42189.
9. Shen H, Goodall JC, Hill GJ. Frequency and phenotype of peripheral blood Th17 cells in ankylosing spondylitis and rheumatoid arthritis. Arthritis Rheum. 2009;60(6):1647–56.
10. Wang C, Liao Q, Hu Y, Zhong D. T lymphocyte subset imbalances in patients contribute to ankylosing spondylitis. Exp Ther Med. 2015;9(1):250–6.
11. Gabrilovich DI, Nagaraj S. Myeloid-derived suppressor cells as regulators of the immune system. Nat Rev Immunol. 2009;9(3):162–74.
12. Rabinovich GA, Gabrilovich D, Sotomayor EM. Immunosuppressive strategies that are mediated by tumor cells. Annu Rev Immunol. 2007;25:267–96.
13. Pan T, Zhong L, Wu S, Cao Y, Yang Q, Cai Z, Cai X, Zhao W, Ma N, Zhang W, et al. 17beta-Oestradiol enhances the expansion and activation of myeloid-derived suppressor cells via signal transducer and activator of transcription (STAT)-3 signalling in human pregnancy. Clin Exp Immunol. 2016;185(1):86–97.
14. Liu YF, Chen YY, He YY, Wang JY, Yang JP, Zhong SL, Jiang N, Zhou P, Jiang H, Zhou J. Expansion and activation of granulocytic, myeloid-derived suppressor cells in childhood precursor B cell acute lymphoblastic leukemia. J Leukoc Biol. 2017;102(2):449–58.
15. Bronte V, Brandau S, Chen SH, Colombo MP, Frey AB, Greten TF, Mandruzzato S, Murray PJ, Ochoa A, Ostrand-Rosenberg S, et al. Recommendations for myeloid-derived suppressor cell nomenclature and characterization standards. Nat Commun. 2016;7:12150.
16. Peranzoni E, Zilio S, Marigo I, Dolcetti L, Zanovello P, Mandruzzato S, Bronte V. Myeloid-derived suppressor cell heterogeneity and subset definition. Curr Opin Immunol. 2010;22(2):238–44.
17. Dumitru CA, Moses K, Trellakis S, Lang S, Brandau S. Neutrophils and granulocytic myeloid-derived suppressor cells: immunophenotyping, cell biology and clinical relevance in human oncology. Cancer Immunol Immunother. 2012;61(8):1155–67.
18. Bronte V, Zanovello P. Regulation of immune responses by L-arginine metabolism. Nat Rev Immunol. 2005;5(8):641–54.
19. Zea AH, Rodriguez PC, Atkins MB, Hernandez C, Signoretti S, Zabaleta J, McDermott D, Quiceno D, Youmans A, O'Neill A, et al. Arginase-producing myeloid suppressor cells in renal cell carcinoma patients: a mechanism of tumor evasion. Cancer Res. 2005;65(8):3044–8.
20. Guo C, Hu F, Yi H, Feng Z, Li C, Shi L, Li Y, Liu H, Yu X, Wang H, et al. Myeloid-derived suppressor cells have a proinflammatory role in the pathogenesis of autoimmune arthritis. Ann Rheum Dis. 2016;75(1):278–85.
21. Moret FM, van der Wurff-Jacobs KM, Bijlsma JW, Lafeber FP, van Roon JA. Synovial T cell hyporesponsiveness to myeloid dendritic cells is reversed by preventing PD-1/PD-L1 interactions. Arthritis Res Ther. 2014;16(6):497.
22. Wang Y, Tian J, Wang S. The potential therapeutic role of myeloid-derived suppressor cells in autoimmune arthritis. Semin Arthritis Rheum. 2016; 45(4):490–5.
23. van der Linden S, Valkenburg HA, Cats A. Evaluation of diagnostic criteria for ankylosing spondylitis. A proposal for modification of the New York criteria. Arthritis Rheum. 1984;27(4):361–8.
24. Garrett S, Jenkinson T, Kennedy LG, Whitelock H, Gaisford P, Calin A. A new approach to defining disease status in ankylosing spondylitis: the bath ankylosing spondylitis disease activity index. J Rheumatol. 1994;21(12):2286–91.
25. Liu YF, Wei JY, Shi MH, Jiang H, Zhou J. Glucocorticoid induces hepatic steatosis by inhibiting activating transcription factor 3 (ATF3)/S100A9 protein signaling in granulocytic myeloid-derived suppressor cells. J Biol Chem. 2016;291(41):21771–85.
26. Srivastava MK, Sinha P, Clements VK, Rodriguez P, Ostrand-Rosenberg S. Myeloid-derived suppressor cells inhibit T-cell activation by depleting cystine and cysteine. Cancer Res. 2010;70(1):68–77.
27. Kortylewski M, Kujawski M, Wang T, Wei S, Zhang S, Pilon-Thomas S, Niu G, Kay H, Mule J, Kerr WG, et al. Inhibiting Stat3 signaling in the hematopoietic system elicits multicomponent antitumor immunity. Nat Med. 2005;11(12):1314–21.
28. Condamine T, Gabrilovich DI. Molecular mechanisms regulating myeloid-derived suppressor cell differentiation and function. Trends Immunol. 2011; 32(1):19–25.
29. Thevenot PT, Sierra RA, Raber PL, Al-Khami AA, Trillo-Tinoco J, Zarreii P, Ochoa AC, Cui Y, Del VL, Rodriguez PC. The stress-response sensor chop regulates the function and accumulation of myeloid-derived suppressor cells in tumors. Immunity. 2014;41(3):389–401.
30. Fujii W, Ashihara E, Hirai H, Nagahara H, Kajitani N, Fujioka K, Murakami K, Seno T, Yamamoto A, Ishino H, et al. Myeloid-derived suppressor cells play crucial roles in the regulation of mouse collagen-induced arthritis. J Immunol. 2013;191(3):1073–81.
31. Crook KR, Jin M, Weeks MF, Rampersad RR, Baldi RM, Glekas AS, Shen Y, Esserman DA, Little P, Schwartz TA, et al. Myeloid-derived suppressor cells regulate T cell and B cell responses during autoimmune disease. J Leukoc Biol. 2015;97(3):573–82.
32. Gabrilovich DI, Bronte V, Chen SH, Colombo MP, Ochoa A, Ostrand-Rosenberg S, Schreiber H. The terminology issue for myeloid-derived suppressor cells. Cancer Res. 2007;67(1):425. 426

33. Marigo I, Bosio E, Solito S, Mesa C, Fernandez A, Dolcetti L, Ugel S, Sonda N, Bicciato S, Falisi E, et al. Tumor-induced tolerance and immune suppression depend on the C/EBPbeta transcription factor. Immunity. 2010;32(6):790–802.
34. Ioannou M, Alissafi T, Lazaridis I, Deraos G, Matsoukas J, Gravanis A, Mastorodemos V, Plaitakis A, Sharpe A, Boumpas D, et al. Crucial role of granulocytic myeloid-derived suppressor cells in the regulation of central nervous system autoimmune disease. J Immunol. 2012;188(3):1136–46.
35. Nefedova Y, Nagaraj S, Rosenbauer A, Muro-Cacho C, Sebti SM, Gabrilovich DI. Regulation of dendritic cell differentiation and antitumor immune response in cancer by pharmacologic-selective inhibition of the janus-activated kinase 2/signal transducers and activators of transcription 3 pathway. Cancer Res. 2005;65(20):9525–35.
36. Poschke I, Mougiakakos D, Hansson J, Masucci GV, Kiessling R. Immature immunosuppressive CD14+HLA-DR−/low cells in melanoma patients are Stat3hi and overexpress CD80, CD83, and DC-sign. Cancer Res. 2010;70(11):4335–45.
37. Marigo I, Bosio E, Solito S, Mesa C, Fernandez A, Dolcetti L, Ugel S, Sonda N, Bicciato S, Falisi E, et al. Tumor-induced tolerance and immune suppression depend on the C/EBPbeta transcription factor. Immunity. 2010;32(6):790–802.
38. Corzo CA, Condamine T, Lu L, Cotter MJ, Youn JI, Cheng P, Cho HI, Celis E, Quiceno DG, Padhya T, et al. HIF-1alpha regulates function and differentiation of myeloid-derived suppressor cells in the tumor microenvironment. J Exp Med. 2010;207(11):2439–53.

9

The relationship between ferritin and urate levels and risk of gout

Tahzeeb Fatima[1], Cushla McKinney[1], Tanya J. Major[1], Lisa K. Stamp[2], Nicola Dalbeth[3], Cory Iverson[4], Tony R. Merriman[1*] ⓘ and Jeffrey N. Miner[5]

Abstract

Background: Ferritin positively associates with serum urate and an interventional study suggests that iron has a role in triggering gout flares. The objective of this study was to further explore the relationship between iron/ferritin and urate/gout.

Methods: European (100 cases, 60 controls) and Polynesian (100 cases, 60 controls) New Zealand (NZ) males and 189 US male cases and 60 male controls participated. The 10,727 participants without gout were from the Jackson Heart (JHS; African American = 1260) and NHANES III (European = 5112; African American = 4355) studies. Regression analyses were adjusted for age, sex, body mass index and C-reactive protein. To test for a causal relationship between ferritin and urate, bidirectional two-sample Mendelian randomization analysis was performed.

Results: Serum ferritin positively associated with gout in NZ Polynesian (OR (per 10 ng ml^{-1} increase) = 1.03, p = 1.8E–03) and US (OR = 1.11, p = 7.4E–06) data sets but not in NZ European (OR = 1.00, p = 0.84) data sets. Ferritin positively associated with urate in NZ Polynesian (β (mg dl^{-1}) = 0.014, p = 2.5E–04), JHS (β = 0.009, p = 3.2E–05) and NHANES III (European β = 0.007, p = 5.1E–11; African American β = 0.011, p = 2.1E–16) data sets but not in NZ European (β = 0.009, p = 0.31) or US (β = 0.041, p = 0.15) gout data sets. Ferritin positively associated with the frequency of gout flares in two of the gout data sets. By Mendelian randomization analysis a one standard deviation unit increase in iron and ferritin was, respectively, associated with 0.11 (p = 8E–04) and 0.19 mg dl^{-1} (p = 2E–04) increases in serum urate. There was no evidence for a causal effect of urate on iron/ferritin.

Conclusions: These data replicate the association of ferritin with serum urate. Increased ferritin levels associated with gout and flare frequency. There was evidence of a causal effect of iron and ferritin on urate.

Keywords: Urate, Gout, Ferritin, Iron, Association, Causal, Mendelian randomization

Background

Ferritin stores excess iron in a nontoxic form. Urate is a byproduct of purine catabolism in humans. In some hyperuricemic individuals, supersaturation of urate (> 0.41 mmol/L) can result in deposition of monosodium urate (MSU) crystals in the synovium with gout arising due to an innate immune response [1]. Urate acts as a chelator for iron and, in turn, iron can modulate the activity of xanthine oxidase and the production of urate [2]. Indeed, ferritin has been positively associated with serum urate in both the US National Health and Nutrition Examination Survey (NHANES) [3] and the China Health and Nutrition Survey

[4] with elevation in serum urate suggested as an indicator of iron overload [5]. Iron could contribute to gouty inflammation by forming complexes with MSU crystals, stimulating oxidative stress through the generation of reactive oxygen species, and contributing to granulocyte and complement activation [6]. A decrease in gout flares following phlebotomy to attain near iron-deficient levels in hyperuricemic patients [7] is also suggestive of a role in gout.

Food is the primary source of iron, providing heme and nonheme iron through animal and plant sources, respectively. Diet is also a key source of purines. Interestingly, purine-rich foods from an animal-based diet have been associated with increased risk of recurrent gout attacks while purine-rich foods from a plant-based diet are not [8]. These observations, combined with the

* Correspondence: tony.merriman@otago.ac.nz
[1]Department of Biochemistry, University of Otago, Dunedin, New Zealand
Full list of author information is available at the end of the article

other observational and intervention data [3, 5, 7], are consistent with the hypothesis that iron in purine-rich foods (e.g., red meat) could be a causal factor for gout and flare frequency.

Despite a positive association of iron/ferritin with urate, no data are yet available investigating a possible causal association. The positive association between urate and iron/ferritin could result from unmeasured confounders [9, 10]. Mendelian randomization can be used to explore the causal association between an exposure and an outcome [11]. This approach exploits random assignment of alleles at conception to disentangle cause and effect in the presence of confounding. Genetic variants that predict an observational exposure are used as unconfounded proxy instruments for the exposure itself to provide evidence of causation for the outcome of interest.

In this study, we first aimed to replicate the observational association of serum ferritin with serum urate and to test for association of serum ferritin with gout and flare frequency. The second aim was to assess a possible causal relationship between iron/ferritin and urate using Mendelian randomization.

Methods
Biochemical analyses
Study participants
The NZ participants were recruited during 2006–2014 from community-based settings and primary and secondary health care. The NZ sample set comprised male NZ European (100 cases and 60 controls) and Polynesian (Māori and/or Pacific Island ancestry; 100 cases and 60 controls) individuals. All NZ gout cases were intercritical and had a clinically confirmed diagnosis of gout by the 1977 American Rheumatology Association (ARA) preliminary classification criteria [12]. New Zealand gout cases were not screened for current use of anti-inflammatory therapy. New Zealand control participants without self-reported gout were convenience sampled from the Auckland, Otago and Canterbury regions. The US group comprised a mixture of people of Latino, African American and European ancestry (189 male gout cases and 60 male controls) and serum samples were purchased from Bioreclamation Inc. (New Cassel, NY, USA). All US gout cases had crystal-proven or clinically diagnosed gout, no active acute gout at the time of sample draw, and no nonsteroidal anti-inflammatory drug or colchicine usage within 2 weeks of the sample draw. The US control group comprised sex-matched and ancestrally-matched volunteers. Individuals with a history of liver damage or disease were excluded from the NZ and US case group and US control participants were included if they had never been diagnosed with gout and were not currently taking any nonsteroidal anti-inflammatory drug or colchicine. The Lower South Ethics Committee (OTA/

99/11/098) and the NZ Multi-region Ethics Committee (MEC/05/10/130) granted ethical approval for the NZ arm. In the US, recruitment of participants for the study had applicable local regulatory requirements (including Institutional Review Board approval). Written informed consent was obtained from all subjects.

Publicly available data from two cohorts were used for serum ferritin versus urate association analyses. A total of 1260 African American individuals were included from the Jackson Heart Study (JHS) [13] via the Database of Genotypes and Phenotypes (approval #834: The Genetic Basis of Gout). The second data set was The Third National Health and Nutrition Examination Survey (NHANES III) cohort (https://wwwn.cdc.gov/nchs/nhanes/nhanes3/Default.aspx) [14], comprised of 4355 African American and 5112 European individuals. Subjects who self-reported as taking any diuretic or other urate-lowering medication(s), or had kidney disease or gout, or had first-degree relatives with gout were excluded. This categorization was made to assess urate association only in non gout subjects and to minimize bias due to gout or other potential factors affecting urate levels and thus differed from the criteria applied to the previous study that used the same NHANES III data [3]. Also, in contrast to Ghio et al. [3], we analyzed the NHANES III European and African American participants separately and adjusted by C-reactive protein (CRP) levels. Additional file 1: Tables S1 and S2 report the demographic and clinical data for all of the study groups.

Serum biomarker measurements
Additional file 1 describes the determination of biochemical markers (serum urate, iron, transferrin, ferritin and CRP) for this study.

Statistical analyses
Differences in the means for intergroup and intragroup comparisons were calculated using an unpaired t test in R (v3.3.2). Logistic and linear regression analyses were carried out using R v3.3.2 [15] to test for an association of serum ferritin (explanatory variable) with gout (binary response variable) and urate (continuous response variable), respectively. Individuals with missing data for any variable were excluded. Adjusted odds ratios (ORs) and β estimates were obtained by including age (in years), sex, body mass index (BMI) and CRP, and the number of self-reported Polynesian grandparents for the Polynesian sample set, as covariates in the regression models. Ferritin is a marker of inflammation [16] and therefore CRP was included as a covariate in the regression models to control for the possibility that association between ferritin/iron and risk of gout and flare frequency was a consequence of elevated ferritin levels in hyperuricemia [17] and gout [18] per se owing to the increased inflammatory milieu. The urate-producing enzyme xanthine oxidase also releases

iron from ferritin [19]. Therefore, the average levels of ferritin (and other iron measures) were also compared within the NZ and US gout cases by stratifying the data sets according to the usage of the xanthine oxidase inhibitor allopurinol. Odds ratios for logistic models and β estimates for linear regression models were meta-analyzed using the meta package in R (v3.3.2). A Q statistic was calculated to measure the heterogeneity; if the heterogeneity was significant ($p < 0.05$) the fixed-effect model was replaced with a random-effect model.

Mendelian randomization analysis
Selection of instrumental variable
Mendelian randomization (MR) analysis in this study was based on publicly available summary estimate data for European individuals from the Genetics of Iron Status Consortium ($n = 48,978$) [20] and the Global Urate Genetics Consortium ($n = 110,347$) [21]. The genetic variants were selected as instruments for iron/ferritin and urate from these GWAS and $p \leq 5 \times 10^{-8}$ was set as a threshold for a variant to be a valid instrument, corresponding to an F statistic of 30 and considered an adequately powered instrument for MR analysis [22]. To minimize pleiotropy, a priori literature searches and eQTL (expression quantitative trait locus) data available online (https://gtexportal.org/home/) and Haploreg v4.1(https://pubs.broadinstitute.org/mammals/haploreg/haploreg.php) were used to test for association of genetic variants to be included in instruments with expression of genes implicated in iron/ferritin and urate metabolism (as appropriate)—if there was evidence for association then the genetic variant was excluded.

Statistical analyses
Two-sample Mendelian randomization analysis was performed using the MR-Base (Mendelian Randomization-Base) platform (www.mrbase.org) [23]. The files for exposure instruments were manually uploaded into MR-Base. To eliminate linkage disequilibrium (LD) of $r^2 > 0.6$ between the instruments, the 'LD clumping' command was used. To ensure that the effect estimate of the exposure instrument corresponds to the same allele as the outcome effect, the 'allele harmonization' command was used. The Wald ratio method [24, 25] was used to separately calculate the Mendelian randomization estimate for each instrument. With a single instrument, the Wald ratio method is as robust to detect a causal effect as a two-stage least squares method [26, 27]. The effect estimates were combined together in multiple-instrument MR via the inverse-variance weighted method [22], while the Egger-regression method [28] was applied as a sensitivity test for a posteriori adjustment for horizontal pleiotropy within multiple-instrument Mendelian randomization. To determine whether any individual instrument was an outlier, leave-one-out permutation analysis [29]

was used as a sensitivity test. A power calculation (for a continuous outcome) was performed using the online calculator for Mendelian randomization studies (https://sb452.shinyapps.io/power) [30].

Results
Demographic and biochemical information on the study cohorts is presented in Additional file 1: Tables S1 and S2.

Biochemical observational association analysis
Association with serum urate concentration
Serum ferritin concentration was positively associated with serum urate concentration in nongout African American individuals from the JHS (males β per 10 ng ml^{-1} increase (mg dl^{-1}) = 0.007, $p = 9.3E–03$; females β = 0.014, $p = 1.7E–03$) and NHANES III (males β = 0.006, $p = 5.1E–04$; females β = 0.016, $p = 1.8E–15$) as well as Europeans (males β = 0.004, $p = 6.6E–03$; females β = 0.012, $p = 3.4E–10$) from the NHANES III study (Table 1). It was interesting to observe the consistently stronger association in females than males (2-fold to 3-fold greater effect size in females; P_Q by meta-analysis of males and females was 0.27 in JHS, 1E–04 in NHANES III African American and 1.5E–03 in NHANES III European). A positive association between ferritin and SU was also observed in NZ Polynesian (β = 0.014, $p = 2.5E–04$) individuals, but not in NZ European (β = 0.009, $p = 0.31$) or US (β = 0.041, $p = 0.15$) individuals from the gout control sample sets (Table 1).

Association with gout
The average levels of ferritin were elevated in both NZ Polynesian ($p = 2.3E–04$) and US ($p = 6.6E–17$) gout cases compared to controls, but not between NZ European gout cases and controls ($p = 0.21$) (Table 2). An increase in serum ferritin of 10 ng ml^{-1} was associated with an increased risk of developing gout in NZ Polynesian (OR (CI) =1.03 (1.01; 1.05), $p = 1.8E–03$) and US (OR (CI) =1.11 (1.07; 1.17), $p = 7.4E–06$) individuals. However, ferritin was not associated with increased risk of gout in the NZ European sample set (OR (CI) =1.00 (0.97; 1.02), $p = 0.84$) (Table 2). Exclusion of gout patients on allopurinol treatment from the US sample set did not influence the association of ferritin levels with gout (OR (CI) =1.11 (1.06; 1.16), $p = 2.4E–05$).

Association of ferritin with flare frequency
We also tested for an association of serum ferritin, CRP and serum urate with self-reported frequency of gout flares (per year). Each 10 ng ml^{-1} increase in ferritin was associated with an increased frequency of gout flares in the US (β = 0.02 flares/year, $p = 2E–03$) and NZ European (β = 0.09, $p = 0.04$) individuals but not in NZ Polynesian (β = – 0.11, $p = 0.14$) individuals. C-reactive protein and

Table 1 Association of ferritin (per 10 ng ml^{-1} increment) with serum urate (mg dl^{-1})

Population	n^a	β (95% CI)^b	p^b	β (95% CI)^c	p^c
NZ European	60	0.011 (− 0.006; 0.027)	0.24	0.009 (− 0.009; 0.027)	0.31
NZ Polynesian	60	0.015 (0.007; 0.023)	1.4E−04	0.014 (0.007; 0.022)	2.5E−04
US	60	0.048 (− 0.006; 0.102)	0.079	0.041 (− 0.015; 0.097)	0.15
JHS (males)	567	0.008 (0.002; 0.014)	9.6E−03	0.007 (0.002; 0.014)	9.3E−03
JHS (females)	693	0.023 (0.015; 0.032)	1.6E−07	0.014 (0.005; 0.022)	1.7E−03
JHS (combined)	1260	0.027 (0.023; 0.033)	1.8E−27	0.009 (0.005; 0.014)	3.2E−05
NHANES III African American (males)	1925	0.010 (0.007; 0.014)	7.2E−09	0.006 (0.003; 0.009)	5.1E−04
NHANES III African American (females)	2430	0.028 (0.027; 0.032)	1.3E−42	0.016 (0.012; 0.020)	1.8E−15
NHANES III African American (combined)	4355	0.029 (0.026; 0.031)	2.0E−97	0.011 (0.008; 0.013)	2.1E−16
NHANES III European (males)	2460	0.006 (0.003; 0.009)	1.0E−04	0.004 (0.001; 0.007)	6.6E−03
NHANES III European (females)	2652	0.019 (0.015; 0.023)	1.3E−22	0.012 (0.008; 0.015)	3.4E−10
NHANES III European (combined)	5112	0.025 (0.023; 0.028)	6.9E−84	0.007 (0.005; 0.009)	5.1E−11
Meta-analyzed data	10,907	0.025 (0.021; 0.028)	9.3E−34	0.009 (0.007; 0.011)	3.9E−32

Beta values represent change in serum urate in mg dl^{-1} per 10 ng ml^{-1} increase in concentration of serum ferritin

CI confidence interval, *NZ* New Zealand, US United States, JHS Jackson Heart Study, NHANES National Health and Nutrition Examination Survey

[a]Number of nongout (control) individuals

[b]Unadjusted

[c]Adjusted for age, body mass index, C-reactive protein and number of self-reported Polynesian grandparents in the NZ Polynesian analyses. Combined analyses are additionally adjusted for sex

urate concentrations were not associated with frequency of gout flares in all three data sets (Table 3).

Association of ferritin levels with allopurinol use

Significantly increased serum ferritin levels were observed among participants with gout who reported taking allopurinol in the NZ Polynesian ($p = 0.005$) and US ($p = 0.02$) sample sets; however, the average levels of ferritin were not significantly different in the NZ European sample set when the same stratification was done ($p = 0.47$) (Table 4).

Analysis with log-transformed ferritin

The ferritin distribution deviated from normality for all study groups (Additional file 1: Figure S1, S2), therefore the data were log transformed. Results for the log-transformed (normalized) data are presented

in Additional file 1: Tables S3–S5. The results were similar to those from the untransformed data.

Mendelian randomization analysis

The Mendelian randomization analysis had 100% power to detect a causal effect (change in outcome in SD units per SD change in exposure) of 0.1 at $p < 0.05$. The two GWASs selected for two-sample MR (84,978 for iron measures [20] and 110,347 for serum urate [21]) had an overlap of 20,160 individuals; this overlap is considered sufficiently low to avoid any potential bias in Mendelian randomization estimates [31].

Additional file 1: Table S6 provides the list of genetic variants evaluated as instrumental variables for iron ($n = 3$), ferritin ($n = 5$) and urate ($n = 3$). Details of selection of these instruments, along with approaches to minimize pleiotropy, are outlined in Additional file 1 and Additional file 1: Figure S3.

Table 2 Comparison of average values of serum ferritin (ng ml^{-1}) in gout case–control groups and the association with gout

Population	Comparison of average		Association analysis			
	p	(95% CI)$_{for\ difference}$	OR (95% CI)^a	p^a	OR (95% CI)^b	p^b
NZ European	0.21	(−97.46; 22.02)	1.01 (0.99; 1.03)	0.22	1.00 (0.97; 1.02)	0.84
NZ Polynesian	2.3E−04	(− 211.88; − 66.31)	1.03 (1.01; 1.05)	1.7E−03	1.03 (1.01; 1.06)	1.8E−03
US	6.6E−17	(− 167.19; − 107.16)	1.25 (1.07; 1.17)	1.5E−06	1.11 (1.07; 1.17)	7.4E−06
US no allopurinol	6.6E−17	(−167.19; − 107.16)	1.11 (1.07; 1.16)	4.5E−06	1.11 (1.06; 1.16)	2.4E−05
Meta-analysis^c	–	–	1.04 (1.01; 1.08)	0.02	1.04 (0.99; 1.09)	0.09

All OR values represent change in risk per 10 ng ml^{-1} increase in serum ferritin

CI confidence interval, *OR* odds ratio, *NZ* New Zealand, *US* United States

[a]Unadjusted

[b]Adjusted for age, body mass index, C-reactive protein and number of self-reported Polynesian grandparents in the NZ Polynesian analyses

[c]Only sample sets not stratified for allopurinol exposure were included in the meta-analysis

Table 3 Association of serum ferritin, CRP and serum urate with gout flares/year

Population	Ferritin (ng ml^{-1})				C-reactive protein (mg dl^{-1})		Serum urate (mg dl^{-1})	
	β (95% CI)[a]	p[a]	β (95% CI)[b]	p[b]	β (95% CI)[a]	p[a]	β (95% CI)[a]	p[a]
NZ European	0.09 (0.003; 0.17)	0.042	0.069 (− 0.01; 0.14)	0.067	1.75 (− 3.85; 7.37)	0.54	− 0.61 (− 1.48; 0.25)	0.16
NZ Polynesian	− 0.11 (− 0.24; 0.03)	0.14	−0.091 (− 0.22; 0.03)	0.15	−9.95 (− 23.75; 3.84)	0.16	−1.59 (− 3.88; 0.71)	0.17
US	0.02 (0.01; 0.04)	0.002	0.018 (0.001; 0.04)	0.043	0.10 (− 0.13; 0.35)	0.38	0.13 (− 0.04; 0.30)	0.13

Values represent change in the annual frequency of flares per 10 ng ml^{-1} increase in serum ferritin. Levels of urate are at the time of subject recruitment
CRP C-reactive protein, *CI* confidence interval, *NZ* New Zealand, *US* United States
[a]Adjusted for age, body mass index and number of self-reported Polynesian grandparents in the NZ Polynesian analyses
[b]Additionally adjusted for allopurinol usage

Iron biomarkers as exposures for urate as outcome

The strongest signal for iron and ferritin at *HFE rs1800562* (allele A) in the exposure data was found to causally increase urate levels in Europeans (iron β = 0.11 mg dl^{-1} increase in serum urate per standard deviation unit increase in iron, p = 0.0008; ferritin β = 0.19, p = 0.0002) (Table 5). A causal effect of ferritin levels on urate levels was also observed when *ABO rs651007* (allele T) was used as a single instrument in the Mendelian randomization model (β = 0.32, p = 0.02) (Table 5). However multiple-instrument Mendelian randomization using the inverse-variance weighted method did not indicate any causal effect of iron (β = 0.056, p = 0.15, P_Q = 0.18) or ferritin (β = 0.089, p = 0.17, P_Q = 0.06) on urate (Table 5). The nonsignificant effect remained consistent after a posteriori adjustment for horizontal pleiotropy, with effects across the variants showing heterogeneity, via MR-Egger for both iron (β = 0.064, p = 0.61, P_Q = 0.01) and ferritin (β = 0.16, p = 0.32, P_Q = 0.01) (Table 5). MR-Egger did not indicate high pleiotropy for an effect on urate using all three instruments for iron ($p_{intercept}$ = 0.95) and five instruments for ferritin ($p_{intercept}$ = 0.58) (Table 5). However, leave-one-out sensitivity analysis indicated *TMPRSS6 rs855791* and *SLC40A1 rs12693541* to be potential outliers driving a noncausal observed effect of iron and ferritin on urate, respectively (Table 6). Leaving these two variants out in a subsequent combined inverse-variance weighted analysis demonstrated iron (β = 0.11, p = 1.96E−04) and

ferritin (β = 0.14, p = 0.03) to causally increase urate levels in Europeans (Table 6).

Urate as exposure for iron biomarkers as outcome

None of the urate instruments (*SLC2A9 rs12498742*, *SLC16A9 rs1171614* and *SLC22A12 rs478607*) indicated causality for serum urate levels on iron and ferritin levels when tested individually (Additional file 1: Table S7). The noncausal relationship remained consistent when analyzed using multiple-instrument inverse-variance weighting and a posteriori adjustment for horizontal pleiotropy using MR-Egger (Additional file 1: Table S7). By leave-one-out analysis, none of the urate instruments was an outlier for a causal effect on iron or ferritin (Additional file 1: Table S8).

Discussion

We extended the previously reported associations of serum ferritin with serum urate [3, 4] using adjustment by CRP to exclude the possibility that the relationship is a consequence of the association of ferritin with inflammatory states, particularly since there is evidence that serum urate levels drop in acute inflammation in hospitalized patients [32]. The association of serum ferritin with serum urate has now been reported in European, Chinese, African American, and NZ Māori and Pacific (Polynesian) sample sets. We associated increased serum ferritin with the risk of gout and gout flares, although

Table 4 Self-reported allopurinol use and iron profile comparison in gout patients

Population/marker	No allopurinol	Allopurinol	p	(95% CI)$_{for\ difference}$
NZ European (*n*)	23	66	–	
Serum iron (μmol L^{-1})	100.44	98.65	0.77	(− 10.661; 14.258)
Serum ferritin (ng ml^{-1})	253.71	284.31	0.48	(− 115.787; 54.597)
NZ Polynesian (*n*)	22	74		
Serum iron (μmol L^{-1})	91.21	85.08	0.26	(− 4.592; 16.816)
Serum ferritin (ng ml^{-1})	373.81	494.32	0.005	(− 204.466; − 36.548)
US (*n*)	155	34		
Serum ferritin (ng ml^{-1})	158.57	248.21	0.02	(− 164.816; 14.451)

CI confidence interval, *NZ* New Zealand, *US* United States

Table 5 Association between iron/ferritin and urate using two-sample Mendelian randomization

MR analysis	Phenotype		Gene/ locus	Genetic variant	estimate	SE	(95% CI)	p-causal	Q–p	MR Egger_HP	
	Exposure	Outcome								intercept	p value
Wald ratio	Iron	Urate	TF	rs1525892	0.127	0.076	(− 0.02; 0.28)	0.093	–	–	–
–	Iron	Urate	HFE	rs1800562	0.107	0.032	(0.04; 0.17)	0.0008	–	–	–
–	Iron	Urate	TMPRSS6	rs855791	− 0.001	0.031	(− 0.06; 0.06)	0.99	–	–	–
IVW	Iron	Urate	–	All	0.056	0.039	(− 0.02; 0.13)	0.15	0.179	–	–
MR Egger	Iron	Urate	–	All	0.064	0.109	(− 0.15; 0.28)	0.61	0.011	− 0.0016	0.95
Wald ratio	Log ferritin	Urate	SLC40A1	rs12693541	− 0.068	0.076	(− 0.22; 0.08)	0.37	–	–	–
–	Log ferritin	Urate	HFE	rs1800562	0.190	0.057	(0.08; 0.30)	0.0002	–	–	–
–	Log ferritin	Urate	TMPRSS6	rs2413450	0.011	0.106	(− 0.20; 0.22)	0.92	–	–	–
–	Log ferritin	Urate	TEX14	rs411988	− 0.048	0.123	(− 0.29; 0.19)	0.70	–	–	–
–	Log ferritin	Urate	ABO	rs651007	0.320	0.140	(0.05; 0.59)	0.022	–	–	–
IVW	Log ferritin	Urate	–	All	0.089	0.066	(− 0.04; 0.22)	0.18	0.063	–	–
MR Egger	Log ferritin	Urate	–	All	0.160	0.134	(− 0.10; 0.42)	0.32	0.014	− 0.0067	0.58

All beta estimates presented as an effect of per standard deviation unit change in iron and ferritin on change in urate (mg dl^{-1})

MR Mendelian randomization, *SE* standard error, *CI* confidence interval, p-*causal p* value using MR analysis, Q–p Cochran's heterogeneity test showing *p* value for heterogeneity, *MR Egger_HP* Egger test for horizontal pleiotropy, *IVW* meta-analysis using inverse-variance method, *MR Egger* Mendelian randomization using Egger regression

for both relationships an association was observed in only two of the three data sets used. Given that allopurinol exposure raises ferritin levels and given the limited number of gout patients not exposed to allopurinol available to us, we cannot conclude that the gout–ferritin association is independent of allopurinol exposure. Mendelian randomization single instrument analysis (Table 5) and multiple instrument leave-one-out analysis (Table 6) provided evidence for a causal role of iron and ferritin in increasing urate levels in Europeans. In single instrument analysis, *HFE rs1800562* provided evidence of causality. In multiple instrument 'leave-one-out' sensitivity analysis, excluding two variants (*TMPRSS6 rs855791* and *SLC40A1 rs12693541*) also provided evidence of causality. These variants may obscure a causal effect because they mediate an unidentified link between urate and ferritin metabolism.

Metal ions can potentially cause oxidative stress when bound to storage or transport proteins [33] and urate is a well-known antioxidant in humans, by scavenging oxygen radicals, singlet oxygen and oxo-heme oxidants [34–36]. Thus it has been proposed that urate could reduce iron-catalyzed oxidative stress by acting as a metal chelator [37]. Xanthine oxidase acts as the sole enzymatic source of urate in humans and exposure to iron may enhance its activity [2, 38, 39]. This may explain a causal

Table 6 Leave-one-out sensitivity analysis for association between iron/ferritin and urate using inverse-variance weighted two-sample Mendelian randomization

Phenotype		Instrumental variant excluded from IVW analysis	β estimate	(95% CI)	p-causal
Exposure	Outcome				
Iron	Urate	TF rs1525892	0.050	(− 0.06; 0.16)	0.35
Iron	Urate	HFE rs1800562	0.017	(− 0.07; 0.10)	0.70
Iron	Urate	TMPRSS6 rs855791	0.110	(0.05; 0.17)	2.0E−04
Iron	Urate	All	0.050	(− 0.02; 0.13)	0.15
Log ferritin	Urate	SLC40A1 rs12693541	0.141	(0.02; 0.27)	0.027
Log ferritin	Urate	HFE rs1800562	0.007	(− 0.14; 0.15)	0.93
Log ferritin	Urate	TMPRSS6 rs2413450	0.101	(− 0.05; 0.26)	0.20
Log ferritin	Urate	TEX14 rs411988	0.103	(− 0.04; 0.25)	0.17
Log ferritin	Urate	ABO rs651007	0.070	(− 0.06; 0.20)	0.30
Log ferritin	Urate	All	0.089	(− 0.04; 0.22)	0.18

All beta estimates presented as an effect of per standard deviation unit change in iron and ferritin on change in urate (mg dl^{-1})

IVW meta-analysis using inverse-variance method, *CI* confidence interval, p-*causal p* value using IVW meta-analysis, *HFE* human hemochromatosis protein, *TMPRSS6* transmembrane protease serine-6, *ABO* alpha 1–3-*N*-acetylgalactosaminyltransferase

effect of iron on serum urate levels. A Mendelian randomization analysis demonstrated causality of iron/ferritin on renal function with increased levels being protective [40]. Given that reduced renal function is causal of hyperuricemia, it is unlikely that our Mendelian randomization data, supporting a causal role for iron/ferritin increasing serum urate levels, is mediated via an effect on kidney function. An increase in urate in both rodents [41, 42] and humans [43] in response to acute exposure to iron also supports a direct link between levels of iron and urate. Elevated serum urate is sometimes used as a cue to screen for hemochromatosis [5]. Our study, however, did not provide any evidence supporting a causal effect of urate on iron/ferritin levels.

We found a positive correlation between the number of gout flares and ferritin. Iron deposits have been reported to be consistently present in the synovial membrane of people with rheumatoid arthritis but not those with other joint pathologies [44]. Some rodent studies have also demonstrated an improvement in joint-related inflammation following the removal of iron by chelation treatment [45, 46]. Maintenance of near iron deficiency by depleting the levels via phlebotomy in people with gout induces either complete or marked reduction in incidence and severity of gout flares in humans [7].

Iron-rich foods are top triggers for gout flares: 62.5% people with gout reporting seafood/fish, 35.2% red meat [47]. There is a positive correlation between the consumption of red meat and incident gout risk in a study of 28,990 men [48], and another study in 47,150 men associated the consumption of meat and seafood, but not purine-rich vegetables, with an increased risk of incident gout [49]. A Turkish retrospective study indicated that higher consumption of total meat (including fish) acts as a precipitating factor for gout flares [50]. Also, purines from animal-based, but not plant-based, food have been associated with increased risk of recurrent gout attacks [8]. In line with these findings there is an association of increased consumption of red meat with hyperuricemia in NHANES III [51]. It is possible that, additional to purines, the iron content of animal-based foods contributes to the risk of gout and flares.

There was elevation of serum ferritin levels in individuals on allopurinol treatment. This is of interest as xanthine oxidase is involved in the release of iron from ferritin and facilitating cellular stress through the production of hydroxyl radicals [19]. Use of allopurinol as a xanthine oxidase inhibitor has been attributed to an increased iron overload in rodent liver cells and elevated serum iron in patients with secondary gout [52]. Although a possible influence of allopurinol in iron metabolism in human is unclear, our results are consistent with previous reports [53, 54], namely that our data imply higher serum ferritin levels in gout patients on allopurinol therapy. Confirming the possible effect of allopurinol on iron metabolism in gout patients, using cohorts that are matched for clinical features of gout, could assist decision-making in treatment options for patients with a risk of iron overload. It is interesting to observe that a possible consequence of allopurinol exposure in gout could be an increase in serum urate levels via a possible causal effect of increased ferritin levels, although any increase would be considerably smaller than the decrease exacted by inhibition of xanthine oxidase by allopurinol.

There are several limitations to our study. Firstly, the gout cases were ascertained differently between the NZ and US cohorts (by clinical diagnosis only and by a combination of clinical diagnosis and crystal-proven gout, respectively). Furthermore, the NZ gout cases were not screened for current exposure to anti-inflammatory medication, a potential confounder. Secondly, only a limited number of possible confounders were adjusted for in the serum ferritin versus serum urate/gout/flares analyses. Other possible confounders could be alcohol (and other dietary exposures), liver steatosis and diabetes. The primary reason for using a limited set of confounders was the limited data available in the US gout sample set. Therefore, our observational epidemiological data can only support the observation that increased ferritin levels associate with serum urate levels, the risk of gout and the number of self-reported flares and cannot be used to claim that this association is independent of known confounders. Certainly, our data support a role for allopurinol in raising ferritin levels (Table 4). We do note, however, that the Mendelian randomization analysis supported a causal role for increased serum ferritin levels in increasing serum urate levels. Thirdly, self-report of gout flares can be regarded as an inaccurate method of flare frequency ascertainment, although it is the only practical way of collecting these data in large cohorts for epidemiological studies. However, it has been reported that, compared to the gold standard of physician assessment of flare, self-reported flares have a high sensitivity of 91% [55]. Finally, the Mendelian randomization data are unreplicated and only performed using cohorts of European ancestry. Currently it is not possible to replicate owing to the unavailability of suitable independent sample sets.

The consistency of our observational findings with previously reported experimental and clinical intervention studies and the positive causal association via Mendelian randomization analysis, albeit unreplicated, support the argument that there is a causal relationship between serum iron/ferritin and urate. This could have clinical implications with respect to causing gout. (We are unaware of any studies investigating links between hemochromatosis and gout.) Furthermore, our data support investigation of the possibility of an iron-rich diet as a trigger for gout flares that may ultimately improve flare avoidance advice given to people with gout.

Conclusions

This study further confirmed the observational relationship between increased serum ferritin and iron levels and serum urate levels. We provide the first evidence for positive association of serum ferritin levels with the risk of gout and with the frequency of gout flares. By Mendelian randomization there was evidence for a causal relationship for ferritin and iron in increasing urate levels, but not for urate increasing ferritin and iron levels. Clinically, our data suggest that consideration of avoidance of iron-rich foods could improve flare avoidance advice given to people with gout.

Abbreviations

ABO: Alpha 1–3-N-acetylgalactosaminyltransferase; ARA: American Rheumatology Association; BMI: Body mass index; CI: Confidence interval; CRP: C-reactive protein; eQTL: Expression quantitative trait locus; GWAS: Genome-wide association study; HFE: Human hemochromatosis protein; JHS: Jackson Heart Study; LD: Linkage disequilibrium; MR: Mendelian randomization; MSU: Monosodium urate; NHANES: National Health and Nutrition Examination Survey; NY: New York; NZ: New Zealand; OR: Odds ratio; SD: Standard deviation; SLC: Solute carrier; TMPRSS6: Transmembrane protease serine-6; US: United States

Acknowledgements

The Health Research Council of New Zealand, Arthritis New Zealand, New Zealand Lottery Health and the University of Otago supported this work. The authors would like to thank Jill Drake (Canterbury District Health Board), Roddi Laurence, Chris Franklin, Meaghen House, Jordyn Allen (all University of Auckland) and Gabrielle Sexton (University of Otago) for recruitment. The authors would also like to thank Vivienne Trethowen from Southern Community Laboratory, Dunedin Hospital, New Zealand for iron profile measurements for the New Zealand sample sets. The Jackson Heart Study is supported and conducted in collaboration with Jackson State University (HHSN268201300049C and HHSN268201300050C), Tougaloo College (HHSN268201300048C) and the University of Mississippi Medical Center (HHSN268201300046C and HHSN268201300047C) with contracts from the National Heart, Lung, and Blood Institute (NHLBI) and the National Institute for Minority Health and Health Disparities (NIMHD). The authors thank the participants and data collection staff of the Jackson Heart Study. The views expressed in this manuscript are those of the authors and do not necessarily represent the views of the National Heart, Lung, and Blood Institute; the National Institutes of Health; or the US Department of Health and Human Services.

Funding

The study was funded by the Health Research Council of NZ and Ardea Biosciences. Neither of the funders had influence over the interpretation of results and writing of the manuscript.

Authors' contributions

TF and TRM helped to design the study, oversee its execution and write the manuscript. ND and LKS helped to provide clinical data and write the manuscript. CM and TJM helped to analyze and/or interpret data and write the manuscript. CI and JNM helped to generate data and write the manuscript. All authors read and approved the final manuscript.

Consent for publication

Not applicable.

Competing interests

The authors declare that they have no competing interests.

Author details

[1]Department of Biochemistry, University of Otago, Dunedin, New Zealand. [2]Department of Medicine, University of Otago, Christchurch, New Zealand. [3]Department of Medicine, University of Auckland, Auckland, New Zealand. [4]Medical Scientific Affairs, Ironwood Pharmaceuticals, Cambridge, MA, USA. [5]Biology, Ardea Biosciences, Inc., San Diego, CA, USA.

References

1. Dalbeth N, Merriman TR, Stamp LK. Gout. Lancet. 2016;388:2039–52.
2. Ghio AJ, Kennedy TP, Stonehuerner J, Carter JD, Skinner KA, Parks DA, Hoidal JR. Iron regulates xanthine oxidase activity in the lung. Am J Physiol Lung Cell Mol Physiol. 2002;283:L563–72.
3. Ghio AJ, Ford ES, Kennedy TP, Hoidal JR. The association between serum ferritin and uric acid in humans. Free Rad Res. 2005;39:337–42.
4. Li X, He T, Yu K, Lu Q, Alkasir R, Guo G, Xue Y. Markers of iron status are associated with risk of hyperuricemia among Chinese adults: nationwide population-based study. Nutrients. 2018;10:E191.
5. Mainous AG, Knoll ME, Everett CJ, Matheson EM, Hulihan MM, Grant AM. Uric acid as a potential cue to screen for iron overload. J Am Board Fam Med. 2011;24:415–21.
6. Ghio AJ, Kennedy TP, Rao G, Cooke CL, Miller MJ, Hoidal JR. Complexation of iron cation by sodium urate crystals and gouty inflammation. Arch Biochem Biophys. 1994;313:215–21.
7. Facchini FS. Near-iron deficiency-induced remission of gouty arthritis. Rheumatol. 2003;42:1550–5.
8. Zhang Y, Chen C, Choi H, Chaisson C, Hunter D, Niu J, Neogi T. Purine-rich foods intake and recurrent gout attacks. Ann Rheum Dis. 2012;71:1448–52.
9. Hayden JA, van der Windt DA, Cartwright JL, Cote P, Bombardier C. Assessing bias in studies of prognostic factors. Ann Intern Med. 2013;158:280–6.
10. Shrank WH, Patrick AR, Brookhart MA. Healthy user and related biases in observational studies of preventive interventions: a primer for physicians. J Gen Intern Med. 2011;26:546–50.
11. Robinson P, Choi H, Do R, Merriman TR. Insight into rheumatological cause and effect through the use of Mendelian randomization. Nat Rev Rheumatol. 2016;12:486–96.
12. Wallace SL, Robinson H, Masi AT, Decker JL, McCarty DJ, Yu TF. Preliminary criteria for the classification of the acute arthritis of primary gout. Arthr Rheum. 1977;20:895–900.
13. Taylor HA Jr. The Jackson Heart Study: an overview. Ethn Dis. 2005;15:S6-1-3.
14. Burt VL, Harris T. The Third National Health and Nutrition Examination Survey: contributing data on aging and health. Gerontologist. 1994;34:486–90.
15. Team RC. R: a language and environment for statistical computing. Vienna: R Foundation for Statistical Computing; 2016.
16. Kell DB, Pretorius E. Serum ferritin is an important inflammatory disease marker, as it is mainly a leakage product from damaged cells. Metallomics. 2014;6:748–73.
17. Ruggiero C, Cherubini A, Ble A, Bos AJ, Maggio M, Dixit VD, et al. Uric acid and inflammatory markers. Eur Heart J. 2006;27:1174–81.
18. Roseff R, Wohlgethan J, Sipe J, Canoso JJ. The acute phase response in gout. J Rheumatol. 1987;14:974–7.
19. Bolann BJ, Ulvik R. Release of iron from ferritin by xanthine oxidase. Role of the superoxide radical. Biochem J. 1987;243:55–9.
20. Benyamin B, Tonu E, Ried JS, Radhakrishnan A, Vermeulen SH, Traglia M, et al. Novel loci affecting iron homeostasis and their effects in individuals at risk for hemochromatosis. Nat Commun. 2014;5:4926.
21. Köttgen A, Albrecht E, Teumer A, Vitart V, Krumsiek J, Hundertmark C, et al. Genome-wide association analyses identify 18 new loci associated with serum urate concentrations. Nat Genet. 2013;45:145–54.
22. Burgess S, Butterworth A, Thompson SG. Mendelian randomization analysis with multiple genetic variants using summarized data. Genet Epidemiol. 2013;37:658–65.
23. Hemani G, Zheng J, Wade KH, Laurin C, Elsworth B, Burgess S, et al. MR-Base: a platform for systematic causal inference across the phenome using billions of genetic associations, bioRxiv; 2016. p. 078972.

24. Lawlor DA, Harbord RM, Sterne JA, Timpson N, Davey Smith G. Mendelian randomization: using genes as instruments for making causal inferences in epidemiology. Stat Med. 2008;27:1133–63.

25. Burgess S, Small DS, Thompson SG. A review of instrumental variable estimators for Mendelian randomization. Stat Methods Med Res. 2015;26:2333–55.

26. Burgess S. Identifying the odds ratio estimated by a two-stage instrumental variable analysis with a logistic regression model. Stat Med. 2013;32:4726–47.

27. Didelez V, Meng S, Sheehan NA. Assumptions of IV methods for observational epidemiology. Stat Sci. 2010;25:22–40.

28. Bowden J, Smith GD, Burgess S. Mendelian randomization with invalid instruments: effect estimation and bias detection through egger regression. Int J Epidemiol. 2015;44:512–25.

29. Corbin LJ, Richmond RC, Wade KH, Burgess S, Bowden J, Davey Smith G, Timpson NJ. Body mass index as a modifiable risk factor for type 2 diabetes: refining and understanding causal estimates using Mendelian randomisation. Diabetes. 2016;65:3002–7.

30. Burgess S. Sample size and power calculations in Mendelian randomization with a single instrumental variable and a binary outcome. Int J Epidemiol. 2014;43:922–9.

31. Burgess S, Davies NM, Thompson SG. Bias due to participant overlap in two-sample Mendelian randomization. Genet Epidemiol. 2016;40:597–608.

32. Sivera F, Andrés M, Pascual E. Serum uric acid drops during acute inflammatory episodes. Ann Rheum Dis. 2010;69(Suppl 3):122.

33. Aust SD, Morehouse LA, Thomas CE. Role of metals in oxygen radical reactions. J Free Radic Biol Med. 1985;1:3–25.

34. Howell RR, Wyngaarden JB. On the mechanism of peroxidation of uric acids by hemoproteins. J Biol Chem. 1960;235:3544–50.

35. Kellogg EW, Fridovich I. Liposome oxidation and erythrocyte lysis by enzymically generated superoxide and hydrogen peroxide. J Biol Chem. 1977;252:6721–8.

36. Ames BN, Cathcart R, Schwiers E, Hochstein P. Uric acid provides an antioxidant defense in humans against oxidant-and radical-caused aging and cancer: a hypothesis. Proc Natl Acad Sci U S A. 1981;78:6858–62.

37. Davies K, Sevanian A, Muakkassah-Kelly S, Hochstein P. Uric acid-iron ion complexes. A new aspect of the antioxidant functions of uric acid. Biochem J. 1986;235:747–54.

38. Stonehuerner J, Ghio AJ, Kennedy TP, Skinner KA. Elevations in xanthine oxidase (XO) activity after silica exposure corresponds to complexed iron concentrations. Am J Respir Crit Care Med. 1998;157:A232.

39. Martelin E, Lapatto R, Raivio KO. Regulation of xanthine oxidoreductase by intracellular iron. Am J Physiol Cell Physiol. 2002;283:C1722–8.

40. del Greco F, Foco L, Pichler I, Eller P, Eller K, Benyamin B, et al. Serum iron level and kidney function: a Mendelian randomization study. Nephrol Dial Transplant. 2017;32:273–8.

41. Muntane J, Puig-Parellada P, Fernandez Y, Mitjavila S, Mitjavila MT. Antioxidant defenses and its modulation by iron in carrageenan-induced inflammation in rats. Clin Chim Acta. 1993;214:185–93.

42. Ward V, McGinty J, Church W. Iron (III) chloride injection increases nigral uric acid in Guinea-pig. Neuroreport. 1993;4:787–90.

43. Livrea M, Tesoriere L, Pintaudi A, Calabrese A, Maggio A, Freisleben HJ, et al. Oxidative stress and antioxidant status in beta-thalassemia major: iron overload and depletion of lipid-soluble antioxidants. Blood. 1996;88:3608–14.

44. Muirden K, Senator G. Iron in the synovial membrane in rheumatoid arthritis and other joint diseases. Ann Rheum Dis. 1968;27:38–48.

45. Blake DR, Hall ND, Bacon P, Dieppe PA, Halliwell B, Gutteridge JM. Effect of a specific iron chelating agent on animal models of inflammation. Ann Rheum Dis. 1983;42:89–93.

46. Andrews F, Morris C, Kondratowicz G, Blake DR. Effect of iron chelation on inflammatory joint disease. Ann Rheum Dis. 1987;46:327–33.

47. Flynn TJ, Cadzow M, Dalbeth N, Jones PB, Stamp LK, Harre Hindmarsh J, et al. Positive association of tomato consumption with serum urate: support for tomato consumption as an anecdotal trigger of gout flares. BMC Musculoskelet Disord. 2015;16:196.

48. Williams PT. Effects of diet, physical activity and performance, and body weight on incident gout in ostensibly healthy, vigorously active men. Am J Clin Nutr. 2008;87:1480–7.

49. Choi HK, Atkinson K, Karlson EW, Willett W, Curhan G. Purine-rich foods, dairy and protein intake, and the risk of gout in men. N Engl J Med. 2004; 350:1093–103.

50. Öztürk MA, Kaya A, Şenel S, Dönmez S, Cobankara V, Erhan C, et al. Demographic and clinical features of gout patients in Turkey: a multicenter study. Rheumatol Int. 2013;33:847–52.

51. Choi HK, Liu S, Curhan G. Intake of purine-rich foods, protein, and dairy products and relationship to serum levels of uric acid: the Third National Health and Nutrition Examination Survey. Arthr Rheum. 2005;52:283–9.

52. Powell L, Emmerson B. Haemosiderosis associated with xanthine oxidase inhibition. Lancet. 1966;287:239–40.

53. Emmerson B. Effects of allopurinol on iron metabolism in man. Ann Rheum Dis. 1966;25:700–3.

54. Powell LW. Changing concepts in haemochromatosis. Postgrad Med J. 1970;46:200–9.

55. Gaffo AL, Schumacher HR, Saag KG, Taylor WJ, Dinella J, Outman R, et al. Developing a provisional definition of flare in patients with established gout. Arthritis Rheum. 2012;64:1508–17.

10

Prediction of primary non-response to methotrexate therapy using demographic, clinical and psychosocial variables: results from the UK Rheumatoid Arthritis Medication Study (RAMS)

Jamie C. Sergeant[1,2], Kimme L. Hyrich[2,3], James Anderson[2], Kamilla Kopec-Harding[2], Holly F. Hope[2], Deborah P. M. Symmons[2], RAMS Co-Investigators, Anne Barton[3,4] and Suzanne M. M. Verstappen[2,3*]

Abstract

Background: Methotrexate (MTX) remains the disease-modifying anti-rheumatic drug of first choice in rheumatoid arthritis (RA) but response varies. Predicting non-response to MTX could enable earlier access to alternative or additional medications and control of disease progression. We aimed to identify baseline predictors of non-response to MTX and combine these into a prediction algorithm.

Methods: This study included patients recruited to the Rheumatoid Arthritis Medication Study (RAMS), a UK multi-centre prospective observational study of patients with RA or undifferentiated polyarthritis, commencing MTX for the first time. Non-response to MTX at 6 months was defined as "no response" using the European League Against Rheumatism (EULAR) response criteria, discontinuation of MTX due to inefficacy or starting biologic therapy. The association of baseline demographic, clinical and psychosocial predictors with non-response was assessed using logistic regression. Predictive performance was assessed using the area under the receiver operating characteristic curve (AUC) and calibration plots.

Results: Of 1050 patients, 449 (43%) were classified as non-responders. Independent multivariable predictors of MTX non-response (OR (95% CI)) were rheumatoid factor (RF) negativity (0.62 (0.45, 0.86) for RF positivity versus negativity), higher Health Assessment Questionnaire score (1.64 (1.25, 2.15)), higher tender joint count (1.06 (1.02, 1.10)), lower Disease Activity score in 28 joints (0.29 (0.23, 0.39)) and higher Hospital Anxiety and Depression Scale anxiety score (1.07 (1.03, 1.12)). The optimism-corrected AUC was 0.74.

Conclusions: This is the first model for MTX non-response to be developed in a large contemporary study of patients commencing MTX in which demographic, clinical and psychosocial predictors were considered. Patient anxiety was a predictor of non-response and could be addressed at treatment commencement.

Keywords: Rheumatoid arthritis, Methotrexate, Response, Prediction model

* Correspondence: suzanne.verstappen@manchester.ac.uk
[2]Arthritis Research UK Centre for Epidemiology, Centre for Musculoskeletal Research, Manchester Academic Health Science Centre, University of Manchester, Manchester, UK
[3]NIHR Manchester Biomedical Research Centre, Central Manchester University Hospitals NHS Foundation Trust, Manchester Academic Health Science Centre, Manchester, UK
Full list of author information is available at the end of the article

Background

Methotrexate (MTX) is now the conventional synthetic disease-modifying antirheumatic drug (csDMARD) of first choice, either as monotherapy or combination therapy, for most patients with rheumatoid arthritis (RA) [1]. This is emphasised in a number of international and national guidelines [2–5]. However, response to MTX, although better than to most other csDMARDs, is not universal. In observational studies approximately 30% of patients discontinue MTX in the medium term - around half due to inefficacy and half due to adverse events [6, 7]. Patient-related factors such as female gender and current smoking are associated with MTX non-response [6, 7]. Disease related factors such as disease duration, disease activity, rheumatoid factor (RF) and anti-citrullinated protein antibody (ACPA) status are moderately predictive of inefficacy [6, 7]. Psychosocial factors may also be important but have received little attention to date [8]. Response to treatment may be influenced by the patient's social background [9, 10], by their existing beliefs about their illness and the likely efficacy of the drug, and by whether they have actually taken the medication (adherence) [11]. Genetic or other biological factors may also influence drug response [6, 7].

Many previous studies have attempted to identify independent predictors of response to MTX, although frequently without assessing the ability to assign probabilities of response to individual patients [12–14]. Those prediction models that have been developed have used data from the restricted populations and rigid treatment regimens of clinical trials [15, 16]; have used only small numbers of participants (fewer than 100) from observational studies [17, 18]; or have analysed the outcome of treatment discontinuation rather than a broader assessment of patient condition [19]. The value of predictions from such models for "real world" patients with RA about to start MTX for the first time is uncertain. More likely to be of use is a model developed in an observational study including patients seen in routine clinical practice using readily available or easily measurable demographic, clinical and psychosocial factors. If such a model could identify those unlikely to respond to MTX prior to starting therapy, with sufficient accuracy to be clinically useful, it could enable earlier access to alternative medications such as biologic therapy and the avoidance of disease progression for some patients.

The objectives of this study were, in a large national multi-centre observational study of patients with RA or undifferentiated polyarthritis (UP) commencing MTX for the first time, to (1) describe the pattern of 6-month treatment response, (2) identify patient-specific, disease-specific and psychosocial predictors of primary non-response to MTX, (3) combine predictors of non-response in a model that could be used to assign probability of non-response at the individual patient level and (4) test the accuracy of the model.

Methods

Study design and study population

The Rheumatoid Arthritis Medication Study (RAMS) is a large national (UK) multi-centre (n = 38 centres) study. To be eligible for RAMS, patients had to (1) be aged 18 years or over, (2) have a physician diagnosis of RA or UP and (3) be about to start MTX for the first time, either as monotherapy or in combination with other csDMARDs, including oral steroids. Patients were not eligible if they had current or previous exposure to a biological DMARD (bDMARD). RAMS was approved by the Central Manchester NHS Research Ethics Committee (reference 08/H1008/25) and all patients provided written consent.

The decision to start MTX, the dosage and mode of administration, and whether to use MTX as monotherapy or in combination were made by the patient's rheumatologist based on clinical need, local practice and national guidelines [3]. Patients were generally recruited following the drug education visit and prior to taking their first dose of MTX.

Baseline assessments

Demographic and lifestyle data collected at baseline, and relevant to this analysis, included age, gender, height and weight to calculate body mass index (BMI), smoking status (current/former/never), current alcohol intake (units/fortnight) and current caffeinated tea and coffee consumption (cups/day). Socio-economic status was assigned using the Index of Multiple Deprivation (IMD) 2010 based on the patient's postcode, where a higher IMD score represents a more deprived area [20].

Disease-specific data were collected from the patient by a research nurse and supplemented with information obtained from medical records, including symptom duration; 28 tender and swollen joint count; individual 1987 American College of Rheumatology (ACR) classification criteria for RA [21]; previous csDMARD history; current oral steroid use; intramuscular or intra-articular steroid injections in the past week; current use of non-steroidal anti-inflammatory drugs (NSAIDs); duration of morning stiffness; and serum creatinine. Self-reported comorbidities were selected from a list of predefined conditions (high blood pressure, angina, heart attack, transient ischaemic attack, stroke, epilepsy, asthma, chronic bronchitis/emphysema, bronchiectasis, peptic ulcer disease, liver disease, renal disease, tuberculosis, diabetes mellitus, hyperthyroidism, depression and cancer).

Patients also completed a questionnaire, including pain, fatigue and general well-being visual analogue scales (VAS) (0–100 mm, with 100 mm the worst score);

the British version of the Health Assessment Questionnaire (HAQ) (score range 0–3) [22]; the Hospital Anxiety and Depression Scale (HADS) (score ranges 0–21) [23] and the Beliefs about Medicines Questionnaire (BMQ) (score ranges 5–25) [24], with higher values of the HAQ, HADS and BMQ representing reduced physical function, greater indication of anxiety or depression and stronger beliefs about medication necessity or concerns, respectively. The brief Illness Perception Questionnaire (IPQ-brief) [25] was used to categorise patients' illness representations as positive or negative [26].

Blood samples were taken at baseline and sent to the UK Biobank, Stockport, UK for the measurement of C-reactive protein (CRP) (Beckman Coulter AU5400, CRP assay OSR6147; mg/l) and RF (Beckman Coulter AU5400, RF latex assay OSR61105; IU/ml). RF values in excess of 14 IU/ml were taken to indicate RF positivity. If blood samples were not available to measure CRP, recorded CRP values from medical notes were used. The DAS28 was calculated using the CRP, 28-joint counts and VAS for general well-being [27].

Follow-up assessments

Patients were followed up at 3 and 6 months. Changes in DMARD therapy, including MTX, were recorded and the DAS28-CRP was measured at each visit. If MTX therapy had been stopped, the reason for stopping and whether treatment would be restarted were also recorded.

Outcome: European League Against Rheumatism (EULAR) non-response

Non-response to treatment at 6 months was defined as "no response" using the EULAR response criteria [28], i.e. Disease Activity Score in 28 joints (DAS28) improvement ≤ 0.6, or DAS28 improvement > 0.6 but ≤ 1.2 and 6-month DAS28 > 5.1. In addition, patients who had discontinued MTX by 6 months, i.e. had stopped MTX and did not plan to restart, due to inefficacy were classified as non-responders, as were patients who commenced bDMARD treatment by 6 months. "Moderate" or "good" responders by the EULAR criteria were considered responders, as were patients who discontinued MTX by 6 months due to remission.

Participant selection

To allow for sufficient follow-up time, the current analysis included RAMS participants recruited by 30 September 2015. Patients without a 6-month follow-up record were excluded, unless they had discontinued MTX by their 3-month follow up and so could be classified as non-responders. Also excluded were patients with unknown MTX exposure status at 6 months, those who had discontinued MTX by 6 months for reasons other

than inefficacy or remission (e.g. adverse events), and those who had not discontinued MTX by 6 months but for whom the 6-month EULAR response was unavailable (see Fig. 1). If MTX or restart status at 6 months was unknown, 3-month records were checked for evidence of having discontinued at this time point before excluding a patient.

Statistical analysis

All variables were assessed for their univariable and multivariable association with non-response to MTX at 6 months using logistic regression. Backward selection was used to successively remove non-significant terms ($p \geq 0.05$) from a full multivariable model containing all variables. Forwards selection was also used to successively add significant predictors ($p < 0.05$) into an empty model to validate the list of predictors derived by backwards selection. If the backwards and forwards selection processes delivered different sets of predictors, backwards selection was applied again on the pooled set of predictors derived from both approaches to produce a final model. The ability of the final model to discriminate between responders and non-responders was assessed using the area under the receiver operating characteristic curve (AUC). Agreement between predicted probabilities and observed outcomes was assessed using a calibration plot of the observed proportions of non-responders in each decile of predicted probability of non-response plotted against the mean predicted probabilities for the deciles. As performance was assessed using the same data used to build the model, an estimate of the optimism in the AUC value was produced using 200 bootstrapped datasets. The modelling procedure was followed afresh in each bootstrap dataset and the estimate of optimism was calculated as the average difference between the AUC achieved by a model in its own bootstrap dataset and the AUC achieved by that model in the original dataset [29]. How the model might perform in clinical practice was explored by calculating the sensitivity, specificity, positive predictive value (PPV) and negative predictive value (NPV) when using different cut-offs of predicted probabilities of non-response as thresholds for classifying individuals as having a high risk of non-response.

Rates of missing data were calculated for all potential predictor variables and an analysis using multiple imputation with chained equations to impute missing values in all candidate predictor variables in 50 imputed datasets was performed. All analyses were performed in Stata 13.1 [30].

Results

Of 1656 patients recruited by 30 September 2015, 1050 were included in the current analysis (Fig. 1): 707 (67%)

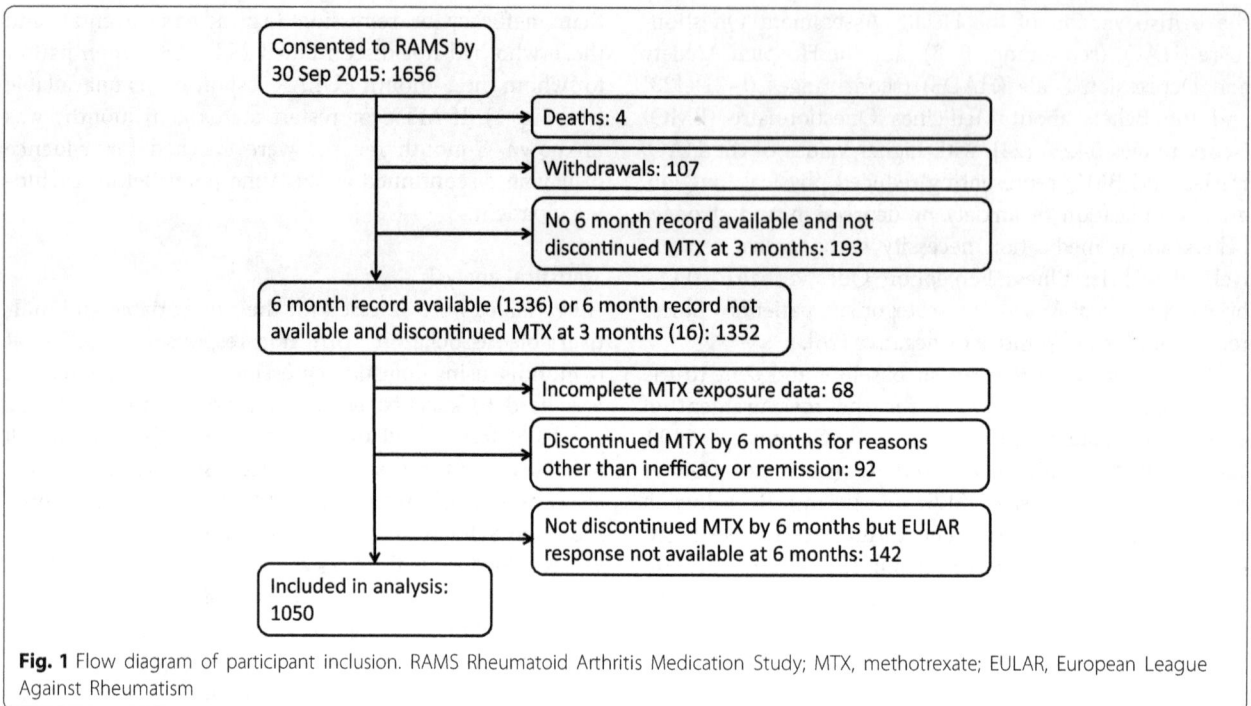

Fig. 1 Flow diagram of participant inclusion. RAMS Rheumatoid Arthritis Medication Study; MTX, methotrexate; EULAR, European League Against Rheumatism

female, median age 59 (IQR 49–68) years and median symptom duration 9 (IQR 4–28) months (Table 1). Of the patients, 66% (584/889) were RF positive and 82% (787/962) satisfied the 1987 ACR criteria for RA at baseline; 77% of patients were starting MTX as their first csDMARD; 18% were currently on another csDMARD; and 4% had prior but not current exposure to one or more csDMARDs (Table 1): 41% were taking oral corticosteroids and/or had recently (within the last week) received an intramuscular corticosteroid injection, and 3% of patients had received an intra-articular steroid injection in the previous week (Table 1). Almost all participants (1003/1005) were starting folic acid at baseline. Starting doses of MTX were recorded at baseline for 1042 (99%) participants and ranged from 2.5 to 25 mg/week, with plans to incrementally increase the dose in 43% (422/984) of cases; 98% (963/978) of participants were starting orally administered MTX.

Outcome: non-response

At 6 months 449/1050 patients (43%) were classified as non-responders. Table 1 gives baseline characteristics stratified by response status at 6 months. In the univariable analysis, significant predictors of MTX non-response (OR (95% CI)) included higher BMI (1.02 (1.00, 1.05) per kg/m^2), current smoking (1.78 (1.28, 2.48) compared to never smoking), longer symptom duration (1.00 (1.00, 1.00) per month); not being RF positive (0.66 (0.50, 0.88) for RF positive compared to not); not satisfying the 1987 ACR criteria (0.59 (0.43, 0.83) for satisfying the 1987 ACR criteria compared to not); lower HAQ score (0.76 (0.64,

0.90) per unit increase in HAQ) and lower DAS28 (0.54 (0.48, 0.60) per unit increase in DAS28) (Table 2). In the multivariable model, not being RF positive (0.62 (0.45, 0.86) for RF positive compared to not), higher HAQ score (1.64 (1.25, 2.15) per unit increase in HAQ), higher tender joint count (1.06 (1.02, 1.10) per additional tender joint), lower DAS28 score (0.29 (0.23, 0.39) per unit increase in DAS28) and higher HADS anxiety score (1.07 (1.03, 1.12) per unit increase in HADS anxiety) were independent predictors of MTX non-response (Table 2). The results using 50 multiple imputation datasets to account for missing values were almost identical (results not shown).

Sensitivity analysis

The most surprising result was the relationship between a lower DAS28 score and non-response. This may be an inevitable consequence of the method of calculating non-response. In order to be classified as a responder to MTX by achieving a moderate or good EULAR response, it is necessary for a patient's DAS28 score to fall by at least 0.6. If patients start with a relatively low DAS28 score they have less potential for achieving such a response. Indeed, since the DAS28-CRP(4) formula includes a constant of 0.96, a DAS28 of 1.56 is the minimum that can fall by 0.6 or more and be classified as response. At baseline, 226 (22%) patients had low disease activity (LDA) (DAS28-CRP ≤ 3.2), including 102 (10%) patients in remission (DAS28-CRP ≤ 2.6). Of these, 72% (162/226) and 88% (90/102), respectively, were non-responders, compared to 43% of all patients (Table 1). 40% (88/219) of those with LDA and 38%

Table 1 Baseline characteristics of the whole cohort and divided by responder status

Characteristic	Data availability	All patients ($n = 1050$)	Responders ($n = 601$)	Non-responders ($n = 449$)
Demographic and lifestyle factors				
Female sex	1050 (100)	707 (67)	398 (66)	309 (69)
Age (years)	1050 (100)	59 (49, 68)	60 (49, 68)	58 (48, 67)
BMI (kg/m^2)	959 (91)	27.5 (24.2, 31.6)	27.4 (24.1, 31.1)	27.9 (24.3, 33.0)
Smoking: never	1042 (99)	420 (40)	260 (44)	160 (36)
Smoking: former		404 (39)	232 (39)	172 (39)
Smoking: current		218 (21)	104 (17)	114 (26)
Alcohol consumption: current	1030 (98)	710 (69)	401 (68)	309 (71)
Alcohol consumption: (units/fortnight)	1009 (96)	2 (0, 10)	2 (0, 10)	2 (0, 12)
Coffee/tea consumption: (cups/day)	815 (78)	4 (3, 6)	4 (2, 6)	4 (3, 6)
IMD score	990 (94)	13.9 (8.9, 24.5)	13.7 (8.5, 23.7)	14.8 (9.5, 27.2)
Disease-specific factors				
Symptom duration (months)	1042 (99)	9 (4, 28)	8 (4, 24)	10 (4, 33)
RF positive	889 (85)	584 (66)	354 (70)	230 (60)
Satisfied the 1987 ACR criteria	962 (92)	787 (82)	470 (85)	317 (77)
HAQ score	989 (94)	1.1 (0.5, 1.6)	1.1 (0.5, 1.8)	1.0 (0.4, 1.5)
Co-morbidities: 0	1050 (100)	392 (37)	240 (40)	152 (34)
Co-morbidities: 1		345 (33)	189 (31)	156 (35)
Co-morbidities: 2+		313 (30)	172 (29)	141 (31)
Creatinine (mg/dl)	970 (92)	67 (59, 77)	66 (58, 76)	67 (60, 79)
Disease activity				
Morning stiffness (minutes)	1000 (95)	60 (15, 120)	60 (20, 120)	60 (10, 90)
TJC28	1050 (100)	6 (2, 13)	8 (4, 15)	4 (1, 10)
SJC28	1050 (100)	5 (2, 10)	6 (3, 12)	3 (1, 7)
CRP (mg/l)	1050 (100)	5.6 (2.0, 16.2)	8.2 (2.8, 21.4)	3.8 (1.5, 9.9)
Patient VAS (mm)	1050 (100)	41 (23, 60)	47 (26, 66)	32 (19, 50)
DAS28-CRP	1050 (100)	4.3 (3.3, 5.3)	4.7 (3.9, 5.7)	3.7 (2.8, 4.6)
DAS28-CRP ≤ 3.2	1050 (100)	226 (22)	64 (11)	162 (36)
DAS28-CRP ≤ 2.6	1050 (100)	102 (10)	12 (2)	90 (20)
Pain VAS (mm)	971 (92)	50 (28, 71)	53 (30, 73)	46 (25, 68)
Fatigue VAS (mm)	974 (93)	54 (27, 73)	54 (28, 74)	53 (27, 72)
Medication				
Oral steroids: current	1048 (100)	210 (20)	119 (20)	91 (20)
Intramuscular steroids: recent	1028 (98)	234 (23)	137 (23)	97 (22)
Intra-articular steroids: recent	882 (84)	27 (3)	14 (3)	13 (3)
Oral or intramuscular steroids: current/recent	1031 (98)	423 (41)	244 (41)	179 (40)
NSAIDs: current	942 (90)	520 (55)	296 (55)	224 (55)
csDMARDs: current	1050 (100)	193 (18)	100 (17)	93 (21)
csDMARDs: ever	1050 (100)	238 (23)	120 (20)	118 (26)
MTX starting dose (mg/week)	1042 (99)	10 (10, 15)	10 (10, 15)	10 (10, 15)
Psychosocial factors				
HADS anxiety	986 (94)	6 (3, 9)	6 (3, 9)	6 (3, 10)
HADS depression	987 (94)	6 (3, 9)	6 (3, 9)	5 (2, 8)
BMQ medication necessity	942 (90)	19 (17, 22)	20 (17, 23)	19 (17, 22)

Table 1 Baseline characteristics of the whole cohort and divided by responder status *(Continued)*

Characteristic	Data availability	All patients (*n* = 1050)	Responders (*n* = 601)	Non-responders (*n* = 449)
BMQ medication concerns	949 (90)	15 (13, 18)	15 (12, 17)	16 (13, 18)
BMQ necessity-concerns	923 (88)	4 (1, 8)	5 (1, 8)	4 (1, 8)
IPQ negative illness representation	967 (92)	560 (58)	330 (59)	230 (56)

Values are frequency (%) or median (IQR)

Abbreviations: BMI body mass index, *IMD* Index of Multiple Deprivation, *RF* rheumatoid factor, *HAQ* Health Assessment Questionnaire, *TJC28* tender 28-joint count, *SJC28* swollen 28-joint count, *CRP* C-reactive protein, *VAS* visual analogue scale, *DAS28* Disease Activity Score based on the 28-joint count, *NSAIDs* non-steroidal anti-inflammatory drugs, *csDMARDs* conventional synthetic disease-modifying anti-rheumatic drugs, *HADS* Hospital Anxiety and Depression Scale, *BMQ* Beliefs about Medicines Questionnaire, *IPQ* Illness Perception Questionnaire

(38/99) of those in remission were on oral corticosteroids at baseline or had received an intramuscular corticosteroid injection in the past week, similar to the 41% of the whole cohort.

To further explore the role of baseline DAS28, we conducted two sensitivity analyses, first excluding patients in remission and second excluding patients with LDA but otherwise following the modelling procedure described above. The multivariable models excluding those in remission and those with LDA contained the same predictors as the main model except for the addition of BMI and the removal of HAQ score and TJC28 (Table 2 and Additional file 1: Table S1). Hence the predictors common to all three multivariable models were RF status, DAS28-CRP and HADS anxiety score.

Additionally, a model was developed to predict failure to achieve LDA (i.e. DAS28-CRP > 3.2) at 6 months (not requiring a minimum improvement in DAS28). Higher BMI, higher HAQ score, higher TJC28 and higher HADS anxiety score, but not lower baseline DAS28, were predictive of failing to achieve LDA at 6 months (Additional file 1: Table S2).

Model assessment

The model predicting non-response in all patients had an AUC of 0.77 (95% CI (0.73, 0.80)) (Table 2), reduced to 0.74 when correcting for optimism. Excluding those in remission or with LDA reduced the AUC to 0.72 (0.68, 0.76) (Table 2) and 0.71 (0.66, 0.75) (Additional file 1: Table S1), respectively. Calibration plots in Fig. 2 and Additional file 1: Figures S1 and S2 indicate that the models have similar properties across the deciles of predicted probabilities. For the outcome of "failure to achieve LDA at 6 months", the AUC was 0.73 (0.70, 0.77) (Additional file 1: Table S2) and the calibration plot is shown in Additional file 1: Figure S3.

Table 3 shows the sensitivity, specificity, PPV and NPV when predicted probability cut-offs ranging from 0.5 to 0.9 are used as thresholds for classifying individuals as being at high risk of non-response. Using a cut-off of 0.8 to indicate high risk, 49 patients (6%) would be predicted to be at high risk of non-response and 98% of these would indeed fail to respond (PPV); 61% of those predicted to respond would do so (NPV). On average

the model would need to be applied to 17 patients to identify one individual at high risk of non-response ("number needed to test").

Discussion

In this large observational study investigating response to MTX among patients with RA in the current era, 43% of patients were classified as non-responders by 6 months after starting treatment, with those discontinuing MTX due to adverse events excluded from the analysis. Baseline predictors of non-response in a multivariable logistic regression model were RF negativity, higher HAQ score, higher tender joint count, higher HADS anxiety score and lower disease activity. The AUC was 0.77 (0.74 optimism-corrected). The AUC was lower in models that excluded either all those in remission or all those with LDA at baseline when attempting to address the fact that it was harder for those with lower baseline DAS28 scores to achieve the definition of response. All models included RF negativity, lower baseline DAS28-CRP and higher HADS anxiety score as predictors of non-response. This is the first study to explore potential psychological factors in prediction of individual MTX non-response and all models retained HADS anxiety score as an independent predictor. Hence this psychological predictor added significant additional predictive information once the clinical predictors in the multivariable model had been accounted for. While the design of the current study does not allow us to examine the mechanism by which anxiety is associated with non-response, and this relationship requires further research, anxiety could be considered a modifiable risk factor, suggesting that the shared decision-making between patient and rheumatologist [2] should be mindful of anxiety issues, and that patient education prior to starting MTX should address anxiety. Although the literature on the association between patient anxiety and response to treatment in RA is limited, a recent study [31] did report that depression and anxiety (without differentiating between the two) may reduce likelihood of remission in those treated with MTX or tumour necrosis factor inhibitors.

While previous attempts have been made to develop models to predict response to MTX [15–19], this is the

Table 2 Univariable and multivariable analysis of predictors of MTX non-response in all subjects and excluding those in remission at baseline

Characteristic	All subjects				Excluding those in remission			
	Univariable		Stepwise multivariable $n = 833$, AUC = 0.77 (95% CI (0.73, 0.80))		Univariable		Stepwise multivariable $n = 700$, AUC − 0.72 (95% CI (0.68, 0.76))	
	OR (95% CI)	p	OR (95% CI)	p	OR (95% CI)	p	OR (95% CI)	p
Demographic and lifestyle factors								
Female sex	1.13 (0.87, 1.46)	0.37			1.20 (0.90, 1.59)	0.22		
Age (years)	0.99 (0.98, 1.00)	0.06			0.99 (0.98, 1.00)	0.04		
BMI (kg/m^2)	1.02 (1.00, 1.05)	0.04			1.04 (1.02, 1.06)	< 0.01	1.05 (1.02, 1.08)	< 0.01
Smoking: never	ref		ref		ref		ref	
Smoking: former	1.20 (0.91, 1.59)	0.19			1.23 (0.91, 1.65)	0.18		
Smoking: current	1.78 (1.28, 2.48)	< 0.01			1.74 (1.22, 2.48)	< 0.01		
Alcohol consumption: current	1.14 (0.87, 1.49)	0.34			1.13 (0.85, 1.51)	0.40		
Alcohol consumption: (units/fortnight)	1.01 (1.00, 1.02)	0.08			1.01 (1.00, 1.02)	0.21		
Coffee/tea consumption: (cups/day)	1.03 (0.98, 1.09)	0.20			1.04 (0.99, 1.10)	0.12		
IMD score (units)	1.01 (1.00, 1.02)	0.02			1.01 (1.00, 1.02)	0.05		
Disease-specific factors								
Symptom duration (months)	1.00 (1.00, 1.00)	< 0.01			1.00 (1.00, 1.01)	< 0.01		
RF positive	0.66 (0.50, 0.88)	< 0.01	0.62 (0.45, 0.86)	< 0.01	0.57 (0.42, 0.76)	< 0.01	0.52 (0.37, 0.73)	< 0.01
Satisfied the 1987 ACR criteria	0.59 (0.43, 0.83)	< 0.01			0.66 (0.46, 0.94)	0.02		
HAQ score (units)	0.76 (0.64, 0.90)	< 0.01	1.64 (1.25, 2.15)	< 0.01	0.92 (0.77, 1.11)	0.39		
Co-morbidities: 0	ref		ref		ref		ref	
Co-morbidities: 1	1.30 (0.97, 1.75)	0.08			1.45 (1.06, 2.00)	0.02		
Co-morbidities: 2+	1.29 (0.96, 1.75)	0.09			1.50 (1.08, 2.07)	0.01		
Creatinine (mg/dl)	1.01 (1.00, 1.01)	0.10			1.01 (1.00, 1.01)	0.18		
Disease activity								
Morning stiffness (minutes)	1.00 (1.00, 1.00)	0.01			1.00 (1.00, 1.00)	0.18		
TJC28 (joints)	0.94 (0.92, 0.96)	< 0.01	1.06 (1.02, 1.10)	< 0.01	0.96 (0.95, 0.98)	< 0.01		
SJC28 (joints)	0.92 (0.90, 0.94)	< 0.01			0.94 (0.92, 0.96)	< 0.01		
CRP (mg/l)	0.98 (0.97, 0.99)	< 0.01			0.99 (0.98, 0.99)	< 0.01		
Patient VAS (mm)	0.98 (0.97, 0.99)	< 0.01			0.99 (0.98, 0.99)	< 0.01		
DAS28-CRP (units)	0.54 (0.48, 0.60)	< 0.01	0.29 (0.23, 0.39)	< 0.01	0.63 (0.55, 0.71)	< 0.01	0.49 (0.41, 0.58)	< 0.01
Pain VAS (mm)	0.99 (0.99, 1.00)	< 0.01			1.00 (0.99, 1.00)	0.26		
Fatigue VAS (mm)	1.00 (0.99, 1.00)	0.29			1.00 (1.00, 1.01)	0.21		
Medication								
Oral or intramuscular steroids: current/recent	0.96 (0.75, 1.24)	0.76			0.97 (0.74, 1.27)	0.82		
NSAIDs: current	1.02 (0.78, 1.32)	0.90			1.08 (0.82, 1.43)	0.58		
csDMARDs: current	1.31 (0.96, 1.79)	0.09			1.37 (0.99, 1.91)	0.06		
csDMARDs: ever	1.43 (1.07, 1.91)	0.02			1.50 (1.11, 2.04)	0.01		
MTX starting dose (mg/week)	0.97 (0.94, 1.02)	0.22			0.98 (0.94, 1.02)	0.30		
Psychosocial factors								
HADS Anxiety (units)	1.02 (0.99, 1.05)	0.21	1.07 (1.03, 1.12)	< 0.01	1.04 (1.01, 1.07)	0.01	1.11 (1.07, 1.15)	< 0.01
HADS Depression (units)	0.98 (0.95, 1.01)	0.19			1.01 (0.98, 1.05)	0.57		
BMQ medication necessity (units)	0.98 (0.94, 1.01)	0.23			0.99 (0.95, 1.03)	0.50		

Table 2 Univariable and multivariable analysis of predictors of MTX non-response in all subjects and excluding those in remission at baseline *(Continued)*

Characteristic	All subjects				Excluding those in remission			
	Univariable		Stepwise multivariable $n = 833$, AUC = 0.77 (95% CI (0.73, 0.80))		Univariable		Stepwise multivariable $n = 700$, AUC = 0.72 (95% CI (0.68, 0.76))	
	OR (95% CI)	p	OR (95% CI)	p	OR (95% CI)	p	OR (95% CI)	p
BMQ medication concerns (units)	1.03 (0.99, 1.06)	0.14			1.03 (0.99, 1.07)	0.14		
BMQ necessity-concerns (units)	0.98 (0.95, 1.00)	0.08			0.98 (0.95, 1.01)	0.16		
IPQ negative illness representation	0.88 (0.68, 1.14)	0.33			1.14 (0.86, 1.51)	0.37		

Abbreviations: BMI body mass index, *IMD* Index of Multiple Deprivation, *RF* rheumatoid factor, *HAQ* Health Assessment Questionnaire, *TJC28* tender 28-joint count, *SJC28* swollen 28-joint count, *CRP* C-reactive protein, *VAS* visual analogue scale, *DAS28* Disease Activity Score based on the 28-joint count, *NSAIDs* non-steroidal anti-inflammatory drugs, *csDMARDs* conventional synthetic disease-modifying anti-rheumatic drugs, *HADS* Hospital Anxiety and Depression Scale, *BMQ* Beliefs about Medicines Questionnaire, *IPQ* Illness Perception Questionnaire

first model to be developed using a large cohort of patients with RA starting MTX for the first time and recruited from routine clinical care with few exclusions, i.e. representative of the setting in which such a model might be applied. That is, our model is designed to be applied in the real-world population of those about to commence MTX, which includes individuals with disease activity lower than might be expected. Final sets of predictor variables vary between published models, with only some measure of patient condition at baseline, be it TJC [15], DAS [16, 17] or HAQ [19], common to most studies. While lower baseline DAS28 was found to be associated with non-response to MTX when defined primarily using the EULAR response criteria, higher baseline DAS28 was associated with failure to achieve LDA (although significant only univariably, with higher TJC being retained in the multivariable model), which matches findings elsewhere [16]. This is a reminder that

models are outcome-specific and that the clinical relevance of outcomes should be considered.

If a predicted probability of 0.9 or above from the model was used to identify patients at high risk of non-response, 100% of those meeting this criterion would go on to be non-responders. However, only 4% of non-responders would be identified in this way. Reducing the cut-off to 0.8 would identify 14% of non-responders, but at the expense of 2% of those labelled as high risk actually being patients who would respond to MTX. The trade-off between the delay in accessing alternative medications for those who will not respond to MTX but are predicted to do so, and the over-treatment with alternative medications of those who would respond to MTX but are predicted not to, is unlikely to be an equally weighted one. Deciding where to draw an appropriate threshold for a label of high risk for clinical practice requires consideration of the treatment options available in a particular setting, their benefits and risks for individual patients, and their health economic implications. Of course, even with perfect prediction of non-response to MTX therapy, there is no guarantee that a better response would be achieved with alternative treatments. Truly informed decision-making by clinicians and their patients would require personalised predictions of patient outcomes for a range of treatment options, a scenario which is still some way off.

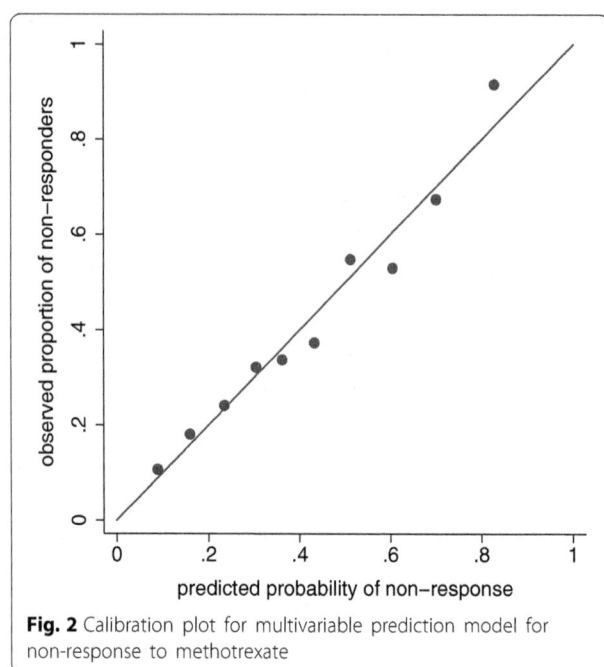

Fig. 2 Calibration plot for multivariable prediction model for non-response to methotrexate

Table 3 Sensitivity (Sen), specificity (Spec), positive predictive value (PPV) and negative predictive value (NPV) for a range of probability cut-offs for classifying those at high risk of non-response (main model)

Cut-off	Predicted non-responders	Sen	Spec	PPV	NPV
0.5	303 (36%)	59%	80%	68%	72%
0.6	210 (25%)	45%	89%	75%	69%
0.7	123 (15%)	30%	96%	86%	65%
0.8	49 (6%)	14%	100%	98%	61%
0.9	13 (2%)	4%	100%	100%	59%

The strengths of this analysis include the large sample size and the fact that it reflects use of MTX according to current guidelines and so supersedes earlier work [12–19]. The definition of non-response at 6 months embraced those who remained on the drug but had not exhibited enough improvement to be classified as moderate or good EULAR responders and also those who had discontinued the drug due to inefficacy or started a bDMARD. Other strengths were the inclusion of potential psychological predictors and using multiple imputation to provide reassurance of the robustness of the results to missing predictor data.

This study also has some limitations. The non-response rate was high. This may, in part, be due to suboptimal dosing or route of administration. Although the study did not dictate the treatment protocol, all patients should have been managed according to national guidelines [3] in which escalation of MTX is permitted and combination therapy is encouraged. We do not know the reasons for any deviations from treatment guidelines, but this prediction model may help guide clinicians as to which patients are less likely to respond as they are currently practicing and encourage them to consider treating more intensively. As we have attempted to predict non-response using only information available before the commencement of MTX, we have not considered the relationship between time-varying MTX dose and non-response. Titration is highly influenced by starting dose and patient response to treatment. The goal of the current work is to try and predict response prior to the start of MTX and, although maximum MTX dose and rate of titration may also be associated with response, that information would not be available pre-treatment. Further research is required to specifically investigate how rate and characteristics of MTX titration may also influence response, taking early response and adverse events into account. It seems likely that the observed association between lower DAS28 at baseline and subsequent non-response is explained by less scope for improvement (the key component of response) for those with lower disease activity. Since patients were recruited from routine clinical care, a high proportion of patients (41%) received oral or intramuscular steroids between the decision to prescribe MTX and the baseline assessment. We therefore performed sensitivity analysis, stratifying by steroid use, and the results were very similar (results not shown). The aim of this study was to use demographic, clinical and psychosocial variables that are readily available or easily measurable, to predict non-response. In future we aim to add genetic and metabolic predictors with the hope of improving the accuracy and clinical applicability of the model. Finally, these models were only validated internally. RAMS continues to recruit new patients so there will be an opportunity for further internal validation ("temporal validation") in the future. However, external validation in an independent dataset, which includes information on the relevant predictor variables that would be needed before the models could be considered for clinical use.

It might be reasonable to consider by-passing MTX therapy altogether in patients predicted to be very unlikely to respond. This model assigns $\geq 90\%$ probability of non-response to only a tiny proportion (2%) of patients. Would it be reasonable to accept a lower probability of non-response as a guide to MTX prescription - or a guide to starting combination therapy? This depends to some extent on the alternative forms of treatment and their efficacy in individuals predicted not to respond to MTX, and their cost. In the current situation it seems reasonable to continue to prescribe MTX for most patients in whom it is not contra-indicated but with a low threshold to move on to stronger combination or biological therapy if there is non-response at 6 months.

Conclusions

We have developed a model to predict non-response to MTX using data from a large contemporary observational study of patients with RA and UP commencing MTX for the first time. This is the first such model to consider patient-specific, disease-specific and psychosocial predictors. Using a high predicted probability to classify patients as at high risk of non-response would identify a small proportion of such individuals with perfect specificity. Patient anxiety was a multivariable predictor of non-response to MTX, a relationship that requires further research and which could be addressed prior to treatment commencement.

Abbreviations
ACPA: Anti-citrullinated protein antibody; ACR: American College of Rheumatology; AUC: Area under the curve; bDMARD: Biological disease-modifying antirheumatic drug; BMI: Body mass index; BMQ: Beliefs about Medicines Questionnaire; CRP: C-reactive protein; csDMARD: Conventional synthetic disease-modifying antirheumatic drug; DAS28: Disease Activity Score in 28 joints; DMARD: Disease-modifying antirheumatic drug; EULAR: European League Against Rheumatism; HADS: Hospital Anxiety and Depression Scale; HAQ: Health Assessment Questionnaire; IMD: Index of Multiple Deprivation; IPQ: Illness Perception Questionnaire; LDA: Low disease activity; MTX: Methotrexate; NPV: Negative predictive value; NSAIDs: Non-steroidal anti-inflammatory drugs; PPV: Positive predictive value; RA: Rheumatoid arthritis; RAMS: Rheumatoid Arthritis Medication Study; RF: Rheumatoid factor; SJC: Swollen joint count; TJC: Tender joint count; UP: Undifferentiated polyarthritis; VAS: Visual analogue scale

Acknowledgements
RAMS Co-Investigators: Ade Adebajo; Khalid Ahmed; Atheer Al-Ansari; Roshan Amarasena; Marwan Bukhari; Margaret Callan; Easwaradhas G Chelliah; Hector Chinoy; Annie Cooper; Bhaskar Dasgupta; Martin Davis; James Galloway;

Andrew Gough; Michael Green; Nicola Gullick; Jennifer Hamilton; Waji Hassan; Samantha Hider; Kimme Hyrich; Sanjeet Kamath; Susan Knight; Suzanne Lane; Martin Lee; Sarah Levy; Lizzy Macphie; Christopher Marguerie; Tarnya Marshall; Catherine Mathews; Frank McKenna; Sophia Naz; Mark Perry; Louise Pollard; Brian Quilty; Lindsay Robertson; Dipak Roy; Paul Sanders; Vadivelu Saravanan; David Scott; Gillian Smith; Richard Smith; Deborah Symmons; Lee-Suan Teh; Nick Viner.

Funding

This report includes independent research supported by the National Institute for Health Research Biomedical Research Unit Funding Scheme (NIHR Manchester Musculoskeletal Biomedical Research Unit). The views expressed in this publication are those of the authors and not necessarily those of the NHS, the National Institute for Health Research or the Department of Health. We thank Arthritis Research UK for their support: Arthritis Research UK grant number 20380.

Authors' contributions

Study concept and design: KLH, AB, SMMV. Data acquisition: JA, RAMS Co-Investigators. Data preparation: JCS, JA, KKH, HFH. Data analysis: JCS. Data interpretation: JCS, KLH, DPMS, SMMV. Manuscript writing: JCS, DPMS. Manuscript review: JCS, KLH, JA, KKH, HFH, DPMS, AB, SMMV. All authors read and approved the final manuscript.

Consent for publication

Not applicable.

Competing interests

The authors declare that they have no competing interests.

Author details

[1]Centre for Biostatistics, Manchester Academic Health Science Centre, University of Manchester, Manchester, UK. [2]Arthritis Research UK Centre for Epidemiology, Centre for Musculoskeletal Research, Manchester Academic Health Science Centre, University of Manchester, Manchester, UK. [3]NIHR Manchester Biomedical Research Centre, Central Manchester University Hospitals NHS Foundation Trust, Manchester Academic Health Science Centre, Manchester, UK. [4]Arthritis Research UK Centre for Genetics and Genomics, Centre for Musculoskeletal Research, Manchester Academic Health Science Centre, University of Manchester, Manchester, UK.

References

1. Lopez-Olivo MA, Siddhanamatha HR, Shea B, Tugwell P, Wells GA, Suarez-Almazor ME. Methotrexate for treating rheumatoid arthritis. Cochrane Database Syst Rev. 2014;6:CD000957.

2. Combe B, Landewe R, Daien CI, et al. 2016 update of the EULAR recommendations for the management of early arthritis. Ann Rheum Dis. 2017;76:948-59.

3. National Institute for Health and Care Excellence. Rheumatoid arthritis in adults: management. NICE guideline (CG79). London: NICE; 2009.

4. Singh JA, Saag KG, Bridges SL Jr, Akl EA, Bannuru RR, Sullivan MC, Vaysbrot E, McNaughton C, Osani M, Shmerling RH, et al. 2015 American College of Rheumatology Guideline for the treatment of rheumatoid arthritis. Arthritis Care Res (Hoboken). 2016, 68(1):1-25.

5. Visser K, Katchamart W, Loza E, Martinez-Lopez JA, Salliot C, Trudeau J, Bombardier C, Carmona L, van der Heijde D, Bijlsma JW, et al. Multinational evidence-based recommendations for the use of methotrexate in rheumatic disorders with a focus on rheumatoid arthritis: integrating systematic literature research and expert opinion of a broad international panel of rheumatologists in the 3E initiative. Ann Rheum Dis. 2009;68(7):1086-93.

6. Romao VC, Canhao H, Fonseca JE. Old drugs, old problems: where do we stand in prediction of rheumatoid arthritis responsiveness to methotrexate and other synthetic DMARDs? BMC Med. 2013;11:17.

7. Verstappen SM, Owen S-A, Hyrich KL. Prediction of response and adverse events to methotrexate treatment in patients with rheumatoid arthritis. Int J Clin Rheumtol. 2012;7(5):559-67.

8. Cook MJ, Diffin J, Scire CA, Lunt M, MacGregor AJ, Symmons DP, Verstappen SM. Predictors and outcomes of sustained, intermittent or never achieving remission in patients with recent onset inflammatory polyarthritis: results from the Norfolk arthritis register. Rheumatology (Oxford). 2016;55(9):1601-9.

9. Jiang X, Sandberg ME, Saevarsdottir S, Klareskog L, Alfredsson L, Bengtsson C. Higher education is associated with a better rheumatoid arthritis outcome concerning for pain and function but not disease activity: results from the EIRA cohort and Swedish rheumatology register. Arthritis Res Ther. 2015;17:317.

10. Norton S, Fu B, Scott DL, Deighton C, Symmons DP, Wailoo AJ, Tosh J, Lunt M, Davies R, Young A, et al. Health assessment questionnaire disability progression in early rheumatoid arthritis: systematic review and analysis of two inception cohorts. Semin Arthritis Rheum. 2014;44(2):131-44.

11. Hope HF, Bluett J, Barton A, Hyrich KL, Cordingley L, Verstappen SM. Psychological factors predict adherence to methotrexate in rheumatoid arthritis: findings from a systematic review of rates, predictors and associations with patient-reported and clinical outcomes. RMD Open. 2016; 2(1):e000171.

12. Hoekstra M, van Ede AE, Haagsma CJ, van de Laar MA, Huizinga TW, Kruijsen MW, Laan RF. Factors associated with toxicity, final dose, and efficacy of methotrexate in patients with rheumatoid arthritis. Ann Rheum Dis. 2003;62(5):423-6.

13. Lima A, Monteiro J, Bernardes M, Sousa H, Azevedo R, Seabra V, Medeiros R. Prediction of methotrexate clinical response in Portuguese rheumatoid arthritis patients: implication of MTHFR rs1801133 and ATIC rs4673993 polymorphisms. Biomed Res Int. 2014;2014:368681.

14. Saevarsdottir S, Wallin H, Seddighzadeh M, Ernestam S, Geborek P, Petersson IF, Bratt J, van Vollenhoven RF, Group STI. Predictors of response to methotrexate in early DMARD naive rheumatoid arthritis: results from the initial open-label phase of the SWEFOT trial. Ann Rheum Dis. 2011;70(3):469-75.

15. Ma MH, Ibrahim F, Walker D, Hassell A, Choy EH, Kiely PD, Williams R, Walsh DA, Young A, Scott DL. Remission in early rheumatoid arthritis: predicting treatment response. J Rheumatol. 2012;39(3):470-5.

16. Wessels JA, van der Kooij SM, le Cessie S, Kievit W, Barerra P, Allaart CF, Huizinga TW, Guchelaar HJ, Pharmacogenetics Collaborative Research G. A clinical pharmacogenetic model to predict the efficacy of methotrexate monotherapy in recent-onset rheumatoid arthritis. Arthritis Rheum. 2007; 56(6):1765-75.

17. Fransen J, Kooloos WM, Wessels JA, Huizinga TW, Guchelaar HJ, van Riel PL, Barrera P. Clinical pharmacogenetic model to predict response of MTX monotherapy in patients with established rheumatoid arthritis after DMARD failure. Pharmacogenomics. 2012;13(9):1087-94.

18. Maillefert JF, Puechal X, Falgarone G, Lizard G, Ornetti P, Solau E, Legre V, Liote F, Sibilia J, Morel J, et al. Prediction of response to disease modifying antirheumatic drugs in rheumatoid arthritis. Joint Bone Spine. 2010;77(6):558-63.

19. Hider SL, Silman AJ, Thomson W, Lunt M, Bunn D, Symmons DP. Can clinical factors at presentation be used to predict outcome of treatment with methotrexate in patients with early inflammatory polyarthritis? Ann Rheum Dis. 2009;68(1):57-62.

20. Department for Communities and Local Government: The English indices of deprivation 2010. 2011.

21. Arnett FC, Edworthy SM, Bloch DA, McShane DJ, Fries JF, Cooper NS, Healey LA, Kaplan SR, Liang MH, Luthra HS, et al. The American rheumatism association 1987 revised criteria for the classification of rheumatoid arthritis. Arthritis Rheum. 1988;31(3):315-24.

22. Wolfe F, Michaud K, Pincus T. Development and validation of the health assessment questionnaire II: a revised version of the health assessment questionnaire. Arthritis Rheum. 2004;50(10):3296-305.

23. Zigmond AS, Snaith RP. The hospital anxiety and depression scale. Acta Psychiatr Scand. 1983;67(6):361-70.

24. Horne R, Weinman J, Hankins M. The beliefs about medicines questionnaire: the development and evaluation of a new method for assessing the cognitive representation of medication. Psychol Health. 1999;14(1):1-24.

25. Broadbent E, Petrie KJ, Main J, Weinman J. The brief illness perception questionnaire. J Psychosom Res. 2006;60(6):631–7.
26. Norton S, Hughes LD, Chilcot J, Sacker A, van Os S, Young A, Done J. Negative and positive illness representations of rheumatoid arthritis: a latent profile analysis. J Behav Med. 2014;37(3):524–32.
27. Prevoo ML, van 't Hof MA, Kuper HH, van Leeuwen MA, van de Putte LB, van Riel PL. Modified disease activity scores that include twenty-eight-joint counts. Development and validation in a prospective longitudinal study of patients with rheumatoid arthritis. Arthritis Rheum. 1995;38(1):44–8.
28. van Gestel AM, Prevoo ML, van 't Hof MA, van Rijswijk MH, van de Putte LB, van Riel PL. Development and validation of the European league against rheumatism response criteria for rheumatoid arthritis. Comparison with the preliminary American College of Rheumatology and the World Health Organization/International League against Rheumatism criteria. Arthritis Rheum. 1996;39(1):34–40.
29. Steyerberg EW, Harrell FE Jr, Borsboom GJ, Eijkemans MJ, Vergouwe Y, Habbema JD. Internal validation of predictive models: efficiency of some procedures for logistic regression analysis. J Clin Epidemiol. 2001;54(8):774–81.
30. StataCorp. Stata statistical software: release 13.1. College Station: StataCorp LP; 2013.
31. Michelsen B, Kristianslund EK, Sexton J, et al. Do depression and anxiety reduce the likelihood of remission in rheumatoid arthritis and psoriatic arthritis? Data from the prospective multicentre NOR-DMARD study. Ann Rheum Dis. 2017;76:1906-10.

11

Adipocyte-specific Repression of PPAR-gamma by NCoR Contributes to Scleroderma Skin Fibrosis

Benjamin Korman[1,2]* ⓘ, Roberta Goncalves Marangoni[1], Gabriel Lord[1], Jerrold Olefsky[3], Warren Tourtellotte[4] and John Varga[1,5]

Abstract

Background: A pivotal role for adipose tissue homeostasis in systemic sclerosis (SSc) skin fibrosis is increasingly recognized. The nuclear receptor PPAR-γ is the master regulator of adipogenesis. Peroxisome proliferator activated receptor-γ (PPAR-γ) has antifibrotic effects by blocking transforming growth factor-β (TGF-β) and is dysregulated in SSc. To unravel the impact of dysregulated PPAR-γ in SSc, we focused on nuclear corepressor (NCoR), which negatively regulates PPAR-γ activity and suppresses adipogenesis.

Methods: An NCoR-regulated gene signature was measured in the SSc skin transcriptome. Experimental skin fibrosis was examined in mice with adipocyte-specific NCoR ablation.

Results: SSc skin biopsies demonstrated deregulated NCoR signaling. A 43-gene NCoR gene signature showed strong positive correlation with PPAR-γ signaling ($R = 0.919$, $p < 0.0001$), whereas negative correlations with TGF-β signaling ($R = -0.796$, $p < 0.0001$) and the modified Rodnan skin score ($R = -0.49$, $p = 0.004$) were found. Mice with adipocyte-specific NCoR ablation demonstrated significant protection from experimental skin fibrosis and inflammation. The protective effects were mediated primarily through endogenous PPAR-γ.

Conclusions: Our results implicate, for the first time, to our knowledge, deregulated NCoR/PPAR-γ pathways in SSc, and they support a role of adipocyte modulation of skin fibrosis. Pharmacologic restoration of NCoR/PPAR-γ signaling may represent a novel strategy to control skin fibrosis in SSc.

Keywords: NCoR, Adipocyte, Skin fibrosis, Scleroderma, PPAR-γ, Adipogenesis, Fibrogenesis

Background

Systemic sclerosis (SSc) is a poorly understood multisystem disorder characterized by autoimmunity, vasculopathy, and fibrosis [1, 2]. A distinguishing hallmark of SSc is simultaneous fibrosis in multiple organs [3]. SSc has high mortality and no effective therapy. Myofibroblasts originating from distinct tissue-resident progenitors are key drivers of organ fibrosis in SSc and other fibrotic conditions [4]. Recent studies have demonstrated that aberrant adipose tissue homeostasis and dysregulated adipogenesis play vital roles in SSc by contributing to myofibroblast accumulation in the fibrotic dermis [5]. Targeting the cellular transition from adipocyte to myofibroblast therefore represents a potential therapeutic approach to reduce fibrosis.

Peroxisome proliferator-activated receptor-γ (PPAR-γ) is a pleiotropic nuclear hormone receptor that is the master regulator of adipogenesis and is required for adipocyte differentiation [6]. Intriguingly, recent studies have shown that PPAR-γ has an important antifibrotic role in SSc and other fibrosing disorders [7]. PPAR-γ counteracts profibrotic TGF-β signaling [8, 9] and has been shown to have antifibrotic activities in several organs relevant to SSc, including skin, lung, and heart [10–12]. Importantly, SSc skin biopsies and explanted fibroblasts demonstrate reduced PPAR-γ expression and activity [5, 11, 13, 14]). In mice, ablation of PPAR-γ in fibroblasts promotes cutaneous fibrogenesis [15]. Moreover, genetic studies

* Correspondence: benjamin_korman@urmc.rochester.edu
[1]Northwestern Scleroderma Program, Division of Rheumatology, Northwestern University Feinberg School of Medicine, Chicago, IL, USA
[2]Division of Allergy, Immunology and Rheumatology, University of Rochester Medical Center, Rochester, NY, USA
Full list of author information is available at the end of the article

demonstrate significant associations of PPAR-γ variants with SSc, and transcriptomic studies have implicated the PPAR-γ pathway as fundamentally dysregulated in SSc skin biopsies [16–18]. Together, these findings provide strong support for the role of PPAR-γ deregulation in the pathogenesis of SSc, and they suggest that targeting PPAR-γ signaling could represent a rational therapeutic approach in fibrosis. Indeed, PPAR-γ agonists, including rosiglitazone and a novel pan-PPAR agonist IVA337, have been shown to have antifibrotic effects in mice [13, 19]. However, because PPAR-γ agonists have off-target and ligand-independent effects [6, 20–24], approaches designed to selectively target the PPAR-γ pathway may provide an alternative way to modulate fibrogenesis in SSc without the adverse side effects of PPAR-γ agonists.

The expression of PPAR-γ is tightly regulated by nuclear coreceptors (NCoRs) [25]. In the absence of ligand, PPAR-γ is complexed to retinoid X receptors (RXRs) and two corepressors, NCoR and SMRT (silencing mediator of retinoid and thyroid receptors), which prevent DNA binding and transcriptional activity [26]. Upon ligation, corepressors are displaced from the PPAR-γ/RXR complex and coactivators are recruited, allowing sequence-specific binding to conserved PPAR-γ response elements in target gene promoters [27]. NCoR is a ubiquitously expressed nuclear corepressor with potent tissue-specific effects on lipid metabolism and mitochondrial energy homeostasis [27]. In adipose tissue, the dominant function of NCoR is inhibition of PPAR-γ activity, and mice with adipocyte-specific NCoR knockout show unrestrained PPAR-γ activity [28].

In light of the fundamental role of PPAR-γ and its regulation of adipogenesis in SSc, we sought to investigate the contribution of NCoR as a key regulator of PPAR-γ in SSc skin fibrosis. We found that an NCoR-regulated gene signature is aberrantly expressed in SSc skin biopsies and correlates with PPAR-γ and TGF-β signaling as well as extent of skin disease. Mice with adipocyte-specific NCoR ablation showed amelioration of skin fibrosis that was mediated via endogenous PPAR-γ. Together, these results support a vital role for the NCoR/PPAR-γ pathways in SSc skin fibrosis. Furthermore, these findings also implicate adipocytes as a key cell type in modulating fibrosis and indicate that restoration of adipose NCoR/PPAR-γ signaling could serve as a novel approach for treating skin fibrosis.

Methods
Measurement of NCoR pathway score in SSc skin biopsies
To assess NCoR pathway activation in SSc, we defined an NCoR-responsive gene signature comprised of 101 genes previously shown to be specifically repressed by NCoR [29]. The expression of this signature was then queried in a microarray dataset [GEO:GSE76886] of SSc ($n = 70$) and healthy control ($n = 22$) skin biopsies. All

biopsies were obtained prior to starting immunomodulatory therapy. There were 43 transcripts out of 101, with a coefficient of variation > 0.5 and a false discovery rate (FDR) < 0.05, and these transcripts were included in subsequent analyses. An NCoR pathway score was calculated on the basis of previously described approaches, and scores were normalized to the mean of the controls [30]. The standardized gene expression levels were summed for each biopsy to provide an NCoR signature score based on the following formula: $\sum_{i=1}^{n} = \frac{GENEi_{SSc} - MEANi_{ctr}}{SDctr} * k$,

where i = each NCoR-regulated gene, Gene i_{SSc} = gene expression level in each SSc biopsy, and Mean i_{ctr} = the average gene expression in controls. For NCoR-induced genes, $k = 1$; for NCoR-suppressed genes, $k = -1$.

In subsequent analyses, the NCoR pathway score in each skin biopsy was correlated with previously defined PPAR-γ and TGF-β gene signatures [5, 31]. In SSc biopsies with sufficient clinical data ($n = 36$), NCoR pathway scores were correlated with the modified Rodnan skin score (MRSS). Because expression data were collected from publicly available sources, detailed clinical information was available for 36 of the patients with SSc and 11 control individuals. The age of patients was 48.0 ± 11.6 (mean ± SD) years, as compared with control individuals, who were aged 39.9 ± 11.8 (mean ± SD) years. Among patients with SSc, 86.1% female, compared with 63.6% of control individuals. Among patients with SSc, 30 had diffuse cutaneous disease (83.3%), 5 had limited cutaneous disease, and 1 had overlap SSc, and the MRSS was 17 ± 10 (mean ± SD). Twelve patients (33%) had early disease (< 2 years disease duration since onset of first non-Raynaud's symptom), and 24 (67%) had late disease (> 2 years disease duration since onset of first non-Raynaud's symptom).

Animals
Mice carrying floxed alleles of NCoR on a C57BL/6J background were backcrossed to mice harboring Cre recombinase driven by the adipocyte protein 2 promoter to create NCoR$^{flx/flx}$ (wild-type [WT]) and NCoR$^{flx/flx}$-ap2Cre (adipocyte nuclear corepressor-knockout [AKO]) animals [28]. Genotypes of all animals were confirmed. All experimental procedures complied with the Public Health Service Policy on Humane Care and Use of Laboratory Animals, and protocols were approved by the institutional animal care and use committee of Northwestern University.

Diets
Mice were fed a standard chow diet (LM-485, 17% kcal from fat; Harlan Teklad, Madison, WI, USA) until 8–12 weeks of age and were subsequently switched to a high-fat diet containing 60% fat

(D12492; Research Diets Inc., New Brunswick, NJ, USA).

Bleomycin-induced fibrosis

Mice were treated with bleomycin (1 mg/ml in PBS; 10 mg/kg/d) or PBS by daily subcutaneous injection for 14 days and killed at 21 days [32, 33]. In some experiments, mice received concurrent daily intraperitoneal injections of the PPAR-γ inhibitor GW9662 (Sigma-Aldrich, St. Louis, MO, USA) (1 mg/kg) for 21 days. At the time mice were killed, skin, gonadal and perirenal fat, and 16-hour fasting serum samples were harvested and processed for analysis. Each experimental group consisted of three to five mice per group, and experiments were repeated two or three times with consistent results. In other experiments, old (> 40 weeks) and young adult (< 20 weeks) mice and male and female mice were used.

RNA isolation and qRT-PCR

Upon harvest, tissues (skin, adipose, lung, liver) were immersed in Ambion RNA*later* (Life Technologies, Carlsbad, CA, USA) and stored at – 80 °C. The samples were homogenized; RNA was isolated using the RNeasy Micro Kit or RNeasy Fibrous Mini Kit (Qiagen, Valencia, CA, USA); and quantification of gene expression was performed as previously described [34].

Serum assays

Fasting serum was assayed for glucose by spectrophotometry (K606-100; BioVision Inc., Milpitas, CA, USA) and for insulin by ELISA (EZRMI-13K; MilliporeSigma, Burlington, MA, USA). Homeostatic model assessment of insulin resistance (HOMA-IR) was calculated using the formula HOMA-IR = glucose × insulin/400. Fasting serum levels of leptin, adiponectin, resistin, and plasminogen activator inhibitor-1 (PAI-1) were determined by multiplex Luminex assays according to the manufacturer's instructions (MADKMAG-71K and MADPNMAG-70K-01; MilliporeSigma).

Adipocyte size and numbers

The number and size of the adipocytes in the perirenal and intradermal adipose depots were evaluated in H&E-stained sections at 100 × magnification [28]. Adipocyte diameters ($n = 250$ [perirenal] and $n = 100$ [intradermal]) were determined in three noncontiguous high-power fields (HPFs) per mouse from three or four mice per group using Fiji software [35], and data were used to generate frequency distribution histograms of adipocyte diameters.

Histopathological analysis

Tissues were fixed in 4% phosphate-buffered paraformaldehyde (pH 7.4) and embedded in paraffin, and 4-μm-thick sections were stained with H&E. Dermal thickness (distance from the epidermis-dermis junction to the dermis-fat junction) and intradermal adipose layer thickness (distance from the dermis-fat junction to the fat-muscle junction) were determined at five randomly selected regions per HPF using Fiji software [32, 34]. To evaluate collagen deposition and organization in the dermis, sections were stained with Masson's trichrome and Picrosirius red, and intensity was measured from two HPFs per mouse and two mice per group using Fiji software.

IHC

Paraffin-embedded sections of lesional skin were incubated with rabbit anti-NCoR (1:100, PA1-844A; Thermo Fisher Scientific, Waltham, MA, USA) rabbit anti-α-smooth muscle actin (α-SMA, 1:200; Sigma-Aldrich), rat anti-F4/80 (1:1000; eBioscience, San Diego, CA, USA), and rat anti-phosho-SMAD2 (1:200; Sigma-Aldrich) primary antibodies [36]. Secondary mouse antibodies were used to localize primary antibody binding. Negative controls without primary antibody were used to confirm specificity. Staining intensity of F4/80-immunopositive cells was determined from two randomly chosen regions of the dermis and the intradermal adipose layer using Fiji software.

Determination of collagen content

Lesional skin was hydrolyzed in HCl, and hydroxyproline content was determined using a colorimetric assay kit (BioVision, Inc.).

Statistical analysis

Data are presented as mean ± SEM. Statistical analyses were performed using Prism 6 software (GraphPad Software, La Jolla, CA, USA). For in vivo studies, statistical significance was assessed by Wilcoxon-Mann-Whitney test for two-group comparisons, and analysis of variance was used for multiple group comparisons. $p < 0.05$ was considered statistically significant.

Results
Deregulated NCoR signaling in SSc skin biopsies
NCoR-regulated genes

We first sought to examine the pattern of genes whose expression was modulated by the PPAR-γ corepressor NCoR in SSc skin biopsies. Forty-three NCoR-specific transcripts (defined in the Methods section above and referred to in this paper as the *NCoR gene signature*) were found to be differentially regulated (FDR < 0.05) in SSc skin biopsies relative to controls. Hierarchical clustering of biopsies based on this NCoR gene signature identified three clusters that robustly discriminated SSc from control biopsies (chi-square = 33.9, $p < 0.0001$ for cluster identity) (Fig. 1a). Among patients with SSc, no

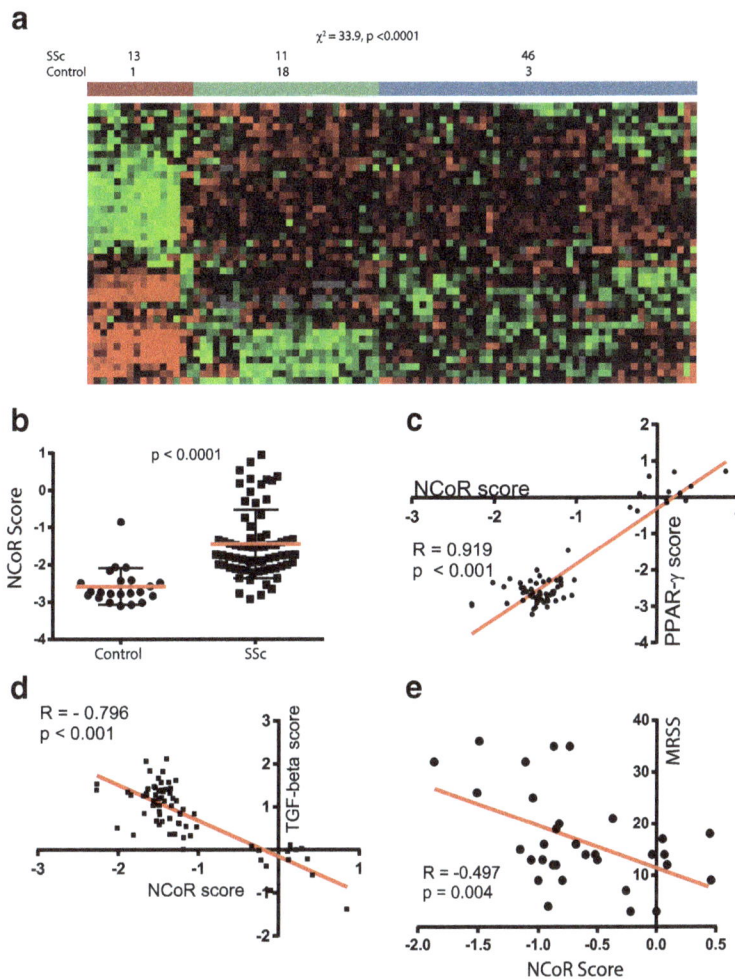

Fig. 1 Differential expression of nuclear corepressor (NCoR)-modulated genes in systemic sclerosis (SSc). **a** Skin biopsy transcriptomes from 70 patients with SSc and 22 healthy control subjects [GEO:GSE76886] were queried for expression of genes negatively regulated by NCoR. Hierarchical clustering identified three subsets: cluster 1, a small subset with significant NCoR upregulation and comprised mostly of patients with SSc; cluster 2, a subset made mostly of control individuals; and cluster 3, a group of patients with SSc with decreased NCoR-mediated expression. These clusters distinguish SSc biopsies from controls ($p < 0.0001$ by chi-square test). The number and percentage of biopsies are denoted for each group. *Red* indicates gene upregulation; *green* indicates downregulation. **b** NCoR pathway scores were determined (*see* the Methods section for derivation). Note the significantly elevated scores in SSc skin biopsies. **c** and **d** NCoR pathway scores correlate significantly with peroxisome proliferator activated receptor-γ (PPAR-γ) and transforming growth factor-β (TGF-β) pathway scores. **e** Correlation of NCoR pathway scores and the modified Rodnan skin score (MRSS)

differences across the three clusters were found in age, sex, disease duration, or MRSS.

In an orthogonal approach, we identified a 45-gene lipid metabolism gene module (defined using KEGG pathway terms) selected from 400 genes coexpressed with NCoR (Spearman's $r > 0.5$), and we used this module to query skin transcriptomes [GEO:GSE76886]. This set of genes used for classification identified two groupings that significantly discriminated SSc from control skin biopsies (chi-square for group identity = 10.5, $p < 0.0001$). NCoR score did not differ in either the limited vs diffuse SSc groups ($p = 0.48$) or the early vs late disease groups ($p = 0.16$). On the basis of these observations using complementary analytic approaches, we

conclude that deregulated NCoR signaling is a hallmark of SSc skin.

NCoR signaling is correlated with PPAR-γ and TGF-β signaling

We found that NCoR pathway scores were significantly elevated in SSc biopsies compared with controls (Fig. 1b). Importantly, the NCoR pathway score showed strong positive correlation with a previously defined PPAR-γ gene signature ($R = 0.919$, $p < 0.0001$) (Fig. 1c). In sharp contrast, the NCoR pathway score was negatively correlated with a TGF-β gene signature score defined using two complementary approaches. The first TGF-β signature was defined on the basis of a clinical trial with genes showing significant change in expression in skin biopsies from patients with SSc treated with anti-TGF-β monoclonal antibody ($R = -0.796, p < 0.0001$) (Fig. 1d) [37]. An alternative TGF-β-regulated gene signature derived from normal and SSc skin fibroblasts treated with TGF-β showed a similar significant correlation with the NCoR pathway ($R = -0.594$, $p = 0.02$) (data not shown) [31]. These findings indicate that NCoR-regulated gene expression positively correlated with antifibrotic PPAR-γ signaling and negatively correlated with fibrotic TGF-β signaling in the skin of patients with SSc.

NCoR signaling is associated with extent of SSc skin disease

To pursue the clinical relevance of these changes, we examined their association with MRSS, a validated measure of global skin involvement. Although local MRSS may be a better predictor of local gene expression, total-body MRSS correlates closely with forearm MRSS and has been used widely as a surrogate for disease severity [38–42]. As shown in Fig. 1e, NCoR pathway scores were negatively correlated with MRSS ($R = -0.49$, $p = 0.004$). The alternate NCoR pathway score (defined using the 45-gene NCoR coexpressed lipid metabolism module) demonstrated similar correlation with MRSS ($R = 0.46$, $p = 0.01$). Together, these orthogonal approaches indicate that NCoR-modulated gene expression is biologically relevant to pathways fundamental to fibrosis in SSc and has clinically significant associations. These findings prompted us to seek experimental evidence to define the role of NCoR in skin fibrosis.

Mice with NCoR adipocyte-specific knockout show PPAR-γ activation

In order to investigate the potential role of NCoR in the development of fibrosis, we took advantage of a mouse model with adipocyte-specific ablation of NCoR: the ap2-Cre-NCoR$^{flx/flx}$ (AKO) mouse [28]. On a high-fat diet, AKO mice demonstrated > 90% lower NCoR levels in adipose tissue than control mice; most other tissues, including lung and liver, showed no significant decrease (Fig. 2a). Skin from AKO mice demonstrated a 30% decrease in NCoR expression, reflecting the loss of intradermal fat. Adipose tissue-specific loss of NCoR in AKO mice was confirmed by IHC of perirenal (visceral) and intradermal white adipose depots (Fig. 2b, c). The size of adipocytes in these fat depots was markedly decreased ($p = 0.0006$), whereas the number of adipocytes was increased ($p = 0.008$), in AKO mice compared with littermate controls, consistent with increased adipogenesis in both visceral and intradermal adipose tissues (Fig. 2d and e) [43]. Skin biopsies from AKO mice demonstrated upregulation of PPAR-γ target genes perilipin, PEPCK, GLUT4, and adiponectin and downregulation of RGS2, a negative regulatory target, in the adipose layer (Fig. 2f).

Furthermore, AKO mice showed improved insulin sensitivity (HOMA-IR), whereas circulating levels of the adipokines leptin, resistin, and PAI-1 were reduced in the serum (Fig. 2g). The ratio of leptin/adiponectin, considered a marker of healthy adipose tissue [44], was reduced in serum from AKO mice (Fig. 2h). Together, these findings indicate that ablation of NCoR in adipose tissue is associated with de-repression of PPAR-γ and enhanced cell-autonomous PPAR-γ activity.

NCoR AKO mice are resistant to skin fibrosis

To evaluate the impact of adipocyte-specific NCoR loss on fibrogenesis, we used the well-characterized bleomycin model [45]. AKO mice and littermate controls maintained on a high-fat diet were challenged with subcutaneous bleomycin or PBS. Under high-fat diet conditions, control mice showed a dramatic enhancement of the intradermal adipose tissue, with increased adipocyte size and number, as expected (Figs. 2d and 3a). In contrast, AKO mice were almost completely resistant to high-fat diet-induced intradermal adipocyte hypertrophy. At day 21 of bleomycin treatment, WT mice showed a significant increase in dermal thickness ($p < 0.001$) and collagen deposition, as well as attenuation of the intradermal adipose layer ($p = 0.02$), compared with vehicle-treated mice (Fig. 3a). Identically treated NCoR-deficient mice showed significantly attenuated increases in dermal thickening ($p = 0.02$) and intradermal adipocyte loss ($p = 0.04$) (Fig. 3b). Consistent results were obtained in three independent experiments, demonstrating reproducible amelioration of dermal fibrosis and maintenance of intradermal adipose tissue in both young (< 20 weeks old) and old (> 40 weeks old) mice, as well as in male and female mice (data not shown) lacking adipocyte NCoR. The extent of dermal collagen deposition and myofibroblast numbers were both reduced in AKO mice (Fig. 3c). Further analysis of the lesional skin demonstrated significant reduction in the expression of numerous fibrotic genes (Col1A2, Col 5A1, fibronectin-EDA, and TGF-β) (Fig. 3d). Together, these results indicate that loss of NCoR in adipocytes is sufficient to protect mice against experimentally induced skin fibrosis.

Pharmacologic inhibition of PPAR-γ reverses the antifibrotic phenotype of AKO mice

In view of the pleiotropic and cell-type-specific functions of NCoR regulating multiple signaling pathways [27], we sought to identify whether the antifibrotic effects observed in mice lacking adipocyte NCoR were mediated through PPAR-γ, a primary target regulated by NCoR. For this purpose, we used the irreversible PPAR-γ antagonist 2-chloro-5-nitrobenzanilide (GW9662) [46]. GW9662 was administered by intraperitoneal injection (1 mg/kg/d)

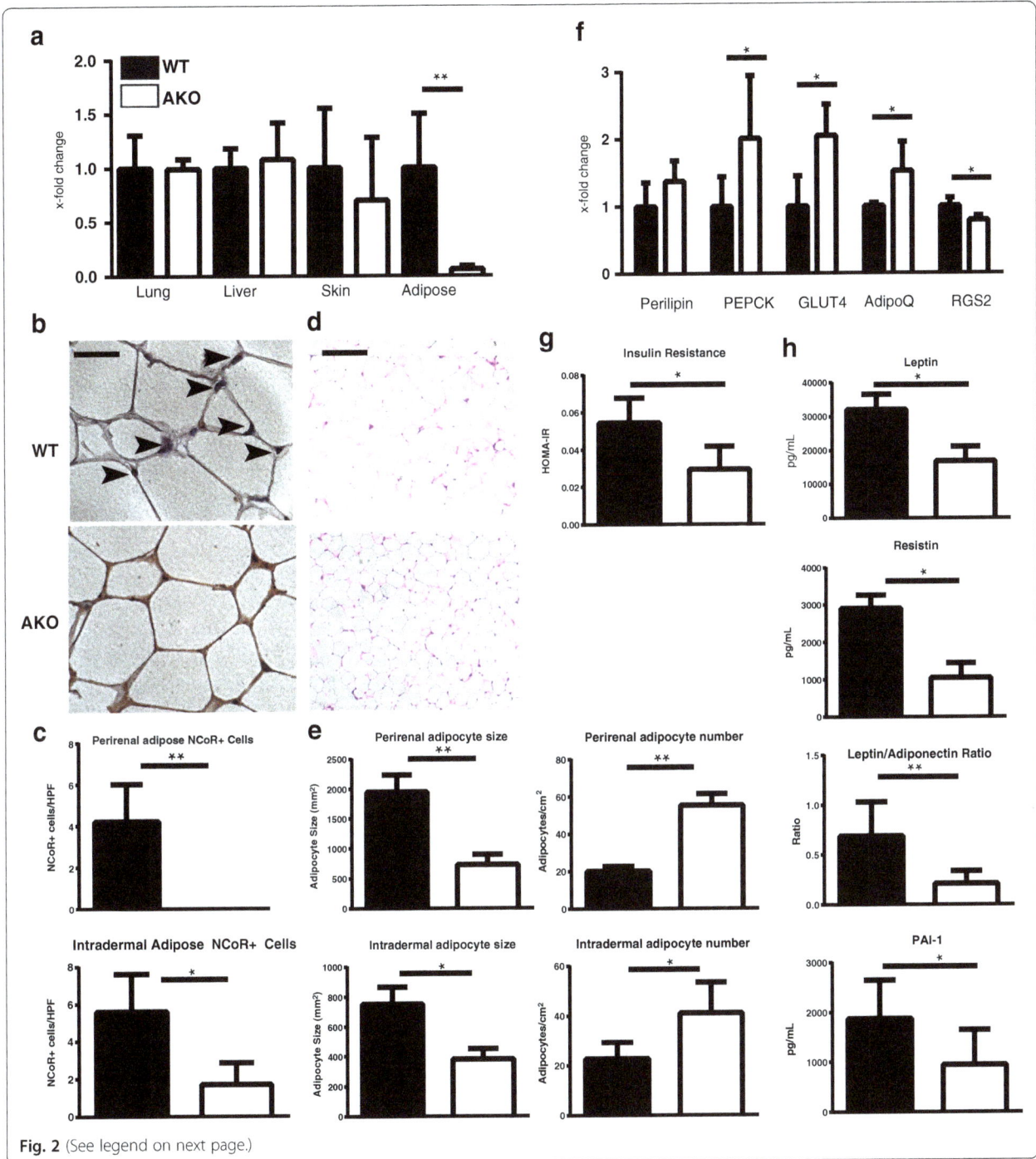

Fig. 2 (See legend on next page.)

(See figure on previous page.)

Fig. 2 Characterization of adipocyte nuclear corepressor-knockout (ap2-NCoR^flx/flx; AKO) mice. Skin, serum, lung, liver, and adipose tissues were harvested from untreated AKO and littermate control mice on a high-fat diet. Tissues were assessed for histologic and biochemical changes suggestive of alterations in adipocyte function. **a** Nuclear corepressor (NCoR) expression is significantly reduced in adipose tissue but not in lung, liver, or skin. Tissue was harvested from 3- to 4-week-old mice, and messenger RNA (mRNA) levels were determined by qPCR. The results represent fold changes in triplicate determinations from three or four mice per group and normalized to GAPDH. ** $p < 0.01$ by Mann-Whitney U test. *Black bars*, wild-type (WT) mice; *white bars*, AKO mice. **b** NCoR IHC staining of perirenal adipose tissue evident in WT mice was not detectable in AKO mice. *Arrowheads* indicate nuclei with positive staining for NCoR. Representative images are shown. Scale bars = 100 μm. **c** Quantification of NCoR+ cells in perirenal and intradermal adipose tissue (cells per high-power field [HPF]). The results are derived from 5 HPFs from two or three mice per group. * $p < 0.05$ by Mann-Whitney U test. **d** AKO mice have reduced expansion of adipocyte size and increased adipocyte number. Representative images of H&E staining of perirenal adipose tissue from mice fed a high-fat diet. Scale bars = 100 μm. **e** Quantification of adipocyte size (left) and number (right) in perirenal (top) and intradermal (bottom) adipocytes. Adipocyte diameter and number (area results derived from > 200 adipocytes/mouse and number quantified from 2 to 4 HPF/mouse from three or four mice per treatment group). Data presented are mean ± SD. * $p < 0.05$ by Mann-Whitney U test. **f** Ablation of NCoR is associated with increased expression of PPAR-γ-responsive genes. Gonadal adipose tissue was harvested, and mRNA levels were analyzed by qRT-PCR. The results represent fold changes compared with littermate controls. Data were obtained in triplicate determinations from three or four mice per group and normalized to GAPDH. * $p < 0.05$ by Mann-Whitney U test. **g** AKO mice have improved insulin sensitivity. The homeostatic model assessment of insulin resistance (HOMA-IR) was calculated from fasting serum insulin and glucose measurements in mice fed high fat diet for 15 weeks, * $p < 0.05$ by Mann-Whitney U test. **h** AKO mice have altered circulating adipokine levels. Adipokines were measured in serum of fasting mice using multiplex Luminex assays (n = 4–5 mice/group; * $p < 0.05$ by Mann-Whitney U test). *PEPCK* Phosphoenolpyruvate carboxykinase, *GLUT4* Glucose transporter type 4, *RGS2* Regulator of G-protein signaling 2, *PAI-1* Plasminogen activator inhibitor -1

concurrently with bleomycin or vehicle. In AKO mice, GW9662 largely abrogated protection from bleomycin-induced fibrosis, whereas on its own GW9662 had no effect. GW9662 on its own had no effect on skin fibrosis in WT mice (Fig. 4a). Moreover, bleomycin-treated AKO mice demonstrated a reduction in F4/80-positive macrophage accumulation compared with similarly treated WT mice, which was reversed by cotreatment with GW9662 (Fig. 4b). We conclude that the fibrotic impact of adipocyte NCoR involves repression of PPAR-γ and that protection from fibrosis seen in NCoR-deficient mice is mediated via antifibrotic activities of endogenous PPAR-γ.

Discussion

In this study, we investigated the effect of adipocyte-specific loss of the PPAR-γ corepressor NCoR on skin fibrosis and its expression in patients with SSc. The results indicate that adipose-specific NCoR ablation ameliorates the development of dermal fibrosis in mice. Moreover, skin fibrosis in SSc is accompanied by increased NCoR activity and decreased expression of PPAR-γ-regulated genes. The antifibrotic effect of NCoR ablation involves cell-autonomous increased PPAR-γ signaling, blockade of TGF-β-dependent fibroblast activation, and attenuation of the cutaneous inflammatory response. Furthermore, loss of NCoR in adipocytes counteracts the depletion of dermal adipose tissue via augmented PPAR-γ activity. Together, these findings indicate that loss of NCoR repression and consequent PPAR-γ activation in adipocytes protect against skin fibrosis. These findings are consistent with the notion that PPAR-γ plays an endogenous antifibrotic role in the skin and suggest that therapies targeting the NCoR/PPAR- γ pathway and adipogenesis represent novel therapeutic approaches for SSc.

Analysis of skin biopsy transcriptomes suggested a link between NCoR signaling and skin fibrosis in SSc. We used two distinct approaches to ascertain NCoR signaling and found that both differentiated SSc biopsies from healthy controls and identified novel SSc subsets with aberrant NCoR signaling. When measured as a pathway score, NCoR activation demonstrated a strong positive correlation with PPAR-γ signaling in SSc skin biopsies ($R = 0.919$) and a strong negative correlation with TGF-β signaling ($R = 0.792$). These correlations are consistent with the idea that in addition to its role as a PPAR-γ corepressor, NCoR downregulates the expression of genes involved in TGF-β signaling. The correlation of NCoR pathway activity with the MRSS potentially implicates NCoR/PPAR-γ in SSc fibrosis and importantly suggests that these molecular findings have implications for the extent of clinical skin disease in SSc.

Mice deficient in adipocyte NCoR demonstrate the importance of this corepressor in dermal fibrosis. NCoR exerts diverse effects that are pleiotropic and tissue-specific. Previous work has demonstrated that NCoR plays a primary role in repressing the expression PPAR-γ in adipose tissue [28]. We ablated NCoR in adipose tissue to assess whether consequent PPAR-γ gain of function could modulate dermal fibrosis. We recently demonstrated a critical role of intradermal adipose tissue homeostasis in the pathogenesis of fibrosis and implicated dermal adipocytes as progenitors of fibrotic myofibroblasts [32]. We therefore hypothesized that de-repression of PPAR-γ could promote adipogenesis in the skin and attenuate dermal fibrosis. Indeed, we found that AKO mice treated with bleomycin showed consistent and significant reductions in dermal thickness and collagen accumulation. Consistent with prior studies that showed a role for adipocytes in skin fibrosis, we found that reduced skin fibrosis resulted from an adipocyte-specific NCoR ablation, therefore further supporting the notion that NCoR signaling in adipocytes

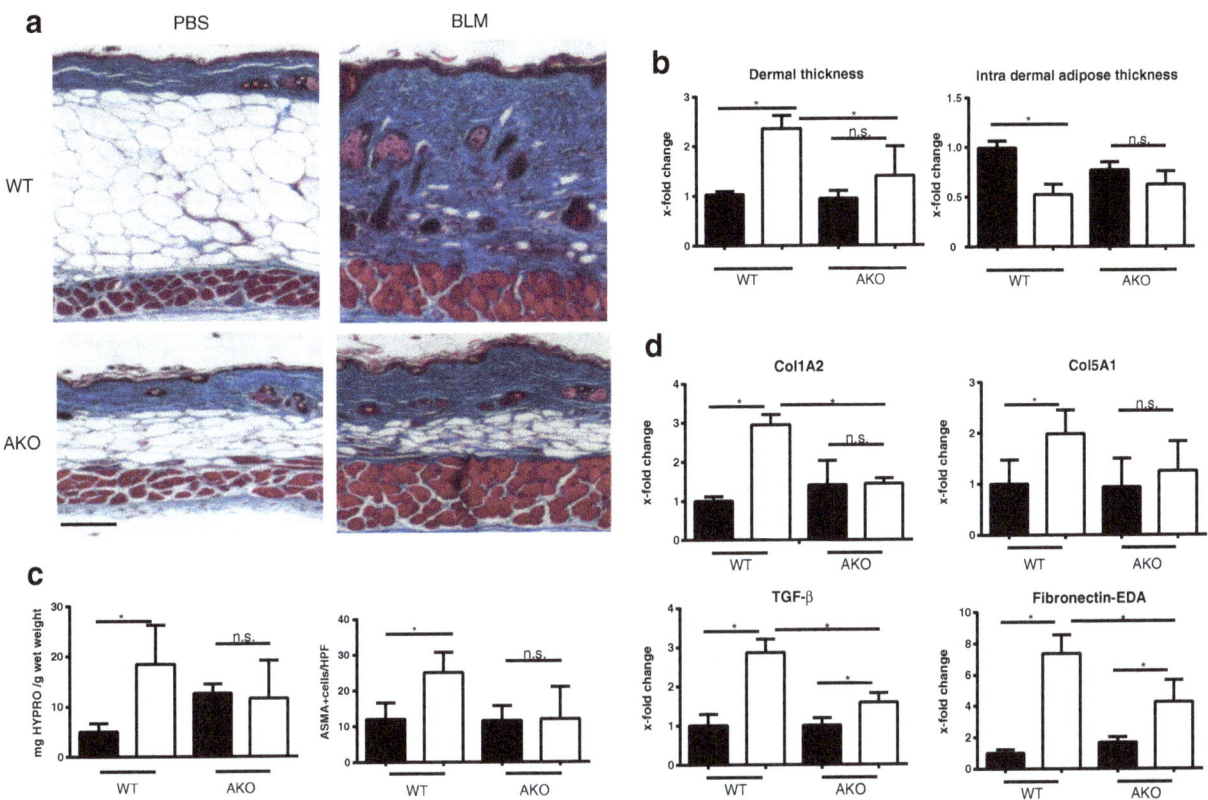

Fig. 3 Adipocyte nuclear corepressor-knockout (AKO) mice are protected from skin fibrosis. Twenty-eight- to 32-week-old AKO mice and littermate controls (wild type [WT]) on a high-fat diet for 20 weeks were given daily subcutaneous injections of bleomycin (BLM) or PBS for 14 days, and skin was harvested at 21 days. **a** Increased dermal collagen deposition and loss of intradermal fat are attenuated in AKO mice. Masson's trichrome stain. Representative images. Scale bars = 100 μm. **b** Quantification of dermal and intradermal adipose layer thickness. Assessments (fold change relative to controls) were performed in four or five mice per group and in five high-power fields per mouse. Data presented are mean ± SD, * $p ≤ 0.05$ by analysis of variance (ANOVA). **c** Reduced collagen accumulation. Left, hydroxyproline (HYPRO) assays, adjusted for wet weight; right, IHC for α-smooth muscle actin (ASMA). ASMA+ cells in the dermis were counted by a blinded observer in three randomly selected high-power fields in three mice per group. Results represent mean ± SEM. * $p < 0.05$ by ANOVA. **d** Fibrotic gene expression in PBS-treated (*black bars*) or BLM-treated (*white bars*) mice. Messenger RNA levels were determined by qRT-PCR. Results represent fold changes compared with control in triplicate determinations from three to five mice per group and normalized to *GAPDH*. * $p < 0.05$ by Mann-Whitney *U* test. *EDA* Extra domain A, *TGF-β* Transforming growth factor-β, *Col1A2* Collagen type I, α2 chain, *Col5A1* Collagen type V, α1 chain

is sufficient to limit fibrosis. These findings support the hypothesis that adipocytes play a central regulatory role in cutaneous fibrosis [32, 47].

NCoR is a transcriptional coregulatory protein that recruits histone deacetylases to DNA promoter regions and functions as a key regulator of nuclear receptors in the downregulation of gene expression [27]. This repression is relevant to multiple processes in cellular homeostasis, including control of blood sugar, muscle metabolism, and cell cycle regulation [26]. Whereas NCoR regulates many other molecules, including other PPAR family members in other tissues, and is more specific to PPAR-β and PPAR-δ in muscle, in adipose tissue NCoR is PPAR-γ-specific [28, 48, 49]. To confirm whether the antifibrotic effect of NCoR was PPAR-γ-specific in this model, we used a specific PPAR-γ inhibitor. This finding that GW9662 reversed the effects of NCoR ablation reiterates the importance of

the PPAR-γ pathway in SSc, confirms that NCoR's antifibrotic effect in SSc skin fibrosis is mediated primarily by PPAR-γ, and confirms that the PPAR-γ pathway is necessary to resisting fibrogenesis.

The exact mechanisms underlying the antifibrotic effects of NCoR remain unclear. Our data suggest that NCoR deficiency reduces macrophage accumulation in the dermis (Fig. 4c). Additionally, NCoR increases omega-3 fatty acids [50]. This effect may explain why NCoR deficiency in our AKO mice did not add additional protection from fibrosis when fed a fish oil-based high-fat diet (data not shown). Further functional studies to characterize NCoR's molecular interactions are needed to describe how corepression and altered PPAR-γ signaling may lead to an altered antifibrotic phenotype. Moreover, whether NCoR modulates fibrosis in other organs such as the lung, where there is no adipose tissue, remains unknown and should be further

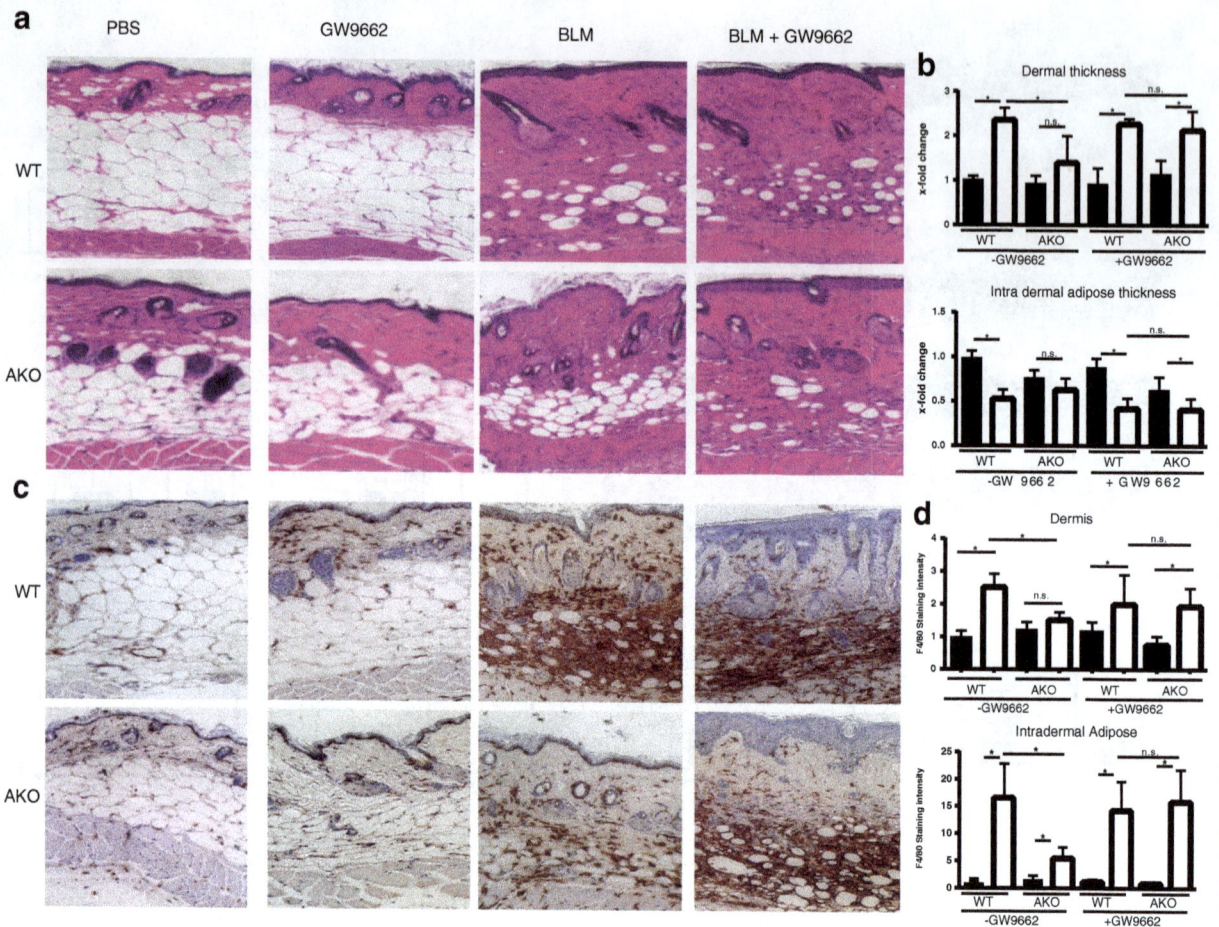

Fig. 4 Protection from fibrosis in adipocyte nuclear corepressor-knockout (AKO) mice is mediated by peroxisome proliferator activated receptor-γ (PPAR-γ). Twenty- to 30-week-old AKO and wild-type (WT) littermate control mice were administered PBS or bleomycin (BLM) for 14 days, and lesional skin was harvested for analysis. The selective PPAR-γ inhibitor GW9662 (Sigma-Aldrich) was coadministered by intraperitoneal injection for 21 days. Injections were given as previously described (Refs [19] and [45]) as daily is not quite accurate. **a** Inhibition of PPAR-γ reversed the nuclear corepressor's antifibrotic effect. H&E stain; representative images are shown. Scale bars = 100 μm. **b** Quantification of dermal (top) and intradermal adipose layer thickness (bottom). Results represent fold changes relative to control mice in two three mice per treatment condition and five high-power field areas per mouse; mean ± SD. * $p \leq 0.05$ by analysis of variance. Results were consistent across two different experiments. **c** IHC was performed for macrophages; F4/80 staining is shown. **d** Relative F4/80 staining intensity in the dermis and intradermal adipose tissue was determined in two randomly chosen regions using Fiji software. Results represent mean ± SEM. * $p < 0.05$

investigated. Although this study demonstrates that adipose tissue is of primary importance, NCoR's role in repressing PPAR-γ in other cell populations should also be investigated.

Despite the theoretical advantages of activating PPAR-γ directly for therapy, the ubiquitous expression and multiple off-target and ligand-independent effects of PPAR agonists have resulted in multiple adverse effects in clinical trials [6]. These include fluid retention, weight gain, bone loss, and congestive heart failure, all of which could be particularly deleterious in patients with SSc [6, 23]. In view of these concerns, targeting PPAR-γ by de-repressing its expression in adipocytes represents an attractive alternative antifibrotic strategy in SSc without causing unwanted side effects. On the basis of our

results, targeting adipogenesis represents an innovative approach to control skin fibrosis in SSc. Molecules that target PPAR-γ in a ligand-independent fashion may be able to promote antifibrotic properties while avoiding some of the PPAR-γ side effects seen with current thiazolidinedione drugs. Moreover, NCoR interacts significantly with histone deacetylase 3 (HDAC3), and this study suggests that targeting the NCoR/HDAC3 complex may have beneficial and antifibrotic effects without some of the nonspecific side effects associated with pan-HDAC inhibitors [51].

Conclusions

This work demonstrates, for the first time, to our knowledge, that the corepressor NCoR, which negatively regulates the activity of adipocyte PPAR-γ, is altered in SSc skin. Loss of NCoR corepression in adipocytes is associated PPAR-γ-mediated protection from skin fibrosis in a mouse model. Our findings highlight the important role of adipocytes in modulating SSc skin fibrosis and the vital antifibrotic role of PPAR-γ signaling. Targeting the NCoR and PPAR-γ pathways may represent a novel and rational treatment strategy for patients with SSc with alterations in these vital pathways.

Abbreviations

AKO: Adipocyte nuclear corepressor-knockout mice; ANOVA: Analysis of variance; ASMA: α-Smooth muscle actin; BLM: Bleomycin; FDR: False discovery rate; GLUT4: Glucose transporter type 4; HOMA-IR: Homeostatic model assessment of insulin resistance; HPF: High-power field; HYPRO: Hydroxyproline; mRNA: Messenger RNA; MRSS: Modified Rodnan skin score; NCoR: Nuclear corepressor; PAI-1: Plasminogen activator inhibitor -1; PEPCK: Phosphoenolpyruvate carboxykinase; PPAR-γ: Peroxisome proliferator activated receptor-γ; RGS2: Regulator of G-*protein* signaling 2; RXR: Retinoid X receptor; SSc: Systemic sclerosis; SMRT: Silencing mediator of retinoid and thyroid receptors; TGF-β: Transforming growth factor-β; WT: Wild type

Acknowledgements
We acknowledge Mitra Bhattacharyya and Wenxia Wang for their technical assistance, members of the Varga laboratory for helpful discussions, and the Northwestern Mouse Histopathology & Phenotyping Laboratory Core and the Northwestern Comprehensive Metabolic Core for their valuable services.

Funding
This study was supported by (NIAMS) grant K08-AR070285-01 (to BK), Eunice Kennedy Shriver National Institute of Child Health and Human Development grant K12 HD055884 (to BK), NIAMS grant 5R03AR066343–02 (to RGM), and NIAMS grant R01 AR42309 (to JV).

Authors' contributions
BK helped to conceive of the study, analyzed the human data, carried out mouse studies, and drafted the manuscript. RGM carried out mouse studies, participated in the design of the study, and critically revised the manuscript. GL performed mouse experiments and interpreted histological images. JO and WT participated in the design of the study and critically revised the manuscript. JV helped to conceive of the study, participated in its design and coordination, and helped to draft the manuscript. All authors read and approved the final manuscript.

Ethics approval
All animal studies were approved by the institutional animal care and use committee of Northwestern University.

Competing interests
The authors declare that they have no competing interests.

Author details
[1]Northwestern Scleroderma Program, Division of Rheumatology, Northwestern University Feinberg School of Medicine, Chicago, IL, USA. [2]Division of Allergy, Immunology and Rheumatology, University of Rochester Medical Center, Rochester, NY, USA. [3]Division of Endocrinology, University of California, San Diego, La Jolla, CA, USA. [4]Department of Pathology, Cedars Sinai Medical Center, Los Angeles, CA, USA. [5]Department of Dermatology, Northwestern University Feinberg School of Medicine, Chicago, IL, USA.

References
1. Varga J, Abraham D. Systemic sclerosis: a prototypic multisystem fibrotic disorder. J Clin Invest. 2007;117(3):557–67.
2. Varga J, Trojanowska M, Kuwana M. Pathogenesis of systemic sclerosis: recent insights of molecular and cellular mechanisms and therapeutic opportunities. J Scleroderma Relat Disord. 2017;2(3):137–52.
3. Bhattacharyya S, Wei J, Varga J. Understanding fibrosis in systemic sclerosis: shifting paradigms, emerging opportunities. Nat Rev Rheumatol. 2011;8(1):42–54.
4. El Agha E, Kramann R, Schneider RK, Li X, Seeger W, Humphreys BD, Bellusci S. Mesenchymal stem cells in fibrotic disease. Cell Stem Cell. 2017;21(2):166–77.
5. Wei J, Ghosh AK, Sargent JL, Komura K, Wu M, Huang QQ, Jain M, Whitfield ML, Feghali-Bostwick C, Varga J. PPAR γ downregulation by TGF-β in fibroblasts and impaired expression and function in systemic sclerosis: a novel mechanism for progressive fibrogenesis. PLoS One. 2010;5(11):e13778.
6. Ahmadian M, Suh JM, Hah N, Liddle C, Atkins AR, Downes M, Evans RM. PPARγ signaling and metabolism: the good, the bad and the future. Nat Med. 2013;19(5):557–66.
7. Wei J, Bhattacharyya S, Varga J. Peroxisome proliferator-activated receptor γ: innate protection from excessive fibrogenesis and potential therapeutic target in systemic sclerosis. Curr Opin Rheumatol. 2010;22(6):671–6.
8. Wei J, Ghosh AK, Sargent JL, Komura K, Wu M, Huang QQ, Jain M, Whitfield ML, Feghali-Bostwick C, Varga J. PPARγ downregulation by TGFβ in fibroblast and impaired expression and function in systemic sclerosis: a novel mechanism for progressive fibrogenesis. PLoS One. 2010;5(11):e13778.
9. Ghosh AK, Bhattacharyya S, Lakos G, Chen SJ, Mori Y, Varga J. Disruption of transforming growth factor β signaling and profibrotic responses in normal skin fibroblasts by peroxisome proliferator-activated receptor γ. Arthritis Rheum. 2004;50(4):1305–18.
10. Burgess HA, Daugherty LE, Thatcher TH, Lakatos HF, Ray DM, Redonnet M, Phipps RP, Sime PJ. PPARγ agonists inhibit TGF-β induced pulmonary myofibroblast differentiation and collagen production: implications for therapy of lung fibrosis. Am J Physiol Lung Cell Mol Physiol. 2005;288(6):L1146–53.
11. Shi-wen X, Eastwood M, Stratton RJ, Denton CP, Leask A, Abraham DJ. Rosiglitazone alleviates the persistent fibrotic phenotype of lesional skin scleroderma fibroblasts. Rheumatology (Oxford). 2010;49(2):259–63.
12. Kis A, Murdoch C, Zhang M, Siva A, Rodriguez-Cuenca S, Carobbio S, Lukasik A, Blount M, O'Rahilly S, Gray SL, et al. Defective peroxisomal proliferators activated receptor γ activity due to dominant-negative mutation synergizes with hypertension to accelerate cardiac fibrosis in mice. Eur J Heart Fail. 2009;11(6):533–41.
13. Ruzehaji N, Frantz C, Ponsoye M, Avouac J, Pezet S, Guilbert T, Luccarini JM, Broqua P, Junien JL, Allanore Y. Pan PPAR agonist IVA337 is effective in prevention and treatment of experimental skin fibrosis. Ann Rheum Dis. 2016;75(12):2175–83.
14. Lee R, Reese C, Carmen-Lopez G, Perry B, Bonner M, Zemskova M, Wilson CL, Helke KL, Silver RM, Hoffman S, et al. Deficient Adipogenesis of scleroderma patient and healthy African American monocytes. Front Pharmacol. 2017;8:174.
15. Kapoor M, McCann M, Liu S, Huh K, Denton CP, Abraham DJ, Leask A. Loss of peroxisome proliferator-activated receptor γ in mouse fibroblasts results in increased susceptibility to bleomycin-induced skin fibrosis. Arthritis Rheum. 2009;60(9):2822–9.
16. Marangoni RG, Korman BD, Allanore Y, Dieude P, Armstrong LL, Rzhetskaya M, Hinchcliff M, Carns M, Podlusky S, Shah SJ, et al. A candidate gene study reveals association between a variant of the peroxisome proliferator-activated receptor γ (PPAR-γ) gene and systemic sclerosis. Arthritis Res Ther. 2015;17:128.
17. Lopez-Isac E, Bossini-Castillo L, Simeon CP, Egurbide MV, Alegre-Sancho JJ, Callejas JL, Roman-Ivorra JA, Freire M, Beretta L, Santaniello A, et al. A genome-wide association study follow-up suggests a possible role for PPARG in systemic sclerosis susceptibility. Arthritis Res Ther. 2014;16(1):R6.
18. Johnson ME, Mahoney JM, Taroni J, Sargent JL, Marmarelis E, Wu MR, Varga J, Hinchcliff ME, Whitfield ML. Experimentally-derived fibroblast gene

signatures identify molecular pathways associated with distinct subsets of systemic sclerosis patients in three independent cohorts. PLoS One. 2015; 10(1):e0114017.

19. Wu M, Melichian DS, Chang E, Warner-Blankenship M, Ghosh AK, Varga J. Rosiglitazone abrogates bleomycin-induced scleroderma and blocks profibrotic responses through peroxisome proliferator-activated receptor-γ. Am J Pathol. 2009;174(2):519–33.

20. Choi JH, Banks AS, Estall JL, Kajimura S, Bostrom P, Laznik D, Ruas JL, Chalmers MJ, Kamenecka TM, Bluher M, et al. Anti-diabetic drugs inhibit obesity-linked phosphorylation of PPARγ by Cdk5. Nature. 2010;466(7305):451–6.

21. Feinstein DL, Spagnolo A, Akar C, Weinberg G, Murphy P, Gavrilyuk V, Dello Russo C. Receptor-independent actions of PPAR thiazolidinedione agonists: is mitochondrial function the key? Biochem Pharmacol. 2005;70(2):177–88.

22. Mughal RS, Warburton P, O'Regan DJ, Ball SG, Turner NA, Porter KE. Peroxisome proliferator-activated receptor γ-independent effects of thiazolidinediones on human cardiac myofibroblast function. Clin Exp Pharmacol Physiol. 2009;36(5–6):478–86.

23. Bortolini M, Wright MB, Bopst M, Balas B. Examining the safety of PPAR agonists - current trends and future prospects. Expert Opin Drug Saf. 2013; 12(1):65–79.

24. Huang JV, Greyson CR, Schwartz GG. PPAR-γ as a therapeutic target in cardiovascular disease: evidence and uncertainty. J Lipid Res. 2012;53(9): 1738–54.

25. Tontonoz P, Spiegelman BM. Fat and beyond: the diverse biology of PPARγ. Annu Rev Biochem. 2008;77:289–312.

26. Yu C, Markan K, Temple KA, Deplewski D, Brady MJ, Cohen RN. The nuclear receptor corepressors NCoR and SMRT decrease peroxisome proliferator-activated receptor γ transcriptional activity and repress 3T3-L1 adipogenesis. J Biol Chem. 2005;280(14):13600–5.

27. Mottis A, Mouchiroud L, Auwerx J. Emerging roles of the corepressors NCoR1 and SMRT in homeostasis. Genes Dev. 2013;27(8):819–35.

28. Li P, Fan W, Xu J, Lu M, Yamamoto H, Auwerx J, Sears DD, Talukdar S, Oh D, Chen A, et al. Adipocyte NCoR knockout decreases PPARγ phosphorylation and enhances PPARγ activity and insulin sensitivity. Cell. 2011;147(4):815–26.

29. Ghisletti S, Huang W, Jepsen K, Benner C, Hardiman G, Rosenfeld MG, Glass CK. Cooperative NCoR/SMRT interactions establish a corepressor-based strategy for integration of inflammatory and anti-inflammatory signaling pathways. Genes Dev. 2009;23(6):681–93.

30. Zien A, Kuffner R, Zimmer R, Lengauer T. Analysis of gene expression data with pathway scores. Proc Int Conf Intell Syst Mol Biol. 2000;8:407–17.

31. Sargent JL, Milano A, Bhattacharyya S, Varga J, Connolly MK, Chang HY, Whitfield ML, TGFβ-responsive A. gene signature is associated with a subset of diffuse scleroderma with increased disease severity. J Invest Dermatol. 2010;130(3):694–705.

32. Marangoni RG, Korman B, Wei J, Wood TA, Graham L, Whitfield ML, Scherer PE, Tourtellotte WG, Varga J. Myofibroblasts in cutaneous fibrosis originate from adiponectin-positive intradermal progenitors. Arthritis Rheumatol. 2015;67(4):1062–73.

33. Bhattacharyya S, Wang W, Morales-Nebreda L, Feng G, Wu M, Zhou X, Lafyatis R, Lee J, Hinchcliff M, Feghali-Bostwick C, et al. Tenascin-C drives persistence of organ fibrosis. Nat Commun. 2016;7:11703.

34. Bhattacharyya S, Tamaki Z, Wang W, Hinchcliff M, Hoover P, Getsios S, White ES, Varga J. Fibronectin[EDA] promotes chronic cutaneous fibrosis through Toll-like receptor signaling. Sci Transl Med. 2014;6(232):232ra250.

35. Schindelin J, Arganda-Carreras I, Frise E, Kaynig V, Longair M, Pietzsch T, Preibisch S, Rueden C, Saalfeld S, Schmid B, et al. Fiji: an open-source platform for biological-image analysis. Nat Methods. 2012;9(7):676–82.

36. Bhattacharyya S, Kelley K, Melichian DS, Tamaki Z, Fang F, Su Y, Feng G, Pope RM, Budinger GR, Mutlu GM, et al. Toll-like receptor 4 signaling augments transforming growth factor-β responses: a novel mechanism for maintaining and amplifying fibrosis in scleroderma. Am J Pathol. 2013; 182(1):192–205.

37. Rice LM, Padilla CM, McLaughlin SR, Mathes A, Ziemek J, Goummih S, Nakerakanti S, York M, Farina G, Whitfield ML, et al. Fresolimumab treatment decreases biomarkers and improves clinical symptoms in systemic sclerosis patients. J Clin Invest. 2015;125(7):2795–807.

38. Furst DE, Clements PJ, Steen VD, Medsger TA Jr, Masi AT, D'Angelo WA, Lachenbruch PA, Grau RG, Seibold JR. The modified Rodnan skin score is an accurate reflection of skin biopsy thickness in systemic sclerosis. J Rheumatol. 1998;25(1):84–8.

39. Verrecchia F, Laboureau J, Verola O, Roos N, Porcher R, Bruneval P, Ertault M, Tiev K, Michel L, Mauviel A, et al. Skin involvement in scleroderma–where histological and clinical scores meet. Rheumatology (Oxford). 2007;46(5): 833–41.

40. Rice LM, Ziemek J, Stratton EA, McLaughlin SR, Padilla CM, Mathes AL, Christmann RB, Stifano G, Browning JL, Whitfield ML, et al. A longitudinal biomarker for the extent of skin disease in patients with diffuse cutaneous systemic sclerosis. Arthritis Rheumatol. 2015;67(11):3004–15.

41. Rice LM, Stifano G, Ziemek J, Lafyatis R. Local skin gene expression reflects both local and systemic skin disease in patients with systemic sclerosis. Rheumatology (Oxford). 2016;55(2):377–9.

42. Hinchcliff M, Huang CC, Wood TA, Matthew Mahoney J, Martyanov V, Bhattacharyya S, Tamaki Z, Lee J, Carns M, Podlusky S, et al. Molecular signatures in skin associated with clinical improvement during mycophenolate treatment in systemic sclerosis. J Invest Dermatol. 2013; 133(8):1979–89.

43. Parlee SD, Lentz SI, Mori H, MacDougald OA. Quantifying size and number of adipocytes in adipose tissue. Methods Enzymol. 2014;537:93–122.

44. Inoue M, Maehata E, Yano M, Taniyama M, Suzuki S. Correlation between the adiponectin-leptin ratio and parameters of insulin resistance in patients with type 2 diabetes. Metab Clin Exp. 2005;54(3):281–6.

45. Marangoni RG, Lu TT. the roles of dermal white adipose tissue loss in scleroderma skin fibrosis. Curr Opin Rheumatol. 2017;29(6):585–90.

46. Leesnitzer LM, Parks DJ, Bledsoe RK, Cobb JE, Collins JL, Consler TG, Davis RG, Hull-Ryde EA, Lenhard JM, Patel L, et al. Functional consequences of cysteine modification in the ligand binding sites of peroxisome proliferator activated receptors by GW9662. Biochemistry. 2002;41(21):6640–50.

47. Wei J, Fang F, Lam AP, Sargent JL, Hamburg E, Hinchcliff ME, Gottardi CJ, Atit R, Whitfield ML, Varga J. Wnt/β-catenin signaling is hyperactivated in systemic sclerosis and induces Smad-dependent fibrotic responses in mesenchymal cells. Arthritis Rheum. 2012;64(8):2734–45.

48. Krogsdam AM, Nielsen CA, Neve S, Holst D, Helledie T, Thomsen B, Bendixen C, Mandrup S, Kristiansen K. Nuclear receptor corepressor-dependent repression of peroxisome-proliferator-activated receptor δ-mediated transactivation. Biochem J. 2002;363(Pt 1):157–65.

49. Yamamoto H, Williams EG, Mouchiroud L, Canto C, Fan W, Downes M, Heligon C, Barish GD, Desvergne B, Evans RM, et al. NCoR1 is a conserved physiological modulator of muscle mass and oxidative function. Cell. 2011; 147(4):827–39.

50. Li P, Spann NJ, Kaikkonen MU, Lu M, Oh DY, Fox JN, Bandyopadhyay G, Talukdar S, Xu J, Lagakos WS, et al. NCoR repression of LXRs restricts macrophage biosynthesis of insulin-sensitizing omega 3 fatty acids. Cell. 2013;155(1):200–14.

51. Phelps MP, Bailey JN, Vleeshouwer-Neumann T, Chen EY. CRISPR screen identifies the NCOR/HDAC3 complex as a major suppressor of differentiation in rhabdomyosarcoma. Proc Natl Acad Sci U S A. 2016; 113(52):15090–5.

12

Biologics and cardiovascular events in inflammatory arthritis: a prospective national cohort study

Joshua L. Lee[1], Premarani Sinnathurai[1,2,3]* (iD), Rachelle Buchbinder[4,5], Catherine Hill[6,7], Marissa Lassere[8,9] and Lyn March[1,2,3]

Abstract

Background: Inflammatory arthritides including rheumatoid arthritis (RA), psoriatic arthritis (PsA) and ankylosing spondylitis (AS) are associated with increased risk of cardiovascular disease. This process may be driven by systemic inflammation, and the use of tumour necrosis factor (TNF) inhibitors could therefore potentially reduce cardiovascular risk by reducing this inflammatory burden. The aims of this study were to evaluate whether the risk of cardiovascular events (CVEs) in patients with inflammatory arthritis is associated with treatment with anti-TNF therapy, compared with other biologics or non-biologic therapy, and to compare the CVE risk between participants with RA, PsA and AS.

Methods: Data from consecutive participants in the Australian Rheumatology Association Database with RA, PsA and AS from September 2001 to January 2015 were included in the study. The Cox proportional hazards model using the counting process with time-varying covariates tested for risk of having CVEs, defined as angina, myocardial infarction, coronary artery bypass graft, percutaneous coronary intervention, other heart disease, stroke/transient ischaemic attack or death from cardiovascular causes. The model was adjusted for age, sex, diagnosis, methotrexate use, prednisone use, non-steroidal anti-inflammatory use, smoking, alcohol consumption, hypertension, hyperlipidaemia, diabetes and functional status (Health Assessment Questionnaire Disability Score).

Results: There were 4140 patients included in the analysis, totalling 19,627 patient-years. After multivariate adjustment, the CVE risk was reduced with anti-TNF use (HR 0.85, 95% CI 0.76–0.95) or other biologic therapies (HR 0.81, 95% CI 0.70–0.95), but not in those who had ceased biologic therapy (HR 0.96, 95% CI 0.83–1.11). After adjustment, no significant difference in CVE risk was observed between participants with RA and PsA (HR 0.92, 95% CI 0.77–1.10) or AS (HR 1.14, 95% CI 0.96–1.36).

Conclusions: Current biologic use was associated with a reduction in major CVEs. No reduction in CVE risk was seen in those who had ceased biologic therapy. After adjustment, the CVE risk was not significantly different between RA, AS or PsA.

Keywords: Biologicals, Cardiovascular disease, Rheumatoid arthritis, Psoriatic arthritis, Ankylosing spondylitis

* Correspondence: Premarani.Sinnathurai@health.nsw.gov.au
[1]Sydney Medical School, University of Sydney, Sydney, Australia
[2]Institute of Bone and Joint Research, Kolling Institute, Northern Sydney Local Health District, St Leonards, NSW, Australia
Full list of author information is available at the end of the article

Background

Inflammatory arthritides such as rheumatoid arthritis (RA), ankylosing spondylitis (AS) and psoriatic arthritis (PsA) impose a heavy burden of morbidity and mortality on populations worldwide. A significant component of this is the two-fold increased risk of cardiovascular events (CVEs) [1], with some evidence for increasing risk with longer disease duration [2–4]. It has been proposed that this is due to inflammatory processes driven by cytokines such as tumour necrosis factor (TNF), with a high inflammatory burden driving autoantibody production and apoptosis of endothelial cells to cause vascular damage [5] and a pro-thrombotic state [6].

The use of TNF inhibitors could therefore potentially reduce cardiovascular risk by controlling systemic inflammation. A recent study demonstrated that an RA cohort with disease onset after the year 2000 did not have an increased mortality risk compared to the general population, whereas those with disease onset prior to 2000 were at increased risk [7]. Several studies have demonstrated that treatment of inflammatory arthritis with TNF inhibitors is associated with an improvement in surrogate markers of cardiovascular health such as endothelial stiffness, biochemical lipid profile and carotid intima-media thickness [8–13].

There is conflicting evidence regarding clinical cardiovascular endpoints such as rate of myocardial infarction, stroke and cardiovascular-related death after treatment with biologics in patients with RA. Some studies report a lower risk of CVEs [14, 15], while others report no significant difference [16, 17]. Studies assessing cardiovascular risk in RA have been performed in locations including North America [14, 18, 19], Britain [20] and Sweden [21], but as yet no studies have been undertaken in the Australian context where there are stringent criteria for accessing biologic therapy. Furthermore, little research has been done to establish the effect of biologics on the CVE rate for inflammatory arthritis apart from RA. Thus, wider research is warranted in a range of arthritic conditions to examine whether biologic therapy is helpful beyond direct arthritic control in these patients.

The aim of this study was to determine whether the risk of CVEs in patients with RA, AS or PsA was associated with treatment with anti-TNF therapy, compared with other biologics or non-biologic therapy, and to compare the CVE risk between arthritis diagnoses.

Methods

The Australian Rheumatology Association Database (ARAD) is a national voluntary registry for patients with inflammatory arthritis (RA, AS, PsA and juvenile idiopathic arthritis). Details regarding the ARAD methodology have been described previously [22]. Briefly, participants with inflammatory arthritis complete self-reported questionnaires in paper or online format. Initially, these were completed biannually; however, from January 2014, the frequency of questionnaires was decreased to annually after the first 2 years of follow-up. The participant questionnaires include self-reported demographic details, current and past use of medications for arthritis, and current and past co-morbid medical conditions. Participants also complete patient-reported outcome measures including the Health Assessment Questionnaire Disability Score (HAQ)—a measure of functional status with scores ranging from 0 to 3 where higher scores indicate greater disability [23].

The majority of participants are referred by their treating rheumatologist (98.5%) and a small proportion is self-referred. Rheumatologists complete basic information at baseline including demographics and diagnosis. Cause of death is validated by data linkage to the Australian National Death Index, which provides verified International Statistical Classification of Diseases and Related Health Problems, 10th revision (ICD-10) coding for cause of death [24]. Skilled data-entry personnel review inputs and correct errors, contacting participants for clarification as required.

Consecutive participants with RA, PsA or AS who had completed at least two separate ARAD questionnaires from database inception on 12 September 2001 to 28 January 2015 were included in the analysis. Demographic details, diagnosis, date of questionnaire, medications, medical history, HAQ score and, when applicable, cause of death were extracted from the ARAD on 28 January 2015. The primary outcome of interest was the composite rate of CVEs. CVEs were defined as any stable/unstable angina, myocardial infarction, coronary artery bypass graft, percutaneous coronary intervention, other heart disease (e.g. valvular), stroke/transient ischaemic attack or death from cardiovascular causes. This was in line with definitions commonly used in the literature [25–28]. Identification of CVEs, other than cardiovascular-related death, was based upon participants' self-report. Based on ICD-10 codes obtained via data linkage with the Australian National Death Index, any cause of death in Chapter IX (Blocks I00–I99, "Diseases of the circulatory system") was identified as a cardiovascular-related death and included in the composite measure of CVEs [24, 29].

Statistical methods

Survival analysis was conducted in SAS 9.4 using the Cox proportional hazards model and the counting process method to estimate hazard ratios (HRs) and corresponding 95% confidence intervals (95% CIs) for the rate of CVEs in patients who had anti-TNF biologic treatment, as compared to those with other biologic therapy or no biologic therapy. A repeated-events counting process model was utilised rather than a time-to-first-event model in order to account for the increased risk from multiple events during follow-up [30–32]. Participants who did not experience any CVE were right censored at the end of follow-up.

The main predictor of interest was biologic therapy use. The ARAD codes individual biologic therapies as current, previous, never or unknown, at each reported time point. For this analysis, biologic therapies were coded by conflation into anti-TNF (infliximab, etanercept, adalimumab, golimumab, certolizumab pegol) or other (anakinra, rituximab, abatacept, tocilizumab) to form the mutually exclusive groups of current anti-TNF use, current other biologic use, previous biologic use (any) or biologic-naïve. Data points where participants reported unknown biologic use were treated as missing and were excluded from the analysis. Medication use was coded as a time-varying variable to account for participants being put on different treatment across the longitudinal cohort study. Included participants were assumed to continue their reported biologic therapy for the interval between surveys.

Other participant characteristics included in the model as explanatory variables were age, sex, arthritis diagnosis, disease duration, alcohol usage and smoking status. Treatment status for non-steroidal anti-inflammatory drugs (NSAIDs), methotrexate and prednisone/prednisolone was coded as never, current, past or unknown. Co-morbid medical illnesses which are known cardiac risk factors (hyperlipidaemia, hypertension or diabetes) were also included as explanatory variables. These were self-reported in the ARAD as current, past, never or unknown. Those that were reported as current or past were coded as a positive history while those reported as never were coded as negative. Data points where participants reported an unknown history were treated as missing data and dropped from the analysis. The HAQ was included as a continuous variable. Univariate analyses were conducted and continuous variables were checked for linearity. Variables with a p value less than 0.25 in the univariate analysis were included in the multivariate model. Multi-collinearity in the multivariate model was evaluated using variance inflation factors (VIFs).

Multivariate analysis was performed using the backwards elimination method and the χ^2 likelihood ratio test. Hazard ratios (HRs) with 95% confidence intervals (95% CIs) were reported using an α value of 0.05. The risk of CVEs was compared between RA, AS and PsA using the HR for each diagnosis from the final adjusted multivariate model. The results were reported in accordance with the "Strengthening the Reporting of Observational Studies in Epidemiology" (STROBE) guidelines [33].

Results

Between 2001 and 2015, there were 4787 participants enrolled in the ARAD with a diagnosis of RA, AS or

PsA (Fig. 1). Participants with only a single completed questionnaire (n = 647) were excluded. Thus, 4140 participants were included in the analysis, totalling 32,844 completed questionnaires. Participant demographics at the time of enrolment in the ARAD are presented in Table 1. The median age was 56 years (interquartile range (IQR) 46–64 years), and 33.6% were male. The majority of participants had a diagnosis of RA (n = 3167, 76.5%), 561 (13.6%) had AS and 412 (10.0%) had PsA. The median time since diagnosis was 10 years (IQR 4–19 years) and the median (IQR) HAQ was 1.13 (0.50–1.75). Participants who had ever smoked regularly comprised 37.2% of the sample. In terms of alcohol use, 13.2% of participants were daily users, 54.4% occasional users and 32.4% non-users. Self-reported co-morbidities included hypertension (34.9%), hyperlipidaemia (19.1%) and diabetes (7.6%).

Table 2 presents disease-modifying anti-rheumatic drug (DMARD) use at the time of enrolment in the ARAD: the majority of participants were recruited on current anti-TNF biologic therapy (56.8%), with some on alternative biologics (3.1%), and 36.8% of participants were biologic-naïve at ARAD enrolment. At baseline, 1776 (56.3%) participants with RA, 265 (64.5%) participants with PsA and 437 (78.0%) participants with AS were taking a biologic therapy. Current methotrexate use was reported by 55.6% of participants at enrolment, 39.0% were currently taking prednisone or prednisolone and 51.4% were currently taking NSAIDs.

The study period comprised a total of 19,627 patient-years. Therapy was primarily anti-TNF (12,555 patient-years, 64.0%) or other biologics (1963 patient-years, 10.1%), while 10.0% (1955 patient-years) had ceased biologic therapy and 15.9% (3116 patient-years) were biologic-naïve. Only 29 patient-years (0.1%) included unknown DMARD therapy. Across the study period, 552 participants (13.3%) experienced a composite cardiac event and 10 died secondary to cardiovascular causes, with only one of these 10 participants reporting a CVE during the study period before dying of a cardiovascular cause.

Univariate Cox proportional hazards regression analyses for the whole group showed that increased age, male gender, RA diagnosis, disease duration, greater disability (higher HAQ), ever smoking regularly, ever using methotrexate, current prednisone/prednisolone or NSAIDs, or a medical history of hypertension, hyperlipidaemia and diabetes were all significant predictors of CVEs at the 0.25 level of significance (Table 3). Use of biologic therapy, past but not current use of prednisone/prednisolone and any level of alcohol use were inversely associated with CVEs. Continuous variables of age and disease duration were evaluated for linearity, and there was no evidence of multi-collinearity.

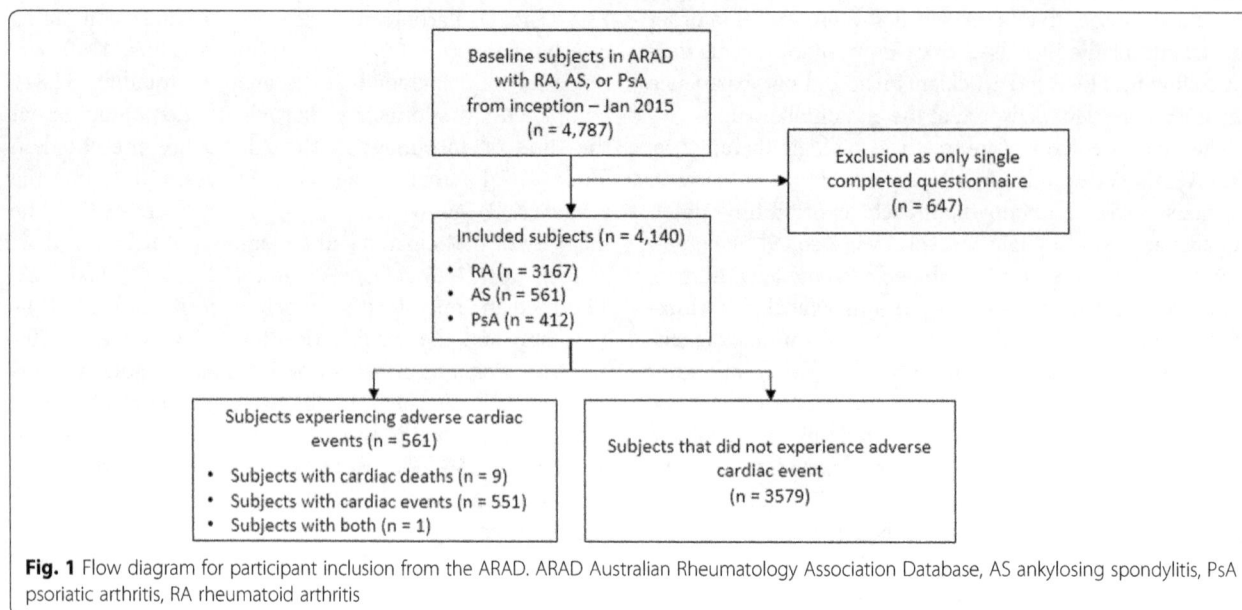

Fig. 1 Flow diagram for participant inclusion from the ARAD. ARAD Australian Rheumatology Association Database, AS ankylosing spondylitis, PsA psoriatic arthritis, RA rheumatoid arthritis

Multivariate analysis for the whole group (Table 4) found that, following adjustment for potential confounders, compared to the biologic-naïve, the CVE risk was reduced with anti-TNF use (HR 0.85, 95% CI 0.76–0.95) as well as use of other biologic therapies (HR 0.81, 95% CI 0.70–0.95), but was not reduced when biologic use was ceased (HR 0.96, 95% CI 0.83–1.11). After adjustment, no significant difference in the CVE rate was observed between RA and PsA (HR 0.92, 95% CI 0.77–1.10) or AS (HR 1.14, 95% CI 0.96–1.36). Co-morbid hypertension, hyperlipidaemia and diabetes were all significant positive predictors of major adverse CVEs, as were increased age, male sex, ever smoking regularly, greater disability (higher HAQ) and current treatment with methotrexate or current use of NSAIDs. Alcohol use was associated with a decreased risk of CVEs. After adjusting for other variables, disease duration was not a significant predictor of major adverse CVEs.

Discussion

This study has demonstrated a reduction in CVEs associated with biologic use for both anti-TNF and other biologic agents in ARAD participants with RA, PsA or AS, compared with ARAD participants who were biologic-naïve. However, this protective effect for the CVE rate was not observed in those who had ceased using biologic agents. Previous studies have shown that people with any inflammatory arthritis have increased rates of both cardiovascular morbidity and cardiovascular mortality compared to the general population [4, 34–36]. However, there are few primary studies directly comparing event rates between different forms of inflammatory arthritis.

Our study explored the relationship between anti-TNF use and CVEs in the Australian context and was also able to examine three different types of inflammatory arthritis in the same cohort. A reduced risk of myocardial infarction for RA patients treated with anti-TNF agents compared with conventional DMARDs was also reported in a recently updated analysis of the British Society for Rheumatology Biologic Register (BSRBR-RA) [37]. The baseline characteristics of patients entered in the ARAD are similar to the biologic-exposed population in the BSRBR-RA [20]. A similar reduction in acute coronary syndrome events for patients with RA using anti-TNF therapy was also found in a recent Swedish cohort study [38]. A recent systematic review reported a decreased risk of CVEs in patients with RA treated with TNF inhibitors or with methotrexate, and an increased risk in those using glucocorticoids or NSAIDs [39]. This review also reported that treatment with systemic therapy decreased the risk of CVEs in patients with PsA or psoriasis. However, there was insufficient data to compare the CVE risk between individual therapies.

In the multivariate model, while current methotrexate use was not associated with any difference in CVE risk, those who had ceased methotrexate had an increased risk of CVEs compared to those who had never taken the medication. Conversely, participants who had ceased taking prednisone or prednisolone were at lower risk of CVEs compared with those who had never taken prednisone. The reasons for these associations are unclear, but there may be confounding by indication for these medications. There may also be confounders which are not accounted for, including socioeconomic factors which may influence the prescription of different therapies, or some associations may have occurred by chance.

Strengths of this study include the large database of prospective longitudinal data, which was fully utilised

Table 1 Patient characteristics at ARAD enrolment (*n* = 4140)

	Median (interquartile range)	Number	Percentage
Age (years)	56 (46–64)		
< 40		569	13.7
40–49		779	18.8
50–59		1182	28.6
60–69		1067	25.8
≥ 70		543	13.1
Sex			
Male		1393	33.6
Female		2747	66.4
Disease duration (years)	10 (4–19)		
≤ 5		1075	26.0
6–10		833	20.1
11–20		694	16.8
21–30		536	12.9
> 30		986	23.8
Unknown[a]		16	0.4
Diagnosis			
RA		3167	76.5
AS		561	13.5
PsA		412	10.0
Health Assessment Questionnaire Disability Score[b]	1.13 (0.50–1.75)		
Smoking regularly			
Current or past		1540	37.2
Never		2129	51.4
Unknown[a]		471	11.4
Alcohol consumption			
Never		1342	32.4
Sometimes		2253	54.4
Every day		545	13.2
History of co-morbid medical conditions			
Diabetes			
No		3826	92.4
Yes		313	7.6
Unknown[a]		1	0.0
Hypertension			
No		2654	64.1
Yes		1446	34.9
Unknown[a]		40	1.0
Hyperlipidaemia			
No		3263	78.8
Yes		791	19.1
Unknown[a]		86	2.1

Table 1 Patient characteristics at ARAD enrolment (*n* = 4140) (Continued)

	Median (interquartile range)	Number	Percentage
Angina			
No		3949	95.4
Yes		171	4.1
Unknown[a]		20	0.5
Myocardial infarction			
No		3984	96.2
Yes		149	3.6
Unknown[a]		7	0.2
Coronary artery bypass graft			
No		4084	98.6
Yes		52	1.3
Unknown[a]		4	0.1
Percutaneous coronary intervention			
No		4031	97.4
Yes		105	2.5
Unknown[a]		4	0.1
Other heart disease (e.g. valve disease)			
No		3914	94.5
Yes		216	5.2
Unknown[a]		10	0.2
Stroke/TIA			
No		4042	97.6
Yes		92	2.2
Unknown[a]		6	0.1

ARAD Australian Rheumatology Association Database, *AS* ankylosing spondylitis, *PsA* psoriatic arthritis, *RA* rheumatoid arthritis, *TIA* transient ischaemic attack
[a]Participant reports that they do not know, or are unsure
[b]Range 0–3 where a higher score indicates greater disability

with the counting process method of survival analysis which counts multiple events, and contrasts with the time-to-first-event analyses which has been used in previous studies [17, 35, 40]. Our study also had a moderate mean follow-up time of 5 years, and made a direct comparison between several forms of inflammatory arthritis. Additionally, the continual reporting of participant biologic use at each questionnaire significantly reduced the potential for misclassification bias.

This article also has some limitations due to the type of study and the structure of the database. This is an observational cohort study with the choice of therapy being made by the rheumatologists and patients, and as such is only able to show an association and not causation. Therefore, there are two possible explanations for the reduction in the CVE rate. There may be an intrinsic causative benefit of biologic therapy theoretically due to

Table 2 DMARD usage at ARAD enrolment ($n = 4140$)

	Number	Percentage
Biologic use		
Never taken	1525	36.8
Currently taking anti-TNF biologics	2350	56.8
Currently taking other biologics	128	3.1
Abatacept	32	0.8
Anakinra	7	0.2
Rituximab	66	1.6
Tocilizumab	23	0.6
Previous use	121	2.9
Unknown[a]	16	0.4
Methotrexate status		
Never taken	977	23.6
Currently taking	2302	55.6
Stopped taking	856	20.7
Unknown[a]	5	0.1
Prednisone/prednisolone status		
Never taken	1529	36.9
Currently taking	1613	39.0
Stopped taking	969	23.4
Unknown[a]	29	0.7
NSAID status		
Not currently taking	2011	48.6
Currently taking	2129	51.4

ARAD Australian Rheumatology Association Database, *DMARD* disease-modifying anti-rheumatic drug, *TNF* tumour necrosis factor, *NSAID* non-steroidal anti-inflammatory drug
[a]Participant reports that they do not know, or are unsure of the answer

Table 3 Unadjusted univariate Cox proportional hazards regression for factors predicting cardiovascular events in patients with inflammatory arthritis ($n = 4140$)

Factor	HR	95% CI	p value
Increased age (years)	1.05	1.06–1.07	< 0.0001
Greater disease duration (years)	1.02	1.02–1.02	< 0.0001
Sex (males vs females)	1.44	1.33–1.55	< 0.0001
Biologic use (referent: biologic naïve)			< 0.0001
Current TNF biologics	0.63	0.58–0.70	< 0.0001
Current other biologics	0.69	0.60–0.80	< 0.0001
Stopped taking biologics	0.97	0.85–1.10	0.59
Diagnosis (referent: rheumatoid arthritis)			< 0.0001
Ankylosing spondylitis	0.61	0.53–0.70	< 0.0001
Psoriatic arthritis	0.75	0.64–0.88	0.0004
Methotrexate treatment (referent: never)			< 0.0001
Currently taking methotrexate	1.37	1.18–1.59	< 0.0001
Stopped taking methotrexate	1.56	1.34–1.82	< 0.0001
Prednisone/prednisolone treatment (referent: never)			< 0.0001
Currently taking prednisone	1.35	1.22–1.49	< 0.0001
Stopped taking prednisone	0.85	0.76–0.95	0.003
NSAID treatment vs not currently taking	1.19	1.10–1.28	< 0.0001
Smoking regularly ever	1.50	1.39–1.62	< 0.0001
Alcohol use (referent: never)			< 0.0001
Sometimes	0.64	0.59–0.69	< 0.0001
Every day	0.85	0.76–0.95	0.01
Hypertension (referent: no)			< 0.0001
Positive history for hypertension	2.21	2.04–2.41	< 0.0001
Hyperlipidaemia (referent: no)			< 0.0001
Positive history for hyperlipidaemia	2.39	2.22–2.59	< 0.0001
Diabetes (referent: no)			< 0.0001
Positive history for diabetes	1.98	1.80–2.18	< 0.0001
Higher HAQ[a]	1.83	1.74–1.92	< 0.0001

HR hazard ratio, *CI* confidence interval, *HAQ* Health Assessment Questionnaire Disability Score, *NSAID* non-steroidal anti-inflammatory drug, *TNF* tumour necrosis factor
[a]Range 0–3, where higher scores indicate greater functional impairment

anti-inflammatory properties. Alternatively, it may be due to selection bias or bias by indication: rheumatologists choose to prescribe biologics for healthier patients, or to patients with higher levels of education or socioeconomic status who are consequently at lower risk of cardiovascular disease. While it is possible that patients with higher levels of co-morbidities may not have been offered biologics given higher thresholds for general health before treatment, patients that qualify for subsidy under the Australian Pharmaceutical Benefits Scheme must have more severe or resistant disease—overall, the net direction of any bias is therefore unclear [22]. Furthermore, disease activity measures such as active joint counts or inflammatory markers are not collected in the ARAD. It was therefore not possible to account for disease activity in this analysis and it is possible that it is tighter disease control achieved by biologic therapy which led to a reduction of CVEs, rather than an intrinsic effect of the biologics themselves acting on vascular inflammation.

There were only 10 deaths from cardiovascular causes observed in our study, which is lower than that which might be expected from the general Australian population. The rate of cardiovascular death in Australia in 2015 was 151 per 100,000 persons [41]. Therefore, approximately 30 deaths might have been expected in our study which included a total of 19,627 patient-years of follow-up. This low mortality rate may reflect a recruitment bias in the ARAD—most participants are Caucasian and speak English as their first language, and approximately one third have a tertiary-level education. Higher socioeconomic status and education levels are associated with reduced risk of cardiovascular death.

Table 4 Multivariate Cox proportional hazards regression for factors predicting cardiovascular events in patients with inflammatory arthritis ($n = 4140$)

Factor	HR	95% CI	p value
Increased age (years)	1.05	1.05–1.06	< 0.0001
Sex (males vs females)	1.72	1.57–1.88	< 0.0001
Biologic use (referent: biologic naïve)			0.006
Current TNF biologics	0.85	0.76–0.95	
Current other biologics	0.81	0.70–0.95	
Stopped taking biologics	0.96	0.83–1.11	
Diagnosis (referent: rheumatoid arthritis)			0.18
Ankylosing spondylitis	1.14	0.96–1.36	
Psoriatic arthritis	0.92	0.77–1.10	
Methotrexate treatment (referent: never)			0.0001
Currently taking methotrexate	1.08	0.90–1.29	
Stopped taking methotrexate	1.28	1.07–1.53	
Prednisone/prednisolone treatment (referent: never)			0.02
Currently taking prednisone/prednisolone	0.96	0.85–1.08	
Stopped taking prednisone/prednisolone	0.86	0.76–0.97	
NSAID treatment vs not currently taking	1.22	1.13–1.32	< 0.0001
Smoking regularly ever	1.17	1.07–1.27	0.0003
Alcohol use (referent: never)			< 0.0001
Sometimes	0.77	0.70–0.84	
Everyday	0.77	0.68–0.87	
Hypertension (referent: no)			< 0.0001
Positive history for hypertension	1.27	1.16–1.39	
Hyperlipidaemia (referent: no)			< 0.0001
Positive history for hyperlipidaemia	1.65	1.52–1.80	
Diabetes (referent: no)			< 0.0001
Positive history for diabetes	1.28	1.16–1.42	
Higher HAQ[a]	1.48	1.40–1.57	< 0.0001

HR hazard ratio, *CI* confidence interval, *HAQ* Health Assessment Questionnaire Disability Score, *NSAID* non-steroidal anti-inflammatory drug, *TNF* tumour necrosis factor

[a]Range 0–3, where higher scores indicate greater functional impairment

The results may not be generalisable to the broader population with these conditions.

Apart from cardiovascular death, in this study CVEs were identified through participant self-report and it is possible that there was under-reporting of events. It is not possible to directly compare the incidence of CVEs in our study with data for the general population in Australia due to differences in the definitions of CVEs used in the Australian Institute of Health and Welfare (AIHW) analysis of the AIHW National Hospital Morbidity Database and AIHW National Mortality Database [41].

The majority of ARAD participants have RA. The ARAD was founded in 2001 for the purpose of monitoring the benefits and safety of new therapies, particularly biologics. At that time in Australia, biologics were only subsidised by the Pharmaceutical Benefits Scheme for RA, so these patients made up the bulk of initial recruitment until biologics were subsidised for AS in 2004 and PsA in 2006 [22]. However, this should not materially affect the analysis, as comparison is between biologic therapies and biologic-naïve patients. We did not find any difference in the CVE risk between RA, PsA and AS, after adjustment for other risk factors. However, as the number of participants with PsA and AS is small relative to the number of RA participants, a false negative finding is possible. The prevalence of biologics use in the ARAD population is higher than would be expected for the Australian population of patients with these rheumatic diseases. This likely reflects recruitment bias as patients commencing biologic therapy were targeted in the early recruitment process.

Furthermore, we used a composite measure for biologic use due to the small numbers of patients treated with each individual agent. It was therefore not possible to ascertain whether there was any difference in the CVE risk between individual biologic therapies. Although the ARAD collects information on reasons for biologic cessation, it was difficult to isolate a single cause to explain the finding that the CVE risk in the group who had ceased using biologic agents was not significantly different from the biologic-naïve group. This could be because those who had ceased biologic therapy were generally resistant to biologic therapy and thus did not derive any improvement in either disease status or the CVE rate, or it could be because any protective effect from biologic use is not sustained after biologic cessation and participants returned to their previous level of cardiovascular risk. Medication use was self-reported and dosages of glucocorticoid and DMARDs were not collected. Furthermore, some participants reported they were unsure if they had certain medical conditions, or had taken some medications. However, this made up only a small proportion of data points, and is unlikely to have affected the overall results.

Conclusions

Current use of biologics, whether anti-TNF or another mechanism of action, is associated with a reduction in the CVE rate compared to the rate among people with inflammatory arthritis who are biologic-naïve. This event reduction was no longer observed in those who had ceased biologic use. There was no difference in the CVE risk between RA, PsA and AS. These findings support the hypothesis that control of systemic inflammation in these conditions may reduce the cardiovascular risk.

Abbreviations
ARAD: Australian Rheumatology Association Database; AS: Ankylosing spondylitis; BSRBR-RA: British Society for Rheumatology Biologic Register; CI: Confidence interval; CVE: Cardiovascular event; DMARD: Disease-modifying anti-rheumatic drug; HAQ: Health Assessment Questionnaire Disability Score; HR: Hazard ratio; ICD-10: International Statistical Classification of Diseases and Related Health Problems, 10th revision; IQR: Interquartile range; NSAID: Non-steroidal anti-inflammatory drug; PsA: Psoriatic arthritis; RA: Rheumatoid arthritis; TNF: Tumour necrosis factor

Acknowledgements
The authors would like to thank Jillian Patterson, Kolling Institute of Medical Research Statistics Clinic, Royal North Shore Hospital for assistance with the recommended models of statistical analyses. They would like to acknowledge the contributions of Joan McPhee, Vibhasha Chand, Lyndall Henderson and the ARAD Steering Committee with special thanks to Graeme Carroll and Claire Barrett. The authors also thank Australian rheumatologists and patients for contributing data to the ARAD.

Funding
PS is supported by a Commonwealth Government of Australia National Health & Medical Research Council (NHMRC) postgraduate scholarship. RB is funded by an NHMRC Senior Principal Research Fellowship.
The ARAD is currently supported by unrestricted educational grants administered through the Australian Rheumatology Association from AbbVie Pty Ltd, Pfizer Australia, Sanofi Australia, Celgene Australian & NZ and Bristol-Myers Squibb Australia Pty Ltd. Previous sponsorship for the ARAD included an NHMRC Enabling Grant (384330), Amgen Australia Pty Ltd, Aventis, AstraZeneca, Roche, Monash University and Cabrini Health. Infrastructure support for the ARAD was received from Cabrini Health, Monash University, Royal North Shore Hospital and the Australian Rheumatology Association.

Authors' contributions
JLL, PS and LM analysed and interpreted the data. JLL and PS drafted the manuscript. All authors were substantially involved in study concept and design, critically reviewed the manuscript and approved the final version to be published.

Consent for publication
Not applicable.

Competing interests
The authors declare that they have no competing interests.

Author details
[1]Sydney Medical School, University of Sydney, Sydney, Australia. [2]Institute of Bone and Joint Research, Kolling Institute, Northern Sydney Local Health District, St Leonards, NSW, Australia. [3]Department of Rheumatology, Royal North Shore Hospital, Reserve Road, St Leonards, NSW 2065, Australia. [4]Monash Department of Clinical Epidemiology, Cabrini Institute, Melbourne, VIC, Australia. [5]Centre of Cardiovascular Research & Education in Therapeutics, School of Public Health and Preventive Medicine, Monash University, Melbourne, VIC, Australia. [6]Department of Rheumatology, The Queen Elizabeth Hospital, Adelaide, SA, Australia. [7]University of Adelaide, Adelaide, SA, Australia. [8]School of Public Health and Community Medicine, University of New South Wales, Sydney, NSW, Australia. [9]Rheumatology Department, St George Hospital, Sydney, NSW, Australia.

References
1. Perk J, De Backer G, Gohlke H, Graham I, Reiner Ž, Verschuren M, et al. European guidelines on cardiovascular disease prevention in clinical practice (version 2012). Eur Heart J. 2012;33:1635–701.
2. Solomon DH, Goodson NJ, Katz JN, Weinblatt ME, Avorn J, Setoguchi S, et al. Patterns of cardiovascular risk in rheumatoid arthritis. Ann Rheum Dis. 2006;65:1608–12.
3. Wolfe F, Mitchell DM, Sibley JT, Fries JF, Bloch DA, Williams CA, et al. The mortality of rheumatoid arthritis. Arthritis Rheum. 1994;37:481 94.
4. Han C, Robinson DW, Hackett MV, Paramore LC, Fraeman KH, Bala MV. Cardiovascular disease and risk factors in patients with rheumatoid arthritis, psoriatic arthritis, and ankylosing spondylitis. J Rheumatol. 2006;33:2167–72.
5. Ferraccioli G, Gremese E. Thrombogenicity of TNF alpha in rheumatoid arthritis defined through biological probes: TNF alpha blockers. Autoimmun Rev. 2004;3:261–6.
6. Beinsberger J, Heemskerk JW, Cosemans JM. Chronic arthritis and cardiovascular disease: altered blood parameters give rise to a prothrombotic propensity. Semin Arthritis Rheum. 2014;44:345–52.
7. Lacaille D, Avina-Zubieta JA, Sayre EC, Abrahamowicz M. Improvement in 5-year mortality in incident rheumatoid arthritis compared with the general population—closing the mortality gap. Ann Rheum Dis. 2017;76:1057.
8. Shen J, Shang Q, Tam LS. Targeting inflammation in the prevention of cardiovascular disease in patients with inflammatory arthritis. Transl Res. 2016;167:138–51.
9. Di Minno MN, Iervolino S, Zincarelli C, Lupoli R, Ambrosino P, Pizzicato P, et al. Cardiovascular effects of Etanercept in patients with psoriatic arthritis: evidence from the cardiovascular risk in rheumatic diseases database. Expert Opin Drug Saf. 2015;14:1905–13.
10. Choy E, Ganeshalingam K, Semb AG, Szekanecz Z, Nurmohamed M. Cardiovascular risk in rheumatoid arthritis: recent advances in the understanding of the pivotal role of inflammation, risk predictors and the impact of treatment. Rheumatology (Oxford). 2014;53:2143–54.
11. Peters MJ, van Sijl AM, Voskuyl AE, Sattar N, Smulders YM, Nurmohamed MT. The effects of tumor necrosis factor inhibitors on cardiovascular risk in rheumatoid arthritis. Curr Pharm Des. 2012;18:1502–11.
12. Brezinski EA, Follansbee MR, Armstrong EJ, Armstrong AW. Endothelial dysfunction and the effects of TNF inhibitors on the endothelium in psoriasis and psoriatic arthritis: a systematic review. Curr Pharm Des. 2014; 20:513–28.
13. Daien CI, Duny Y, Barnetche T, Daures JP, Combe B, Morel J. Effect of TNF inhibitors on lipid profile in rheumatoid arthritis: a systematic review with meta-analysis. Ann Rheum Dis. 2012;71:862–8.
14. Greenberg JD, Kremer JM, Curtis JR, Hochberg MC, Reed G, Tsao P, et al. Tumour necrosis factor antagonist use and associated risk reduction of cardiovascular events among patients with rheumatoid arthritis. Ann Rheum Dis. 2011;70:576–82.
15. Bili A, Tang X, Pranesh S, Bozaite R, Morris SJ, Antohe JL, et al. Tumor necrosis factor alpha inhibitor use and decreased risk for incident coronary events in rheumatoid arthritis. Arthritis Care Res (Hoboken). 2014;66:355–63.
16. Desai RJ, Rao JK, Hansen RA, Fang G, Maciejewski M, Farley J. Tumor necrosis factor-alpha inhibitor treatment and the risk of incident cardiovascular events in patients with early rheumatoid arthritis: a nested case-control study. J Rheumatol. 2014;41:2129–36.
17. Solomon DH, Avorn J, Katz JN, Weinblatt ME, Setoguchi S, Levin R, et al. Immunosuppressive medications and hospitalization for cardiovascular events in patients with rheumatoid arthritis. Arthritis Rheum. 2006;54:3790–8.
18. Al-Aly Z, Pan H, Zeringue A, Xian H, McDonald JR, El-Achkar TM, et al. Tumor necrosis factor-alpha blockade, cardiovascular outcomes, and survival in rheumatoid arthritis. Transl Res. 2011;157:10–8.
19. Solomon DH, Curtis JR, Saag KG, Lii J, Chen L, Harrold LR, et al. Cardiovascular risk in rheumatoid arthritis: comparing TNF-alpha blockade with nonbiologic DMARDs. Am J Med. 2013;126:730. e9–730.e17
20. Dixon WG, Watson KD, Lunt M, Hyrich KL, British Society for Rheumatology Biologics Register Control Centre Consortium, Silman AJ, et al. Reduction in the incidence of myocardial infarction in patients with rheumatoid arthritis who respond to anti-tumor necrosis factor alpha therapy: results from the British Society for Rheumatology Biologics Register. Arthritis Rheum. 2007; 56:2905–12.
21. Ljung L, Askling J, Rantapaa-Dahlqvist S, Jacobsson L, Group AS. The risk of acute coronary syndrome in rheumatoid arthritis in relation to tumour necrosis factor inhibitors and the risk in the general population: a national cohort study. Arthritis Res Ther. 2014;16:R127.
22. Buchbinder R, March L, Lassere M, Briggs A, Portek I, Reid C, et al. Effect of treatment with biological agents for arthritis in Australia: the Australian rheumatology association database. Intern Med J. 2007;37:591–600.
23. Fries JF, Spitz P, Kraines RG, Holman HR. Measurement of patient outcome in arthritis. Arthritis Rheum. 1980;23:137–45.
24. World Health Organization. International Statistical Classification of Diseases and Related Health Problems, 10th Revision. World Health Organization. 2016. http://apps.who.int/classifications/icd10/browse/2016/en. Accessed 4 Jan 2018.

25. Gulati AM, Semb AG, Rollefstad S, Romundstad PR, Kavanaugh A, Gulati S, et al. On the HUNT for cardiovascular risk factors and disease in patients with psoriatic arthritis: population-based data from the Nord-Trøndelag Health Study. Ann Rheum Dis. 2016;75:819–24.

26. Husted JA, Thavaneswaran A, Chandran V, Eder L, Rosen CF, Cook RJ, et al. Cardiovascular and other comorbidities in patients with psoriatic arthritis: a comparison with patients with psoriasis. Arthritis Care Res (Hoboken). 2011; 63:1729–35.

27. Westlake SL, Colebatch AN, Baird J, Kiely P, Quinn M, Choy E, et al. The effect of methotrexate on cardiovascular disease in patients with rheumatoid arthritis: a systematic literature review. Rheumatology (Oxford). 2010;49:295–307.

28. Fowkes FGR, Price JF, Stewart MC, Butcher I, Leng GC, Pell AC, et al. Aspirin for prevention of cardiovascular events in a general population screened for a low ankle brachial index: a randomized controlled trial. JAMA. 2010;303: 841–8.

29. Mozaffarian D, Benjamin E, Go A, Arnett D, Blaha M, Cushman M, et al. AHA statistical update heart disease and stroke statistics—2015 update. Circulation. 2015;131:e29–e322.

30. UCLA: Statistical Consulting Group. How can I model repeated events survival analysis in PROC PHREG? https://stats.idre.ucla.edu/sas/faq/how-can-i-model-repeated-events-survival-analysis-in-proc-phreg/. Accessed 12 Aug 2016.

31. Montemezzani S, Muller S, Sbardella C. Recurrent event survival analysis. Swiss Federal Institute of Technology. 2011. https://stat.ethz.ch/education/semesters/ss2011/seminar/contents/presentation_10.pdf. Accessed 12 Aug 2016.

32. Thomas L, Reyes EM. Tutorial: survival estimation for Cox regression models with time-varying coefficients using SAS and R. J Stat Softw. 2014;61:1–23.

33. von Elm E, Altman DG, Egger M, Pocock SJ, Gotzsche PC, Vandenbroucke JP. Strengthening the Reporting of Observational Studies in Epidemiology (STROBE) statement: guidelines for reporting observational studies. J Clin Epidemiol. 2008;61:344–9.

34. Peters MJ, van der Horst-Bruinsma IE, Dijkmans BA, Nurmohamed MT. Cardiovascular risk profile of patients with spondylarthropathies, particularly ankylosing spondylitis and psoriatic arthritis. Semin Arthritis Rheum. 2004;34: 585–92.

35. Li L, Hagberg KW, Peng M, Shah K, Paris M, Jick S. Rates of cardiovascular disease and major adverse cardiovascular events in patients with psoriatic arthritis compared to patients without psoriatic arthritis. J Clin Rheumatol. 2015;21:405–10.

36. Mathieu S, Motreff P, Soubrier M. Spondyloarthropathies: an independent cardiovascular risk factor? Joint Bone Spine. 2010;77:542–5.

37. Low ASL, Symmons DPM, Lunt M, Mercer LK, Gale CP, Watson KD, et al. Relationship between exposure to tumour necrosis factor inhibitor therapy and incidence and severity of myocardial infarction in patients with rheumatoid arthritis. Ann Rheum Dis. 2017;76:654–60.

38. Ljung L, Rantapää-Dahlqvist S, Jacobsson LTH, Askling J. Response to biological treatment and subsequent risk of coronary events in rheumatoid arthritis. Ann Rheum Dis. 2016;75:2087–94.

39. Roubille C, Richer V, Starnino T, McCourt C, McFarlane A, Fleming P, et al. The effects of tumour necrosis factor inhibitors, methotrexate, non-steroidal anti-inflammatory drugs and corticosteroids on cardiovascular events in rheumatoid arthritis, psoriasis and psoriatic arthritis: a systematic review and meta-analysis. Ann Rheum Dis. 2015;74:480–9.

40. Ljung L, Simard JF, Jacobsson L, Rantapaa-Dahlqvist S, Askling J, Anti-Rheumatic Therapy in Sweden Study Group. Treatment with tumor necrosis factor inhibitors and the risk of acute coronary syndromes in early rheumatoid arthritis. Arthritis Rheum. 2012;64:42–52.

41. Australian Institute of Health and Welfare. Cardiovascular Health Compendium. 2017. https://www.aihw.gov.au/reports/heart-stroke-vascular-disease/cardiovascular-health-compendium/data. Accessed 29 Apr 2018.

13

Serum levels of B-cell activating factor of the TNF family (BAFF) correlate with anti-Jo-1 autoantibodies levels and disease activity in patients with anti-Jo-1positive polymyositis and dermatomyositis

Olga Kryštůfková[1,2]* [iD], Hana Hulejová[1], Heřman F. Mann[1,2], Ondřej Pecha[3], Ivana Půtová[1], Louise Ekholm[4], Ingrid E. Lundberg[4] and Jiří Vencovský[1,2]

Abstract

Background: B-cell activating factor of the tumour necrosis factor family (BAFF) plays a role in autoantibody production and is elevated in dermatomyositis (DM) and anti-Jo-1-positive polymyositis (PM). We investigated the inter-relationships between serum levels of BAFF, anti-Jo-1 autoantibodies, and disease activity.

Methods: Serum levels of BAFF and anti-Jo-1 antibodies measured by enzyme-linked immunosorbent assay (ELISA) were compared to levels of myoglobin, creatine kinase (CK), aminotransferases (alanine (ALT) and aspartate (AST)), C-reactive protein (CRP), and disease activity assessed by the Myositis Disease Activity Assessment Tool in 63 anti-Jo-1 antibody-positive DM/PM patients. Serial serum samples collected at 2 (46 cases) and 3–5 time points (23 cases) were included. Relationships between BAFF, anti-Jo-1, disease activity, CRP, and their longitudinal changes were evaluated using correlation analysis, multiple regression (MR), path analysis (PA), and hierarchical linear models (HLM).

Results: Cross-sectional assessment demonstrated significant correlations between the levels of BAFF and anti-Jo-1 antibodies which were associated with levels of CK, myoglobin, AST, and CRP, as well as multivariate associations between BAFF, anti-Jo-1 antibodies, and CK levels. PA revealed direct effects of anti-Jo-1 antibodies on CK ($\beta = 0.41$) and both direct ($\beta = 0.42$) and indirect (through anti-Jo-1 antibodies; $\beta = 0.17$) effects of BAFF on CK. Changes in levels of both BAFF and anti-Jo-1 between two time points (Δ) were associated with Δmyoglobin and Δaminotransferases and changes of BAFF correlated with ΔCK, Δcutaneous, Δmuscle, Δglobal, and Δskeletal disease activities.

The longitudinal analysis showed a high intra-individual variability of serum levels of BAFF over time (97%) which could predict 79% of the variance in anti-Jo-1 levels. The anti-Jo-1 variability was explained by inter-individual differences (68%). The close longitudinal relationship between levels of BAFF, anti-Jo-1, and disease activity was supported by high proportions of their variance explained with serum levels of CK and CRP or pulmonary and muscle activities.

Conclusion: Our findings of associations between levels of BAFF and anti-Jo-1 antibodies in serum and myositis activity suggest a role of this cytokine in disease-specific autoantibody production as part of disease mechanisms, and support BAFF as a potential target for intervention in anti-Jo-1-positive myositis patients.

Keywords: BAFF, Anti-Jo-1 autoantibodies, ILD, Myositis

* Correspondence: krystufkova@revma.cz
[1]Institute of Rheumatology, Prague, Czech Republic
[2]Department of Rheumatology, First Faculty of Medicine, Charles University, Prague, Czech Republic
Full list of author information is available at the end of the article

Background

Polymyositis (PM) and dermatomyositis (DM) are chronic, inflammatory disorders characterised by muscle weakness and by the presence of inflammatory infiltrates in the skeletal muscle [1]. Other organs such as the skin and lungs are frequently involved. Myositis-specific antibodies (MSA) or myositis-associated antibodies are present in up to 80% of PM/DM patients [2]. The anti-histidyl-tRNA synthetase (anti-Jo-1) autoantibodies are the most frequent MSA (present in 20–30% of DM/PM patients) [3] and are associated with a distinct clinical phenotype (i.e. anti-synthetase syndrome), characterised by myositis, Raynaud's phenomenon, interstitial lung disease (ILD), arthritis, and skin changes of the hands [4]. The observation that anti-Jo-1 antibodies could be present before the onset of clinical symptoms may suggest a possible role of the antibody in the pathogenesis of this subset of myositis [5, 6].

B-cell activating factor of the tumour necrosis factor family (BAFF; also known as B lymphocyte stimulator, or BLyS) is crucial for B-cell maturation and survival. BAFF is also believed to play a role in autoantibody production [7]. High serum levels of BAFF have been reported in patients with autoimmune diseases [8–15] and are associated with disease activity and the presence or levels of autoantibodies [9, 10, 12–14, 16]. In patients with myositis, elevated serum levels of BAFF were found to correlate with serum levels of creatine kinase (CK). In addition, the linear regression analysis of variance (ANOVA) model confirmed that anti-Jo-1 antibodies and ILD are the main influencing factors for levels of BAFF, particularly in PM patients [17]. Based on this observation and on the previously reported correlations between serum levels of anti-Jo-1 antibodies and disease activity [18], we aimed to study associations between BAFF and anti-Jo-1 antibody levels in longitudinally collected serum samples and their relation to standardised clinical measures and laboratory markers of disease activity in patients with DM/PM, with a focus on early cases and the subgroup defined by the presence of ILD. C-reactive protein (CRP) is currently not used as a biomarker of disease activity in myositis. However, correlations between serum levels of CRP and lung function tests among anti-Jo-1-positive myositis patients with ILD have been reported [19], and elevated CRP levels have been described as a risk factor for developing ILD in patients with myositis [20, 21]. Moreover, an association between increased BAFF and CRP levels in the serum was reported in patients with systemic lupus erythematosus (SLE) [13, 22]. Therefore, we also included analysis of associations with serum levels of CRP.

Methods

Patients and controls

All patients with myositis who had tested positive for anti-Jo-1 antibodies over a period of 9 years in the Institute of Rheumatology Prague, Czech Republic ($n = 53$), and ten patients from the Rheumatology Clinic at Karolinska University Hospital, Stockholm, Sweden, with available longitudinally collected clinical data and paired serum samples were included in the study. Of these, 41 patients were diagnosed as probable or definite PM and 22 as DM based on the Bohan and Peter criteria [23, 24] and 48 of them (76%) had myositis-associated ILD defined by pathological chest x-ray or computed tomography (CT), and abnormal pulmonary function tests.

Clinical data and serum samples were collected prospectively at consecutive clinical visits over 9 years using a disease register in both hospitals. The prospectively collected disease activity assessments were available in 58 patients (20 DM and 38 PM) in the form of the Myositis Disease Activity Assessment Tool (MDAAT) according to the International Myositis Assessment and Clinical Studies (IMACS) Group, including extramuscular, muscular, and physician's global score of disease activity by visual analogue scale (VAS) and MYOACT score [25]. The Swedish and Czech cohorts had comparable demographic and clinical characteristics, but Swedish patients were older and had longer disease duration (data not shown). Sera from 41 age- (mean 51.1 ± 11.7 years) and gender (female:male = 28:13)-comparable Czech healthy individuals without any known inflammatory disease or recent infection were used as controls. Ethics committees of both institutions approved the study and informed consent was obtained from the participants.

Altogether, 143 serum samples were collected within the study. The earliest available serum sample obtained from each patient was used for the cross-sectional analysis. Paired samples obtained during regular clinic appointments (median 1.5 years, range 0.4 – 7.2) with clinical activity assessment by MDAAT at both visits were available in 46 cases (36 Czech and 10 Swedish, 17 DM and 29 PM patients). Sera from three to five time points collected from 23 patients were included to analyse longitudinal associations between BAFF and anti-Jo-1 antibody levels and their relation with disease activity. Intervals between the first and last sample ranged from 0.6 to 8.9 years and the time flow of individual visits is represented in Additional file 1: Figure S1.

Laboratory measurements

Serum levels of CK, myoglobin, alanine aminotransferase (ALT), aspartate aminotransferase (AST), and CRP were routinely measured in local laboratories with comparable reference levels for Czech and Swedish cohorts

(Table 1). All other laboratory analyses were performed in the same laboratory at the Institute of Rheumatology in Prague in serum samples stored at −80 °C until analysis.

The levels of BAFF were measured in serum samples by an enzyme-linked immunosorbent assay (ELISA) according to the manufacturer's instructions (R&D Systems, Inc., Minneapolis, MN, USA). The cut-off was defined as the mean plus two standard deviations of the control subjects.

Anti-Jo-1 levels were measured in the same patient's serum samples with the use of ELISA according to the manufacturer's instructions (Orgentec, Mainz, Germany). The declared cut-off range for positivity was < 15 kU/l with borderline values 15–25 kU/l. To confirm anti-Jo-1 positivity, patient samples were tested using myositis Western blot (Anti-Myositis–Antigen EUROLINE-WB, Euroimmun, Lubeck, Germany) and line blot assay (Myositis-LIA, IMTEC, Berlin, Germany).

The ELISA test revealed levels of anti-Jo-1 antibodies above the upper detection limit of the assay in six out of 143 serum samples that were not available for further titration; therefore, they were excluded from parametric statistical analyses. Six patients had initial levels of anti-Jo-1 antibodies below the cut-off 15 kU/l, but samples were found to be confirmed positive using line blot and/or Western blot assays.

Statistical analyses

Statistical analyses were performed using GraphPad Prism 5 (GraphPad Software, Inc., San Diego, CA, USA) and SPSS 17.0 (SPSS, Inc., Chicago, IL, USA). With respect to non-normal distribution of data, non-parametric tests were used or the logarithmical transformation to normality was applied where appropriate. For analysis of differences between groups, Mann-Whitney U test and for comparison of changes between two time-points Wilcoxon's signed rank test were performed. Spearman's rank order test (correlation coefficient rho abbreviated here as r) was used for correlations of parameters in cross-sectional evaluation and changes between two time points (Δ; computed by subtraction of values at the second visit from values obtained at first visit). Contingency tables were evaluated with Fisher's exact test. The p values below 0.05 were considered as statistically significant. The Bonferroni correction of alpha values was introduced where appropriate. Based on the distribution, data are presented as median (range; minimum−maximum) values or (for age) as mean ± SD.

Multivariate analysis

Multiple regression (MR) of serum levels of BAFF, anti-Jo-1 antibodies, and CRP (as independent variables), and CK (as dependent variable) was performed using

SPSS package 17.0 (SPSS, Inc., Chicago, Illinois, USA). The path analysis (PA) of these variables was performed with use of the software package LISREL 8.8 (Scientific Software International, Inc., Lincolnwood, IL, USA) [26] on a covariance matrix derived from the logarithmically transformed variables with function $\ln(1 + x)$, due to their positively skewed distributions [27]. The maximum likelihood (ML) method was selected to estimate correct standard errors and the associated goodness-of-fit statistics [28, 29]. Models and their variants were evaluated by several fit indices: the chi-square statistics, root mean square error of approximation (RMSEA), comparative fit index (CFI), and parsimony normed fit index (PNFI). RMSEA < 0.05 and CFI > 0.95 were considered as acceptable model fit. Lower values of chi-square statistics and higher values of PNFI also indicate a good fit. Only significant standardised path coefficients (β) were accepted.

Analysis of longitudinal data

None of the traditional ANOVA-like models is appropriate for the analysis of repeated measures over time of the unbalanced design of longitudinal collection of samples (as illustrated in Additional file 1: Figure S1). Therefore, the two-level hierarchical linear model (HLM) was designed separately for BAFF, anti-Jo-1, and CK using the HLM 6 package [30]. The principles of HLM are explained in detail in Additional file 2 [31].

A sequence of three consecutive models was accomplished. Firstly, the unconditional model was used for evaluation of the variance components situated within patients (lower level 1; 3 and more time points) and between patients (higher level 2; 23 cases) [32]. Their ratio, the intra-class correlation coefficient (ICC), described the proportion of the total variance between patients. Next, the unconditional growth model with time as the independent variable was applied as an indicator of intensity of associations over time. Finally, the model with one time-varying independent variable was used to assess the percentage of the variance of either BAFF, anti-Jo-1, or CK explained by a relevant variable measured repeatedly over time along with a given dependent variable (pseudo R^2).

Since the limited sample size of longitudinally collected samples entered the HLM, only few variables representing the hypothesis were included to keep it in proportion with the sample size and to let the path-analytic model and HLM to be identified.

Results

Patient group characteristics

Patient demographic, laboratory, and clinical characteristics at initial assessment are summarised in Table 1. DM and PM cohorts had comparable disease activity (except for cutaneous VAS), descriptive characteristics, and

Table 1 Demographic characteristics, clinical, and laboratory data of patients at time of blood sampling at initial evaluation

	DM (n = 22)		PM (n = 41)		All (n = 63)	
Female:male	15:7		28:13		43:20	
Age (years), mean ± SD	52.5 ± 10.9		52 ± 12.6		52.2 ± 11.9	
Years of symptoms	5.9 (0.1–31.0)		3.8 (0.2–23.8)		4.1 (0.1–31.0)	
Years from diagnosis	1.3 (0–29.0)		0.8 (0–23.3)		1.0 (0–29.0)	
Early cases[a], n (%)	10 (45%)		20 (49%)		30 (48%)	
ILD, n (%)	15 (68%)		33 (80.5%)		48 (76%)	
Medication, n (%)						
GC	20 (91%)		36 (88%)		56 (89%)	
DMARDs	11 (50%)		23 (56%)		34 (54%)	
No therapy	1 (4.5%)		4 (10%)		5 (8%)	
Dose of GC (mg/day)[b]	15 (0–80)		17.5 (0–85)		17.5 (0–85)	
MDAAT visual analogue scale (mm)	(n = 20)		(n = 38)		(n = 58)	
Constitutional	1 (0–35)		0 (0–25)		0 (0–35)	
Cutaneous	10 (0–30)		0 (0–21)		1 (0–30)	
Skeletal	0 (0–43)		0 (0–63)		0 (0–63)	
Gastrointestinal	0 (0–17)		0 (0–27)		0 (0–27)	
Pulmonary	11 (0–86)		13 (0–66)		12.5 (0–86)	
Cardiac	0 (0–10)		0 (0–36)		0 (0–36)	
Other	0 (0–17)		0 (0–29)		0 (0–29)	
Extramuscular global	11.5 (0–64)		17.5 (0–44)		15 (0–64)	
Muscle	7.5 (0–82)		11.3 (0–71)		11 (0–82)	
Global	21 (0–79)		16.5 (0–59)		17.5 (0–79)	
MYOACT score[c]	0.07 (0–0.26)		0.05 (0–0.23)		0.06 (0–0.26)	
	n		n		n	
BAFF (ng/ml)	22	2.1 (0.8–20.9)	41	1.7 (0.3–18.7)	63	1.8 (0.3–20.9)
anti-Jo-1 (kU/l)	22	127 (0.6–2135)	41	178 (0.8–3605)	63	162 (0.6–3605)
CK (µkat/l)	22	1.8 (0.25–94.5)	41	3.6 (0.3–78.4)	63	2.6 (0.25–94.5)
Myoglobin (µg/l)	19	80 (24 - 5313)	34	115 (10.6–3498)	53	94 (10.6–5313)
ALT (µkat/l)	22	0.4 (0.1–6.7)	40	0.5 (0.1–3.6)	62	0.5 (0.1–6.7)
AST (µkat/l)	21	0.5 (0.1–5.1)	40	0.4 (0.2–6.5)	61	0.4 (0.1–6.5)
CRP (mg/l)	22	3.0 (0.2–29.4)	38	3.5 (0.5–54.8)	60	3.25 (0.2–54.8)

Data are shown as median (range; minimum–maximum) unless otherwise stated

Myoglobin normal levels < 92 µg/l for men and < 76 µg/l for women

ALT alanine aminotransferase (normal levels < 0.75 µkat/l for men and < 0.57 µkat/l for women), AST aspartate aminotransferase (normal levels < 0.58 µkat/L for men and < 0.52 µkat/L for women), BAFF B-cell activating factor of the tumour necrosis factor family, CK creatine kinase (normal levels for Swedish cohort < 2.5 µkat/L for men and < 2.0 µkat/L for women, and for Czech cohort < 2.85 µkat/l and < 2.42 µkat/l), CRP= C-reactive protein (normal levels < 5 mg/l), DM dermatomyositis, DMARD disease-modifying anti-rheumatic drug, GC glucocorticoids, ILD interstitial lung disease (ever present), MDAAT Myositis Disease Activity Assessment Tool, PM polymyositis

[a]Early case = disease duration up to 6 months

[b]Equivalent of prednisone

[c]MYOACT score is the sum of the 10-cm visual analogue scale scores for each of the six individual organ systems divided by the total maximum possible score

frequency of treatment with glucocorticoids (GC) or disease-modifying anti-rheumatic drugs (DMARDs), with comparable daily doses of GC. Patients with ILD had higher pulmonary activity, extramuscular global assessment and global disease activity VAS, and MYOACT score compared with non-ILD patients (median values in ILD: 20, 19, 19 mm and 0.75 index; non-ILD: 0, 4, 6.5 mm

and 0.27 index; $p < 0.05$ for all) but otherwise comparable disease activity, laboratory parameters, and clinical characteristics. A shorter duration of symptoms ($p = 0.04$) and time from diagnosis ($p = 0.006$) at inclusion was seen in patients with ILD.

Early cases (up to 6 months after diagnosis of myositis) constituted 48% of the total cohort ($n = 30$). These had higher disease activity as assessed by MYOACT score (median 0.87 vs 0.31), extramuscular global assessment, global, muscle and pulmonary activity VAS or serum levels of ALT (23.0, 25.0, 16.5, 23.0 mm and 0.57 µkat/l) when compared with patients with longer disease duration (7.5, 8.0, 6.5, 6.5 mm, 0.35 µkat/l; $p < 0.05$ for all after Bonferroni correction).

Serum levels of BAFF and anti-Jo-1 antibodies and their mutual correlation at initial evaluation

Patients with PM/DM had higher serum levels of BAFF (median 1.8, range 0.3–20.9 ng/ml) compared with healthy individuals (0.8, 0.4–2.0 ng/ml, $p < 0.0001$), and elevated levels were documented in 54% of patients.

The serum levels of anti-Jo-1 antibodies had a high variability between individual patients with a wide range (Table 1) and the distribution was skewed towards lower values.

Serum levels of both BAFF and anti-Jo-1 were comparable between subgroups of patients with DM and PM (Table 1; BAFF, $p = 0.30$; anti-Jo-1, $p = 0.13$), and with or without ILD (median and range of BAFF: ILD = 1.8, 0.5–20.9, and non-ILD = 1.5, 0.3–8.6 ng/ml; $p = 0.56$; or anti-Jo-1: ILD = 173.6, 0.8–3604, and non-ILD = 151.8, 0.55–2063 kU/l; $p = 0.36$).

Positive correlations were found in the whole patient cohort between serum levels of BAFF and anti-Jo-1 antibodies ($r = 0.42$, $p = 0.0006$, $n = 63$), as well as in subgroups with DM or PM and with or without ILD (Table 2).

Associations of serum levels of BAFF and anti-Jo-1 antibodies with laboratory and clinical parameters of disease activity and CRP at initial evaluation

Serum levels of BAFF or anti-Jo-1 were positively associated with serum markers of muscle involvement (levels of CK, myoglobin, and AST; Table 2 and Additional file 3), particularly in patients with early disease.

When analysing the disease activity measures, a positive correlation was found between levels of BAFF and cutaneous activity (Spearman's correlation coefficient $r = 0.46$, $p = 0.04$, $n = 20$) in patients with DM.

A significant correlation of serum levels of CRP with levels of BAFF ($p = 0.0004$) and anti-Jo-1 antibodies ($p = 0.003$; Table 2) was recorded. Therefore, we incorporated associations of CRP into further analyses. The baseline levels of CRP in the serum were significantly higher in patients compared with healthy individuals (median 3.25 mg/l, range 0.2–54.8 mg/l vs 1.3 mg/l, 0.4–3.5 mg/l; $p < 0.001$). Elevation of CRP levels above the reference limit (5 mg/l) occurred in 38% of the entire patient group and in 47% of patients with early disease. CRP levels were associated with muscle involvement (serum levels of CK ($r = 0.30$; $p = 0.02$, $n = 60$) and myoglobin ($r = 0.42$, $p = 0.002$, n = 60)0 as analysed in the whole group of patients and in subsets with PM or with ILD (CK: $r = 0.42$ or 0.30, $p = 0.009$ or 0.045, $n = 38$ or 45; myoglobin: $r = 0.53$ or 0.40; $p = 0.008$ or 0.01, $n = 33$ or 40, respectively). No correlation was found between CRP levels and clinical assessments of disease activity, including constitutional and skeletal VAS.

Multivariate analysis of the cross-sectional relationships between serum levels of BAFF, anti-Jo-1 antibodies, CK, and CRP

The associations among bivariate correlated variables were analysed with multiple regression in the entire cohort of patients ($n = 63$). Serum levels of BAFF, anti-Jo-1 antibodies, and CRP were included as independent variables, and serum levels of CK as a dependent variable. This analysis showed significant associations both for serum levels of CK and BAFF (with

Table 2 Correlations between serum levels of BAFF and anti-Jo-1 antibodies with serum levels of muscle enzymes (CK and AST), myoglobin, and CRP at baseline evaluation in myositis patients and in subgroups with dermatomyositis/polymyositis, with or without lung involvement, and in patients with short disease duration

		anti-Jo-1		CK		Myoglobin		AST		CRP	
		r	p	r	p	r	p	r	p	r	p
All (n = 63)	BAFF	0.42	0.0006**	0.50	< 0.0001***	0.39	0.004*	0.45	0.0003**	0.44	0.0004**
	anti-Jo-1	–	–	0.47	0.0001***	0.46	0.0006**	0.28	0.03	0.38	0.003*
PM (n = 41)	BAFF	0.43	0.005*	0.63	< 0.0001***	0.42	0.01	0.43	0.006*	0.48	0.002*
	anti-Jo-1	–	–	0.44	0.004*	0.46	0.006*	0.18	0.26	0.41	0.01
ILD (n = 48)	BAFF	0.38	0.008	0.49	< 0.0001***	0.40	0.01	0.46	0.001*	0.44	0.003*
	anti-Jo-1	–	–	0.49	< 0.0001***	0.58	< 0.0001***	0.30	0.04	0.47	0.001*
Early (n = 30)	BAFF	0.57	0.001*	0.63	0.0002**	0.55	0.0025*	0.61	0.0003**	0.41	0.03
	anti-Jo-1	–	–	0.69	< 0.0001***	0.74	< 0.0001***	0.56	0.001*	0.34	0.06

AST aspartate aminotransferase, *BAFF* B-cell activating factor of the tumour necrosis factor family, *CK* creatine kinase, *CRP* C-reactive protein, *Early* early case, defined as duration up to 6 months from diagnosis, *ILD* interstitial lung disease, *PM* polymyositis
$p = p$ value; *alfa = 0.05 (0.006 after Bonferroni correction); **alfa = 0.01 (0.001 after Bonferroni correction); ***alfa = 0.001 (0.0001 after Bonferroni correction)

path coefficient $\beta = 0.38$; $p = 0.005$) and levels of CK and anti-Jo-1 antibodies ($\beta = 0.28$; $p = 0.02$).

The possible causal relationships among these variables were further evaluated with the path analysis (PA) as shown by the path diagram (Fig. 1a). The modification of the MR model (explained in detail in Additional file 4) resulted in the PA model (Fig. 1b) where the dependence of anti-Jo-1 levels on BAFF levels ($\beta = 0.42$) appeared. Also, the positive effect of serum levels of anti-Jo-1 antibodies ($\beta = 0.41$) and BAFF on serum CK levels was recorded. The effect of BAFF on CK was both direct ($\beta = 0.29$) and indirect through anti-Jo-1 antibodies (following multiplicative rules: $\beta = 0.42 \times 0.41 = 0.17$). The effect of CRP on CK was only indirectly mediated by BAFF and anti-Jo-1, but was significant ($\beta = (0.52 \times 0.29) + (0.52 \times 0.42 \times 0.41) = 0.24$; $p = 0.001$). Modification of this model for subgroups of patients with DM and PM also supported direct effects of BAFF and anti-Jo-1 antibodies on CK and of CRP to BAFF (data not shown).

Alternative models testing whether CRP levels could result from the muscular or lung activity did not exhibit acceptable fit.

Time changes in serum levels of BAFF, anti-Jo-1 antibodies, and disease activity, their mutual associations, and effect of treatment with glucocorticoids

A time-related decrease in disease activity and BAFF levels was documented by a negative correlation of time elapsed from diagnosis until sampling with laboratory markers of muscle involvement (CK, myoglobin, LDH, ALT, and AST; $r = -0.32, -0.32, -0.30, -0.40$, and -0.32, respectively; $p < 0.05$ for all; $n = 63, 53, 55, 62$, and 61, respectively) and clinical disease activity (cutaneous, skeletal, pulmonary, extramuscular global, muscle, physician's global disease activity and MYOACT Score; $r = -0.34, -0.36, -0.41, -0.62, -0.40, -0.65$ and, -0.55 respectively; $p < 0.01$ and $n = 58$ for all). The negative association of serum levels of BAFF ($r = -0.55$, $p = 0.002$, $n = 30$) as well as marginally significant negative association of anti-Jo-1 levels ($r = -0.35$, $p = 0.06$, $n = 30$) with disease duration was documented in early patients.

Between the first two samplings, a significant reduction in myoglobin (median from 94 to 62.8 µg/l; $p = 0.001$) and a borderline significant drop in CK (from 2.62 to 1.22 µcat/l; $p = 0.07$) in the total group was recorded, as well as a significant decrease in other muscle enzymes (LDH, ALT, and AST; $p < 0.05$) in the early patient group. The clinical activity decreased significantly ($p < 0.05$ for all) in cutaneous, pulmonary, global extraskeletal muscle, muscle, and physician's global disease activity between assessments at the first (VAS medians 1, 12.5, 15, 11, and 17.5 mm) and second (0, 4, 5, 6, and 11 mm) time points.

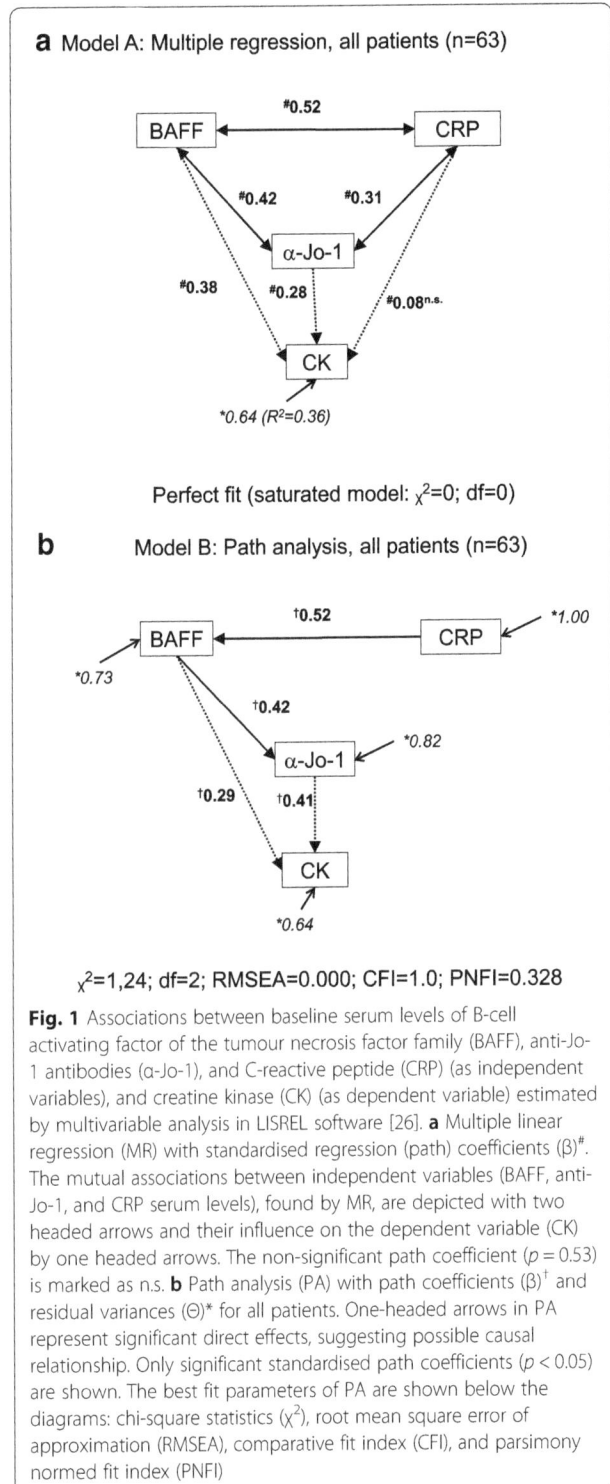

Fig. 1 Associations between baseline serum levels of B-cell activating factor of the tumour necrosis factor family (BAFF), anti-Jo-1 antibodies (α-Jo-1), and C-reactive peptide (CRP) (as independent variables), and creatine kinase (CK) (as dependent variable) estimated by multivariable analysis in LISREL software [26]. **a** Multiple linear regression (MR) with standardised regression (path) coefficients (β)#. The mutual associations between independent variables (BAFF, anti-Jo-1, and CRP serum levels), found by MR, are depicted with two headed arrows and their influence on the dependent variable (CK) by one headed arrows. The non-significant path coefficient ($p = 0.53$) is marked as n.s. **b** Path analysis (PA) with path coefficients (β)† and residual variances (Θ)* for all patients. One-headed arrows in PA represent significant direct effects, suggesting possible causal relationship. Only significant standardised path coefficients ($p < 0.05$) are shown. The best fit parameters of PA are shown below the diagrams: chi-square statistics (χ^2), root mean square error of approximation (RMSEA), comparative fit index (CFI), and parsimony normed fit index (PNFI)

The significant reduction in BAFF levels between the two time points was documented within the entire patient group (from 1.8 to 1.3 ng/ml; $p = 0.04$) and was more pronounced in early patients (from 1.6 to 1.05 ng/ml; $p = 0.02$). In total, serum BAFF levels decreased to below the cut-off in 37.5% of patients with high BAFF, but an increase above the cut-off was recorded in 27% of patients with initially low BAFF levels. This non-linear variability of BAFF levels over time was also seen in a growth model as described below.

No significant change in anti-Jo-1 antibody levels between two time points was found (from 153.9 to 102.8 kU/l, $p = 0.93$). The serum levels of anti-Jo-1 antibodies detected in the first and second samplings were closely correlated ($r = 0.70$, $p < 0.0001$, $n = 46$), which corresponds to lower variability of anti-Jo-1 with time.

We further analysed correlations between changes in serum levels of BAFF or anti-Jo-1 and changes in laboratory markers and clinical disease activity in individual patients (Δ = value at first visit minus value at second visit). The changes in BAFF were associated with ΔCK, Δmyoglobin, ΔALT, and ΔAST, and showed a trend to association with Δcutaneous, Δmuscle, Δglobal, and Δskeletal disease activities (Table 3 and Additional file 5, left panel). The Δanti-Jo-1 antibody levels correlated only with the change in laboratory markers ΔAST and marginally with ΔALT, Δmyoglobin, and ΔCRP (Table 3 and Additional file 5, centre panel).

Changes in BAFF were associated with the daily dose of GC used at the time of first blood sampling. The change in disease activity assessed by Δmyoglobin, ΔALT, ΔAST, Δpulmonary, and Δglobal VAS also reflected the effect of GC therapy (Table 3, right column). Thus, higher doses of GC were followed by a larger decrease of serum levels of BAFF and with a decrease in some indicators of disease activity, but not with change in the anti-Jo-1 levels ($r = 0.10$, $p = 0.54$).

Finally, the changes in levels of anti-Jo-1 and BAFF were not mutually significantly associated, with a trend to improve after the exclusion of a single outlying value of Δanti-Jo-1 (Additional file 5).

The proportion of patients with high serum CRP decreased from an initial 38% to 28% at the second sampling, but no significant quantitative decrease in CRP levels was recorded. However, the changes in CRP were associated with changes in BAFF and anti-Jo-1 (Table 3), Δmyoglobin ($r = 0.33$, $p < 0.05$, $n = 36$) and weakly with Δconstitutional disease activity ($r = 0.31$, $p = 0.07$, $n = 36$).

Longitudinal relations between serum levels of BAFF or anti-Jo-1 antibodies and disease activity markers or CRP

The time variability in serum levels of BAFF, anti-Jo-1, and CK showed comparable trends within time in a majority of patients who were followed from the early period after the diagnosis (illustrated in Fig. 2 with diagrams of 12 patients who had samples from three and more time points and short disease duration at first sampling; 1.0 ± 1.4 months after diagnosis determination). In general, high levels of serum BAFF declined after initial treatment with a high dose of GC, tended to rise in individual cases after GC tapering, and were parallel to CK levels more closely than anti-Jo-1 antibody levels (Fig. 2).

Anti-Jo-1 antibody levels became negative during follow-up in seven out of 40 patients (17.5%) within 0.5–4.3 years, in association with a significant decrease in serum levels of BAFF (median from 1.9 to

Table 3 Correlations of changes between first two visits (Δ = first visit − second visit) in levels of BAFF or anti-Jo-1 antibodies with change of disease activity and their association with prior daily dose of glucocorticoids given at initial assessment

	Change in BAFF			Change in anti-Jo-1			GC daily dose		
	n	r	p	n	r	p	n	r	p
Δ BAFF	–	–	–	44	0.18	0.25	43	0.31	0.04[a]
Δ CK	44	0.75	< 0.0001***	42	0.24	0.13	41	0.23	0.14
Δ Myoglobin	36	0.64	< 0.0001***	34	0.44	0.009	33	0.35	0.04
Δ ALT	45	0.52	0.0003**	43	0.31	0.04	42	0.33	0.03
Δ AST	43	0.63	< 0.0001***	41	0.54	0.0003**	40	0.30	0.05
Δ CRP	42	0.32	0.04	40	0.33	0.04	39	0.27	0.10
Δ Muscle VAS	39	0.33	0.04	37	−0.12	0.49	39	0.28	0.08
Δ Global VAS	39	0.38	0.02	37	−0.05	0.78	39	0.38	0.02
Δ Skeletal VAS	39	0.45	0.004**	37	0.1	0.56	39	0.06	0.72
Δ Cutaneous VAS[b]	12	0.64	0.03[a]	11	−0.03	0.92	12	0.38	0.22
Δ Pulmonary VAS[c]	30	−0.01	0.94	28	−0.30	0.12	30	0.42	0.02[a]

ALT alanine aminotransferase, AST aspartate aminotransferase, BAFF B-cell activating factor of the tumour necrosis factor family, CK creatine kinase, CRP C-reactive protein, GC glucocorticoids, VAS visual analogue scale

$p = p$ value; **alfa = 0.01 (0.001 after Bonferroni correction); ***alfa = 0.001 (0.0001 after Bonferroni correction).

[a]No multiple testing correction applicable

[b]Evaluated within patients with dermatomyositis

[c]Evaluated within patients with interstitial lung disease

0.7 ng/ml; $p = 0.02$) and a decrease in disease activity measured as CK, myoglobin, ALT, and AST ($p < 0.05$). These patients were treated with a combination of GC (median daily dose 27.5 mg) and DMARDs (3 × azathioprine, 2 × methotrexate, 1 × cyclosporine A, and 1 × cyclophosphamide).

At a group level, statistical analysis of repeated measures with HLM showed high intra-individual variability in serum levels of BAFF over time (Table 4). This suggests that the majority (97%) of the variability of BAFF levels depends on time-related changes within the individual patient (ICC = 0.03), whereas 68% of the variability of anti-Jo-1 levels was explained by inter-individual differences between patients (ICC = 0.678).

The percentage of explained variance within patients in the unconditional growth model with time from diagnosis as an independent variable (Table 4) showed that linear regression is a good model for

anti-Jo-1 (62%) and marginally acceptable for CK (31%), but not appropriate for BAFF (0%) levels in serum. BAFF was a good predictor of within-patient variability of anti-Jo-1 (it explained 79% of anti-Jo-1 variance) but the opposite prediction was not found, which corresponds to the dependence of anti-Jo-1 levels on BAFF detected by the PA model as described above (Fig. 1b).

The close longitudinal associations between serum levels of BAFF or anti-Jo-1 antibodies with markers of muscle involvement and clinical disease activity were supported, with a high proportion of their variance explained by CK, CRP, pulmonary, and muscle VAS (BAFF: 76%, 74%, 61%, and 85%; or anti-Jo-1: 74%, 70%, 60%, and 72%). Moreover, anti-Jo-1 antibody levels could be predicted with global disease activity (71%).

The extended interpretation of the further results of HLM is provided in detail in Additional file 2.

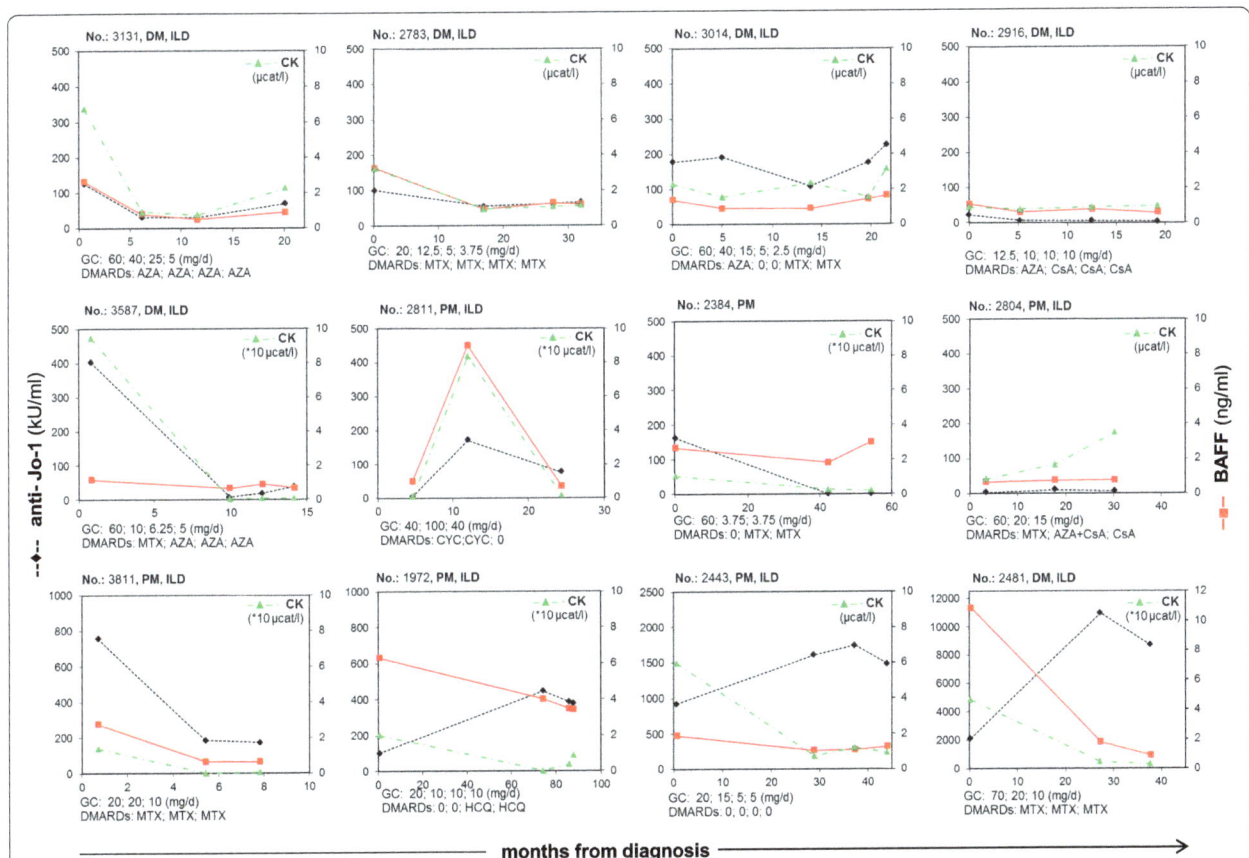

Fig. 2 The time variability monitoring of B-cell activating factor of the tumour necrosis factor family (BAFF), anti-Jo-1-antibodies, and creatine kinase (CK) levels in serum of patients with myositis (dermatomyositis (DM) = 6; polymyositis (PM) = 6) longitudinally followed from an early period of disease (1.0 ± 1.4 months after diagnosis determination) receiving therapy. The dosage of glucocorticoids (GC) or treatment with disease-modifying anti-rheumatic drugs (DMARDs) from respective time points of sampling is listed under each graphical window. All patients except one had interstitial lung disease (ILD) as expressed in the graphical titles. The serum levels of BAFF (plain red lines) show similar course within time with CK (dash-and-dotted green lines) as well as with anti-Jo-1 (broken black lines) in the majority of cases. Left ordinate shows the anti-Jo-1 autoantibody levels in serum and right ordinate shows the serum levels of BAFF or CK. The abscissae show time intervals in months. MTX methotrexate; AZA azathioprine, CsA cyclosporine A, CYC cyclophosphamide, HCQ hydroxychloroquine

Table 4 Hierarchical linear model (HLM) of long-term relations of serum levels of BAFF and anti-Jo-1 antibodies with serum levels of CK, CRP, and disease activity

Predictors	ICC[a]	Explained variance (%)[b]			Intercept						Slope[c]					
		BAFF	anti-Jo-1	CK	BAFF (ng/ml)	p	anti-Jo-1 (kU/l)	p	CK (μkat/l)	p	BAFF (ng/ml)	p	anti-Jo-1 (kU/l)	p	CK (μkat/l)	p
Time from diagnosis[d,e]	–	0	62.3	31.2	1.85	<0.001	340.9	0.04	9.06	0.04	0.01	0.10	11.9	0.21	−0.06	0.63
BAFF[e] (ng/ml)	0.030	–	79.1	49.6	–	–	748.0	0.03	0	0.99	–	–	91.6	0.22	4.34	0.003
anti-Jo-1[e] (kU/l)	0.678	31.6	–	72.3	2.33	<0.001	–	–	1.4	0.34	0.002	0.03	–	–	0.02	0.05
CK[e] (μkat/l)	0.100	75.6	73.8	–	2.30	<0.001	747.1	0.03	–	–	0.14	0.02	7.14	0.59	–	–
CRP[f] (mg/l)	0.107	74.3	70.2	44.1	2.35	<0.001	749.5	0.03	8.7	0.02	0.15	0.08	−21.7	0.76	0.98	0.07
Pulmonary VAS[g] (mm)	0.582	61.7	60.4	ND	2.32	<0.001	785.8	0.03	ND	–	0.11	0.16	−16.5	0.03	ND	–
Muscle VAS[g] (mm)	0.319	84.5	71.9	ND	2.32	<0.001	784.4	0.03	ND	–	−0.12	0.54	−7.8	0.22	ND	–
Global VAS[g] (mm)	0.241	28.3	71.2	ND	1.30	<0.001	939.3	0.07	ND	–	0.06	0.01	−7.4	0.21	ND	–

Dependent variables are situated in columns and predictors in rows

BAFF B-cell activating factor of the tumour necrosis factor family, *CK* creatine kinase, *CRP* C-reactive protein, *ICC* intra-class correlation coefficient, *ND* not done, *VAS* visual analogue scale

[a] ICC; the ratio of the between-individuals variance (level 2) to the total variance

[b] % of variance explained at level 1 (within individuals); pseudo R^2; based on HLM

[c] Average effect of explanatory variables (Slope) was estimated using maximum likelihood method with robust standard errors

[d] Average change over time (months from diagnosis); based on the unconditional growth model

[e] Determined in 80 repeated measures on 23 patients

[f] Determined in 79 repeated measures on 23 patients

[g] Determined in 73 repeated measures on 22 patients

Discussion

The main finding of this study was a strong correlation between serum levels of BAFF and anti-Jo-1 antibodies and their association with disease activity variables and clinical phenotype of myositis-associated ILD. In addition, we characterised differences in time-related variability of BAFF and anti-Jo-1 serum levels during longitudinal follow-up. Whereas serum levels of BAFF were associated with treatment within the same individual, the levels of anti-Jo-1 were more stable and did not reflect currently used therapy. Finally, we recorded associations of the serum levels of CRP with BAFF, anti-Jo-1, and markers of muscle impairment.

Higher serum levels of BAFF compared with healthy individuals confirm previous reports in unselected cohorts of patients with myositis [17, 33–35]. Here, we analysed the whole accessible cohort of anti-Jo-1-positive patients with myositis. The higher proportion of PM patients compared with DM is in accordance with the known higher frequency of anti-Jo-1 in PM [36], and the high proportion of patients with ILD compared with the overall myositis population [37] corresponds with the strong association of ILD with anti-Jo-1 positivity [19, 38]. The numerically more frequent ILD in patients with PM compared with those with DM is in agreement with already published data and, again, can be explained by the anti-Jo-1 status [39].

Contrary to earlier reports in autoantibody heterogeneous [17] or not defined [34] cohorts of myositis patients, we did not find a difference in serum levels of BAFF between patients with DM and PM subgroups or higher BAFF levels in patients with ILD within the current autoantibody homogenous, anti-Jo-1-positive cohort. However, the present findings confirm our previous results of multiple regression analysis showing that diagnosis of PM or DM was less discriminatory for BAFF levels than the presence of anti-Jo-1 antibodies or lung involvement, and explaining higher serum BAFF levels in myositis-associated ILD by the presence of anti-Jo-1 antibodies [17]. We also found a close correlation between serum levels of BAFF and anti-Jo-1, particularly in early cases and in patients with PM or in PM/DM patients with ILD. A similar association between serum levels of BAFF and other disease-specific autoantibodies has been reported, for example anti-dsDNA or anti-Smith antibodies in SLE [9, 10, 13, 16, 22, 40, 41], rheumatoid factor (RF) or anti-CCP antibodies in rheumatoid arthritis (RA) [10, 42], and RF or anti-SSA/B antibodies in Sjögren's syndrome [14], suggesting a close relationship between BAFF and autoantibody production. A biologic association between BAFF and anti-Jo-1 antibody levels was supported by our path analysis which revealed a dependence of anti-Jo-1 levels on BAFF levels in serum. A possible causal relationship was further corroborated by longitudinal analysis with the HLM, where a high proportion of anti-Jo-1 variance was explained by serum levels of BAFF, but the converse was not true. This analysis, together with the reported quantitative association of BAFF with another MSA anti-MDA5 (melanoma differentiation-associated gene 5) in juvenile DM [35], further supports involvement of a disease-specific inflammatory process in the production of autoantibodies triggered by BAFF release into the circulation in inflammatory myopathies.

Studies from other systemic diseases (SLE and RA) reported limited variation of serum levels of BAFF over time and no relation to disease flares [9, 13]. However, our findings of changes in serum levels of BAFF over time in association with changes in disease activity was similar to a longitudinal follow-up in systemic sclerosis (SSc), early RA, and SLE [8, 41, 42], indicating that BAFF may have a higher impact in early disease.

Only 54% of our anti-Jo-1-positive patients had elevated baseline serum levels of BAFF, and the levels varied considerably in association with the laboratory markers of muscle impairment, which confirms previous reports [17, 34]. These correlations were expressed particularly early after the diagnosis and in subgroups of patients with PM or ILD, further supporting the hypothesis that BAFF is more involved in early phases of this disease and that other factors may also influence autoantibody production.

Moreover, serum levels of BAFF were associated with cutaneous disease activity in DM patients. An association of serum BAFF levels with severity of skin sclerosis in SSc, with higher numbers of plaque lesions in localised scleroderma and with malar rash in SLE [8, 12, 40], has been reported previously. All these associations point to a possibility that active skin lesions might be a source of BAFF.

The main variability of serum levels of BAFF was seen in time-related changes within individual patients and a substantial number of patients expressed reduction from high to low levels between two time points, but the opposite, an increase in BAFF levels, also occurred. These changes correlated with changes in markers of muscle impairment and also with changes in cutaneous, muscular, skeletal, and global disease activity. The close longitudinal relationship between disease activity and serum BAFF levels was further supported by a high proportion of its variance being explained by serum CK levels and muscle or pulmonary VAS in analysis with HLM. This, together with the position of BAFF in the PA model, may suggest BAFF as a possible direct mediator of disease mechanisms in patients with anti-Jo-1-positive myositis.

The changes between two samplings in serum levels of BAFF and laboratory and clinical disease activity measures showed a trend towards an association with initial daily glucocorticoid doses. Similar associations were also seen in patients with SLE or SSc [9, 12]. We have previously reported an association of an early decrease of BAFF levels with cumulative glucocorticoid doses at the beginning of treatment in early myositis cases [17], and our current findings provide further support for the sensitivity of BAFF production to glucocorticoid treatment in myositis.

The anti-Jo-1 antibody became negative in patients with a decrease of disease activity (in 18%), which was preceded by intensive treatment and associated with a decrease in serum BAFF levels. This is similar to previous reports of the disappearance of anti Jo-1 autoantibodies in periods of disease inactivity [18, 43, 44]. This could also be an explanation for the low anti-Jo-1 antibody levels in six already treated patients who had positive anti-Jo-1 levels in sera taken before the study start.

Similar to BAFF, the serum levels of anti-Jo-1 antibodies correlated with serum markers of muscle impairment. The results of our unconditional growth model demonstrated associations between variations in anti-Jo-1 antibody levels over time and with muscular, pulmonary, and global disease activity comparable to longitudinal observations analysed with mixed linear regression for repeated measures reported by Stone et al. [18], and supports the role of anti-Jo-1 in disease mechanisms.

An unexpected finding in our study was the association of serum levels of CRP with levels of BAFF and anti-Jo-1 antibodies. Besides the association with change of constitutional activity, CRP also reflected muscle impairment by correlation with CK and myoglobin in serum both at baseline and longitudinal follow-up. These associations were recorded despite the modest elevations in CRP levels. Although CRP is not considered to be a marker of disease activity in most systemic diseases, some studies indicates its role mainly in patients with lung involvement [45], including myositis [19–21, 46]. We recorded more pronounced associations of muscle impairment markers with CRP in a subset of patients with ILD, but no correlation of CRP levels in serum with pulmonary activity. In our PA model, CRP displayed significant effects on serum levels of BAFF, similar to that reported in SLE (Fig. 1b) [13, 22, 47]. This finding could be explained by the described capability of CRP to trigger the release of soluble, biologically active BAFF from myeloid cells by FcγIa receptor engagement [48]. These mechanisms, however, need further exploration.

A limitation of our study is the wide heterogeneity of disease activity with low median values (Table 1), which

may explain the absence of associations between serum levels of BAFF and clinical activity measures or anti-Jo-1 at baseline, as seen by other authors [18, 34]. The low disease activity in some patients could possibly be explained by the intensive treatment that patients received before inclusion in our study.

Conclusion

In summary, levels of anti-Jo-1 in serum are proposed as a biomarker of disease activity in patients with anti-Jo-1-positive myositis. Our study demonstrated that serum levels of BAFF correlate with serum levels of anti-Jo-1 antibodies. Moreover, the longitudinal analysis showed a high intra-individual variability of serum levels of BAFF over time which could predict 79% of anti-Jo-1 level variance, whereas the anti-Jo-1 variability was explained by inter-individual differences. A relationship between serum levels of BAFF, anti-Jo-1, and disease activity was supported by high proportions of their variance being explained by serum levels of CK and CRP or pulmonary and muscle activities. The finding of an association between serum levels of CRP and levels of BAFF, anti-Jo-1 antibodies, or markers of muscle impairment was surprising, although consistent with some reports in other systemic diseases.

Associations between serum levels of BAFF and anti-Jo-1 antibodies with disease activity measures support a possible role of BAFF in the pathogenesis of anti-Jo-1-positive myositis. The anti-Jo-1 autoantibody was recently described as one of the strongest predictors of response in rituximab-treated myositis patients in the RIM trial [49]. Our finding of an association of anti-Jo-1 levels with BAFF, particularly in patients with PM and ILD, also implies that BAFF-blocking therapy could be an attractive novel treatment for these patients.

Abbreviations
ALT: Alanine aminotransferase; ANOVA: Analysis of variance; AST: Aspartate aminotransferase; BAFF: B-cell activating factor of the tumour necrosis factor family; CFI: Comparative fit index; CK: Creatine kinase; CRP: C-reactive protein; DM: Dermatomyositis; DMARD: Disease-modifying anti-rheumatic drug; ELISA: Enzyme-linked immunosorbent assay; GC: Glucocorticoids; HLM: Hierarchical linear model; ICC: Intra-class correlation coefficient; ILD: Interstitial lung disease; IMACS: International Myositis Assessment and Clinical Studies; MDAAT: Myositis Disease Activity Assessment Tool; MR: Multiple regression; MSA: Myositis-specific antibodies; PA: Path analysis; PM: Polymyositis; PNFI: Parsimony normed fit index; RA: Rheumatoid arthritis; RF: Rheumatoid factor; RMSEA: Root mean square error of approximation; SLE: Systemic lupus erythematosus; SSc: Systemic sclerosis; VAS: Visual analogue scale

Acknowledgements
The authors are thankful to Johan Rönnelid, M.D., prof., Uppsala University, Uppsala, Sweden, for kind consultations on methodological issues of autoantibody quantification.

Funding

This study was supported by grant NT/12438–4 of IGA MZCR of the Project for Conceptual Development of Research Organisation 00023728 from the Ministry of Health in the Czech Republic, the Swedish Research Council K2014-52X-14045-14, and through the regional agreement on medical training and clinical research (ALF) between Stockholm County Council and Karolinska Institutet.

Authors' contributions

OK had full access to all the data in the study and takes responsibility for the integrity of the data and the accuracy of the data analysis. OK was responsible for the coordination and participated in the design of the study, clinical data collection, ELISA assay evaluation, statistical analysis, and drafted the manuscript. HH performed ELISA tests and helped to draft the manuscript. HFM carried out clinical data collection and helped to draft the manuscript. OP performed statistical analysis and participated in drafting the manuscript. IP was responsible for detailed autoantibody analysis and helped to draft the manuscript. LE and IEL carried out clinical data collection and helped to draft the manuscript. JV conceived the design of the study, carried out clinical data collection, participated in the evaluation of autoantibody analysis, and drafting the manuscript. All authors read and approved the final manuscript.

Consent for publication

Not applicable as no individual personal data are included.

Competing interests

The authors declare that they have no competing interests.

Author details

[1]Institute of Rheumatology, Prague, Czech Republic. [2]Department of Rheumatology, First Faculty of Medicine, Charles University, Prague, Czech Republic. [3]Technology Centre ASCR, Prague, Czech Republic. [4]Division of Rheumatology, Department of Medicine, Karolinska University Hospital, Solna, Karolinska Institutet, Stockholm, Sweden.

References

1. Plotz PH, Rider LG, Targoff IN, Raben N, O'Hanlon TP, Miller FW. NIH conference. Myositis: immunologic contributions to understanding cause, pathogenesis, and therapy. Ann Intern Med. 1995;122(9):715–24.
2. Gunawardena H, Betteridge ZE, McHugh NJ. Myositis-specific autoantibodies: their clinical and pathogenic significance in disease expression. Rheumatology (Oxford). 2009;48(6):607–12.
3. Ronnelid J, Barbasso Helmers S, Storfors H, Grip K, Ronnblom L, Franck-Larsson K, Nordmark G, Lundberg IE. Use of a commercial line blot assay as a screening test for autoantibodies in inflammatory myopathies. Autoimmun Rev. 2009;9(1):58–61.
4. Love LA, Leff RL, Fraser DD, Targoff IN, Dalakas M, Plotz PH, Miller FW. A new approach to the classification of idiopathic inflammatory myopathy: myositis-specific autoantibodies define useful homogeneous patient groups. Medicine. 1991;70(6):360–74.
5. Yoshifuji H, Fujii T, Kobayashi S, Imura Y, Fujita Y, Kawabata D, Usui T, Tanaka M, Nagai S, Umehara H, et al. Anti-aminoacyl-tRNA synthetase antibodies in clinical course prediction of interstitial lung disease complicated with idiopathic inflammatory myopathies. Autoimmunity. 2006;39(3):233–41.
6. Matsushita T, Hasegawa M, Fujimoto M, Hamaguchi Y, Komura K, Hirano T, Horikawa M, Kondo M, Orito H, Kaji K, et al. Clinical evaluation of anti-aminoacyl tRNA synthetase antibodies in Japanese patients with dermatomyositis. J Rheumatol. 2007;34(5):1012–8.
7. Mackay F, Schneider P, Rennert P, Browning J. BAFF AND APRIL: a tutorial on B cell survival. Annu Rev Immunol. 2003;21:231–64.
8. Matsushita T, Hasegawa M, Matsushita Y, Echigo T, Wayaku T, Horikawa M, Ogawa F, Takehara K, Sato S. Elevated serum BAFF levels in patients with localized scleroderma in contrast to other organ-specific autoimmune diseases. Exp Dermatol. 2007;16(2):87–93.
9. Stohl W, Metyas S, Tan SM, Cheema GS, Oamar B, Xu D, Roschke V, Wu Y, Baker KP, Hilbert DM. B lymphocyte stimulator overexpression in patients with systemic lupus erythematosus: longitudinal observations. Arthritis Rheum. 2003;48(12):3475–86.
10. Pers JO, Daridon C, Devauchelle V, Jousse S, Saraux A, Jamin C, Youinou P. BAFF overexpression is associated with autoantibody production in autoimmune diseases. Ann N Y Acad Sci. 2005;1050:34–9.
11. Vallerskog T, Heimburger M, Gunnarsson I, Zhou W, Wahren-Herlenius M, Trollmo C, Malmstrom V. Differential effects on BAFF and APRIL levels in rituximab-treated patients with systemic lupus erythematosus and rheumatoid arthritis. Arthritis Res Ther. 2006;8(6):R167.
12. Matsushita T, Hasegawa M, Yanaba K, Kodera M, Takehara K, Sato S. Elevated serum BAFF levels in patients with systemic sclerosis: enhanced BAFF signaling in systemic sclerosis B lymphocytes. Arthritis Rheum. 2006;54(1):192–201.
13. Becker-Merok A, Nikolaisen C, Nossent HC. B-lymphocyte activating factor in systemic lupus erythematosus and rheumatoid arthritis in relation to autoantibody levels, disease measures and time. Lupus. 2006;15(9):570–6.
14. Mariette X, Roux S, Zhang J, Bengoufa D, Lavie F, Zhou T, Kimberly R. The level of BLyS (BAFF) correlates with the titre of autoantibodies in human Sjogren's syndrome. Ann Rheum Dis. 2003;62(2):168–71.
15. Szodoray P, Alex P, Jonsson MV, Knowlton N, Dozmorov I, Nakken B, Delaleu N, Jonsson R, Centola M. Distinct profiles of Sjogren's syndrome patients with ectopic salivary gland germinal centers revealed by serum cytokines and BAFF. Clin Immunol. 2005;117(2):168–76.
16. Cheema GS, Roschke V, Hilbert DM, Stohl W. Elevated serum B lymphocyte stimulator levels in patients with systemic immune-based rheumatic diseases. Arthritis Rheum. 2001;44(6):1313–9.
17. Krystufkova O, Vallerskog T, Helmers SB, Mann H, Putova I, Belacek J, Malmstrom V, Trollmo C, Vencovsky J, Lundberg IE. Increased serum levels of B cell activating factor (BAFF) in subsets of patients with idiopathic inflammatory myopathies. Ann Rheum Dis. 2009;68(6):836–43.
18. Stone KB, Oddis CV, Fertig N, Katsumata Y, Lucas M, Vogt M, Domsic R, Ascherman DP. anti-Jo-1 antibody levels correlate with disease activity in idiopathic inflammatory myopathy. Arthritis Rheum. 2007;56(9):3125–31.
19. Richards TJ, Eggebeen A, Gibson K, Yousem S, Fuhrman C, Gochuico BR, Fertig N, Oddis CV, Kaminski N, Rosas IO, et al. Characterization and peripheral blood biomarker assessment of anti-Jo-1 antibody-positive interstitial lung disease. Arthritis Rheum. 2009;60(7):2183–92.
20. Cen X, Zuo C, Yang M, Yin G, Xie Q. A clinical analysis of risk factors for interstitial lung disease in patients with idiopathic inflammatory myopathy. Clin Dev Immunol. 2013;2013:648570.
21. Marie I, Hachulla E, Cherin P, Dominique S, Hatron PY, Hellot MF, Devulder B, Herson S, Levesque H, Courtois H. Interstitial lung disease in polymyositis and dermatomyositis. Arthritis Rheum. 2002;47(6):614–22.
22. Eilertsen GO, Van Ghelue M, Strand H, Nossent JC. Increased levels of BAFF in patients with systemic lupus erythematosus are associated with acute-phase reactants, independent of BAFF genetics: a case-control study. Rheumatology (Oxford). 2011;50(12):2197–205.
23. Bohan A, Peter JB. Polymyositis and dermatomyositis (second of two parts). N Engl J Med. 1975;292(8):403–7.
24. Bohan A, Peter JB. Polymyositis and dermatomyositis (first of two parts). N Engl J Med. 1975;292(7):344–7.
25. Isenberg DA, Allen E, Farewell V, Ehrenstein MR, Hanna MG, Lundberg IE, Oddis C, Pilkington C, Plotz P, Scott D, et al. International consensus outcome measures for patients with idiopathic inflammatory myopathies. Development and initial validation of myositis activity and damage indices in patients with adult onset disease. Rheumatology (Oxford). 2004;43(1):49–54.
26. Jöreskog KG, Sörbom D. LISREL (version 8.8). Lincolnwood: Scientific Software International, Inc; 2006. p. 22–69.
27. Montfort K, Mooijaart A, Meijerink F. Estimating structural equation models with nonnormal variables by using transformations. Statistica Nederlandica. 2009;63(2):213–26.
28. Kaplan DW. Structural equation modeling: foundation and extension. Thousand Oaks: Sage; 2008. p. 13–38.
29. Kline RB. Principles and practice of structural equation modeling. 2nd ed. New York: Guilford Press; 2005. p. 93–161.
30. Raudenbush SW, Bryk AS, Cheong YF, Congon R, duToit M. HLM 6: hierarchical linear and nonlinear modeling. Lincolnwood: Scientific Software International, Inc; 2004. p. 14–64.
31. Hedeker D, Gibbons R. Longitudinal Data Analysis. New Jersey: Wiley; 2006. p. 47.
32. Singer JD, Willett JB. Applied longitudinal data analysis: modeling change and event occurrence. New York: Oxford University Press; 2003. p. 45–74.

33. Szodoray P, Alex P, Knowlton N, Centola M, Dozmorov I, Csipo I, Nagy AT, Constantin T, Ponyi A, Nakken B, et al. Idiopathic inflammatory myopathies, signified by distinctive peripheral cytokines, chemokines and the TNF family members B-cell activating factor and a proliferation inducing ligand. Rheumatology (Oxford). 2010;49(10):1867–77.

34. Peng QL, Shu XM, Wang DX, Wang Y, Lu X, Wang GC. B-cell activating factor as a serological biomarker for polymyositis and dermatomyositis. Biomark Med. 2014;8(3):395–403.

35. Kobayashi N, Kobayashi I, Mori M, Sato S, Iwata N, Shigemura T, Agematsu K, Yokota S, Koike K. Increased serum B cell activating factor and a proliferation-inducing ligand are associated with interstitial lung disease in patients with juvenile dermatomyositis. J Rheumatol. 2015;42(12):2412–8.

36. Brouwer R, Hengstman GJ, Vree Egberts W, Ehrfeld H, Bozic B, Ghirardello A, Grondal G, Hietarinta M, Isenberg D, Kalden JR, et al. Autoantibody profiles in the sera of European patients with myositis. Ann Rheum Dis. 2001;60(2):116–23.

37. Lilleker JB, Vencovsky J, Wang G, Wedderburn LR, Diederichsen LP, Schmidt J, Oakley P, Benveniste O, Danieli MG, Danko K, et al. The EuroMyositis registry: an international collaborative tool to facilitate myositis research. Ann Rheum Dis. 2018;77(1):30–9.

38. Schmidt WA, Wetzel W, Friedlander R, Lange R, Sorensen HF, Lichey HJ, Genth E, Mierau R, Gromnica-Ihle E. Clinical and serological aspects of patients with anti-Jo-1 antibodies—an evolving spectrum of disease manifestations. Clin Rheumatol. 2000;19(5):371–7.

39. Fathi M, Dastmalchi M, Rasmussen E, Lundberg IE, Tornling G. Interstitial lung disease, a common manifestation of newly diagnosed polymyositis and dermatomyositis. Ann Rheum Dis. 2004;63(3):297–301.

40. McCarthy EM, Lee RZ, Ni Gabhann J, Smith S, Cunnane G, Doran MF, Howard D, O'Connell P, Kearns G, Jefferies CA. Elevated B lymphocyte stimulator levels are associated with increased damage in an Irish systemic lupus erythematosus cohort. Rheumatology (Oxford). 2013;52(7):1279–84.

41. Petri M, Stohl W, Chatham W, McCune WJ, Chevrier M, Ryel J, Recta V, Zhong J, Freimuth W. Association of plasma B lymphocyte stimulator levels and disease activity in systemic lupus erythematosus. Arthritis Rheum. 2008;58(8):2453–9.

42. Bosello S, Youinou P, Daridon C, Tolusso B, Bendaoud B, Pietrapertosa D, Morelli A, Ferraccioli G. Concentrations of BAFF correlate with autoantibody levels, clinical disease activity, and response to treatment in early rheumatoid arthritis. J Rheumatol. 2008;35(7):1256–64.

43. Yoshida S, Akizuki M, Mimori T, Yamagata H, Inada S, Homma M. The precipitating antibody to an acidic nuclear protein antigen, the Jo-1, in connective tissue diseases. A marker for a subset of polymyositis with interstitial pulmonary fibrosis. Arthritis and rheumatism. 1983;26(5):604–11.

44. Miller FW, Twitty SA, Biswas T, Plotz PH. Origin and regulation of a disease-specific autoantibody response. Antigenic epitopes, spectrotype stability, and isotype restriction of anti-Jo-1 autoantibodies. J Clin Invest. 1990;85(2):468–75.

45. Muangchan C, Harding S, Khimdas S, Bonner A, Canadian Scleroderma Research Group, Baron M, Pope J. Association of C-reactive protein with high disease activity in systemic sclerosis: results from the Canadian Scleroderma Research Group. Arthritis Care Res. 2012;64(9):1405–14.

46. Xu Y, Yang CS, Li YJ, Liu XD, Wang JN, Zhao Q, Xiao WG, Yang PT. Predictive factors of rapidly progressive-interstitial lung disease in patients with clinically amyopathic dermatomyositis. Clin Rheumatol. 2016;35(1):113–6.

47. Roth DA, Thompson A, Tang Y, Hammer AE, Molta CT, Gordon D. Elevated BLyS levels in patients with systemic lupus erythematosus: associated factors and responses to belimumab. Lupus. 2016;25(4):346–54.

48. Li X, Su K, Ji C, Szalai AJ, Wu J, Zhang Y, Zhou T, Kimberly RP, Edberg JC. Immune opsonins modulate BLyS/BAFF release in a receptor-specific fashion. J Immunol. 2008;181(2):1012–8.

49. Aggarwal R, Bandos A, Reed AM, Ascherman DP, Barohn RJ, Feldman BM, et al. Predictors of clinical improvement in rituximab-treated refractory adult and juvenile dermatomyositis and adult polymyositis. Arthritis Care Res. 2014;66(3):740–9.

14

The role of anti-citrullinated protein antibody reactivities in an inception cohort of patients with rheumatoid arthritis receiving treat-to-target therapy

Maria Karolina Jonsson[1,2*], Aase Haj Hensvold[3], Monika Hansson[3], Anna-Birgitte Aga[4], Joseph Sexton[4], Linda Mathsson-Alm[5], Martin Cornillet[3,6], Guy Serre[6], Siri Lillegraven[4], Bjørg-Tilde Svanes Fevang[1,2], Anca Irinel Catrina[3] and Espen Andre Haavardsholm[4,7]

Abstract

Background: Anti-citrullinated protein antibody (ACPA) reactivities precede clinical onset of rheumatoid arthritis (RA), and it has been suggested that ACPA reactivities towards distinct target proteins may be associated with differences in RA phenotypes. We aimed to assess the prevalence of baseline ACPA reactivities in an inception cohort of patients with early RA, and to investigate their associations with disease activity, treatment response, ultrasound findings and radiographic damage.

Methods: Disease-modifying antirheumatic drug (DMARD)-naïve patients with early RA, classified according to the 2010 American College of Rheumatology (ACR)/European League Against Rheumatism (EULAR) criteria, were included in the ARCTIC trial and assessed in the present analysis. During follow up, patients were monitored frequently and treatment was adjusted according to a predetermined protocol, starting with methotrexate monotherapy with prednisolone bridging. Analysis of 16 different ACPA reactivities targeting citrullinated peptides from fibrinogen, alpha-1 enolase, vimentin, filaggrin and histone was performed using a multiplex chip-based assay. Samples from 0, 3, 12 and 24 months were analysed. Controls were blood donors with similar characteristics to the patients (age, gender, smoking status).

Results: A total of 217 patients and 94 controls were included. Median [25, 75 percentile] number of ACPA reactivities in all patients was 9 [4, 12], and were most prevalent in anti-cyclic citrullinated peptide /rheumatoid factor-positive patients 10 [7, 12]. Disease activity measures and ultrasound scores at baseline were lower in ACPA reactivity-positive compared to ACPA reactivity-negative patients. ACPA reactivity levels decreased after 3 months of DMARD treatment, most pronounced for fibrinogenβ 60–74 to 62% of baseline antibody level, with least change in filaggrin 307–324 to 81% of baseline antibody level, both $p < 0.001$. However, outcomes in disease activity measures, ultrasound and radiographic scores after 12 and 24 months were not associated with baseline levels or changes in ACPA reactivity levels and/or seroreversion after 3 months.

(Continued on next page)

* Correspondence: jonssonmk@gmail.com
[1]Department of Rheumatology, Haukeland University Hospital, Pb 1400, NO-5021 Bergen, Norway
[2]Department of Clinical Science, University of Bergen, Bergen, Norway
Full list of author information is available at the end of the article

(Continued from previous page)

Conclusions: The clinical relevance of analysing ACPA reactivities in intensively treated and closely monitored early RA was limited, with no apparent associations with disease activity, prediction of treatment response or radiographic progression. Further studies in larger patient materials are needed to understand the role of ACPA reactivities in patients with RA classified according to the 2010 ACR/EULAR criteria and treated according to modern treatment strategies.

Keywords: Rheumatoid arthritis, Biomarkers, Inflammation, Imaging, Outcomes

Background

A high level of anti-citrullinated protein antibodies (ACPA) is predictive of radiographic progression in rheumatoid arthritis (RA) [1, 2], and ACPA positivity has been associated with radiographic damage even before RA onset [1] and in early RA [1, 3–7]. Positivity to the anti-cyclic citrullinated peptide (anti-CCP2) test, hereafter referred to as "anti-CCP", reflects presence of antibodies to mixed cyclic citrullinated peptides (i.e. ACPAs) as an artificial mimic of the true autoantigens [8]. The ACPA response against citrullinated antigens in RA, hereafter referred to as "ACPA reactivity", has been shown to be heterogeneous [9–15]. Presence of ACPA reactivities may precede the onset of anti-CCP positivity [16], as several studies have shown that both the number of ACPA reactivities and their individual titres increase before clinical onset of RA [12, 13, 16–19].

RA patients may be characterised by distinct autoantibody profiles, as serum samples from the majority of anti-CCP-positive patients react with one or more specific citrullinated target proteins [12, 13, 16, 17, 20]. ACPA reactivities have also been found in patients who are anti-CCP negative [14, 15, 20–22]. Previous studies have shown that the individual titre of selected ACPA reactivities, such as anti-citrullinated vimentin, declines significantly after initiation of disease-modifying antirheumatic drug (DMARD) treatment, while the presence of anti-CCP antibodies remains stable over time [23, 24]. Higher numbers of specificities have been associated with increased risk of relapse in patients with early RA, who are in clinical remission and tapering DMARDs [25].

ACPA reactivity against citrullinated vimentin has been proposed to be involved in the bone-destructive processes in undifferentiated arthritis [26], early RA [23, 24, 26, 27] and established RA [28]. In early RA, seroreversion of citrullinated vimentin during the first 3 months of treatment has been shown to be associated with significantly less 2-year radiographic progression, compared with patients who remained positive [23]. However, the clinical relevance of measuring ACPA reactivities to obtain prognostic information on treatment response or radiographic damage in early undifferentiated arthritis [22, 29–31] or early RA [32] has not been established.

To our knowledge, the associations between individual ACPA reactivities and disease characteristics have not been studied in patients with early RA classified according to the 2010 American College of Rheumatology (ACR)/European League Against Rheumatism (EULAR) criteria. The aim of this study was to assess the prevalence of selected baseline ACPA reactivities, and to investigate the association between ACPA reactivities and disease activity, ultrasound findings, treatment response and radiographic damage in an inception cohort of patients with early RA.

Methods

Design and setting of the study

We used data from the completed "Aiming for remission in rheumatoid arthritis: a randomized trial examining the benefit of ultrasound in a clinical tight control regimen" (the ARCTIC trial, NCT01205854) [33], a study designed to assess whether incorporation of ultrasound information into treatment decisions would lead to improved patient outcomes. All patients were treated according to a tight-control treat-to-target strategy, with evaluation at baseline and 12 additional study visits during the 2-year follow up. The treatment target was no swollen joints and Disease Activity Score (DAS) < 1.6 [34], and in half of the patients an additional target was no joints with disease activity demonstrated on power Doppler ultrasound [33]. Core disease activity measures were collected at each visit. Initial treatment consisted of methotrexate monotherapy 15 mg/week escalating to 20 mg/week and prednisolone starting at 15 mg with tapering to stop over 7 weeks. If the treatment target was not achieved, treatment was intensified following a predetermined treatment protocol, with escalation to triple therapy and then biologic DMARDs (bDMARDs). Swollen joints and/or joints with power Doppler ultrasound activity could be injected with triamcinolone hexacetonide (up to a maximum of 80 mg per visit). As clinical and radiographic outcomes of the two strategy arms were similar after 2 years, in the current report the data from the two arms were pooled and analysed together.

Patients and controls

In the ARCTIC trial [33], 230 DMARD-naïve patients with early RA classified according to the 2010 ACR/EULAR criteria were recruited at 11 Norwegian rheumatology centres between September 2010 and April 2013. The patients were 18–75 years of age with symptom duration less than 2 years from first patient-reported swollen joint, and DMARD-naïve with indication for DMARD treatment. For the current analyses, all patients with follow-up biobank serum samples were selected (n = 217). Controls were blood donors with similar characteristics to the patients included in the study (age, gender and smoking status (n = 94)). Serum samples were collected at each visit and stored at - 70 °C. The study was approved by the local ethics committee of the South-Eastern Norway Regional Health Authority and was conducted in compliance with the Declaration of Helsinki and the International Conference on Harmonization Guidelines for Good Clinical Practice. All patients provided written informed consent.

Laboratory examinations

Analysis of 16 ACPA reactivities and the corresponding native arginine-containing control peptides targeting citrullinated peptides from fibrinogen (Fib), alpha-1 enolase (citrullinated enolase peptide 1 (CEP-1)), vimentin (Vim), filaggrin (Fil) and histone (H) was performed using a multiplex chip-based assay based on the ImmunoCAP ISAC system (Phadia AB, Uppsala, Sweden) [15, 20]. All samples from 0, 3, 12 and 24 months were analysed. ACPA reactivity titres (AU/ml) were considered positive if above the 98-percentile of values in 619 subjects without RA [20]. Erythrocyte sedimentation rate (ESR) and C-reactive protein (CRP) were analysed locally by in-house standard methodology. Anti-CCP was analysed by fluorometric enzyme immunocapture assay (FEIA) (positive if $\geq$ 10 IU/mL) and rheumatoid factor (RF) by ELISA (positive if $\geq$ 25 IU/mL).

Clinical and imaging assessments

Clinical joint examination was performed using the 44 swollen joint count (SJC44) and Ritchie Articular Index for tender joints [35]. Patients and physicians reported the overall assessment of disease activity and pain on visual analogue scales (VAS), range 0–100. The composite index DAS was calculated [34] and response according to the EULAR criteria [36] and fulfillment of ACR/EULAR Boolean remission criteria were evaluated [37].

Radiographic examinations of the hands and feet from baseline, 12 and 24 months were scored according to the van der Heijde modified Sharp score [38]. Scoring was performed in chronological order by two trained readers blinded to clinical information, and the average of the two scores was used. Presence of erosive disease was defined as van der Heijde modified Sharp erosion score $\geq$ 3, in line with the definition suggested by a EULAR task force [39]. Radiographic progression was defined as a change in van der Heijde modified Sharp total score of $\geq$ 2 units over 2 years, which is above the smallest detectable change (1.94 units).

Ultrasound examination was performed according to a validated semi-quantitative 32-joint protocol with scores of 0–3, separately for grey scale synovitis and power Doppler ultrasound [40]. Half the patients underwent ultrasound examination at all visits, while the patients in the conventional group were examined clinically at every visit and by ultrasound at baseline, 12 and 24 months [33]. Examiners were thoroughly trained and an atlas was available for reference [40].

Statistical analysis

Baseline characteristics were compared using the chi-square test, t test and Mann-Whitney U test, as appropriate. Correlation between anti-CCP/ACPA reactivity levels and number of ACPA reactivities and disease activity measures, ultrasound and radiography scores were assessed using Spearman's rank correlation coefficient. Spearman's correlation was classified as very weak, weak, moderate, strong or very strong [41]. Association between number of ACPA reactivities and treatment response was evaluated using the Mann-Whitney U test. Association between anti-CCP/ACPA reactivity status and continuous variables was evaluated by the Mann-Whitney U test, and association with categorical variables was assessed by the chi-square test. ACPA reactivity median levels at baseline and follow-up visits were compared by paired samples using the Wilcox test, comparing each time point with the baseline level. A p value <0.05 was considered statistically significant. Statistical analyses were performed using Stata Statistical Software, version 14 (StataCorp LLC, TX, USA) and R Statistical Software, version 3.4.0 (copyright 2017, The R Foundation for Statistical Computing).

Results

Patient characteristics

A total of 217 patients and 94 healthy controls were included in the study. Baseline characteristics according to autoantibody subgroups are provided in Table 1. Presence of ACPA reactivities was seen mainly in patients positive for anti-CCP and RF (Table 1), but ACPA reactivities also occurred more frequently in anti-CCP/RF negative patients than in controls (0 (0, 1) vs. 0 (0, 0), p = 0.050; Table 1, Fig. 1). The anti-CCP level significantly correlated with the number of citrullinated antigens recognised (r = 0.76, p < 0.0001). ACPA reactivity presence in the RF-negative subset was generally higher than in the

Table 1 Baseline characteristics and anti-citrullinated protein antibody (ACPA) reactivities in subgroups of patients with rheumatoid arthritis (RA) and controls

	All RA n = 217	Anti-CCP+ n = 178	Anti-CCP- n = 39	RF+ n = 154	RF- n = 63	Anti-CCP+/RF+ n = 147	Anti-CCP-/RF- n = 32	Controls n = 94
Age, years[a]	51.5 (13.6)	50.8 (13.2)	55.0 (14.9)	51.9 (13.3)	50.8 (14.2)	51.7 (13.6)	55.0 (16.1)	52.1 (9.2)
Female[b]	131 (60)	109 (61)	22 (56)	91 (59)	40 (63)	86 (59)	17 (53)	57 (61)
Ever-smoker[b]	148 (68)	122 (69)	26 (67)	109 (71)	39 (62)	103 (70)	20 (62)	60 (64)
DAS[a]	3.5 (1.2)	3.4 (1.1)	4.0 (1.3)	3.5 (1.2)	3.5 (1.2)	3.42 (1.1)	3.9 (1.2)	NA
DAS28[a]	4.4 (1.2)	4.4 (1.2)	4.7 (1.2)	4.5 (1.2)	4.2 (1.3)	4.5 (1.1)	4.5 (1.1)	NA
vdHSS total[c]	4.0 [1.5, 8.0]	4.0 [1.5, 7.9]	4.5 [2.0, 10]	4.5 [2.0, 8.0]	3.5 [1.5, 10]	4.5 [2.0, 8.0]	5.5 [1.8, 12.8]	NA
vdHSS erosion[c]	3.0 [1, 4.5]	3.0 [1, 4.5]	3.0 [1.0, 5.5]	3.0 [1.5, 4.5]	3.0 [1.0, 5.5]	3.0 [1.0, 4.5]	3.0 [1.0, 6.3]	NA
vdHSS JSN[c]	1.0 [0.0, 3.0]	1.0 [0.0, 3.0]	1.5 [0.0, 5.0]	1.0 [0.0, 3.0]	1.0 [0.0, 3.0]	1.0 [0.0, 3.0]	1.5 [0.0, 6.5]	NA
Ultrasound grey scale[c]	18 [10, 28]	16 [9, 24]	33 [20, 51]	17 [10, 26]	21 [12, 36]	16 [9, 25]	33 [21, 52]	NA
Ultrasound power Doppler[c]	7 [3, 14]	6 [2, 12]	14 [6, 28]	6 [2, 13]	8 [3, 15]	6 [2, 12]	13 [6, 29]	NA
Number of ACPA reactivities[c]	9 [4, 12]	10 [7, 12]	0 [0, 1]	10 [7, 12]	2 [0, 10]	10 [7, 12]	0 [0, 1]	0 [0, 0]
ACPA reactivity status, n (%)								
Fibβ 60-74cit	162 (75)	160 (90)	2 (5)	136 (88)	26 (41)	134 (91)	0 (0)	0 (0)
Vim 60-75cit	159 (73)	152 (85)	7 (18)	130 (84)	29 (46)	128 (87)	5 (16)	5 (5)
H4 31-50cit	145 (67)	142 (80)	3 (8)	119 (77)	26 (41)	118 (80)	2 (6)	1 (1)
CEP-1	140 (65)	137 (77)	3 (8)	117 (76)	23 (37)	115 (78)	1 (3)	1 (1)
Fil 307-324cit	136 (63)	134 (75)	2 (5)	113 (73)	23 (37)	112 (76)	1 (3)	0 (0)
Fibα 573cit	123 (57)	121 (68)	2 (5)	99 (64)	24 (38)	99 (67)	2 (6)	0 (0)
Fibβ 36-52cit	117 (54)	116 (65)	1 (3)	96 (62)	21 (33)	96 (65)	1 (3)	2 (2)
H3 1-30cit	107 (49)	106 (60)	1 (3)	93 (60)	14 (22)	92 (63)	0 (0)	0 (0)
H4 14-34cit	105 (48)	103 (58)	2 (5)	90 (58)	15 (24)	88 (60)	0 (0)	3 (3)
H3 21-44cit	96 (44)	94 (53)	2 (5)	80 (52)	16 (25)	79 (54)	1 (3)	1 (1)
Fibα 621-635cit	93 (43)	92 (52)	1 (3)	78 (51)	15 (24)	77 (52)	0 (0)	1 (1)
Vim 2-17cit	88 (41)	87 (49)	1 (3)	80 (52)	8 (13)	79 (54)	0 (0)	0 (0)
Fibα 36-50cit	79 (36)	79 (44)	0 (0)	67 (44)	12 (19)	67 (46)	0 (0)	0 (0)
Fibα 591cit	69 (32)	66 (37)	3 (8)	56 (36)	13 (21)	55 (37)	2 (6)	1 (1)
Fibβ 74cit	66 (30)	60 (34)	6 (15)	54 (35)	12 (19)	51 (35)	3 (9)	3 (3)
Fibβ 72cit	27 (12)	24 (13)	3 (8)	21 (14)	6 (1)	20 (14)	2 (6)	2 (2)

Abbreviations: *RA* rheumatoid arthritis; *anti-CCP* anti-cyclic citrullinated peptide, *RF* rheumatoid factor, *DAS* Disease Activity Score, *vdHSS* van der Heijde modified Sharp score, *JSN* joint space narrowing, *ACPA* anti-citrullinated protein antibody, *Fib* fibrinogen, *cit* citrullinated, *Vim* vimentin, *H* histone, *CEP-1* citrullinated enolase peptide-1, *Fil* filaggrin; numbers referring to amino acid sequence, *NA* not applicable
[a]Mean (SD)
[b]Number (percentage)
[c]Median [25, 75 percentile]

anti-CCP-negative group (Table 1). Among the 63 RF-negative patients, 31 were anti-CCP positive.

ACPA reactivities and disease activity at baseline

The DAS, SJC44 and ultrasound grey scale and power Doppler scores were significantly higher in patients who were negative for anti-CCP. Similarly, lack of the most commonly occurring ACPA reactivities (Fibβ 60–74, Vim 60–75 and H4 31–50) was associated with higher DAS, SJC44 and ultrasound grey scale and power Doppler to a statistically significant level (Table 2).

When performing the same analyses on the anti-CCP positive cohort only, there were no differences in DAS, SJC44 or ultrasound scores between the patients testing positive versus negative for the ACPA reactivities (Additional file 1: Table S1). The DAS, SJC44 and ultrasound grey scale and power Doppler scores were negatively correlated with the majority of the ACPA reactivity levels at baseline (Additional file 1: Table S2). This association was not seen when considering the anti-CCP-positive cohort only (Additional file 1: Table S3). Number of ACPA reactivities was not correlated with ESR and CRP (data not shown).

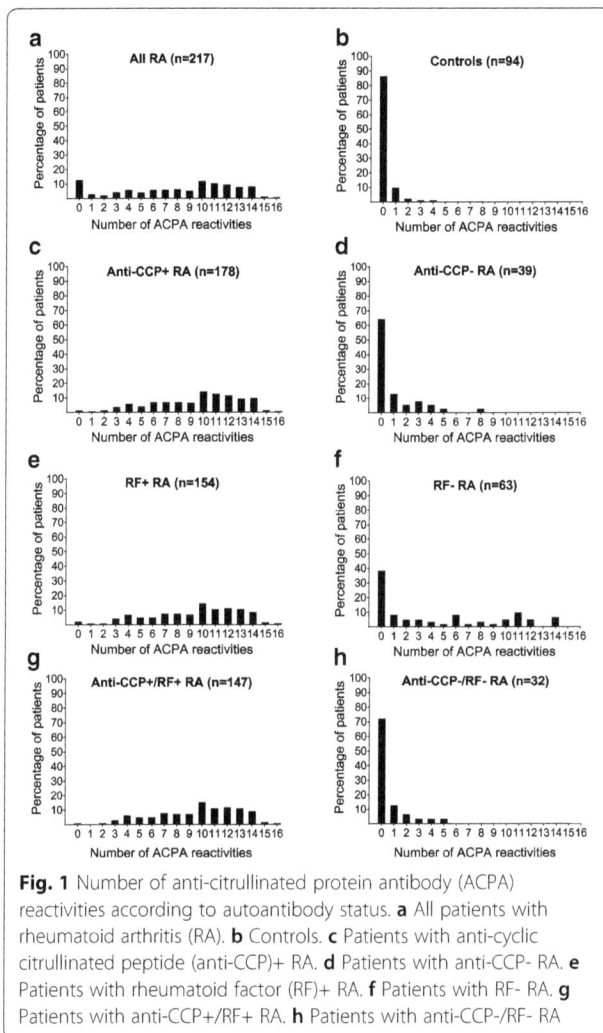

Fig. 1 Number of anti-citrullinated protein antibody (ACPA) reactivities according to autoantibody status. **a** All patients with rheumatoid arthritis (RA). **b** Controls. **c** Patients with anti-cyclic citrullinated peptide (anti-CCP)+ RA. **d** Patients with anti-CCP- RA. **e** Patients with rheumatoid factor (RF)+ RA. **f** Patients with RF- RA. **g** Patients with anti-CCP+/RF+ RA. **h** Patients with anti-CCP-/RF- RA

ACPA reactivities and disease activity after initiation of DMARD treatment

ACPA reactivity levels declined significantly after initiation of DMARD treatment (Fig. 2a) with the most prominent drop in ACPA reactivity levels occuring within the first 3 months. The delta median change in DAS (after 6, 12 and 24 months), ultrasound grey scale and power Doppler (both after 12 and 24 months) was higher in the ACPA reactivity negative patients, with few exceptions (Table 3). However, these differences between the ACPA reactivity negative versus positive patients in DAS, ultrasound grey scale and power Doppler evened out during follow up (data not shown). The most pronounced relative change comparing baseline levels to levels after 3 months was seen for Fibβ 60–74 and the least marked decrease was for Fil 307–324 (38% vs. 19% decrease, both $p < 0.001$; Fig. 2a). We wanted to investigate whether the relative change in ACPA reactivity levels after 3 months differed between patients with

lasting methotrexate treatment response and patients requiring triple treatment and/or bDMARDs over the 2 years of follow up. A greater relative change after 3 months of DMARD treatment was seen in most ACPA reactivities in patients who were methotrexate monotherapy responders, and to a statistically significant degree for Vim 60–75 and H4 31–50 (Fig. 2b).

ACPA reactivities at baseline and prediction of treatment response

There was no difference in median baseline level of the individual ACPA reactivities (data not shown) or baseline median number of ACPA reactivities between patients with successful methotrexate monotherapy according to EULAR good/moderate response and patients with no treatment response after 3 months (9 [4, 12] vs. 10 [4, 11]; $p = 0.80$). Likewise, no difference was seen in median baseline level of the individual ACPA reactivities (data not shown) or median number of ACPA reactivities in patients reaching remission vs. not reaching remission according to DAS (8 [3, 12] vs. 10 [6, 12]; $p = 0.16$) or ACR/EULAR Boolean criteria (9 [4, 12] vs. 9 [5, 11]; $p = 0.74$) after 6 months of methotrexate treatment. Median baseline number of ACPA reactivities for patients reaching vs. not reaching DAS remission at 12 months was 8 [4, 11] vs. 10 [6, 11], $p = 0.26$ and for 24 months 8 [4, 12] vs. 10 [4, 11], $p = 0.87$. For ACR EULAR Boolean remission at 12 months, the corresponding numbers were 7 [3, 11] vs. 10 [5, 11], $p = 0.08$ and at 24 months 8 [3, 11] vs. 9 [6, 12], $p = 0.36$, respectively.

When stratifying by number of ACPA reactivities, there was a trend that patients with no ACPA reactivities present at baseline were more likely to be in methotrexate monotherapy remission according to DAS after 6 months than patients with 1-5, 6-8or ≥9 ACPA reactivities present at baseline (70% vs. 53%, 53%, and 47%, respectively; $p = 0.18$). No such trend was found for DAS remission at 12 months (81% vs. 67%, 77% and 67%, respectively; $p = 0.50$) or 24 months (89% vs. 85%, 78%, and 78%, respectively; $p = 0.71$). When comparing the proportion of patients in remission according to the ACR/EULAR Boolean remission criteria in relation to number of baseline ACPA reactivities, no trend was seen at 6, 12 or 24 months (data not shown).

ACPA and radiographic damage

Anti-CCP positivity was not associated with baseline radiographic scores, and neither of the individual ACPA reactivity levels was associated with baseline radiographic scores or baseline erosive disease (Table 2). Overall median observed change in van der Heijde modified Sharp total score after 12 and 24 months did not differ between ACPA reactivity-positive vs. reactivity-negative patients (Table 3). Baseline presence

Table 2 Baseline disease characteristics (median values) in anti-CCP and ACPA reactivity-positive versus reactivity-negative patients

		ESR	p	CRP	p	DAS	p	SJC44	p	RAI	p	US GS	p	US PD	p	vdHSS E	p	vdHSS JSN	p	vdHSS T	p
Anti-CCP	+ (82%)	21	0.10	7	0.20	3.24	*< 0.01*	8	*< 0.01*	7	0.17	16	*< 0.01*	6	*< 0.01*	3	0.72	1	0.10	4	0.37
	- (18%)	13		7		4.09		18		8		33		14		3		1.5		4.5	
Fibβ 60–74	+ (75%)	20	0.63	7	*0.04*	3.28	*0.02*	7	*< 0.01*	7	0.65	17	*< 0.01*	6	*< 0.01*	3	0.97	1	0.71	4.5	0.73
	- (25%)	19		10		3.87		14		7		28		11		3		0.5		3.5	
Vim 60–75	+ (73%)	18	0.95	7	0.54	3.29	*0.05*	8	*< 0.01*	6	0.83	17	*< 0.01*	6	*0.02*	3	0.96	1	0.26	4.5	0.95
	- (27%)	21		7		3.77		14		7		23		9		3		1		4	
H4 31–50	+ (67%)	21	0.39	8	0.65	3.27	*0.01*	8	*< 0.01*	6	*0.03*	17	*0.01*	6	*0.01*	3	0.88	1	0.94	4.5	0.70
	- (33%)	17		7		3.84		13		10		21		9		3		0.75		3.25	
CEP-1	+ (65%)	21	0.13	8	0.93	3.32	0.35	9	0.06	7	0.47	17	*0.03*	6	0.12	3	0.76	1	0.46	4.5	0.54
	- (35%)	17		6		3.36		11		7		21		7		3		0.5		3.5	
Fil 307–324	+ (63%)	21	0.15	8	0.70	3.29	0.06	7	*< 0.01*	7	0.54	17	*0.01*	6	*< 0.01*	3	0.94	1	0.98	4	0.91
	- (37%)	17		7		3.64		13		7		21		9		3		1		4	
Fibα 573	+ (57%)	22	0.13	8	0.85	3.27	*0.03*	7	*< 0.01*	6	0.14	17	*0.05*	6	0.12	3	0.61	1	0.23	4.5	0.37
	- (43%)	16		7		3.42		12		8		21		8		3		0.5		4	
Fibβ 36–52	+ (54%)	21	0.08	8	0.78	3.26	*0.05*	8	*< 0.01*	6	0.06	17	0.06	6	*0.03*	3	0.58	1	*0.05*	4.5	0.19
	- (46%)	17		7		3.63		11		8		19		8		3		0.5		3.5	
H3 1–30	+ (49%)	18	0.97	7	0.40	3.29	0.48	8	0.09	6	1.00	17	*0.04*	6	0.09	3	0.62	0.5	*0.04*	4	0.16
	- (51%)	20		7		3.37		10		7		19		7		3		1		4.5	
H4 14–34	+ (48%)	21	0.13	8	0.74	3.27	0.28	7	*< 0.01*	7	0.77	17	0.30	7	0.86	3	0.39	1	0.30	4	0.28
	- (52%)	18		7		3.45		11		7		20		6		3		1		4.5	
H3 21–44	+ (44%)	22	0.09	9	0.21	3.31	0.69	9	0.07	7	0.84	17	0.28	6	0.41	3	0.68	0.5	0.14	4	0.32
	- (56%)	18		6		3.36		10		7		19		7		3		1		4.5	
Fibα 621–635	+ (43%)	22	0.36	8	0.84	3.29	0.09	7	*< 0.01*	7	0.54	16	*0.02*	6	0.07	2.5	0.46	0.5	0.30	4	0.34
	- (57%)	18		7		3.37		12		7		20		7		3		1		4.5	
Vim 2–17	+ (41%)	19	0.72	7	0.49	3.29	0.34	7	*< 0.01*	7	0.48	17	0.08	6	0.13	3	0.50	1	0.61	4	0.45
	- (59%)	20		7		3.36		11		7		20		7		3		1		4	
Fibα 36–50	+ (36%)	20	0.73	8	0.86	3.29	0.68	8	*0.04*	7	0.46	17	0.08	6	*0.05*	3	0.84	0.5	0.29	4	0.59
	- (64%)	19		7		3.41		11		7		19		7		3		1		4	
Fibα 591	+ (32%)	19	0.70	6	0.29	3.29	*0.05*	7	*< 0.01*	6	0.28	17	0.53	6	0.88	3	0.86	1	0.33	4.5	0.70
	- (68%)	20		8		3.40		11		7		19		7		3		0.5		4	
Fibβ 74	+ (30%)	22	0.19	8	0.87	3.25	0.53	9	0.12	8	0.74	17	0.08	6	0.67	2.5	0.57	0.5	0.32	4	0.48
	- (70%)	18		7		3.33		10		7		19		7		3		1		4	
Fibβ 72	+ (12%)	21	0.25	5	0.59	3.59	0.37	10	0.48	9	0.52	22	0.19	9	0.06	3	0.73	0.5	0.72	4	0.98
	- (88%)	19		7		3.31		9		7		17		6		3		1		4	

Anti-citrullinated protein antibody (ACPA) reactivities are sorted by decreasing frequency in the cohort: p values (p) were derived from the Mann-Whitney U test; statistically significant differences are in italics

Abbreviations: ESR erythrocyte sedimentation rate (millimetre/hour, 1–140), CRP C-reactive protein (milligram/litre), DAS Disease Activity Score (0–10), SJC swollen joint count (0–44), RAI Ritchie articular index (0–78), US ultrasound, GS grey scale (0–96), PD power Doppler (0–96), vdHSS van der Heijde modified Sharp score, E erosion (0–280), JSN joint space narrowing (0–168), T total (0–448), *anti-CCP* anti-cyclic citrullinated peptide, *Fib* fibrinogen, *Vim* vimentin, *H* histone, *CEP-1* citrullinated enolase peptide-1, *Fil* filaggrin; numbers referring to amino acid sequence

and/or levels of any of the ACPA reactivities were not associated with progression of radiographic damage or change in radiographic score after 12 and 24 months, and seroreversion of any ACPA reactivity after 3 months of treatment was not associated with less radiographic progression after 12 and 24 months (data not shown).

Outcomes did not differ when performing subanalyses on the anti-CCP-positive cohort only. Number of ACPA reactivities was not associated with baseline radiographic scores or presence of baseline erosive disease (Table 4). However, there was a trend towards less radiographic progression after 12 and 24 months in patients with no

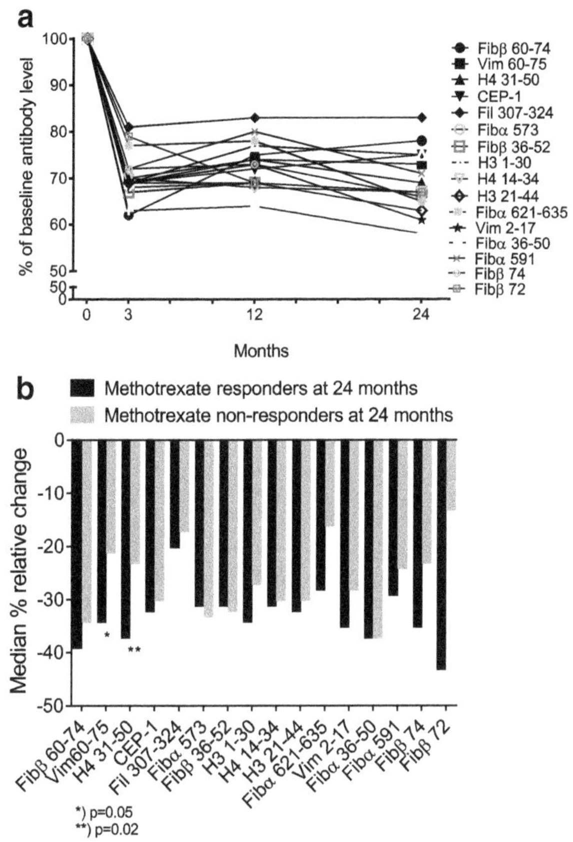

Fig. 2 Relative change in levels of various anti-citrullinated protein antibody (ACPA) reactivities in patients with early rheumatoid arthritis (RA) (only baseline seropositive patients included) **a** Relative change between baseline and 3, 12 and 24 months, **b** Relative change after 3 months, comparing patients on methotrexate monotherapy at 24 months (n = 113) to patients on triple and/or biological disease-modifying antirheumatic drugs (bDMARDs) at 24 months (n = 82). Fib, fibrinogen; Vim, vimentin; H, histone; CEP-1, citrullinated enolase peptide-1; Fil, Filaggrin, numbers referring to amino acid sequence

baseline ACPA reactivities compared with 1–5, 6–8 and ≥ 9 reactivities (Fig. 3), and also when comparing no baseline ACPA reactivities with ≥ 1 reactivities (21% vs. 39% at 12 months, p = 0.10 and 33% vs. 39% at 24 months, p = 0.66).

Discussion

To our knowledge, this is the first study to examine the relationship between ACPA reactivities in patients with early RA classified according to the 2010 ACR/EULAR criteria and imaging and serological and clinical disease activity measures, and their potential use in prediction of treatment response and radiographic progression [42]. The prevalence of ACPA reactivities was associated with anti-CCP/RF positivity, and baseline disease activity measures and ultrasound scores were lower in ACPA

reactivity-positive compared to ACPA reactivity-negative patients. ACPA reactivity levels decreased after initiation of DMARD treatment, but the clinical implications of measuring ACPA reactivities to predict treatment response and radiographic progression in this cohort of intensively treated patients with early RA were limited.

High levels of anti-CCP antibodies have previously been shown to be a risk factor for erosive disease [1, 2], and selected ACPA reactivities have also been shown to be associated with osteoclast activation and radiographic damage [23, 24, 26, 27, 43]. Kastbom et al. have shown that ACPA reactivity levels declined after 3 months of methotrexate treatment, and that disappearance of certain ACPA reactivities was associated with less 2-year radiographic progression [23]. In our study, levels of all ACPA reactivities declined after 3 months of DMARD treatment. None of the individual ACPA reactivities analysed were associated with baseline erosive disease or radiographic progression, nor was seroreversion of individual ACPA reactivities associated with less radiographic progression over the 2 years of follow up in our study. Presence, but not titre, of reactivities to citrullinated fibrinogen was associated with faster joint destruction in the ESPOIR cohort of patients with very early RA fulfilling either the 1987 ACR criteria at inclusion or the 2010 ACR/EULAR criteria within 3 years of inclusion [26]. We identified a trend that patients with ≥ 1 ACPA reactivity at baseline experienced more radiographic progression at 12 and 24 months compared to patients with no ACPA reactivities present, but the findings were not significant. Lack of significant association between number of ACPA reactivities and radiographic progression has previously also been described in the Leiden early arthritis cohort where patients fulfilled the 1987 ACR criteria within 1 year after inclusion [29–31]. Previous studies have not demonstrated association between the individual ACPA reactivities and disease activity measures in early undifferentiated arthritis and early RA [29–32]. ACPA reactivities present in anti-CCP-negative patients with RA have not been shown to be associated with clinical or prognostic parameters [22]. As previously published, seropositive patients in the ARCTIC cohort had significantly lower disease activity compared to seronegative patients [44], similar to what has been reported in other cohorts [45, 46]. The most prevalent ACPA reactivities in our study were negatively correlated with the DAS, SJC44 and ultrasound grey scale and power Doppler scores at baseline, and the disease activity measurements were numerically higher in patients who were negative for the individual ACPA reactivities, which has not been described previously. These differences were no longer present when excluding the anti-CCP-negative subgroup and are thus potentially a consequence of the 2010 ACR/EULAR

Table 3 Change in disease characteristics (delta median values) in ACPA reactivity-positive versus reactivity-negative patients

		Delta DAS 6 months	p	Delta DAS 12 months	p	Delta DAS 24 months	p	Delta US GS 12 months	p	Delta US GS 24 months	p	Delta US PD 12 months	p	Delta US PD 24 months	p	Delta vdHSS T 12 months	p	Delta vdHSS T 24 months	p
Fibβ 60–74	+	−1.9	0.04	−2.0	<0.01	−2.0	0.02	−12	<0.01	−13	<0.01	−6	<0.01	−6	<0.01	0.5	0.92	1.0	0.69
	−	−2.5		−2.6		−2.6		−19		−21		−9		−10		0.5		1.0	
Vim 60–75	+	−1.9	<0.01	−1.9	<0.01	−2.0	0.02	−12	<0.01	−13	<0.01	−6	0.06	−6	0.02	0.5	0.59	1.0	0.68
	−	−2.6		−2.6		−2.6		−17		−17		−8		−8		0.5		1.0	
H4 31–50	+	−1.9	<0.01	−1.9	<0.01	−2.0	<0.01	−12	0.05	−13	<0.01	−6	0.08	−6	0.02	0.5	0.15	1.0	0.81
	−	−2.5		−2.8		−2.7		−15		−17		−7		−8		0.5		1.0	
CEP-1	+	−2.0	0.75	−2.1	0.79	−2.1	0.48	−12	0.23	−14	0.24	−6	0.17	−6	0.14	0.5	0.50	1.0	0.41
	−	−2.1		−2.2		−2.0		−14		−14		−7		−7		0.5		1.0	
Fil 307–324	+	−1.9	0.01	−1.8	<0.01	−1.9	0.01	−12	0.06	−13	0.01	−6	0.03	−5	0.01	0.5	0.75	1.0	0.76
	−	−2.4		−2.5		−2.5		−16		−16		−7		−7		0.5		1.0	
Fibα 573	+	−1.9	<0.01	−1.8	<0.01	−1.9	<0.01	−13	0.36	−14	0.12	−6	0.21	−6	0.08	0.5	0.89	1.0	0.77
	−	−2.5		−2.6		−2.4		−13		−15		−7		−7		0.5		1.5	
Fibβ 36–52	+	−1.9	0.02	−1.9	<0.01	−1.9	<0.01	−12	0.23	−14	0.09	−6	0.08	−5	0.02	0.5	0.89	1.0	0.58
	−	−2.4		−2.5		−2.5		−14		−14		−7		−7		0.5		1.5	
H3 1–30	+	−2.1	0.97	−2.2	0.97	−2.0	0.44	−12	0.31	−13	0.04	−6	0.25	−6	0.09	0.5	0.24	1.0	0.45
	−	−2.0		−2.1		−2.2		−14		−16		−7		−7		0.5		1.2	
H4 14–34	+	−1.9	0.07	−2.0	0.12	−2.0	0.14	−12	0.46	−12	0.02	−7	0.63	−6	0.54	0.5	0.32	1.5	0.10
	−	−2.1		−2.3		−2.2		−14		−16		−6		−6		0.5		1.0	
H3 21–44	+	−2.0	0.48	−2.0	0.31	−2.0	0.37	−12	0.29	−13	0.39	−6	0.28	−6	0.38	0.5	0.39	1.5	0.76
	−	−2.0		−2.2		−2.2		−15		−15		−7		−7		0.5		1.0	
Fibα 621–635	+	−1.7	0.04	−1.8	0.04	−1.9	0.03	−11	0.02	−13	0.01	−6	0.09	−6	0.05	0.5	0.20	1.0	0.22
	−	−2.3		−2.4		−2.2		−15		−16		−7		−7		0.5		1.5	
Vim 2–17	+	−1.9	0.04	−1.8	0.02	−1.8	0.01	−12	0.12	−12	<0.01	−6	0.21	−5	0.04	0.5	0.90	1.0	0.87
	−	−2.2		−2.3		−2.3		−14		−16		−7		−7		0.5		1.0	
Fibα 36–50	+	−2.0	0.83	−2.0	0.74	−2.0	0.45	−11	0.09	−12	0.10	−5	0.02	−5	0.02	0.5	0.61	1.0	0.52
	−	−2.0		−2.2		−2.2		−14		−15		−7		−7		0.5		1.0	
Fibα 591	+	−1.9	0.08	−1.8	0.03	−1.8	0.01	−13	0.69	−16	0.70	−6	0.84	−6	0.77	0.5	0.41	1.0	0.58
	−	−2.2		−2.3		−2.3		−13		−14		−6		−7		0.5		1.5	
Fibβ 74	+	−1.8	0.41	−2.0	0.79	−2.1	0.55	−12	0.36	−13	0.94	−7	0.82	−7	0.98	0.5	0.06	1.5	0.54
	−	−2.1		−2.2		−2.0		−13		−14		−6		−6		0.5		1.0	
Fibβ 72	+	−2.0	0.84	−2.0	0.73	−1.9	0.78	−16	0.19	−17	0.21	−7	0.13	−9	0.11	0.2	0.98	0.5	0.51
	−	−2.0		−2.2		−2.1		−12		−14		−6		−6		0.5		1.0	

Anti-citrullinated protein antibody (ACPA) reactivities are sorted by decreasing frequency in the cohort; p values (p) were derived from the Mann-Whitney U test; statistically significant differences are in italics

Abbreviations: DAS Disease Activity Score (0–10), SJC swollen joint count (0–44), US ultrasound, GS grey scale (0–96), PD power Doppler 0–96), vdHSS van der Heijde modified Sharp score, T total (0–448), Fib fibrinogen, Vim vimentin, H histone, CEP-1 citrullinated enolase peptide-1, Fil filaggrin; numbers referring to amino acid sequence

classification criteria, where the anti-CCP/RF-negative patients require greater joint involvement than the seropositive patients to fulfill the criteria [42, 44].

Current guidelines for treat-to-target emphasise the importance of improvement in disease activity within 3 months (EULAR good/moderate response) and attainment of the treatment target (ACR/EULAR Boolean remission) within 6 months after initiating treatment [47]. A greater decrease in ACPA reactivity levels has been demonstrated in treatment responders compared to non-responders [23]. In our cohort we identified a similar trend whereby reduction in ACPA reactivity levels after 3 months was more pronounced in patients remaining on methotrexate monotherapy after 2 years of follow up, but we did not observe any baseline predictors of treatment response.

Table 4 Association between number of baseline ACPA reactivities and van der Heijde modified Sharp scores (erosion, joint space narrowing and total) and association between number of baseline ACPA reactivities and baseline erosive disease

	Number of ACPA reactivities				
	0 n = 27	1–5 n = 39	6–8 n = 37	≥9 n = 114	p value
vdHSS erosion[a]	3.0 [1.0, 5.8]	3.0 [1.5, 4.0]	3.0 [2.0, 4.0]	3.0 [1.0, 4.5]	0.87
vdHSS joint space narrowing[a]	1.5 [0.0, 4.8]	0.5 [0.0, 2.0]	0.5 [0.0, 3.0]	1.0 [0.0, 3.8]	0.54
vdHSS total[a]	3.0 [1.5, 11.2]	3.5 [1.5, 6.0]	4.5 [2.5, 7.0]	4.2 [1.5, 9.0]	0.83
Erosive disease[b]	15 (56)	21 (54)	21 (57)	60 (53)	0.97

Abbreviations: ACPA Anti-citrullinated protein antibody, vdHSS van der Heijde modified Sharp score
[a]Median [25,75 percentile]
[b]Number (percentage)

Comparison between our results and those of other studies may be limited by the fact that patients in most previous studies were classified by the 1987 ACR criteria or in cohorts of patients treated less intensively. The relatively few anti-CCP-negative patients in comparison with the larger amount of anti-CCP positive patients reflects an effect of implementing the 2010 ACR/EULAR classification criteria [33] and in this study, the number of patients in the subgroups of anti-CCP and ACPA reactivity-negative patients is somewhat small for meaningful comparisons. When applying the 2010 ACR/EULAR criteria as inclusion criteria, the seronegative patients included in the study were required to have more joint involvement with > 10 clinically involved joints [42]. Patients with a clinical seronegative RA diagnosis involving fewer joints were not included. Strengths of the study were that all patients were classified by the 2010 ACR/EULAR criteria, were DMARD and corticosteroid naïve at inclusion and were treated according to a standardised treatment protocol adhering to current treatment recommendations [33]. The treatment regimen of the ARCTIC trial is well in line with current EULAR recommendations for treatment of early RA [47]. Such intensive treatment may suppress the RA disease activity to such a degree that prognostic markers identified in previous less strictly controlled RA cohorts may no longer be present or of clinical relevance. The current study was also strengthened by a relatively large sample size and a broad collection of serological, clinical and imaging data.

Conclusions

New classification criteria and modern intensive treatment strategies have altered the disease course of early RA, and consequently established predictors for treatment response and progression of radiographic damage should be re-evaluated in appropriate cohorts. In this inception cohort of RA patients classified according to the ACR/EULAR 2010 criteria, the prevalence of ACPA reactivities differed in subgroups according to anti-CCP and RF status, and ACPA reactivity levels decreased after initiation of DMARD treatment. There were no apparent associations with disease activity, prediction of treatment response or radiographic progression, and further studies in larger patient samples are needed to understand the role of ACPA reactivities in patients with RA classified according to the 2010 ACR/EULAR criteria.

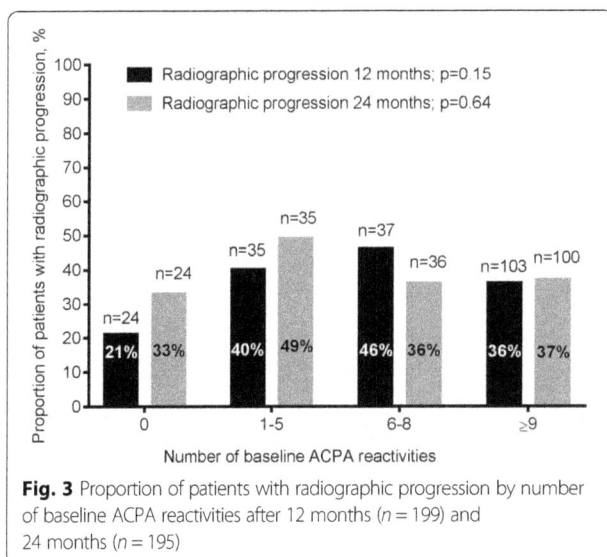

Fig. 3 Proportion of patients with radiographic progression by number of baseline ACPA reactivities after 12 months (n = 199) and 24 months (n = 195)

Abbreviations
ACPA: Anti-citrullinated protein antibody; ACR: American College of Rheumatology; Anti-CCP: Anti-cyclic citrullinated peptide; ARCTIC: Aiming for remission in rheumatoid arthritis: a randomized trial examining the benefit of ultrasound in a clinical tight control regimen; AU: Accredited units; bDMARDs: Biologic disease-modifying antirheumatic drug; CEP-1: Citrullinated enolase peptide-1; CRP: C-reactive protein; DAS: Disease Activity Score; DMARD: Disease-modifying antirheumatic drug; E: Erosion; ELISA: Enzyme-linked immunosorbent assay; ESR: Erythrocyte sedimentation rate; EULAR: European League Against Rheumatism; FEIA: Fluorometric enzyme immunocapture assay; Fib: Fibrinogen; Fil: Filaggrin; H: Histone; JSN: Joint space narrowing; mL: Milliliter; RA: Rheumatoid arthritis; RAI: Ritchie Articular Index; RF: Rheumatoid factor; SJC: Swollen joint count; T: Total; VAS: Visual analogue scale; vdHSS: van der Heijde modified Sharp score; Vim: Vimentin

Acknowledgements

We would like to thank Ellen Moholt and Camilla Fongen at Diakonhjemmet Hospital, Marianne Eidsheim and Kjerstin Jakobsen at the Broegelmann Research Laboratory and the ARCTIC investigators: Hallvard Fremstad, Tor Magne Madland, Åse Stavland Lexberg, Hilde Haukeland, Erik Rødevand, Christian Høili, Hilde Stray, Anne Noraas, Inger Johanne Widding Hansen and Gunnstein Bakland.

Funding

The study has received grants from the Norwegian Research Council, the Southern and Eastern Norway Regional Health Association, the Norwegian Rheumatism Association, the Western Norway Regional Health Authority, the Norwegian ExtraFoundation for Health and Rehabilitation and unrestricted grant support from AbbVie, Pfizer, MSD, UCB and Roche.

Authors' contributions

All authors were involved in drafting the article or revising it critically for important intellectual content and approved the final manuscript to be submitted and agreed to be accountable for all aspects of the work. Conception and design of the study: EAH, SL, MKJ, BTSF, ABA, JS, AHH and AIC. Acquisition of data: MKJ, EAH and ABA. Analysis and interpretation of data: MKJ, AHH, MH, EAH, LMA, SL, BTSF, ABA, GS, MC, AIC and JS.

Competing interests

MKJ reports grants from Norwegian Extra Foundation for Health and Rehabilitation and the Western Norway Regional Health Authority. AHH: none. MH: none. ABA: none. JS: none. LMA is an employee of Thermo Fisher Scientific. MC: none. GS is co-inventor of several international patents for ACPA antigens held by BioMérieux Cy and licensed to Eurodiagnostica Cy and Axis-Shield Cy for commercialization of the CCP2 assays; according to French law he receives a part of the royalties paid to the Toulouse III University and the University Hospital of Toulouse. SL: none. BTSF: none. AIC: none. EAH has received investigator-initiated grants from AbbVie, Pfizer, MSD, UCB Pharma and Roche.

Author details

[1]Department of Rheumatology, Haukeland University Hospital, Pb 1400, NO-5021 Bergen, Norway. [2]Department of Clinical Science, University of Bergen, Bergen, Norway. [3]Center for Molecular Medicine, Karolinska University Hospital, Stockholm, Sweden. [4]Department of Rheumatology, Diakonhjemmet Hospital, Oslo, Norway. [5]Thermo-Fisher Scientific, Uppsala, Sweden. [6]Epithelial Differentation and Rheumatoid Autoimmunity Unit, UMRS 1056 Inserm University of Toulouse, Toulouse, France. [7]Department of Health and Society, Oslo University Hospital, Oslo, Norway.

References

1. Berglin E, Johansson T, Sundin U, Jidell E, Wadell G, Hallmans G, et al. Radiological outcome in rheumatoid arthritis is predicted by presence of antibodies against cyclic citrullinated peptide before and at disease onset, and by IgA-RF at disease onset. Ann Rheum Dis. 2006;65:453–8.
2. Syversen SW, Gaarder PI, Goll GL, Odegard S, Haavardsholm EA, Mowinckel P, et al. High anti-cyclic citrullinated peptide levels and an algorithm of four variables predict radiographic progression in patients with rheumatoid arthritis: results from a 10-year longitudinal study. Ann Rheum Dis. 2008;67:212–7.
3. Forslind K, Ahlmen M, Eberhardt K, Hafstrom I, Svensson B, Group BS. Prediction of radiological outcome in early rheumatoid arthritis in clinical practice: role of antibodies to citrullinated peptides (anti-CCP). Ann Rheum Dis. 2004;63:1090–5.
4. Lindqvist E, Eberhardt K, Bendtzen K, Heinegard D, Saxne T. Prognostic laboratory markers of joint damage in rheumatoid arthritis. Ann Rheum Dis. 2005;64:196–201.
5. Nielen MM, van der Horst AR, van Schaardenburg D, van der Horst-Bruinsma IE, van de Stadt RJ, Aarden L, et al. Antibodies to citrullinated human fibrinogen (ACF) have diagnostic and prognostic value in early arthritis. Ann Rheum Dis. 2005;64:1199–204.
6. Ronnelid J, Wick MC, Lampa J, Lindblad S, Nordmark B, Klareskog L, et al. Longitudinal analysis of citrullinated protein/peptide antibodies (anti-CP) during 5 year follow up in early rheumatoid arthritis: anti-CP status predicts worse disease activity and greater radiological progression. Ann Rheum Dis. 2005;64:1744–9.
7. Machold KP, Stamm TA, Nell VP, Pflugbeil S, Aletaha D, Steiner G, et al. Very recent onset rheumatoid arthritis: clinical and serological patient characteristics associated with radiographic progression over the first years of disease. Rheumatology (Oxford). 2007;46:342–9.
8. Pruijn GJ, Wiik A, van Venrooij WJ. The use of citrullinated peptides and proteins for the diagnosis of rheumatoid arthritis. Arthritis Res Ther. 2010;12:203.
9. Schellekens GA, de Jong BA, van den Hoogen FH, van de Putte LB, van Venrooij WJ. Citrulline is an essential constituent of antigenic determinants recognized by rheumatoid arthritis-specific autoantibodies. J Clin Invest. 1998;101:273–81.
10. Girbal-Neuhauser E, Durieux JJ, Arnaud M, Dalbon P, Sebbag M, Vincent C, et al. The epitopes targeted by the rheumatoid arthritis-associated antifilaggrin autoantibodies are posttranslationally generated on various sites of (pro)filaggrin by deimination of arginine residues. J Immunol. 1999; 162:585–94.
11. Snir O, Widhe M, von Spee C, Lindberg J, Padyukov L, Lundberg K, et al. Multiple antibody reactivities to citrullinated antigens in sera from patients with rheumatoid arthritis: association with HLA-DRB1 alleles. Ann Rheum Dis. 2009;68:736–43.
12. van der Woude D, Rantapaa-Dahlqvist S, Ioan-Facsinay A, Onnekink C, Schwarte CM, Verpoort KN, et al. Epitope spreading of the anti-citrullinated protein antibody response occurs before disease onset and is associated with the disease course of early arthritis. Ann Rheum Dis. 2010;69:1554–61.
13. van de Stadt LA, van der Horst AR, de Koning MH, Bos WH, Wolbink GJ, van de Stadt RJ, et al. The extent of the anti-citrullinated protein antibody repertoire is associated with arthritis development in patients with seropositive arthralgia. Ann Rheum Dis. 2011;70:128–33.
14. Lundberg K, Bengtsson C, Kharlamova N, Reed E, Jiang X, Kallberg H, et al. Genetic and environmental determinants for disease risk in subsets of rheumatoid arthritis defined by the anticitrullinated protein/peptide antibody fine specificity profile. Ann Rheum Dis. 2013;72:652–8.
15. Ronnelid J, Hansson M, Mathsson-Alm L, Cornillet M, Reed E, Jakobsson PJ, et al. Anticitrullinated protein/peptide antibody multiplexing defines an extended group of ACPA-positive rheumatoid arthritis patients with distinct genetic and environmental determinants. Ann Rheum Dis. 2018;77:203–11.
16. Sokolove J, Bromberg R, Deane KD, Lahey LJ, Derber LA, Chandra PE, et al. Autoantibody epitope spreading in the pre-clinical phase predicts progression to rheumatoid arthritis. PLoS One. 2012;7:e35296.
17. Brink M, Hansson M, Mathsson L, Jakobsson PJ, Holmdahl R, Hallmans G, et al. Multiplex analyses of antibodies against citrullinated peptides in individuals prior to development of rheumatoid arthritis. Arthritis Rheum. 2013;65:899–910.
18. Johansson L, Pratesi F, Brink M, Arlestig L, D'Amato C, Bartaloni D, et al. Antibodies directed against endogenous and exogenous citrullinated antigens pre-date the onset of rheumatoid arthritis. Arthritis Res Ther. 2016;18:127.
19. Arkema EV, Goldstein BL, Robinson W, Sokolove J, Wagner CA, Malspeis S, et al. Anti-citrullinated peptide autoantibodies, human leukocyte antigen shared epitope and risk of future rheumatoid arthritis: a nested case-control study. Arthritis Res Ther. 2013;15:R159.
20. Hansson M, Mathsson L, Schlederer T, Israelsson L, Matsson P, Nogueira L, et al. Validation of a multiplex chip-based assay for the detection of autoantibodies against citrullinated peptides. Arthritis Res Ther. 2012;14:R201.
21. Wagner CA, Sokolove J, Lahey LJ, Bengtsson C, Saevarsdottir S, Alfredsson L, et al. Identification of anticitrullinated protein antibody reactivities in a subset of anti-CCP-negative rheumatoid arthritis: association with cigarette smoking and HLA-DRB1 'shared epitope' alleles. Ann Rheum Dis. 2015;74:579–86.
22. van Heemst J, Trouw LA, Nogueira L, van Steenbergen HW, van der Helm-van Mil AH, Allaart CF, et al. An investigation of the added value of an ACPA multiplex assay in an early rheumatoid arthritis setting. Arthritis Res Ther. 2015;17:276.
23. Kastbom A, Forslind K, Ernestam S, Geborek P, Karlsson JA, Petersson IF, et al. Changes in the anticitrullinated peptide antibody response in relation to therapeutic outcome in early rheumatoid arthritis: results from the SWEFOT trial. Ann Rheum Dis. 2016;75:356–61.
24. Hensvold AH, Joshua V, Li W, Larkin M, Qureshi F, Israelsson L, et al. Serum RANKL levels associate with anti-citrullinated protein antibodies in early untreated rheumatoid arthritis and are modulated following methotrexate. Arthritis Res Ther. 2015;17:239.

25. Figueiredo CP, Bang H, Cobra JF, Englbrecht M, Hueber AJ, Haschka J, et al. Antimodified protein antibody response pattern influences the risk for disease relapse in patients with rheumatoid arthritis tapering disease modifying antirheumatic drugs. Ann Rheum Dis. 2017;76:399–407.

26. Cornillet M, Ajana S, Ruyssen-Witrand A, Constantin A, Degboe Y, Cantagrel A et al. Autoantibodies to human citrullinated fibrinogen and their subfamilies to the alpha36-50Cit and beta60-74Cit fibrin peptides similarly predict radiographic damages: a prospective study in the French ESPOIR cohort of very early arthritides. Rheum. 2016;55:1859-70.

27. Harre U, Georgess D, Bang H, Bozec A, Axmann R, Ossipova E, et al. Induction of osteoclastogenesis and bone loss by human autoantibodies against citrullinated vimentin. J Clin Invest. 2012;122:1791–802.

28. Montes A, Perez-Pampin E, Calaza M, Gomez-Reino JJ, Gonzalez A. Association of anti-citrullinated vimentin and anti-citrullinated alpha-enolase antibodies with subsets of rheumatoid arthritis. Arthritis Rheum. 2012;64:3102–10.

29. Willemze A, Bohringer S, Knevel R, Levarht EW, Stoeken-Rijsbergen G, Houwing-Duistermaat JJ, et al. The ACPA recognition profile and subgrouping of ACPA-positive RA patients. Ann Rheum Dis. 2012;71:268–74.

30. van Beers JJ, Willemze A, Jansen JJ, Engbers GH, Salden M, Raats J, et al. ACPA fine-specificity profiles in early rheumatoid arthritis patients do not correlate with clinical features at baseline or with disease progression. Arthritis Res Ther. 2013;15:R140.

31. Scherer HU, van der Woude D, Willemze A, Trouw LA, Knevel R, Syversen SW, et al. Distinct ACPA fine specificities, formed under the influence of HLA shared epitope alleles, have no effect on radiographic joint damage in rheumatoid arthritis. Ann Rheum Dis. 2011;70:1461–4.

32. Fisher BA, Plant D, Brode M, van Vollenhoven RF, Mathsson L, Symmons D, et al. Antibodies to citrullinated alpha-enolase peptide 1 and clinical and radiological outcomes in rheumatoid arthritis. Ann Rheum Dis. 2011;70:1095–8.

33. Haavardsholm EA, Aga AB, Olsen IC, Lillegraven S, Hammer HB, Uhlig T, et al. Ultrasound in management of rheumatoid arthritis: ARCTIC randomised controlled strategy trial. BMJ. 2016;354:i4205.

34. van der Heijde DM, van 't Hof MA, van Riel PL, Theunisse LA, Lubberts EW, van Leeuwen MA, et al. Judging disease activity in clinical practice in rheumatoid arthritis: first step in the development of a disease activity score. Ann Rheum Dis. 1990;49:916–20.

35. Ritchie DM, Boyle JA, McInnes JM, Jasani MK, Dalakos TG, Grieveson P, et al. Clinical studies with an articular index for the assessment of joint tenderness in patients with rheumatoid arthritis. Q J Med. 1968;37:393–406.

36. van Gestel AM, Prevoo ML, van 't Hof MA, van Rijswijk MH, van de Putte LB, van Riel PL. Development and validation of the European league against rheumatism response criteria for rheumatoid arthritis. Comparison with the preliminary American College of Rheumatology and the World Health Organization/international league against rheumatism criteria. Arthritis Rheum. 1996;39:34–40.

37. Felson DT, Smolen JS, Wells G, Zhang B, van Tuyl LH, Funovits J, et al. American College of Rheumatology/European league against rheumatism provisional definition of remission in rheumatoid arthritis for clinical trials. Ann Rheum Dis. 2011;70:404–13.

38. van der Heijde D. How to read radiographs according to the sharp/van der Heijde method. J Rheumatol. 1999;26:743–5.

39. van der Heijde D, van der Helm-van Mil AH, Aletaha D, Bingham CO, Burmester GR, Dougados M, et al. EULAR definition of erosive disease in light of the 2010 ACR/EULAR rheumatoid arthritis classification criteria. Ann Rheum Dis. 2013;72:479–81.

40. Hammer HB, Bolton-King P, Bakkeheim V, Berg TH, Sundt E, Kongtorp AK, et al. Examination of intra and interrater reliability with a new ultrasonographic reference atlas for scoring of synovitis in patients with rheumatoid arthritis. Ann Rheum Dis. 2011;70:1995–8.

41. Swinscow TDV. Statistics at square one, ninth edn. London: BMJ publishing Group; 1997.

42. Aletaha D, Neogi T, Silman AJ, Funovits J, Felson DT, Bingham CO 3rd, et al. 2010 Rheumatoid arthritis classification criteria: an American College of Rheumatology/European league against rheumatism collaborative initiative. Arthritis Rheum. 2010;62:2569–81.

43. Krishnamurthy A, Joshua V, Haj Hensvold A, Jin T, Sun M, Vivar N, et al. Identification of a novel chemokine-dependent molecular mechanism underlying rheumatoid arthritis-associated autoantibody-mediated bone loss. Ann Rheum Dis. 2016;75:721–9.

44. Nordberg LB, Lillegraven S, Lie E, Aga AB, Olsen IC, Hammer HB et al. Patients with seronegative RA have more inflammatory activity compared with patients with seropositive RA in an inception cohort of DMARD-naive patients classified according to the 2010 ACR/EULAR criteria. Ann Rheum Dis. 2016;76:341-5.

45. Barra L, Pope JE, Orav JE, Boire G, Haraoui B, Hitchon C, et al. Prognosis of seronegative patients in a large prospective cohort of patients with early inflammatory arthritis. J Rheumatol. 2014;41:2361–9.

46. Choi ST, Lee KH. Clinical management of seronegative and seropositive rheumatoid arthritis: a comparative study. PLoS One. 2018;13:e0195550.

47. Smolen JS, Landewe R, Bijlsma J, Burmester G, Chatzidionysiou K, Dougados M et al. EULAR recommendations for the management of rheumatoid arthritis with synthetic and biological disease-modifying antirheumatic drugs: 2016 update. Ann Rheum Dis. 2017;76:960-77.

15

A bivalent compound targeting CCR5 and the mu opioid receptor treats inflammatory arthritis pain in mice without inducing pharmacologic tolerance

Raini Dutta[1†], Mary M. Lunzer[2†], Jennifer L. Auger[1†], Eyup Akgün[2], Philip S. Portoghese[2] and Bryce A. Binstadt[1*] (iD)

Abstract

Background: Pain accompanies rheumatoid arthritis and other chronic inflammatory conditions and is difficult to manage. Although opioids provide potent analgesia, chronic opioid use can cause tolerance and addiction. Recent studies have demonstrated functional interactions between chemokine and opioid receptor signaling pathways. Reported heterodimerization of chemokine and opioid receptors led our group to develop bivalent compounds that bind both types of receptors, with the goal of targeting opioids to sites of inflammation. MCC22 is a novel bivalent compound containing a CCR5 antagonist and mu opioid receptor (MOR) agonist pharmacophores linked through a 22-atom spacer. We evaluated the efficacy of MCC22 in the K/B.g7 T-cell receptor transgenic mouse model of spontaneous inflammatory arthritis.

Methods: MCC22 or morphine was administered intraperitoneally at varying doses to arthritic K/B.g7 mice or nonarthritic control mice. Mechanical pain hypersensitivity was measured each day before and after drug administration, using the electronic von Frey test. The potency of MCC22 relative to that of morphine was calculated. Functional readouts of pain included grip strength and nesting behavior. A separate dosing regimen was used to determine whether the drugs induced pharmacologic tolerance.

Results: MCC22 provided ~ 3000-fold more potent analgesia than morphine in this model. Daily treatment with MCC22 also led to a cumulative analgesic effect, reducing the daily baseline pain level. MCC22 produced no observable analgesic effect in nonarthritic control mice. Importantly, repeated administration of MCC22 did not induce pharmacologic tolerance, whereas a similar regimen of morphine did. Both grip strength and nesting behaviors improved among arthritic mice treated with MCC22. Ankle thickness and arthritis scores were not affected by MCC22. The analgesic effect of MCC22 was abolished in K/B.g7 mice genetically lacking CCR5, demonstrating the receptor specificity of the antagonist pharmacophore.

(Continued on next page)

* Correspondence: binstadt@umn.edu
†Raini Dutta, Mary M. Lunzer and Jennifer L. Auger contributed equally to this work.
[1]Department of Pediatrics and Center for Immunology, University of Minnesota, 2-114 Wallin Medical Biosciences Building, 2101 6th Street SE, Minneapolis, MN 55414, USA
Full list of author information is available at the end of the article

A bivalent compound targeting CCR5 and the mu opioid receptor treats inflammatory arthritis pain in mice...

155

(Continued from previous page)

Conclusions: MCC22 is a novel bivalent ligand that targets CCR5 and MOR. Our findings demonstrate that MCC22 provides highly potent analgesia and improved functional outcomes in a model of inflammatory arthritis, without inducing typical opioid tolerance. These findings suggest that MCC22 or similar compounds could be used to treat the pain associated with inflammatory arthritis and related conditions, while minimizing the risks typically associated with chronic opioid use.

Keywords: Analgesia, CCR5, Chemokine receptor, Heteromer, Inflammation, Opioid receptor, Pain, Rheumatoid arthritis

Background

Pain affects nearly all patients with chronic inflammatory conditions, including rheumatoid arthritis (RA). Pain in RA is due to both local factors at the level of the joint as well as central neuronal processing. Pain and inflammation interact at many levels from the molecular to the psychological, making the pain of chronic inflammation challenging to manage [1].

Opioids are potent analgesics. Their use for chronic pain is limited, however, by the fact that they provoke pharmacologic tolerance, meaning that higher doses are needed to achieve effective analgesia. These higher doses lead to problems of overdosing and dependence/addiction [2]. Opioids and their receptors are intimately involved in chronic inflammation [3]. For instance, endogenous opioids released from chronic inflammatory cells can provide local pain relief by acting on opioid receptors whose sensitivity is increased by certain inflammatory compounds. Recent studies have demonstrated that certain opioid receptors can form heterodimers with inflammation-promoting chemokine receptors [4].

Numerous chemokines and their receptors have been implicated in leukocyte infiltration into the inflamed synovium of RA patients [5]. The C-C chemokine-receptor type 5 (CCR5) is abundantly expressed on T cells and macrophages, and its ligand (CCL5) is found in the synovial fluid of patients with RA [5]. In juvenile arthritis, elevated synovial levels of CCL5 predict a more severe disease course [6]. These observations suggest that CCR5 could be mechanistically involved in the pathogenesis of inflammatory arthritis. Several studies have evaluated the efficacy of CCR5 antagonists in patients with RA, alone or in combination with methotrexate. However, none of these compounds has resulted in reduced arthritis severity relative to placebo [7–9].

CCR5 and the mu opioid receptor (MOR) are both expressed on certain neurons as well as on certain leukocytes [4]. CCR5 can heterodimerize with MOR, which can lead to functional desensitization of both receptors [10]. Specifically, opioid treatment of immune cells inhibits the chemotactic response induced by several chemokines; conversely, pretreatment with some chemokines reduces the chemotaxis induced by some opioids [10]. Our group

has developed a novel bivalent pharmacophore, MCC22, comprising a MOR agonist and a CCR5 antagonist (TAK-220) joined by a 22-atom spacer [11, 12] (Additional file 1: Figure S1). The intention of this design was to target the opioid agonist to anatomic sites of increased CCR5 expression, thereby potentially increasing its therapeutic potency. Indeed, in a model of lipopolysaccharide (LPS)-induced inflammation, MCC22 provided ~ 3500-fold more potent analgesia than did a mixture of its monomer constituents when delivered directly to the central nervous system [11]. In that same model, the irreversible MOR antagonist beta-funaltrexamine (beta-FNA) [13] potently inhibited the antinociceptive efficacy of MCC22, implicating the importance of the MOR agonist pharmacophore of MCC22 in antinociception via the MOR protomer in the MOR-CCR5 heterodimer (Akgün et al., manuscript in preparation). A related bivalent ligand MMG22, comprising a MOR agonist and a metabotropic glutamate receptor 5 (mGluR5) antagonist, also connected by a 22-atom spacer, also has much greater potency than its monomer constituents in a murine cancer model, and importantly did not induce opioid tolerance [14]. The 22-atom spacer length of these bivalent pharmacophores appears to be critical. Longer or shorter spacers have resulted in much lower analgesic efficacy, suggesting receptor heteromers as targets for both MCC22 and MMG22 bivalent ligands [11, 14].

We hypothesized that MCC22 administration would provide potent analgesia in the context of inflammatory arthritis. We tested this hypothesis in the K/B.g7 T-cell receptor (TCR) transgenic mouse model of spontaneous inflammatory arthritis. In this model, mice develop symmetric polyarticular arthritis affecting primarily the ankle/wrist equivalents and the digits [15].

Methods

Animals

KRN TCR transgenic mice on the C57BL/6 (B6) background and B6 mice congenic for H-2^{g7} (B6.g7) were gifts from Diane Mathis and Christophe Benoist (Harvard Medical School, Boston, Massachusetts and Institute de Génétique et de Biologie Moléculaire et Cellulaire, Strasbourg, France). *Ccr5*-deficient (B6.129P2-$^{Ccr5tm1Kuz/J}$)

[16] and wild-type B6 mice were purchased from Jackson Laboratory (Bar Harbor, ME, USA). The mice were intercrossed as needed to create the animals used for this study.

Animals were maintained in our specific pathogen-free animal facility at the University of Minnesota (Minneapolis, MN) under protocols approved by the Institutional Animal Care and Use Committee of the University.

Mouse genotyping
Genotypes of mice were determined by polymerase chain reaction (PCR) amplification of genomic DNA extracted from mouse ear punched tissues.

Determination of serum CCL5 levels
Serum concentrations of CCL5/RANTES were measured using a commercially available enzyme-linked immunosorbent assay, according to the manufacturer's instructions (R&D Systems).

Immunohistochemical staining
Tissue sections were prepared as previously described [17, 18]. Briefly, paraffin sections of 10% buffered formalin-fixed and decalcified ankles were deparaffinized and placed in acidic antigen retrieval solution (R&D Systems) at 95 °C for 10 min. Sections were cooled at room temperature for 20 min and rinsed under cold tap water for 5 min. Bloxall (Vector Laboratories) was applied to sections to block endogenous peroxidases for 10 min. Fc receptors were blocked with anti-CD16/32 (clone 70–0161-M001, Tonbo Biosciences) and anti-CD64 (clone 139,302, BioLegend) in 2% bovine serum albumin (BSA). Sections were incubated overnight with anti-CCR5-Biotin (clone 107,003, BioLegend) or control Armenian Hamster IgG-Biotin at 4 °C at 1:100 dilution. Sections were incubated with Vectastain ABC reagent (Vector Laboratories) for 30 min followed by ImmPACT DAB peroxidase substrate (Vector Laboratories) for 10 min. Sections were cleared with Xylene and mounted with Vectamount (Vector Laboratories).

Compound synthesis and administration
MCC22 and MCC14 were synthesized as described previously [11]. Morphine was purchased from Mallinckrodt Pharmaceuticals Company (Mallinckrodt Chemical, St. Louis, Missouri). All the compounds were dissolved in 10% (wt/vol) dimethyl sulfoxide (DMSO) and then diluted to less than 1% DMSO in the final solutions. Vehicle control was 1% DMSO. All the compounds were administrated via intraperitoneal injection.

Mechanical hypersensitivity test
The mechanical pain threshold was quantified by measuring the hind paw withdrawal response using an electronic Von Frey anesthesiometer (IITC Life Science, Woodland Hills, CA). Briefly, animals were placed into enclosures in a test chamber with a metal mesh floor through which the von Frey rigid tip monofilaments were applied, and mechanical pain thresholds (in grams) were measured. The mechanical threshold (in grams) of both hind paws was averaged for each animal. Baseline measurements were recorded before each dose of drug or vehicle. Animals were tested again for their hind paw withdrawal 2 h after drug administration. Drugs were administered once daily for up to 15 consecutive days. Recordings were taken on days indicated in each Figure. After a maximum of 15 days, drug administration was stopped and the animals were monitored to record the accumulative analgesic effect of the administered drug.

Tolerance test
A drug tolerance test was performed by administering the ED_{90} dose (defined as the dose at which 90% of animals experience an analgesic effect) of drug twice daily for 9 days. Electronic Von Frey stimulation was performed on days 1, 3, and 9, and the mechanical thresholds were recorded.

Grip strength measurement
Forelimb grip strength was recorded using a Chatillon Force Gauge DFE II (Ametek) according to the manufacturer's instructions.

Nest-building behavior
Scoring of mouse nest building was performed as described previously [19]. Briefly, nest scores (scale of 1–5) are determined by the wall height of nest/dome made by mice around them in the cage using the same amount of nesting material (1 = nesting material scattered in the cage, 2 = flat nest, 3 = less than half height of nesting dome, 4 = half height of nesting dome, 5 = greater than half height of nesting dome). Double-blinded scoring was performed to measure the height of the nesting dome.

Arthritis assessment
Assessment of ankle thickness and arthritis severity scores were performed as per standard protocols [15]. In brief, ankle thickness measurements were determined by measuring across the malleoli using a Kafer dial thickness gauge with flat anvils (Long Island Indicator Service, Hauppauge, NY). Arthritis severity scores are determined using a scale of 0–3 for each paw, where 0 is normal and 3 is maximum arthritis severity; the maximum total score for a given mouse is 12.

Histopathology of ankles

Paraffin sections of 10% buffered formalin-fixed and decalcified ankles were stained with hematoxylin and eosin. Sections were scored from 0 for normal to 5 for inflammation, fibroplasia, and cartilage injury per the scoring system of Caplazi and Diehl [20].

Statistical analysis

Prism 5.01 (GraphPad Software, Inc., La Jolla, CA) was used for all analysis and graphical representation of data. For tests involving multiple comparisons, one-way or repeated measures two-way analysis of variance (ANOVA) were used followed by post-hoc Tukey's or Sidak's multiple-comparison tests, as appropriate. For comparisons of two groups, the paired t test or Mann-Whitney U test was used as appropriate. The particular statistical tests used for each experiment are indicated in the Figure legends. ED_{50} values with 95% confidence intervals (CIs) were computed with Prism using nonlinear regression methods. For all tests, P values < 0.05 were considered significant.

Results

CCR5/CCL5 expression is increased in K/B.g7 arthritic mice

We first sought to determine whether CCL5 and CCR5 were overexpressed in K/B.g7 mice. Serum levels of the CCR5 ligand CCL5 (RANTES) were higher in K/B.g7

arthritic mice relative to nonarthritic control animals (Fig. 1a). Immunohistochemical staining demonstrated some CCR5 expression near the tendons and blood vessels of nonarthritic control animals; in arthritic animals, infiltrating cells expressing CCR5 are readily identifiable around and within the inflamed ankle joint, including in rests of cells in the subchondral bone (Fig. 1b); cartilage loss and tibiotalar joint space narrowing are also evident.

MCC22 is 3000-fold more potent than morphine, and depends on the 22-atom spacer length

We next asked whether the bivalent pharmacophore, MCC22, comprising a MOR agonist and CCR5 antagonist, would provide effective analgesia in this model. We evaluated the mechanical pain threshold in mice using an electronic Von Frey test. We first determined the time to peak analgesic effect for both MCC22 and the commonly used opioid receptor agonist morphine. MCC22 reached peak analgesic effect at 2 h and morphine at 30 min after administration (Fig. 2a); we therefore used these peak times for all subsequent experiments. We next compared the potency of MCC22 to morphine. A standard dose response experiment revealed that MCC22 was ~ 3000-fold more potent than morphine in alleviating mechanical hyperalgesia in arthritic K/B.g7 mice (Fig. 2b–d). The 22-atom spacer length of MCC22 was crucial—a similar compound with a

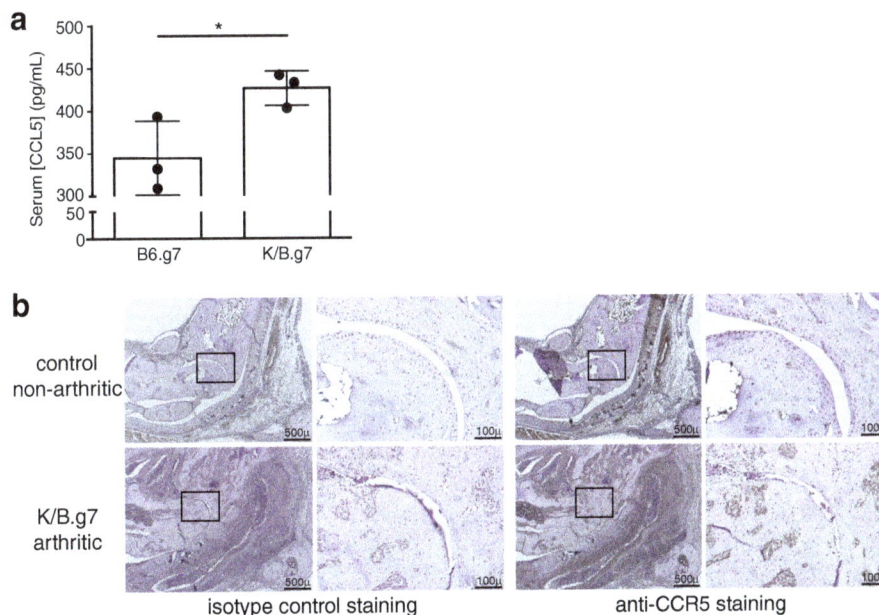

Fig. 1 CCL5 and CCR5 expression are increased in K/B.g7 mice. **a** Serum was collected from 8-week-old control nonarthritic B.g7 mice or arthritic K/B.g7 mice ($n = 3$/group). The concentration of CCL5 was determined by ELISA and data were compared using a Mann Whitney U test. Points represent individual mice; bars indicate mean $\pm$ SEM; *$p < 0.05$. **b** Sections of ankle joints from nonarthritic control mice or K/B.g7 mice were stained with isotype control antibody or anti-CCR5 antibody, as indicated. Brown indicates positive staining. The black box in the lower-power (4× objective) images indicates the region of the tibiotalar joint magnified (20× objective) in the right images. Relative to the control ankles, ankles from the arthritic mice have joint space narrowing, cartilage loss, and numerous CCR5-expressing inflammatory cells

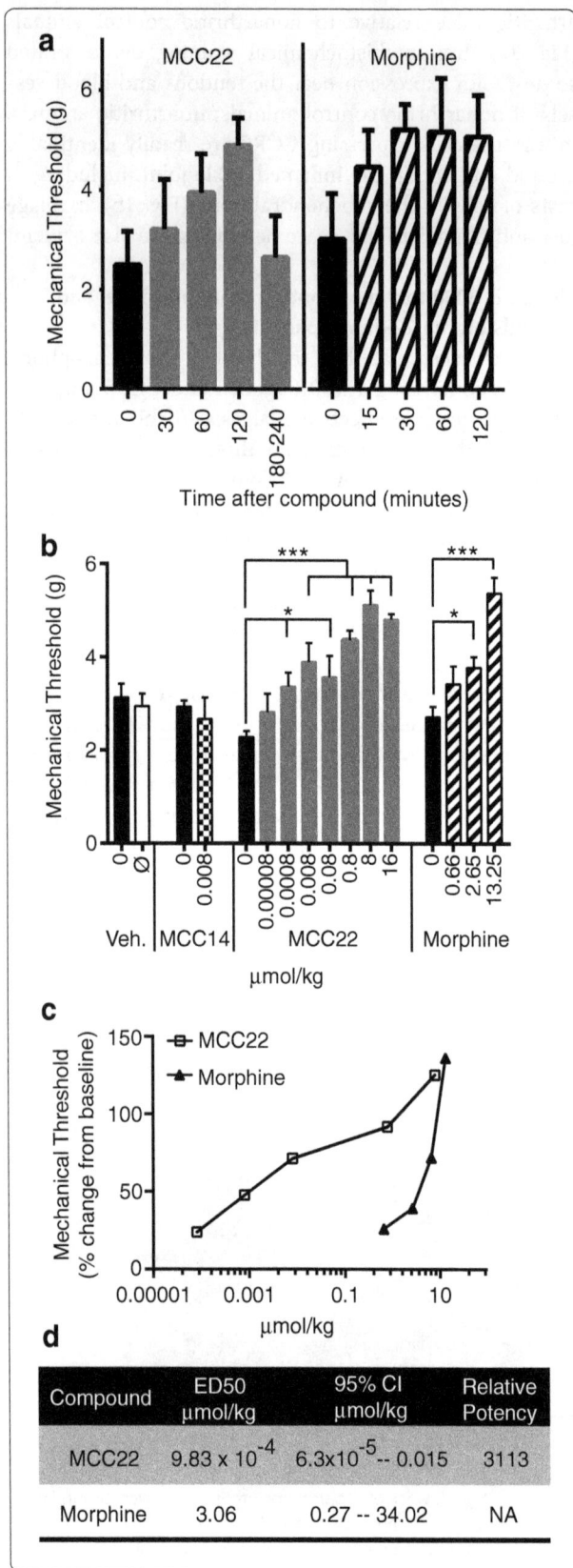

Fig. 2 MCC22 is ~ 3000-fold more potent than morphine. **a** Mechanical thresholds were measured at the indicated times after administration of MCC22 (8 μmol/kg) or morphine (13.25 μmol/kg) to arthritic K/B.g7 mice; n = 4–10 mice/group, bars represent means ± SD. **b** Arthritic K/B.g7 mice received injections of vehicle, MCC22, MCC14, or morphine intraperitoneally at the indicated doses. The mechanical pain threshold was determined 2 hours later for vehicle, MCC22, MCC14, and 30 min later for morphine. Each bar includes data from 5 to 12 mice. The data were compared within each group using either paired t tests (for vehicle and MCC14) or one-way ANOVA followed by post-hoc Tukey's test (for MCC22 and morphine). Data are presented as mean ± SEM; *$p < 0.05$, ***$p < 0.001$, versus the baseline for the group. **c** The mean data are displayed as a percent change from baseline. **d** The calculated ED_{50} of each compound is shown, along with the 95% confidence interval (CI)

shorter 14-atom spacer (MCC14) did not provide analgesia when given at a similar dose (Fig. 2b).

MCC22 produces cumulative analgesia in the setting of chronic inflammation

To determine the efficacy of MCC22 in chronic arthritis pain, we used K/B.g7 mice that were 6 weeks old and had maximum arthritis severity scores of 12. Daily administration of MCC22 to K/B.g7 arthritic mice resulted in higher analgesic potency at days 1 and 3 relative to the daily baseline pain threshold (Fig. 3a). It is noteworthy that the baseline pain threshold in MCC22-treated arthritic mice increased steadily from days 1 to 10, with 110%, 148%, and 173% increases over the day 1 thresholds on days 3, 7, and 10, respectively (Fig. 3a). Arthritic mice that received vehicle had no change in the pain threshold (Fig. 3b). Control nonarthritic mice had higher baseline pain thresholds than arthritic mice, and this was not further increased by MCC22, even with a dose of MCC22 that is 10^4-fold greater than its ED_{50} (Fig. 3c). These findings demonstrate that MCC22 provides effective analgesia in the setting of chronic inflammatory arthritis. Even at this high dose, MCC22 also did not affect arthritis severity scores; all mice continued to have maximum arthritis scores of 12 throughout the duration of the experiment (Fig. 3d). Furthermore, MCC22 treatment did not affect the degree of ankle thickening (Fig. 3d) or histopathologic scoring of arthritis severity (Fig. 3e and Additional file 1: Figure S2).

MCC22 does not induce opioid tolerance

A major limitation to the clinical use of morphine and other opioids is that they induce pharmacologic tolerance. We therefore evaluated whether MCC22 induced tolerance in this model, using morphine as a comparator. MCC22 given at 70% of the maximum pharmacologic effect (MPE) dose retained analgesic efficacy over 9 days of administration, whereas the efficacy of morphine was

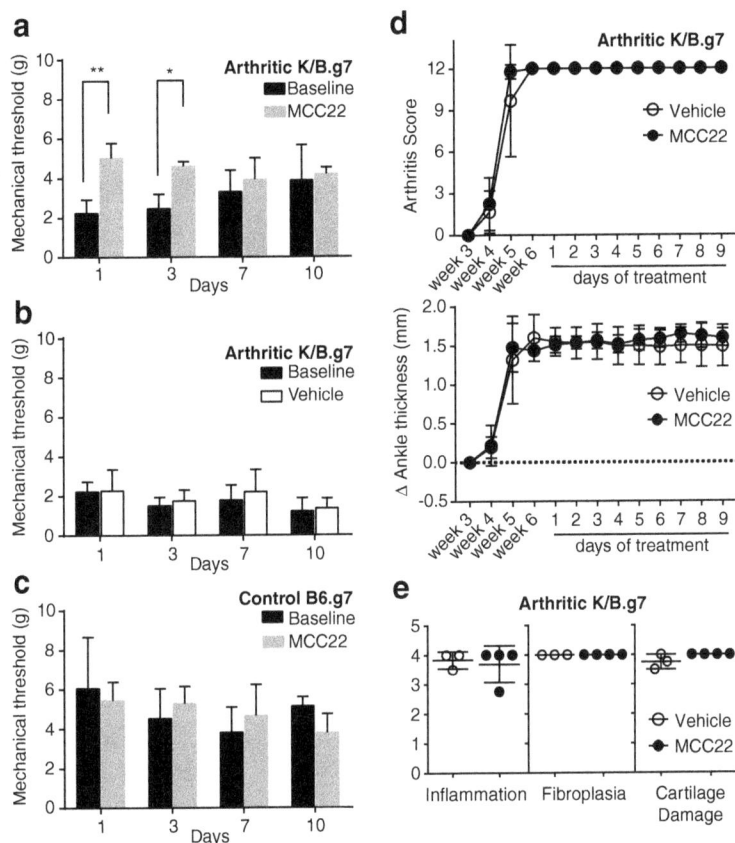

Fig. 3 MCC22 is effective in the setting of inflammation, has an accumulative effect, and depends on the 22-atom spacer length. **a** Six- to 8-week-old K/B.g7 arthritic mice were treated with MCC22 once daily (8 μmol/kg/dose). The baseline mechanical pain threshold was recorded each day. The drug was then administered, and the pain threshold was determined again 2 h later. **b** K/B.g7 arthritic mice that received saline injections showed no increase in mechanical pain threshold. **c** Nonarthritic control B6.g7 mice have higher baseline mechanical pain thresholds than K/B.g7 mice (compare with panels **a** and **b**) and this is not increased by MCC22 (dosed as in panel **a**). Data were analyzed using two-way repeated-measures ANOVA with post-hoc Sidak's multiple comparisons test. Data are displayed as mean ± SEM; $n = 4$–5 mice/group. **d** Arthritic K/B.g7 mice received MCC22 or vehicle once daily starting at 6 weeks of age. MCC22 did not affect arthritis severity or ankle thickness. Data are representative of three experiments with a total of 11–13 mice/group and are displayed as mean ± SD. **e** Histopathologic scoring of ankle inflammation, fibroplasia, and cartilage damage following treatment with vehicle or MCC22. Circles indicate individual mice, bars indicate mean ± SD. $*p < 0.05$, $**p < 0.01$

diminished as early as day 3 of administration (Fig. 4). Furthermore, prolonged administration of morphine did not increase the baseline pain threshold, whereas MCC22 did (Figs. 2a and 4). Thus, MCC22 is substantially more potent than morphine and also does not cause typical opioid tolerance.

MCC22 improves function in arthritic mice

Patients with inflammatory arthritis experience difficulties with routine activities of daily living, due to both pain and restricted mobility of joints. We therefore asked whether MCC22 improved functional measures in K/B.g7 arthritic mice. First, we evaluated forelimb grip strength. Compared to control nonarthritic mice, all of the K/B.g7 mice had lower grip strength. Grip strength improved in K/B.g7 mice treated for 9 days with MCC22, but not in mice treated with morphine (Fig. 5a).

This difference was not apparent at earlier time points in the experiment (data not shown). As a second measure of function, we evaluated nesting behavior. Healthy mice normally build nests when given pressed nesting material, and nesting behavior can be quantified using a standard scoring scale. Indeed, we found that control nonarthritic mice built more robust nests than did arthritic K/B.g7 mice. MCC22 treatment of K/B.g7 mice normalized the nesting behavior, whereas morphine had no effect (Fig. 5b, c). In summary, MCC22 improves functional measures in mice with inflammatory arthritis. These effects were not due to reduced inflammation, as treatment with MCC22 had no effect on arthritis severity (see Fig. 3d, e). Furthermore, these improved functional measures are consistent with our observations that MCC22 did not induce typical opioid side effects (e.g., apnea, sedation), even at higher doses.

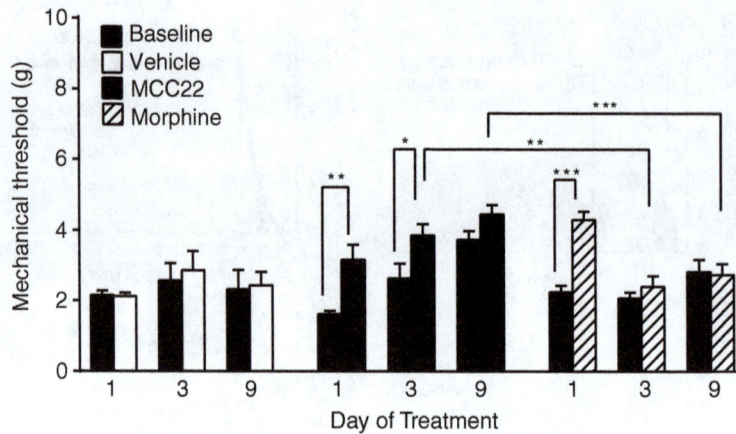

Fig. 4 MCC22 does not induce pharmacologic tolerance. Arthritic K/B.g7 mice were treated daily with vehicle, MCC22 (0.008 μmol/kg/dose), or morphine (6.62 μmol/kg/dose). Mechanical pain thresholds were determined daily before (baseline) and after the administration of the indicated compound. The analgesic effect of MCC22 is apparent at days 1 and 3; in addition, the baseline pain tolerance increases in this group. In contrast, the analgesic efficacy of morphine is lost by day 3. Data are displayed as mean ± SEM; $n = 4$–10 mice/group. Data were analyzed using repeated measures two-way ANOVA with post-hoc Tukey's test for multiple comparisons within treatment groups and Sidak's test for multiple comparisons between treatment groups. $*p < 0.05$, $**p < 0.01$, $***p < 0.001$

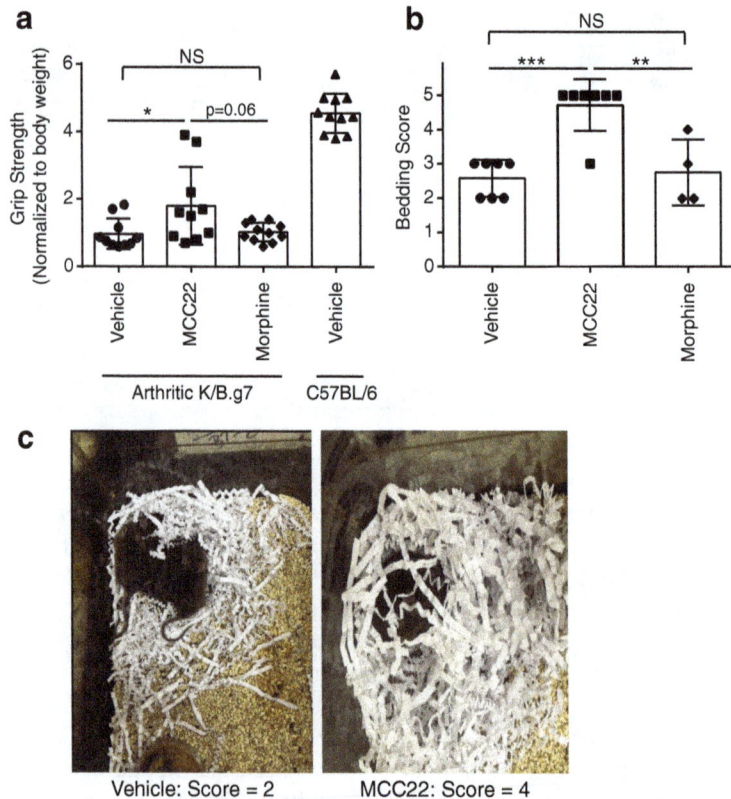

Fig. 5 MCC22 improves grip strength and nest-building behavior. **a** Grip strength was measured in arthritic K/B.g7 mice or nonarthritic control mice. The K/B.g7 mice were treated with the indicated compounds (MCC22 0.008 μmol/kg/dose and morphine 6.62 μmol/kg/dose). Data were compared using one-way ANOVA with post-hoc Tukey's test for multiple comparisons and using the C57BL/6 group as the reference group. The values for the arthritic K/B.g7 mice were all significantly lower than that of the nonarthritic C57BL/6 mice ($p < 0.0001$). **b** Nest-bedding scores were recorded among groups of arthritic K/B.g7 mice treated with the indicated compounds. Data were compared using one-way ANOVA with post-hoc Tukey's test for multiple comparisons. In **a** each point represents one mouse, and in **b** each point represents one cage of mice. Bars represent mean ± SEM. $*p < 0.05$, $**p < 0.01$, $***p < 0.00,1$ NS not significant. **c** Representative photographs of arthritic K/B.g7 mice demonstrating a bedding score of 2 for mice treated with vehicle (left) or and a bedding score of 4 for mice treated with MCC22 (right)

Efficacy of MCC22 depends on CCR5

MCC22 comprises a CCR5 antagonist and MOR agonist pharmacophores. To test its binding specificity, we evaluated the analgesic efficacy of MCC22 in K/B.g7 mice genetically lacking CCR5. Of note, CCR5-deficient K/B.g7 mice developed arthritis equivalently to wild-type K/B.g7 mice (data not shown). In CCR5-deficient K/B.g7 mice, MCC22 provided no analgesic effect, whereas the analgesic efficacy of morphine remained intact (Fig. 6). These data demonstrate that the potent analgesic effect of MCC22 requires CCR5.

Discussion

Opioids are potent analgesics for inflammatory arthritis and other conditions. However, chronic opioid administration promotes downregulation of opioid receptors and hyperalgesia that leads to reduced efficacy. Furthermore, because of their addictive and dependent properties, misuse of prescription opioids has massively increased in recent years. Thus, there is an intense demand to develop safer alternatives to manage pain in patients with arthritis.

Chemokines are known to mediate and modulate pain pathways [21, 22]. Blockade of chemokine-mediated signaling pathways is emerging as a new potential treatment for alleviating chronic pain. A strong correlation has been reported between numerous chemokine pathways and inflammatory arthritis severity, including CCR5 [4]. Consistent with this, we observed increased CCR5 expression in the synovial joints of K/B.g7 arthritic mice, along with an elevated circulating concentration of its ligand CCL5/RANTES. We therefore reasoned that the CCR5 antagonist moiety within MCC22 might direct it specifically to cells mediating inflammatory pain.

We have demonstrated that MCC22 is ~ 3000-fold more potent than morphine, works specifically in the setting of inflammation, and does not induce typical opioid tolerance. We also observed a steady increase in baseline pain thresholds with daily MCC22 administration, but not with morphine. Furthermore, we demonstrated that MCC22 significantly improved the routine functional activities of arthritic mice, with improved grip strength and improved nest-building behavior. Taken together, these findings suggest that MCC22 could be a useful analgesic for patients with chronic inflammatory pain, without inducing tolerance/dependence.

Importantly, MCC22 did not reduce the severity of arthritis in this model. This is consistent with our finding that CCR5-deficient K/B.g7 mice still developed arthritis equivalent to control K/B.g7 mice and prior reports that CCR5 deficiency does not affect the severity of serum-transferred arthritis in mice [23]. It is also consistent with studies of CCR5 antagonists (maraviroc, AZD5672, and SCH351125) in patients with RA, which have failed to demonstrate improvement in disease activity scores [7–9]. Thus, the main benefit of the CCR5 antagonist moiety of MCC22 in this system is to improve the analgesic potency of its MOR agonist moiety, likely by engaging MOR-CCR5 heterodimers. Consistent with this notion, we have demonstrated that the analgesic potency of MCC22 depends specifically on the 22-atom spacer separating the CCR5 antagonist from the MOR agonist, suggesting that MCC22 interacts with MOR and CCR5 heterodimers in a specific orientation [11]. Additional studies of how the interaction of MCC22 with both MOR and CCR5 modulates the function of both receptors will be critical to understanding the basis for its potency.

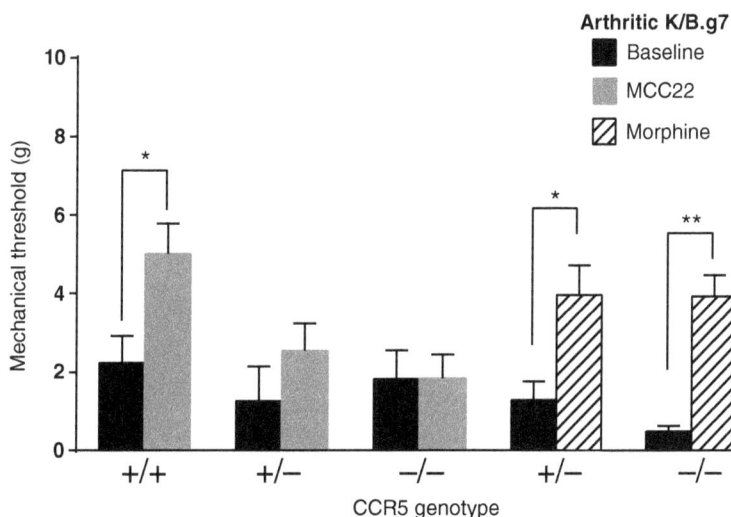

Fig. 6 The activity of MCC22 depends on CCR5 expression. MCC22 (0.008 μmol/kg/dose) or morphine (6.62 μmol/kg/dose) were administered to CCR5$^{+/+}$, CCR5$^{+/-}$ or CCR5$^{-/-}$ K/B.g7 mice, and the mechanical pain threshold was determined before and after administration of the compound. MCC22 is not effective in CCR5-deficient K/B.g7 mice, whereas morphine continues to provide effective analgesia. Data were compared within each group using paired t tests and are displayed as mean ± SEM; n = 4–7 mice/group. $*p < 0.05$, $**p < 0.01$

The question of whether the main cellular targets of MCC22 are present in nociceptive neurons, microglia, or potentially leukocytes remains open. We favor the possibility that MCC22 is acting on neurons on which upregulation of CCR5 has occurred due to chronic inflammation. Further studies will be needed to test this hypothesis. If neurons are the primary cellular target of MCC22, determining whether it acts on peripheral or central neurons will also be of interest.

In addition to MCC22, several other bivalent analgesic compounds have been described recently, including MDAN-21 (MOR agonist:delta opioid receptor antagonist) [24], a series of MOR agonist:cannabinoid receptor 1 (CB1) antagonists [25], and MMG22 (MOR:metabotropic glutamate receptor 5 (mGluR5) antagonist) [14]. Each of these bivalent compounds has demonstrated antinociceptive activity in different murine models of chronic pain. Similar to MCC22, these compounds also provoke less or no tolerance or addictive behaviors when compared with classical opioids.

In a recent study of mice with arthritis induced by injection of complete Freund's adjuvant, a novel modified opioid drug, NFEPP ((±)-N (3-fluoro-1-phenethylpiperidin-4-yl)-N-phenylpropionamide), a fluorinated fentanyl analogue, was reported to have potent analgesic properties [26]. We have observed similar analgesic potency with MCC22 at ~ 1000-fold fold lower dose. Similar to NFEPP, MCC22 also did not exert activity in noninflamed animals. Furthermore, NFEPP did not produce any adverse side effects such as reward-seeking behavior, motor impairment, sedation, respiratory depression, or constipation. MCC22 similarly produced no condition-place preference, a measure of reward-seeking, in a different murine model of pain (our unpublished data). Thus, in the setting of arthritis, MCC22 appears to have a similar analgesic and low side-effect profile to NFEPP, but with greater potency.

Conclusions

In conclusion, MCC22 is a bivalent CCR5 antagonist and MOR agonist compound that provides potent analgesia in mice with inflammatory arthritis without the typical detrimental side effects of opioids. Ongoing studies are directed at understanding its cellular site(s) of action and how its interaction with CCR5 and MOR generates such remarkable potency.

Abbreviations
MOR: Mu opioid receptor; NFEPP: (±)-N (3-fluoro-1-phenethylpiperidin-4-yl)-N-phenylpropionamide; RA: Rheumatoid arthritis; TCR: T-cell receptor

Acknowledgements
The authors thank Diane Mathis and Christophe Benoist for providing mice.

Funding
The study was supported by a Rheumatology Research Foundation (RRF) Pilot Award to BAB. The RRF had no role in the design of the study, collection, analysis and interpretation of data, or in writing the manuscript.

Authors' contributions
RD and BAB drafted and edited the article, and all authors approved the final version to be published. BAB had access to all of the data in the study and takes responsibility for the integrity of the data and the accuracy of the data analysis. Study conception and design: RD, MML, JLA, EA, PSP, and BAB; acquisition of data: RD, MML, and JLA; analysis and interpretation of data: RD, MML, and BAB; generation of pharmacologic compound: EA.

Ethics approval
The studies were approved by the University of Minnesota Institutional Animal Care and Use Committee, protocol 1506-32700A.

Competing interests
The authors declare that they have no competing interests.

Author details
[1]Department of Pediatrics and Center for Immunology, University of Minnesota, 2-114 Wallin Medical Biosciences Building, 2101 6th Street SE, Minneapolis, MN 55414, USA. [2]Department of Medicinal Chemistry, College of Pharmacy, University of Minnesota, Minneapolis, MN, USA.

References
1. McWilliams DF, Walsh DA. Pain mechanisms in rheumatoid arthritis. Clin Exp Rheumatol. 2017;35(Suppl 107):94–101.
2. Volkow ND, McLellan AT. Opioid abuse in chronic pain—misconceptions and mitigation strategies. N Engl J Med. 2016;374:1253–63.
3. Stein C, Kuchler S. Targeting inflammation and wound healing by opioids. Trends Pharmacol Sci. 2013;34:303–12.
4. Melik Parsadaniantz S, Rivat C, Rostene W, Reaux-Le Goazigo A. Opioid and chemokine receptor crosstalk: a promising target for pain therapy? Nat Rev Neurosci. 2015;16:69–78.
5. Koch AE. Chemokines and their receptors in rheumatoid arthritis: future targets? Arthritis Rheum. 2005;52:710–21.
6. Hinks A, Martin P, Flynn E, Eyre S, Packham J, Barton A, Worthington J, Thomson W. Association of the CCR5 gene with juvenile idiopathic arthritis. Genes Immun. 2010;11:584–9.
7. Fleishaker DL, Garcia Meijide JA, Petrov A, Kohen MD, Wang X, Menon S, Stock TC, Mebus CA, Goodrich JM, Mayer HB, Zeiher BG. Maraviroc, a chemokine receptor-5 antagonist, fails to demonstrate efficacy in the treatment of patients with rheumatoid arthritis in a randomized, double-blind placebo-controlled trial. Arthritis Res Ther. 2012;14:R11.
8. Gerlag DM, Hollis S, Layton M, Vencovsky J, Szekanecz Z, Braddock M, Tak PP. Preclinical and clinical investigation of a CCR5 antagonist, AZD5672, in patients with rheumatoid arthritis receiving methotrexate. Arthritis Rheum. 2010;62:3154–60.
9. van Kuijk AW, Vergunst CE, Gerlag DM, Bresnihan B, Gomez-Reino JJ, Rouzier R, Verschueren PC, van der Leij C, Maas M, Kraan MC, Tak PP. CCR5 blockade in rheumatoid arthritis: a randomised, double-blind, placebo-controlled clinical trial. Ann Rheum Dis. 2010;69:2013–6.
10. Chen C, Li J, Bot G, Szabo I, Rogers TJ, Liu-Chen LY. Heterodimerization and cross-desensitization between the mu-opioid receptor and the chemokine CCR5 receptor. Eur J Pharmacol. 2004;483:175–86.
11. Akgun E, Javed MI, Lunzer MM, Powers MD, Sham YY, Watanabe Y, Portoghese PS. Inhibition of inflammatory and neuropathic pain by targeting a mu opioid receptor/chemokine receptor 5 heteromer (MOR-CCR5). J Med Chem. 2015;58:8647–57.
12. Takashima K, Miyake H, Kanzaki N, Tagawa Y, Wang X, Sugihara Y, Iizawa Y, Baba M. Highly potent inhibition of human immunodeficiency virus type 1 replication by TAK-220, an orally bioavailable small-molecule CCR5 antagonist. Antimicrob Agents Chemother. 2005;49:3474–82.
13. Rothman RB, Long JB, Bykov V, Jacobson AE, Rice KC, Holaday JW. Beta-FNA binds irreversibly to the opiate receptor complex: in vivo and in vitro evidence. J Pharmacol Exp Ther. 1988;247:405–16.
14. Akgun E, Javed MI, Lunzer MM, Smeester BA, Beitz AJ, Portoghese PS. Ligands that interact with putative MOR-mGluR5 heteromer in mice with inflammatory pain produce potent antinociception. Proc Natl Acad Sci U S A. 2013;110:11595–9.
15. Monach PA, Mathis D, Benoist C. The K/BxN arthritis model. Curr Protoc Immunol. 2008;Chapter 15(Unit 15):22.

16. Kuziel WA, Dawson TC, Quinones M, Garavito E, Chenaux G, Ahuja SS, Reddick RL, Maeda N. CCR5 deficiency is not protective in the early stages of atherogenesis in apoE knockout mice. Atherosclerosis. 2003;167:25–32.
17. Auger JL, Haasken SS, Binstadt BA. Autoantibody-mediated arthritis in the absence of C3 and activating Fcgamma receptors: C5 is activated by the coagulation cascade. Arthritis Res Ther. 2012;14:R269.
18. Haasken S, Auger JL, Binstadt BA. Absence of beta2 integrins impairs regulatory T cells and exacerbates CD4+ T cell-dependent autoimmune carditis. J Immunol. 2011;187:2702–10.
19. Gaskill BN, Karas AZ, Garner JP, Pritchett-Corning KR. Nest building as an indicator of health and welfare in laboratory mice. J Vis Exp. 2013;82:51012.
20. Caplazi P, Diehl L. Histopathology in mouse models of rheumatoid arthritis. In: Potts SJ, Eberhard DA, Wharton KA, editors. Molecular histopathology and tissue biomarkers in drug and diagnostic development. New York: Springer; 2015. p. 65–78.
21. Rottman JB, Ganley KP, Williams K, Wu L, Mackay CR, Ringler DJ. Cellular localization of the chemokine receptor CCR5. Correlation to cellular targets of HIV-1 infection. Am J Pathol. 1997;151:1341–51.
22. Abbadie C, Bhangoo S, De Koninck Y, Malcangio M, Melik-Parsadaniantz S, White FA. Chemokines and pain mechanisms. Brain Res Rev. 2009;60:125–34.
23. Jacobs JP, Ortiz-Lopez A, Campbell JJ, Gerard CJ, Mathis D, Benoist C. Deficiency of CXCR2, but not other chemokine receptors, attenuates autoantibody-mediated arthritis in a murine model. Arthritis Rheum. 2010; 62:1921–32.
24. Aceto MD, Harris LS, Negus SS, Banks ML, Hughes LD, Akgun E, Portoghese PS. MDAN-21: a bivalent opioid ligand containing mu-agonist and delta-antagonist pharmacophores and its effects in rhesus monkeys. Int J Med Chem. 2012;2012:327257.
25. Le Naour M, Akgun E, Yekkirala A, Lunzer MM, Powers MD, Kalyuzhny AE, Portoghese PS. Bivalent ligands that target mu opioid (MOP) and cannabinoid1 (CB1) receptors are potent analgesics devoid of tolerance. J Med Chem. 2013;56:5505–13.
26. Spahn V, Del Vecchio G, Labuz D, Rodriguez-Gaztelumendi A, Massaly N, Temp J, Durmaz V, Sabri P, Reidelbach M, Machelska H, Weber M, Stein C. A nontoxic pain killer designed by modeling of pathological receptor conformations. Science. 2017;355:966–9.

16

Long noncoding RNA expression profile and association with SLEDAI score in monocyte-derived dendritic cells from patients with systematic lupus erythematosus

Yilun Wang[1†], Shuang Chen[1†], Sunyi Chen[1], Juan Du[1], Jinran Lin[1], Haihong Qin[1], Jie Wang[2], Jun Liang[1*] and Jinhua Xu[1*]

Abstract

Background: Monocyte-derived dendritic cells (moDCs) play important roles in the pathogenesis of systemic lupus erythematosus (SLE). Aberrant expression of long noncoding RNAs (lncRNAs) could affect the function of moDCs. The aim of this study was to explore the lncRNA expression profile in moDCs of SLE patients to provide new insights into SLE.

Methods: LncRNA and mRNA microarrays were performed to identify differentially expressed lncRNAs and mRNAs in moDCs of SLE patients compared with normal controls. Bioinformatics analysis was also performed. Quantitative polymerase chain reaction (qPCR) was used to validate the results, and correlation analysis was used to analyze the relationship between these aberrantly expressed lncRNAs and SLE disease activity index (SLEDAI) scores.

Results: According to the gene expression profiles, 163 lncRNAs were differentially expressed between SLE and normal controls, including 118 that were upregulated and 45 that were downregulated. A total of 137 mRNAs were differentially expressed in moDCs of patients with SLE, including 83 that were upregulated and 54 that were downregulated. Furthermore, qPCR data showed that lncRNA ENST00000604411.1 (18.23-fold, $P < 0.001$) and ENST00000501122.2 (1.96-fold, $P < 0.001$) were upregulated and the other two lncRNAs, lnc-HSFY2–3:3 (0.42-fold, $P < 0.001$) and lnc-SERPINB9–1:2 (0.50-fold, $P = 0.040$), were downregulated in moDCs of SLE patients. The expression levels of ENST00000604411.1 ($r = 0.593$, $P = 0.020$) and ENST00000501122.2 ($r = 0.539$, $P = 0.038$) were positively correlated with the SLEDAI score, respectively.

Conclusions: The results indicate that the abnormal expression of lncRNAs in moDCs may be involved in the pathological processes of SLE. The expression level of ENST00000604411.1 and ENST00000501122.2 may have potential value for the assessment of disease activity in SLE.

Keywords: Systematic lupus erythematosus, Monocyte-derived dendritic cells, Long noncoding RNA, Expression profile

* Correspondence: Liangjun1976@medmail.com.cn; xjhhuashan@126.com
†Yilun Wang and Shuang Chen contributed equally to this work.
[1]Department of Dermatology, Huashan Hospital, Fudan University, 12 Wulumuqi Zhong Road, Shanghai 200040, People's Republic of China
Full list of author information is available at the end of the article

Background

Systematic lupus erythematosus (SLE) is an autoimmune disease that may damage multiple organs by autoantibodies and immune complexes. The precise etiology of SLE is still unclear and it might involve the regulation of genes, environments, and immune imbalance. Experimental evidence suggests that the pathogenesis of SLE is related to the failure of T- and B-cell suppression mediated by defects in cell signaling, immune tolerance, and apoptotic mechanisms promoting autoimmunity [1].

Although T and B cells have been widely studied in SLE, the upper stream cells which could present autoantigens to them have only been emphasized more recently. Autoantigens are released mainly from secondary necrotic cells because of a defective clearance of apoptotic cells in patients with SLE [2]. Dendritic cells (DCs) are the most efficient antigen-presenting cells (APCs) in the human body. Recent research has associated lupus development with changes in the DC compartment, including altered DC subset frequency, localization, phenotype, and functional defects [3]. The dysfunction of DCs is related to the overreaction of T cells and B cells in SLE patients [4], including presenting autoantigens to autoreactive T cells, overproduction of proinflammatory cytokines and chemokines, suppression of Tregs, and promoting B cells to secret autoantibodies [5–8], which results in the loss of self-tolerance and production of autoantibodies.

Recent advances suggest that long noncoding RNAs (lncRNAs) regulate gene expression at the pretranscriptional, transcriptional, and post-transcriptional levels [9]. LncRNAs mediate their molecular functions through a multitude of mechanisms [10]. An lncRNA could interact with proteins in the cytoplasm as a guide, scaffold, or decoy molecule [10]. LncRNAs could also promote or repress the translation of mRNAs in the cytoplasm. For example, the antisense lncRNA BACE1-AS rapidly and reversibly upregulates BACE1 levels in response to a variety of stresses. Since BACE1 and BACE1-AS form an RNA duplex, the duplex may act to alter the secondary or tertiary structure of BACE1 and thereby increase its stability [11]. In the nucleus, lncRNAs can act in *cis* to control local allele-specific functions or in *trans* at one or more genomic loci to regulate gene expression.

LncRNAs are important in regulating the differentiation and function of DCs. Lnc-DC, which is exclusively expressed in human conventional DCs, can affect cellular differentiation (monocytes into dendritic cells) and reduce the capacity of DCs to stimulate T-cell activation by activating the transcription factor STAT3 [12]. The expression of the lncRNA HOTAIRM1 was downregulated when monocytes differentiated into DCs, and silencing of HOTAIRM1 caused changes in the expression of several monocyte differentiation markers such as CD14

and B7H2 [13]. As a result, lncRNAs are able to cause clinical diseases involving the dysfunction of DCs. However, it is largely unknown whether lncRNAs participate in the pathogenesis of SLE by regulating the function of DCs; this is therefore the focus of this study.

Methods

Subjects

Fifteen female SLE patients were recruited from the inpatient service in Huashan Hospital, Fudan University. The diagnostic criteria were in accordance with the 1997 American College Rheumatology revised criteria for the classification of SLE. Relevant clinical and laboratory information regarding the patients is shown in Table 1. Fifteen age-matched female healthy controls were also recruited. The study was approved by the Independent Ethics Committee of Huashan Hospital and written informed consent was obtained from all subjects. All the experiments were carried out in accordance with relevant guidelines and regulations of Huashan Hospital.

Cell culture

In-vitro differentiation of human monocytes into DCs was performed as described previously [8]. Briefly, peripheral blood mononuclear cells (PBMCs) were isolated and $CD14^+$ monocytes were sorted by positive selection using magnetic beads (Miltenyi Biotec, Germany). The cells were then cultured for 5–7 days in RPMI 1640 supplemented with 1000 U/ml granulocyte/macrophage colony-stimulating factor (GM-CSF) and 1000 U/ml interleukin (IL)-4 (PeproTech, Rocky Hill). For monocyte-derived dendritic cell (moDC) maturation, 1 μg/ml lipopolysaccharide (LPS; *Escherichia coli* type 055:B6; Sigma) was added to the medium at day 6. The following antigens were used to identify the phenotype of moDCs: CD11c, HLA-DR, CD40, CD86, CD83, and

Table 1 Clinical and laboratory characteristics of the patients with SLE in the study

Characteristic	SLE ($n = 15$)
Sex, male/female (n)	0/15 (15)
Age (years), median (range)	33 (17–57)
Duration (months), median (range)	3 (1–60)
SLEDAI score, median (range)	15 (10–30)
ANA > 1:320, yes/no (n)	15/0 (15)
Anti-dsDNA (IU/ml), median (range)	391.9 (25.9–800)
Hypocomplementemia, yes/no (n)	12/3 (15)
Organ involvement, yes/no (n)	6/9 (15)
Steroids, yes/no (n)	9/6 (15)
Immunosuppressive drugs, yes/no (n)	15/0 (15)

ANA antinuclear antibody, *SLE* systemic lupus erythematosus, *SLEDAI* systemic lupus erythematosus disease activity index

low expression of CD14. The antibodies were all bought from eBioscience (San Diego).

LncRNA and mRNA microarray
LncRNA expression profiling was determined by Human 4*180 K lncRNA arrays manufactured by Agilent Technologies (Santa Clara, CA), including 63,431 lncRNA probes and 39,887 mRNA probes. Each transcript was represented using 1–5 probes to improve statistical confidence. The lncRNA and mRNA expression data have been deposited into the Gene Expression Omnibus (GEO) under accession number GSE89240.

Gene function analysis
The Database for Annotation, Visualization and Integrated Discovery (DAVID; https://david.ncifcrf.gov) was utilized to identify the molecular function represented in the gene profile. Furthermore, the Kyoto Encyclopedia of Genes and Genomes (KEGG) database (https://www.genome.jp/kegg/) was also used to analyze the potential functions of these target genes in the pathways. The cut-off criterion for false discovery rate (FDR) was set at less than 0.05.

Coexpression network construction
The lncRNA-mRNA coexpression network was constructed based on the correlation between the differentially expressed lncRNAs and mRNAs using Cytoscape. Pearson correlation analysis was used to evaluate the significance of the correlation between the expression levels between each pair of genes. Pearson correlation coefficients were selected for inclusion in the network when they were above 0.95.

Cis and trans target gene analysis of lncRNAs
The gene location for different lncRNAs on the chromosome was determined. Subsequently, the common lncRNA coexpression genes were intersected to identify the genes 10 kbp upstream or downstream of the lncRNAs as potential 'cis' genes. For the trans analyses, we predicted the trans-associated genes of the differentially expressed lncRNAs with RNAplex v0.2. The RNAplex parameters were set as e ≤ –30 in the current study to identify the trans-associated genes, and genes that were found to be located on the same chromosome as the lncRNA were excluded.

Quantitative real-time polymerase chain reaction (qRT-PCR)
Total RNA was reverse transcribed using a PrimeScript RT reagent Kit with gDNA Eraser (Perfect Real Time; TaKaRa, Dalian, China) in accordance with the manufacturer's instructions. The expressions of selected lncRNAs were analyzed using qRT-PCR with an ABI Power SYBR

Green PCR Master Mix (ABI, USA). Glyceraldehyde 3-phosphate dehydrogenase (GAPDH) mRNA was used as an internal control. The primers are listed in Table 2. For quantitative results, expression of each lncRNA was represented as a fold change using the $2^{-\Delta\Delta Ct}$ method and then statistically analyzed.

Statistics
Continuous variables are expressed as means (SD) and categorical variables as frequencies (%). The Student t test or one-way analysis of variance was used to compare continuous variables. All P values were estimated in a two-tailed fashion. Differences were considered to be statistically significant at $P < 0.05$. Data were analyzed using SPSS 13.0 (SPSS Inc., IL, USA). The relationships between the expression levels of lncRNAs and systemic lupus erythematosus disease activity index (SLEDAI) were analyzed by Pearson's correlation coefficient.

Results
Differential expression profile of lncRNAs in moDCs of SLE
Dendritic cells were differentiated from CD14$^+$ monocytes. MoDCs were identified using flow cytometry. The phenotype of moDCs displayed high expression of HLA-DR, CD83, CD11c, CD86, and CD40, and low expression of CD14 (Fig. 1). To profile differentially expressed lncRNAs in moDCs of patients with SLE, we performed a genome-wide analysis of lncRNA expression in moDCs between SLE patients and normal controls. Volcano plot analysis showed that 163 (0.22%) of the lncRNAs were significantly differentially expressed in moDCs of patients with SLE (Fig. 2a), including 118 upregulated and 45 downregulated lncRNAs (fold change ≥ 2.0, $P < 0.05$) (Fig. 2b). We categorized these differentially expressed lncRNAs into six classes: intergenic, intronic sense, intronic antisense, bidirectional, exonic sense, and exonic antisense. We

Table 2 The sequences of quantitative polymerase chain reaction primers

Primer name	Sequence (5' to 3')
gapdh(Hs) forward	TGACTTCAACAGCGACACCCA
gapdh(Hs) reverse	CACCCTGTTGCTGTAGCCAAA
ENST00000604411.1 forward	AGCCCCACTTCACATTAGACC
ENST00000604411.1 reverse	TGATGTTGCAGTCCTGTGAGG
ENST00000501122.2 forward	TTCTGCTTTCTGCCCATGTA
ENST00000501122.2 reverse	GTGGCAGTGACAACCTCTCA
ENST00000568394.1 forward	TCTCTCCCCAGTGACAGTACA
ENST00000568394.1 reverse	GCGATCTGTAGTCCAGGTGT
lnc-HSFY2–3:3 forward	TGATTGGAAGATGGAAGTGGA
lnc-HSFY2–3:3 reverse	GCTCCACCTGAAACTCATTTG
lnc-SERPINB9–1:2 forward	GGGGAAAATAAAAGGGATGGT
lnc-SERPINB9–1:2 reverse	TCTCTCTTAGGGAAGGGCATT

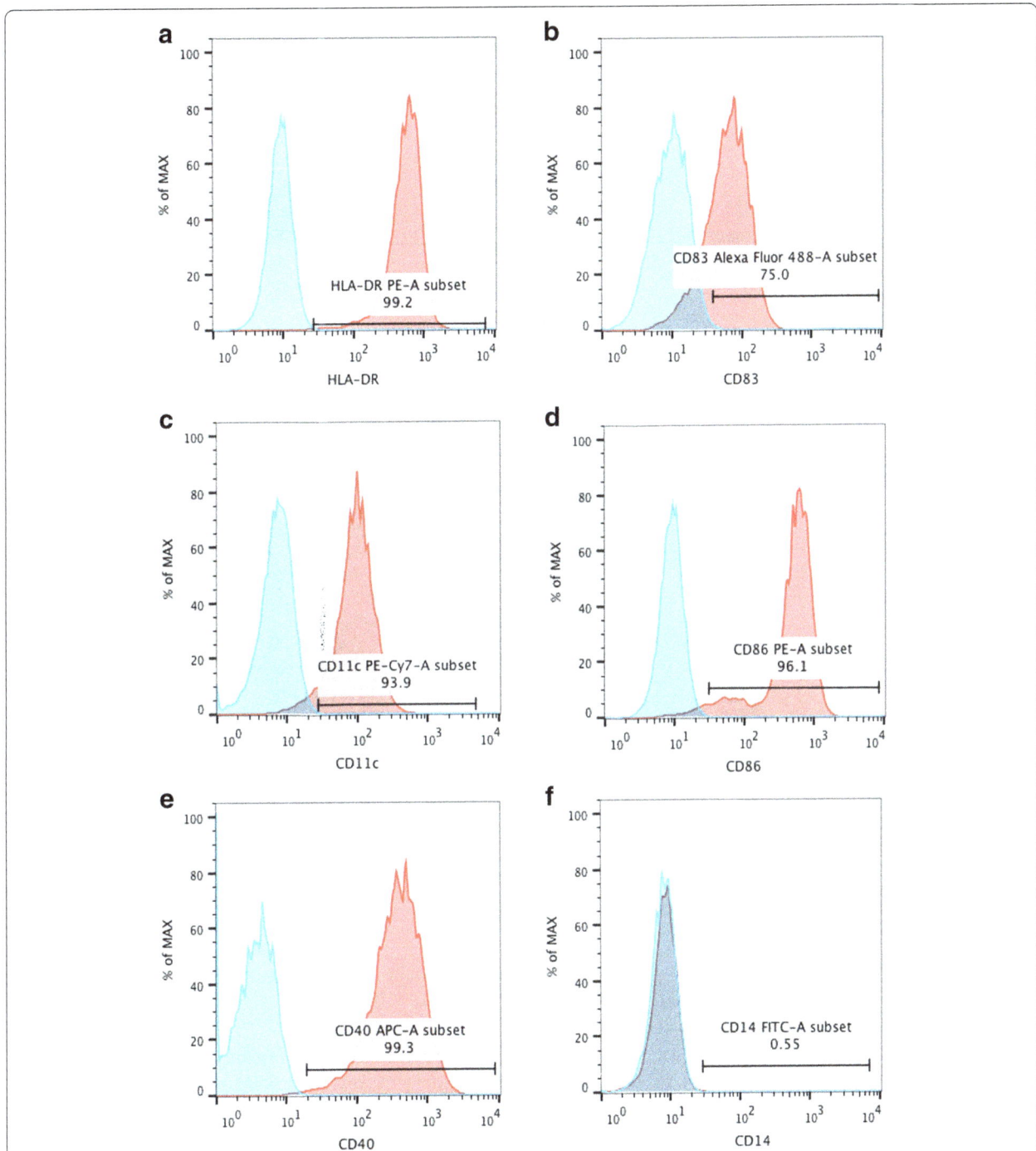

Fig. 1 moDCs were identified using flow cytometry. The phenotype of the cells displayed high expression of **a** HLA-DR, **b** CD83, **c** CD11c, **d** CD86, and **e** CD40, and **f** low expression of CD14

observed 150 intergenic, 2 intronic sense, 1 intronic antisense, 5 bidirectional, 4 exonic sense, and 1 exonic antisense lncRNA (Additional file 1: Table S1).

Differential expression profile of mRNAs in moDCs of SLE

A total of 137 (0.34%) mRNAs were differentially expressed in moDCs of patients with SLE compared with normal controls (fold change ≥ 2.0, $P < 0.05$) (Fig. 2c). Among them, 83 mRNAs were upregulated and 54 mRNAs were downregulated (Fig. 2d, Additional file 2: Table S2). Gene ontology (GO) analysis was performed to classify these differentially expressed mRNAs into three domains: biological process, molecular function, and

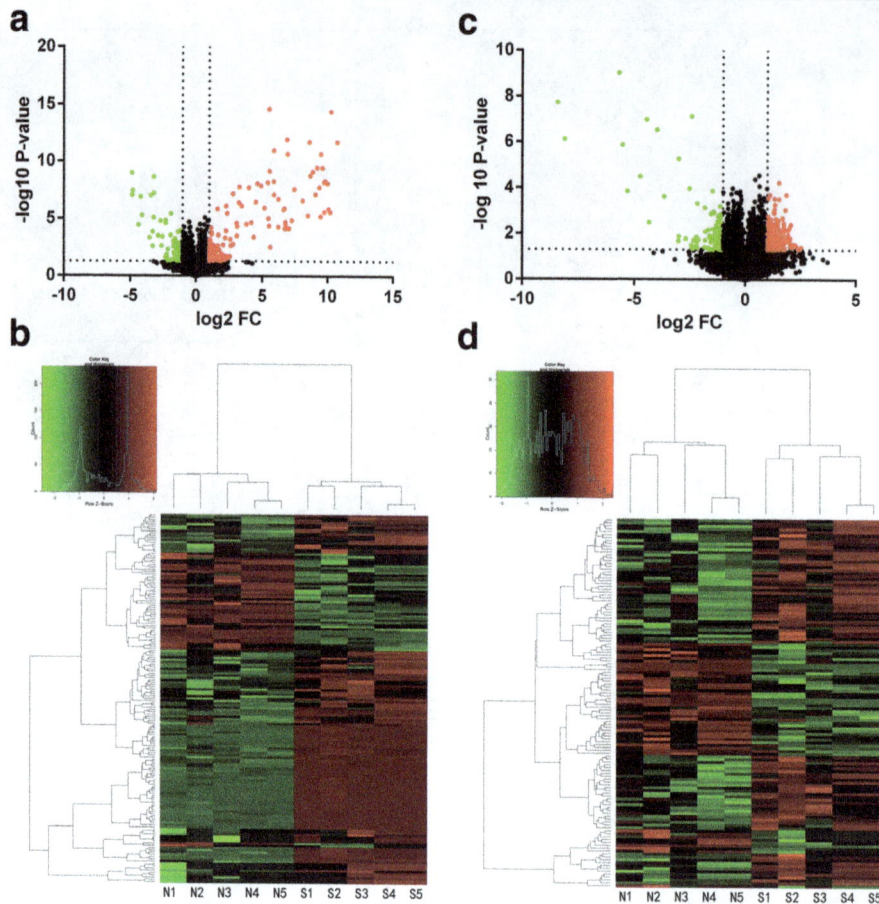

Fig. 2 Volcano plots and hierarchical clusters of differentially expressed lncRNAs and mRNAs. **a** LncRNA volcano plots of SLE patients versus normal controls. **b** A total of 163 lncRNAs were differentially expressed in moDCs of patients with SLE (n = 5) compared with normal controls (n = 5), including 118 upregulated and 45 downregulated lncRNA (fold change (FC) ≥ 2.0, P < 0.05). **c** mRNA volcano plots of SLE patients versus normal controls. **d** A total of 137 mRNAs were differentially expressed in moDCs of patients with SLE (n = 5) compared with normal controls (n = 5), including 83 upregulated and 54 downregulated mRNAs (fold change ≥ 2.0, P < 0.05). In **a** and **c**, each point represents a different transcript. Red points represent genes that were significantly upregulated and green points represent genes that were significantly downregulated. In **b** and **d**, relatively high expression is indicated by red shading and relatively low expression is indicated by green shading. N1–5 represents normal controls and S1–5 represents the patients with SLE

cellular component. In the biological process domain, the GO terms for the differentially expressed mRNAs included cell migration, cell-cell adhesion, and T-cell costimulation, etc. (Fig. 3a). In the cellular component domain, the top five GO terms were extracellular space, protein complex, transcription factor complex, endoplasmic reticulum lumen, and extracellular matrix (Fig. 3b). In the molecular function domain, the GO terms contained signal transducer activity, chemokine activity, and ubiquitin binding (Fig. 3c). KEGG pathway analysis was also conducted to identify the key signaling pathways and the relationships among the differentially expressed mRNAs. We identified 19 signaling pathways that were enriched in moDCs of SLE. The top five pathways were PI3K-Akt signaling pathway, cytokine-cytokine receptor interaction, protein digestion and absorption, extracellular

matrix-receptor interaction, and hematopoietic cell lineage (Fig. 3d).

Construction of the coexpression network with differentially expressed lncRNAs and mRNAs

Next, we constructed a coexpression network of these coding-noncoding genes that included the differentially expressed lncRNAs and mRNAs. Our data showed that the coexpression network was composed of 127 network nodes and 316 connections between 62 lncRNAs and 65 mRNAs. This coexpression network indicated that one lncRNA could target, at most, 16 coding genes and that one coding gene could correlate with at most 12 lncRNAs (Additional file 3: Figure S1). NR_024243 and lnc-BSPH1−2:1 were the most connected lncRNAs. NMT1, NPM3, and UPB1 were the most connected mRNAs.

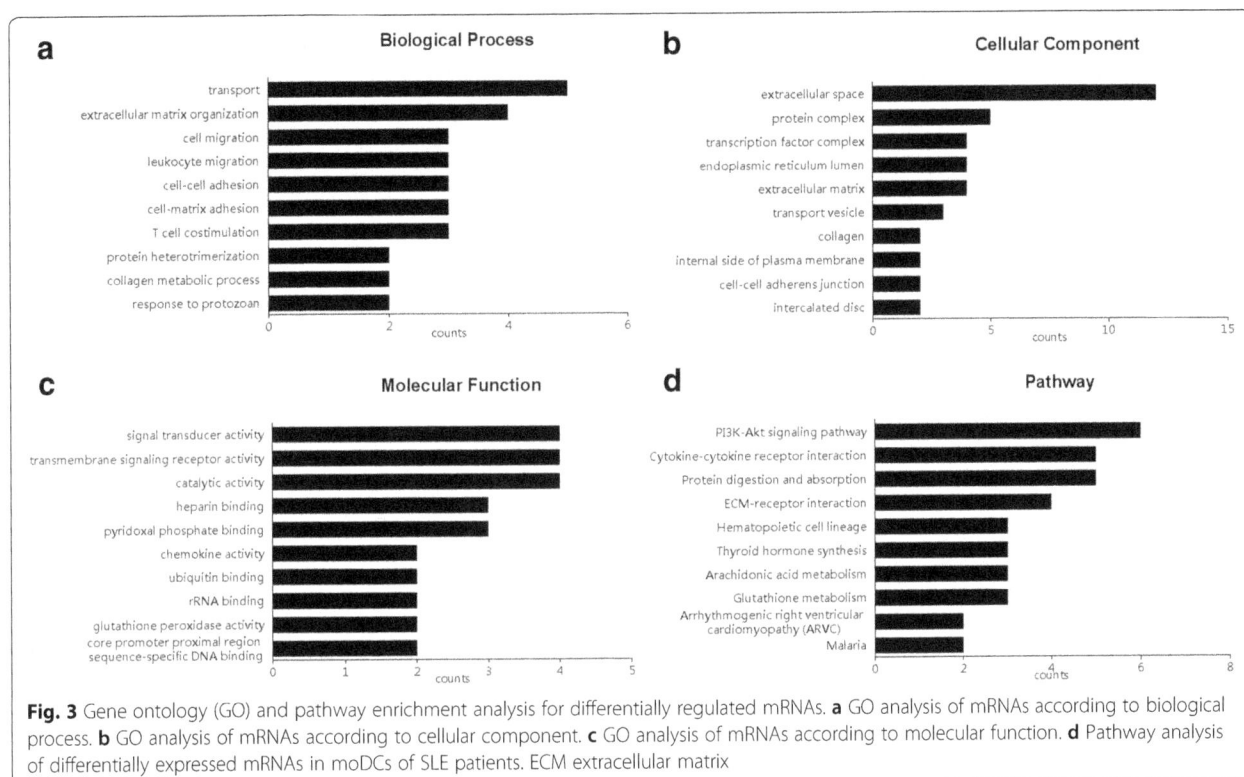

Fig. 3 Gene ontology (GO) and pathway enrichment analysis for differentially regulated mRNAs. **a** GO analysis of mRNAs according to biological process. **b** GO analysis of mRNAs according to cellular component. **c** GO analysis of mRNAs according to molecular function. **d** Pathway analysis of differentially expressed mRNAs in moDCs of SLE patients. ECM extracellular matrix

Analysis of lncRNA-target gene regulatory network

We identified the chromosomal coexpression genes 10 kbp upstream and downstream of the differentially expressed lncRNAs to determine potential lncRNA "cis" genes. The results of the "cis" analyses are shown in Additional file 4 (Table S3). Then we predicted the trans-associated genes of the differentially expressed lncRNAs with RNAplex v0.2, and the results are shown in Additional file 5 (Table S4). Matured moDCs could secrete an abundant source of both inflammatory and lymphoid chemokines, sustaining interaction of naive and activated T cells with antigen-presenting matured moDCs. We then constructed lncRNA-target genes of cytokines and chemokines using Cytoscape software (Additional file 6: Figure S2). Our data show that the lncRNA-target gene network was composed of 83 network nodes and 318 connections between 55 lncRNAs and 28 mRNAs. Within this coexpression network, CXCL10 was the most chemokine connected by lncRNAs and genes and IL-6 was the most cytokine connected by lncRNAs and genes. Lnc-BSPH1–1:1, NR_024214, and ENST00000501122.2 were the most connected lncRNAs.

Confirmation of differentially expressed lncRNAs by qRT-PCR

To confirm the reliability of the microarray data and considering the fold changes and the potential target genes of lncRNAs, we enlarged the sample sizes and selected five

differentially expressed lncRNAs (three upregulated and two downregulated) and measured their expression level using qRT-PCR among 15 patients and 15 healthy controls including those 5 patients and 5 normal controls in the microarray. Consistent with the microarray data, the expression level of ENST00000604411.1 and ENST00000501122.2 were upregulated, and the expression level of lnc-HSFY2–3:3 and lnc-SERPINB9–1:2 were downregulated. However, the expression level of ENST00000568394.1 showed the same changed pattern as seen in the microarray analysis with no statistical significance (Fig. 4).

Correlation between the aberrantly expressed lncRNAs and SLEDAI score of patients with SLE

We further analyzed the correlation between the expression levels of the lncRNAs ENST00000604411.1, ENST00000501122.2, lnc-HSFY2–3:3, lnc-SERPINB9–1:2 and SLEDAI score. The expression levels of ENST00000604411.1 ($r = 0.593$, $P = 0.020$) and ENST00000501122.2 ($r = 0.539$, $P = 0.038$) were positively correlated with the SLEDAI score. However, neither lnc-HSFY2–3:3 nor lnc-SERPINB9–1:2 was significantly correlated with SLEDAI score (Fig. 5).

Discussion

Long noncoding RNAs, more than 200 nucleotides in length, are nonprotein-coding transcripts with a lack of an open reading frame. They can regulate gene expression at

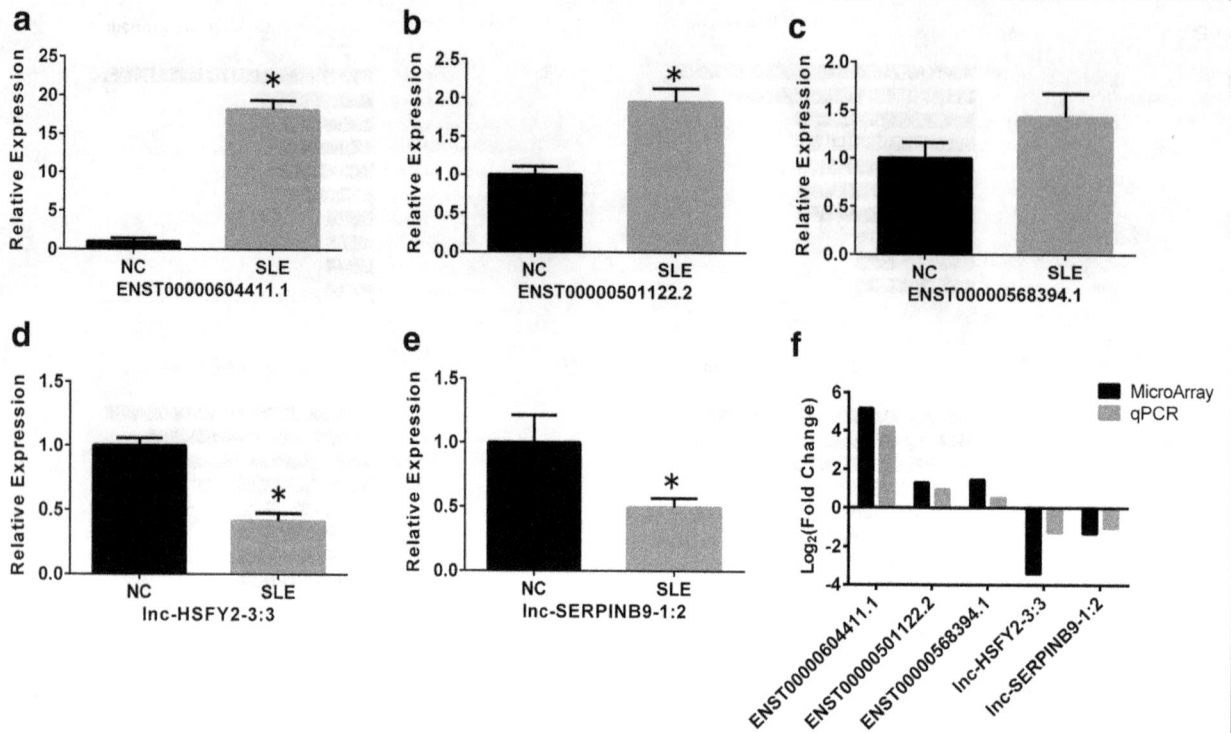

Fig. 4 Validation of selected lncRNAs by qRT-PCR. The levels of ENST00000604411.1 (*$P < 0.001$), ENST00000501122.2 (*$P < 0.001$), ENST00000568394.1 ($P = 0.151$), lnc-HSFY2–3:3 (*$P < 0.001$), and lnc-SERPINB9–1:2 (*$P = 0.040$) were determined in moDCs of 15 normal controls (NC) and 15 patients with systemic lupus erythematosus (SLE) (**a–e**). Data are shown as mean ± SD. **f** The change patterns between microarray analysis and quantitative polymerase chain reaction (qPCR)

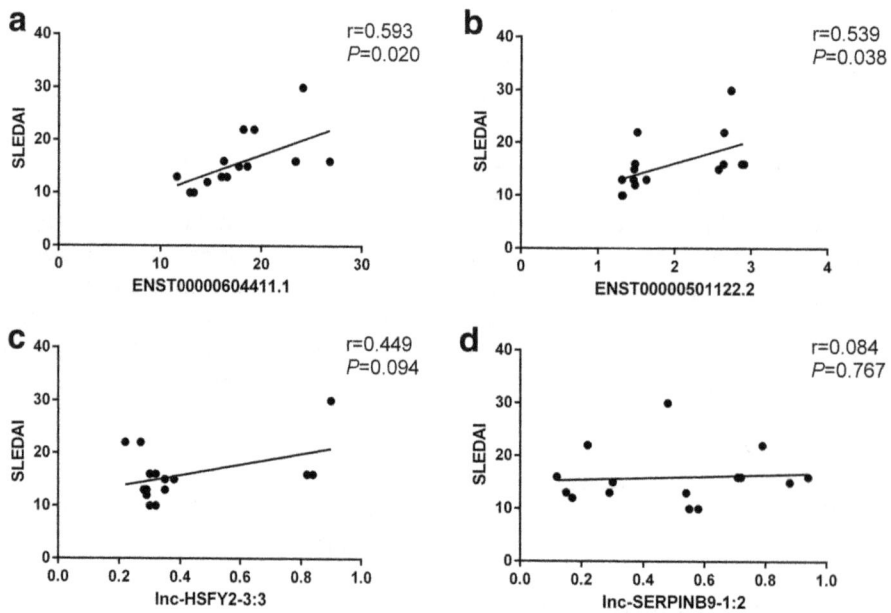

Fig. 5 Correlation between lncRNAs and systemic lupus erythematosus disease activity index (SLEDAI). **a**, **b** ENST00000604411.1 and ENST00000501122.2 expression was positively correlated with SLEDAI score. **c** No significantly correlation was observed between lnc-HSFY2–3:3 and SLEDAI score. **d** No significantly correlation was observed between lnc-SERPINB9–1:2 and SLEDAI score

the level of chromatin remodeling, gene transcription, protein transport, and trafficking [14]. There is increasing interest in the potential involvement of lncRNAs in a number of complex human diseases, including auto-immune diseases, neurological disorders, coronary artery disease, and various cancers [11, 14, 15]. Genetic evidence suggests that lncRNA GAS5, a prime candidate for the chromosome 1q25 SLE locus, is related to susceptibility for SLE [16]. GAS5 also has been linked with an increased susceptibility to SLE in mouse models, presumably as a re-sult of its effect on the immunosuppressant role of gluco-corticoids [17]. The increased lncRNA NEAT1 expression in monocytes is related to the elevated production of a number of cytokines and chemokines in SLE patients [18]. LncRNA MALAT-1 expression was abnormally increased in monocytes of SLE patients, and silencing MALAT-1 significantly reduced the expression of IL-21 in primary monocytes of SLE patients by regulating SIRT1 signaling [19]. This all suggests that lncRNAs could contribute to the pathogenesis of SLE. Furthermore, lncRNAs could also serve as potential biomarkers in SLE. For instance, Linc0949 is decreased in PBMCs of patients with SLE. It can significantly increase following effective treatment for lupus, suggesting its potential as a biomarker for diagno-sis, disease activity, and therapeutic response in SLE [20]. GAS5, linc0597, and lnc-DC in plasma may also specific-ally identify patients with SLE [21].

Published studies involving aberrantly expressed lncRNAs in SLE patients have mainly focused on PBMCs [20, 22], T cells [23], monocytes [18], and plasma [21]. However, there are no current studies regarding lncRNAs of DCs in SLE patients. Since lncRNAs appear to be expressed in a much more cell type-specific man-ner than transcription factors and other protein-coding genes, the aim of our study was to explore aberrant lncRNA expression in moDCs of SLE patients to provide new insight into the pathogenesis of SLE.

We analyzed five moDC samples from individual SLE patients and five moDC samples from normal controls using lncRNA and mRNA microarrays. Based on the microarray data, we found 163 lncRNAs and 137 mRNAs that were differentially expressed. GO and KEGG pathway analyses showed that the differentially expressed mRNAs on moDCs mainly related to T-cell costimulation, chemokine activity, and cytokine-cytokine receptor interaction that are clearly associated with SLE pathogenesis.

We used qRT-PCR to validate the lncRNA microarray results in 15 patients and 15 normal controls, including those in the microarrays. Based on the qRT-PCR results, ENST00000604411.1, ENST00000501122.2, lnc-HSFY2–3:3, and lnc-SERPINB9–1:2 were differentially expressed, which was in agreement with the microarray results. The expression level of ENST00000568394.1 showed the

same change pattern as shown in the microarray analysis with no statistical significance, which is likely due to the fact that the expanded test sample size for the qRT-PCR might have excluded some of the false positive results obtained in the microarray or due to technical limita-tions, such as cross-hybridization, signal saturation, and limited dynamic range in the microarray.

ENST00000604411.1, known as TSIX or LINC00013, expresses a noncoding antisense transcript across the 3′ end of the XIST locus. TSIX was overexpressed in sys-temic sclerosis (SSc) dermal fibroblasts both in vivo and in vitro, and is higher in SSc sera. TSIX is a new regula-tor of collagen expression which stabilizes the collagen mRNA [24]. It also protects the active-X from ectopic si-lencing once X-inactivation has commenced [25]. There is an increased incidence and prevalence of systemic lupus erythematosus in females, which might involve X chromosome inactivation [26]. In our study, we found ENST00000604411.1 was increased in moDCs of SLE patients and the expression level of ENST00000604411.1 was positively correlated with the SLEDAI score. There-fore, the upregulated ENST00000604411.1 might facili-tate X chromosome inactivation through protecting the active-X from ectopic silencing and take part in the pathogenesis of SLE; however, further studies need to be performed to know exactly what role TSIX plays in the processes of the disease.

ENST00000501122.2 is a 22.74-kb intergenic lncRNA transcript, known as NEAT1. This lncRNA is retained in the nucleus where it forms the core structural compo-nent of the paraspeckle suborganelles. Zhang et al. [27] found NEAT1 expression was abnormally increased in SLE patients and predominantly expressed in human monocytes. There was also a positive correlation be-tween NEAT1 and clinical disease activity in SLE pa-tients. Furthermore, silencing NEAT1 significantly reduced the expression of a group of chemokines and cytokines, including IL-6, CXCL10, etc., which were in-duced by LPS continuously and in late stages [27]. NEAT1 is also critical for the expression of IL-8 [28]. In our study, we found NEAT1 expression was increased in moDCs from SLE patients. Therefore, NEAT1 was up-regulated in both moDCs and their parent monocytes in SLE. We have also previously found IL-6 expression was increased in moDCs of SLE patients [8]. Future studies should focus on whether the increased NEAT1 expres-sion in moDCs impact the cells to produce increased cy-tokines and chemokines in SLE patients.

Widespread change in lncRNAs might regulate the gene expression and production of inflammatory media-tors in moDCs. Lnc-DC knockdown impacted the anti-gen uptake function of moDCs, impaired allogenic CD4+ T-cell proliferation, and reduced the strength of cytokine release [12]. A previous study demonstrated that lincRNA-Cox2, a critical inflammation mediator, was induced in bone marrow-derived DCs after stimulation with LPS [29]. A further study revealed that lincRNA-Cox2 mediated both the activation and repression of distinct classes of immune genes, including Irf7, CCL5, and IL-6, etc. [30]. Moreover, lncRNAs, such as THRIL, PACER, and lincRNA-EPS, can also regulate the inducible expression of cytokines following immune activation [31]. In the current study, we found that the predicted target genes of differentially expressed lncRNAs in moDCs included cytokines and chemokines, especially IL-6, CXCL10, IL-10, CXCL2, etc. We also observed that the differentially expressed mRNAs in moDCs of SLE patients were enriched in the process of cell migration and chemokine activity and in the pathways of cytokine-cytokine receptor interaction. This is similar to our previous observation that moDCs in SLE manifested proinflammatory functions such as producing elevated levels of IL-6, CCL2, and CCL5, with the attraction of more CD4$^+$ T cells compared with moDCs of healthy controls [8]. In addition, the majority of patients with SLE display an increased expression of type I interferon (IFN)-regulated genes, also known as an IFN signature [32]. We found that some target genes of the differentially expressed lncRNAs in moDCs are connected to the type I IFN system, such as IRF5 and TREX1. IRF5, the target gene of lncRNA NR_034053.2, is associated with increased serum IFN activity in SLE patients [33]. The target gene of lncRNA n339353 is TREX1, and loss-of-function mutations in this leads to accumulation of intracellular DNA that triggers type I IFN production [34]. The expression level of both lncRNA NR_034053.2 and lncRNA n339353 is elevated in moDCs of SLE patients, which might suggest a regulatory role of moDCs in producing type I IFN in SLE. Since cytokine production is one of the major functions of DCs with great biological importance, more studies are needed to focus on the crosstalk between cytokines and lncRNAs in DCs; the functions of these differentially expressed lncRNAs require further study.

The limitation of our study is that we have not examined lncRNA profiles in circulating myeloid DCs (mDC) and plasmacytoid DCs (pDC) in SLE patients, which is more meaningful in the clinic. However, since the population of mDC and pDC is very small in the peripheral blood, it is difficult to obtain enough cells for study. We therefore utilized the well-accepted model of human DC differentiation from peripheral blood monocytes under inflammatory conditions [12], and we have successfully identified those cells as DCs according to their morphology, phenotype, and function. The potential disadvantage of using moDCs is that it is an artificial system and could be affected by external environments. However, moDCs in our study were differentiated under the same conditions. As a result, the discrepancy between the SLE group and the healthy control group might be due to the intrinsic factors. Another major limitation is that all SLE patients and healthy controls in our study are Chinese females, and so there is gender bias in our findings. Our results may not reflect to male patients and patients of other ethnic backgrounds. Since DCs are the master regulators for initiation, amplification, and perpetuation of SLE [35], targeting DCs may be of benefit for treatment in the future.

Conclusions

Our study provides comprehensive lncRNA and mRNA profiles for moDCs in SLE patients. The differential expression of ENST00000604411.1, ENST00000501122.2, lnc-HSFY2–3:3, and lnc-SERPINB9–1:2 may participate in the pathogenesis of SLE. The expression level of ENST00000604411.1 and ENST00000501122.2 was positively correlated with SLEDAI score and may have disease activity evaluation value for SLE.

Abbreviations

APC: Antigen-presenting cell; DC: Dendritic cell; FDR: False discovery rate; GAPDH: Glyceraldehyde 3-phosphate dehydrogenase; GO: Gene ontology; IFN: Interferon; IL: Interleukin; KEGG: Kyoto Encyclopedia of Genes and Genomes; lncRNA: Long noncoding RNA; LPS: Lipopolysaccharide; moDC: Monocyte-derived dendritic cell; PBMC: Peripheral blood mononuclear cell; qRT-PCR: Quantitative real-time polymerase chain reaction; SLE: Systemic lupus erythematosus; SLEDAI: Systemic lupus erythematosus disease activity index; SSc: Systemic sclerosis

Funding

This research was supported by the National Natural Science Foundation of China (grant no. 81703122, 81773324) and the Natural Science Foundation of Shanghai (16ZR1404900).

Authors' contributions

YW cultured the cells, performed the microarray, and drafted the manuscript. ShC and SuC participated in the design of the study and contributed to the analyses of the results. JD participated in the qPCR experiments. JL and HQ participated in study design and target gene prediction. JW contributed to data interpretation and manuscript revision. JL and JX conceived the study, participated in its design and coordination, and revised the manuscript. All authors read and approved the final version to be published.

Consent for publication

Written informed consents were obtained from the patients for publication of their individual details and accompanying images in this manuscript. The consent form is held by the authors and is available for review by the Editor-in-Chief.

Competing interests

The authors declare that they have no competing interests.

Author details

[1]Department of Dermatology, Huashan Hospital, Fudan University, 12 Wulumuqi Zhong Road, Shanghai 200040, People's Republic of China. [2]Department of Human Anatomy and Histoembryology, School of Basic Medical Science, Fudan University, Shanghai, People's Republic of China.

References

1. Mackern-Oberti JP, Llanos C, Riedel CA, Bueno SM, Kalergis AM. Contribution of dendritic cells to the autoimmune pathology of systemic lupus erythematosus. Immunology. 2015;146(4):497–507.

2. Mahajan A, Herrmann M, Munoz LE. Clearance deficiency and cell death pathways: a model for the pathogenesis of SLE. Front Immunol. 2016;7:1–12.

3. Klarquist J, Zhou Z, Shen N, Janssen EM. Dendritic cells in systemic lupus erythematosus: from pathogenic players to therapeutic tools. Mediat Inflamm. 2016;2016:5045248.

4. Son M, Kim SJ, Diamond B. SLE-associated risk factors affect DC function. Immunol Rev. 2016;269(1):100–17.

5. Chan VS, Nie YJ, Shen N, Yan S, Mok MY, Lau CS. Distinct roles of myeloid and plasmacytoid dendritic cells in systemic lupus erythematosus. Autoimmun Rev. 2012;11(12):890–7.

6. Ding D, Mehta H, McCune WJ, Kaplan MJ. Aberrant phenotype and function of myeloid dendritic cells in systemic lupus erythematosus. J Immunol. 2006;177(9):5878–89.

7. Estrada-Capetillo L, Hernandez-Castro B, Monsivais-Urenda A, Alvarez-Quiroga C, Layseca-Espinosa E, Abud-Mendoza C, Baranda L, Urzainqui A, Sanchez-Madrid F, Gonzalez-Amaro R. Induction of Th17 lymphocytes and Treg cells by monocyte-derived dendritic cells in patients with rheumatoid arthritis and systemic lupus erythematosus. Clin Dev Immunol. 2013;2013:584303.

8. Wang Y, Liang J, Qin H, Ge Y, Du J, Lin J, Zhu X, Wang J, Xu J. Elevated expression of miR-142-3p is related to the pro-inflammatory function of monocyte-derived dendritic cells in SLE. Arthritis Res Ther. 2016;18(1):263.

9. Wu HJ, Zhao M, Yoshimura A, Chang C, Lu QJ. Critical link between epigenetics and transcription factors in the induction of autoimmunity: a comprehensive review. Clinical Reviews in Allergy & Immunology. 2016;50(3):333–44.

10. Atianand MK, Caffrey DR, Fitzgerald KA. Immunobiology of long noncoding RNAs. Annu Rev Immunol. 2017;35:177–98.

11. Faghihi MA, Modarresi F, Khalil AM, Wood DE, Sahagan BG, Morgan TE, Finch CE, Laurent GS, Kenny PJ, Wahlestedt C. Expression of a noncoding RNA is elevated in Alzheimer's disease and drives rapid feed-forward regulation of beta-secretase. Nat Med. 2008;14(7):723–30.

12. Wang P, Xue Y, Han Y, Lin L, Wu C, Xu S, Jiang Z, Xu J, Liu Q, Cao X. The STAT3-binding long noncoding RNA lnc-DC controls human dendritic cell differentiation. Science. 2014;344(6181):310–3.

13. Xin JX, Li J, Feng Y, Wang LY, Zhang Y, Yang RC. Downregulation of long noncoding RNA HOTAIRM1 promotes monocyte/dendritic cell differentiation through competitively binding to endogenous miR-3960. Oncotargets Ther. 2017;10:1–9.

14. Li J, Xuan Z, Liu C. Long non-coding RNAs and complex human diseases. Int J Mol Sci. 2013;14(9):18790–808.

15. Gupta RA, Shah N, Wang KC, Kim J, Horlings HM, Wong DJ, Tsai MC, Hung T, Argani P, Rinn JL, et al. Long non-coding RNA HOTAIR reprograms chromatin state to promote cancer metastasis. Nature. 2010;464(7291):1071–U1148.

16. Kino T, Hurt DE, Ichijo T, Nader N, Chrousos GP. Noncoding RNA Gas5 is a growth arrest- and starvation-associated repressor of the glucocorticoid receptor. Sci Signal. 2010;3(107):ra8.

17. Suarez-Gestal M, Calaza M, Endreffy E, Pullmann R, Ordi-Ros J, Sebastiani GD, Ruzickova S, Santos MJ, Papasteriades C, Marchini M, et al. Replication of recently identified systemic lupus erythematosus genetic associations: a case-control study. Arthritis Res Ther. 2009;11(3):R69.

18. Zhang FF, Wu LL, Qian J, Qu B, Xia SW, La T, Wu YF, Ma JY, Zeng J, Guo Q, et al. Identification of the long noncoding RNA NEAT1 as a novel inflammatory regulator acting through MAPK pathway in human lupus. J Autoimmun. 2016;75:96–104.

19. Yang HX, Liang NX, Wang M, Fei YY, Sun J, Li ZY, Xu Y, Guo C, Cao ZL, Li SQ, et al. Long noncoding RNA MALAT-1 is a novel inflammatory regulator in human systemic lupus erythematosus. Oncotarget. 2017;8(44):77400–6.

20. Wu Y, Zhang F, Ma J, Zhang X, Wu L, Qu B, Xia S, Chen S, Tang Y, Shen N. Association of large intergenic noncoding RNA expression with disease activity and organ damage in systemic lupus erythematosus. Arthritis Res Ther. 2015;17:131.

21. Wu GC, Li J, Leng RX, Li XP, Li XM, Wang DG, Pan HF, Ye DQ. Identification of long non-coding RNAs GAS5, linc0597 and lnc-DC in plasma as novel biomarkers for systemic lupus erythematosus. Oncotarget. 2017;8(14):23650–63.

22. Luo Q, Li X, Xu C, Zeng L, Ye J, Guo Y, Huang Z, Li J. Integrative analysis of long non-coding RNAs and messenger RNA expression profiles in systemic lupus erythematosus. Mol Med Rep. 2018;17(3):3489–96.

23. Li LJ, Zhao W, Tao SS, Li J, Xu SZ, Wang JB, Leng RX, Fan YG, Pan HF, Ye DQ. Comprehensive long non-coding RNA expression profiling reveals their potential roles in systemic lupus erythematosus. Cell Immunol. 2017;319:17–27.

24. Wang ZZ, Jinnin M, Nakamura K, Harada M, Kudo H, Nakayama W, Inoue K, Nakashima T, Honda N, Fukushima S, et al. Long non-coding RNA TSIX is upregulated in scleroderma dermal fibroblasts and controls collagen mRNA stabilization. Exp Dermatol. 2016;25(2):131–6.

25. Gayen S, Maclary E, Buttigieg E, Hinten M, Kalantry S. A primary role for the Tsix lncRNA in maintaining random X-chromosome inactivation. Cell Rep. 2015;11(8):1251–65.

26. McCombe PA, Greer JM, Mackay IR. Sexual dimorphism in autoimmune disease. Curr Mol Med. 2009;9(9):1058–79.

27. Zhang F, Wu L, Qian J, Qu B, Xia S, La T, Wu Y, Ma J, Zeng J, Guo Q et al. Identification of the long noncoding RNA NEAT1 as a novel inflammatory regulator acting through MAPK pathway in human lupus. J Autoimmun. 2016;75:96–104.

28. Imamura K, Imamachi N, Akizuki G, Kumakura M, Kawaguchi A, Nagata K, Kato A, Kawaguchi Y, Sato H, Yoneda M, et al. Long noncoding RNA NEAT1-dependent SFPQ relocation from promoter region to Paraspeckle mediates IL8 expression upon immune stimuli. Mol Cell. 2014;53(3):393–406.

29. Guttman M, Amit I, Garber M, French C, Lin MF, Feldser D, Huarte M, Zuk O, Carey BW, Cassady JP, et al. Chromatin signature reveals over a thousand highly conserved large non-coding RNAs in mammals. Nature. 2009; 458(7235):223–7.

30. Carpenter S, Aiello D, Atianand MK, Ricci EP, Gandhi P, Hall LL, Byron M, Monks B, Henry-Bezy M, Lawrence JB, et al. A long noncoding RNA mediates both activation and repression of immune response genes. Science. 2013;341(6147):789–92.

31. Carpenter S, Fitzgerald KA. Cytokines and long noncoding RNAs. Cold Spring Harb Perspect Biol. 2018;10(6).

32. Bengtsson AA, Ronnblom L. Role of interferons in SLE. Best Pract Res Clin Rheumatol. 2017;31(3):415–28.

33. Niewold TB, Kelly JA, Flesch MH, Espinoza LR, Harley JB, Crow MK. Association of the IRF5 risk haplotype with high serum interferon-alpha activity in systemic lupus erythematosus patients. Arthritis Rheum. 2008;58(2):2481–7.

34. Lee-Kirsch MA, Gong M, Chowdhury D, Senenko L, Engel K, Lee YA, de Silva U, Bailey SL, Witte T, Vyse TJ, et al. Mutations in the gene encoding the 3'-5' DNA exonuclease TREX1 are associated with systemic lupus erythematosus. Nat Genet. 2007;39(9):1065–7.

35. Chan VSF, Nie YJ, Shen N, Yan S, Mok MY, Lau CS. Distinct roles of myeloid and plasmacytoid dendritic cells in systemic lupus erythematosus. Autoimmun Rev. 2012;11(12):890–7.

17

Do ethnicity, degree of family relationship, and the spondyloarthritis subtype in affected relatives influence the association between a positive family history for spondyloarthritis and HLA-B27 carriership? Results from the worldwide ASAS cohort

Miranda van Lunteren[1*], Alexandre Sepriano[1,2], Robert Landewé[3,4], Joachim Sieper[5,6], Martin Rudwaleit[5,7], Désirée van der Heijde[1] and Floris van Gaalen[1]

Abstract

Background: The Assessment of SpondyloArthritis international Society (ASAS) defines a positive family history (PFH) of spondyloarthritis (SpA) as the presence of ankylosing spondylitis (AS), acute anterior uveitis (AAU), reactive arthritis (ReA), inflammatory bowel disease (IBD), and/or psoriasis in first-degree relatives (FDR) or second-degree relatives (SDR). In two European cohorts, a PFH of AS and AAU, but not other subtypes, was associated with human leukocyte antigen B27 (HLA-B27) carriership in patients suspected of axial SpA (axSpA). Because the importance of ethnicity or degree of family relationship is unknown, we investigated the influence of ethnicity, FDR, or SDR on the association between a PFH and HLA-B27 carriership in patients suspected of axSpA.

Methods: Baseline data from the ASAS cohort of patients suspected of axSpA were analyzed. Univariable analyses were performed. Each disease (AS, AAU, psoriasis, IBD, ReA) in a PFH according to the ASAS definition was a determinant in separate models with HLA-B27 carriership as outcome. Analyses were stratified for self-reported ethnicity, FDR, and SDR. Analyses were repeated in multivariable models to investigate independent associations.

Results: A total of 594 patients were analyzed (mean [SD] age 33.7 [11.7] years; 46% male; 52% HLA-B27+; 59% white, 36% Asian, 5% other). A PFH was associated with HLA-B27 carriership in patients with a white (OR, 2.3, 95% CI, 1.4–3.9) or Asian ethnicity (OR, 3.1, 95% CI, 1.6–5.8) and with a PFH in FDR (OR, 2.9, 95% CI, 1.8–4.5), but not with a PFH in SDR (OR, 1.7, 95% CI, 0.7–3.8) or in other ethnicities. A PFH of AS was positively associated with HLA-B27 carriership in all subgroups (white OR, 7.1; 95% CI, 2.9–17.1; Asian OR, 5.7; 95% CI, 2.5–13.2; FDR OR, 7.8; 95% CI, 3.8–16.0; SDR OR, 3.7; 95% CI, 1.2–11.6). A PFH of AAU, ReA, IBD, or psoriasis was never positively associated with HLA-B27 carriership. In the multivariate analysis, similar results were found.

Conclusions: In the ASAS cohort, a PFH of AS, but not of AAU, ReA, IBD, or psoriasis, was associated with HLA-B27 carriership regardless of white or Asian ethnicity or degree of family relationship. This cohort and two European cohorts show that a PFH of AS and possibly a PFH of AAU can be used to identify patients who are more likely to be HLA-B27-positive and therefore may have an increased risk of axSpA.

Keywords: Axial spondyloarthritis, HLA-B27, Positive family history, Ethnicity, Degree of family relationship

* Correspondence: m.van_lunteren@lumc.nl
[1]Department of Rheumatology, Leiden University Medical Center, P.O. Box 9600, 2300 RC Leiden, the Netherlands
Full list of author information is available at the end of the article

Background

Axial spondyloarthritis (axSpA) is a chronic inflammatory disease that causes inflammation mainly in the sacroiliac joints (SI) and spine [1]. In patients with ankylosing spondylitis (AS), also termed radiographic axSpA, susceptibility is thought to be largely genetically determined, and the strongest known genetic risk factor for axSpA is human leukocyte antigen B27 (HLA-B27) [1, 2]. Different prevalence rates of axSpA are reported across geographical regions, which have been related to the varying prevalence of HLA-B27 worldwide [3]. A family history of spondyloarthritis (SpA) is common in patients with AS [4], and HLA-B27-positive first-degree relatives of HLA-B27-positive patients with AS are 16 times more likely to develop AS than HLA-B27-positive individuals in the general population [5]. Additionally, several studies have shown that first-degree relatives of a patient with AS have a higher risk of developing AS than second-degree relatives [6–8]. Therefore, a positive family history (PFH) of SpA, and in particular a PFH in first-degree relatives of patients with SpA, is thought to be a risk factor of axSpA in patients with chronic back pain (CBP), and a PFH of SpA is a component of several SpA classification criteria [9, 10].

The Assessment of SpondyloArthritis international Society (ASAS) defined, by consensus, a PFH of AS, acute anterior uveitis (AAU), reactive arthritis (ReA), inflammatory bowel disease (IBD), and/or psoriasis in first- or second-degree relatives as an SpA feature in the ASAS classification criteria for axSpA [11]. Because a PFH of SpA is thought to increase the risk for axSpA in patients with CBP, it has been incorporated into several referral strategies for patients with CBP suspected of axSpA [12, 13].

So far, only one study has investigated the performance of the definition of a PFH in identifying patients with an increased risk for axSpA. Ez-Zaitouni et al. reported that in two cohorts predominantly Caucasian CBP patients suspected of axSpA, a PFH for AS and AAU was positively associated with HLA-B27 carriership. A PFH for ReA, IBD, or psoriasis was not associated with HLA-B27 carriership and did not point to HLA-B27 carriership in patients with back pain [14]. Unfortunately, this study did not to distinguish between first- or second-degree relatives, and therefore it was unclear if a distinction in a PFH in first- or second-degree relatives matters. Moreover, because the study was performed in two European cohorts, it was unclear if the authors' findings are relevant to populations outside Europe.

The ASAS cohort provides a unique opportunity to study the performance of the current ASAS definition of a PFH in patients of different ethnicities who have CBP and are suspected of axSpA [11, 15, 16]. Therefore, we investigated in this international cohort the impact of ethnicity and degree of family relationship on the association between the current ASAS definition of a PFH and the presence of HLA-B27 in patients suspected of axSpA.

Methods

The ASAS cohort is an international cohort that includes patients with a suspicion of axSpA (> 3 months of back pain, age at onset < 45 years, with or without peripheral symptoms) or peripheral SpA (pSpA; current peripheral arthritis and/or dactylitis and/or enthesitis but without current CBP) [11, 15, 16]. Worldwide, 975 patients were included by 29 ASAS centers between November 2005 and January 2009. Patients were included in a consecutive manner, including all eligible patients or every first to third eligible patient per day. Local ethical committees approved the study, and informed consent was obtained from all study participants before inclusion [11, 15, 16].

Data collection

At baseline, clinical, laboratory, and imaging data were collected from all patients, including HLA-B27 carriership and radiography of the SI. Magnetic resonance imaging of the SI (MRI-SI) was considered obligatory for the first 20 patients of each center. Patients were diagnosed by the treating rheumatologist, and for each patient, the level of confidence regarding the diagnosis on an 11-point numerical rating scale from 0 (not confident at all) to 10 (very confident) was provided. For the current analysis, only patients with a certain diagnosis of axSpA or no axSpA (confidence level ≥ 6) were analyzed.

In addition, patients were asked to report their ethnicity using an open-ended question. Self-reported ethnicities were white, Asian, black, East Indian, Hispanic/Latino, mixed, and Turkish. The self-reported ethnicities were reclassified into white, Asian, and other ethnicities (Hispanic/Latino $n = 11$, black $n = 7$, mixed $n = 4$, Turkish $n = 3$, East Indian $n = 2$, unknown = 5).

The ASAS expert definition was used to assess if patients had a PFH of SpA (ASAS PFH) (i.e., the presence of AS, AAU, psoriasis, IBD, and/or ReA in first- or second-degree relatives) [11]. Patients were asked to report if any family history disease was present in a relative and in which relative(s). In the ASAS expert definition, father, mother, sister, brother, daughter, and son are defined as first-degree relatives and grandmother, grandfather, aunt, uncle, niece, and nephew as second-degree relatives [11]. Furthermore, in addition to the ASAS definition, granddaughter, grandson, half-sister, and half-brother were also considered to be second-degree relatives.

Data analysis

Baseline data were analyzed. Continuous variables were presented as mean and SD and categorical variables as frequencies (proportions). Univariable logistic models, stratified by self-reported ethnicity or degree of family

Table 1 Baseline characteristics of chronic back pain patients suspected of axial spondyloarthritis included in the ASAS cohort

Characteristics	Data (N = 594)
Age at baseline, years	33.7 (11.7)
Male sex	276 (46%)
Duration of back pain, years[a]	7.1 (9.0)
Self-reported ethnicity	
White	348 (59%)
Asian	214 (36%)
Other[b]	32 (5%)
IBP (according to experts' definition)	301/532 (57%)
Good response to NSAIDs[c]	274 (46%)
Peripheral arthritis[d]	197 (33%)
Enthesitis[d]	241 (41%)
AAU[d]	53 (9%)
Dactylitis[d]	23 (4%)
Psoriasis[d]	22 (4%)
IBD[d]	8 (1%)
Positive family history according to ASAS definition	135 (23%)
Positive family history of AS	87 (15%)
Positive family history of AAU	7 (1%)
Positive family history of ReA	8 (1%)
Positive family history of IBD	12 (2%)
Positive family history of Psoriasis	36 (6%)
Total number of SpA-related diseases in first- or second-degree relatives	
Number of patients with one disease	120 (20%)
Number of patients with two diseases	15 (3%)
Total number of family members with SpA-related diseases	
Number of patients with one relative	102 (17%)
Number of patients with two relatives	30 (5%)
Number of patients with three relatives	3 (1%)
Total number of patients with positive family history in	
First-degree relatives only	100 (17%)
Second-degree relatives only	25 (4%)
Both first- and second-degree relatives	10 (2%)
HLA-B27 positivity	310 (52%)
Elevated CRP/ESR	185 (31%)
Definite radiographic sacroiliitis[e]	119/593 (20%)
Presence of active inflammation on MRI-SI	189/424 (45%)

Table 1 Baseline characteristics of chronic back pain patients suspected of axial spondyloarthritis included in the ASAS cohort (Continued)

Characteristics	Data (N = 594)
Number of SpA features[f,g]	2.4 (1.6)
Clinical diagnosis of axSpA[h]	368 (62%)

Abbreviations: AAU Acute anterior uveitis, *AS* Ankylosing spondylitis, *ASAS* Assessment of SpondyloArthritis international Society, *(ax)SpA* (Axial) spondyloarthritis, *CRP* C-reactive protein, *ESR* Erythrocyte sedimentation rate, *HLA-B27* Human leukocyte antigen B27, *IBD* Inflammatory bowel disease, *IBP* Inflammatory back pain, *MRI-SI* Magnetic resonance imaging of the sacroiliac joints, *NSAID* Nonsteroidal anti-inflammatory drug, *ReA* Reactive arthritis, *SI* Sacroiliac joint
Results are presented as mean ± SD unless specified otherwise
[a] < 5% missing values
[b] Self-reported ethnicity was missing for five patients, who are included in this category, and other self-reported ethnicities are black, East Indian, Hispanic/Latino, mixed, or Turkish
[c] Back pain not present anymore or is much better 24–48 hours after a full dose of NSAID
[d] Past or present condition
[e] Grade ≥ 2 bilateral or grade ≥ 3 unilateral
[f] Excluding HLA-B27 carriership and imaging
[g] < 20% missing values
[h] Level of confidence regarding the diagnosis is ≥ 6

relationship (a PFH in first- or only second-degree relatives), were used to assess the association between each disease (AS, AAU, ReA, IBD, psoriasis) in a PFH and HLA-B27 carriership. The analyses were repeated in multivariable logistic models to investigate if each family history disease was associated, independently of other PFH subtypes, with HLA-B27 carriership. Patients with a PFH in both first- and second-degree relatives were classified into the group of patients with PFH in a first-degree relative (n = 11) for both the univariable and multivariable analyses. STATA SE version 14 software (StataCorp, College Station, TX, USA) was used to perform data analyses.

Results

In the ASAS cohort, 642 patients were diagnosed with a confidence level ≥ 6 as axSpA or no axSpA. Patients were excluded from the analysis if the family history was missing (n = 48). For the current analysis, 594 patients were used. Patients had a mean age (SD) of 33.7 (11.7) years, and 46% were male. Mean symptom duration was 7.1 (9.0) years, and a mean of 2.4 (1.6) SpA features, excluding HLA-B27 and imaging, were present. Of the sample, 52% were HLA-B27-positive, 20% had radiographic sacroiliitis, and 45% had active inflammation by MRI-SI (Table 1). Sixty-two percent of the patients were diagnosed as axSpA.

In total, 59% of patients reported to be white, 36% to be Asian, and 5% reported another ethnicity (Table 1). An ASAS PFH was reported by 23% of the patients; a PFH of AS was the most frequently reported family

Table 2 Univariable associations between a positive family history and HLA-B27 carriership in patients suspected of axial spondyloarthritis (n = 594)

	HLA-B27+ (n = 310)	HLA-B27− (n = 284)	OR (95% CI)	p Value
Positive family history according to ASAS definition				
Stratified by self-reported ethnicity				
White	54	26	2.3 (1.4–3.9)	0.001
Asian	38	14	3.1 (1.6–5.8)	0.001
Other ethnicities[a]	2	1	2.3 (0.2–25.0)	0.509
Stratified by degree of family relationship				
First-degree relatives	79	31	2.9 (1.8–4.5)	< 0.001
Only second-degree relatives	15	10	1.7 (0.7–3.8)	0.212
Positive family history of AS				
Stratified by self-reported ethnicity				
White	37	6	7.1 (2.9–17.1)	< 0.001
Asian	35	7	5.7 (2.5–13.2)	< 0.001
Other ethnicities[a]	2	0	n.a.	n.a.
Stratified by degree of family relationship				
First-degree relatives	61	9	7.8 (3.8–16.0)	< 0.001
Only second-degree relatives	13	4	3.7 (1.2–11.6)	0.023
Positive family history of AAU				
Stratified by self-reported ethnicity				
White	4	0	n.a.	n.a.
Asian	2	1	1.9 (0.2–20.7)	0.613
Other ethnicities[a]	0	0	n.a.	n.a.
Stratified by degree of family relationship				
First-degree relatives	5	1	4.7 (0.5–40.1)	0.162
Only second-degree relatives	1	0	n.a.	n.a.
Positive family history of ReA				
Stratified by self-reported ethnicity				
White	2	2	0.9 (0.1–6.5)	0.924
Asian	1	3	0.3 (0.03–2.9)	0.302
Other ethnicities[a]	0	0	n.a.	n.a.
Stratified by degree of family relationship				
First-degree relatives	3	2	1.4 (0.2–8.2)	0.735
Only second-degree relatives	0	3	n.a	n.a

Table 2 Univariable associations between a positive family history and HLA-B27 carriership in patients suspected of axial spondyloarthritis (n = 594) (Continued)

	HLA-B27+ (n = 310)	HLA-B27− (n = 284)	OR (95% CI)	p Value
Positive family history of IBD				
Stratified by self-reported ethnicity				
White	2	7	0.3 (0.05–1.2)	0.089
Asian	0	2	n.a.	n.a.
Other ethnicities[a]	0	1	n.a.	n.a.
Stratified by degree of family relationship				
First-degree relatives	1	7	0.1 (0.02–1.0)	0.054
Only second-degree relatives	1	3	0.3 (0.03–2.9)	0.294
Positive family history of psoriasis				
Stratified by self-reported ethnicity				
White	16	15	1.0 (0.5–2.0)	0.938
Asian	2	2	0.9 (0.1–6.5)	0.926
Other ethnicities[a]	0	1	n.a.	n.a.
Stratified by degree of family relationship				
First-degree relatives	15	14	1.0 (0.5–2.1)	0.949
Only second-degree relatives	3	4	0.7 (0.2–3.1)	0.620

Statistically significant results are printed in bold

Abbreviations: AAU Acute anterior uveitis, *AS* Ankylosing spondylitis, *HLA-B27* Human leukocyte antigen B27, *IBD* Inflammatory bowel disease, *n.a.* Not applicable, *ReA* Reactive arthritis

[a]Self-reported ethnicities was missing for five patients, who are included in this category, and other ethnicities are black, East Indian, Hispanic/Latino, mixed, or Turkish

history, with 15% (64% of all PFH), and a PFH of AAU was the least often reported, with 1% (5% of all PFH), among all patients (Table 1). An ASAS PFH in first-degree relatives only was reported in 17% of patients, in second-degree relatives in 4%, and in both first- and second-degree relatives in 2% of the patients.

An ASAS PFH and a PFH of AS were positively associated with HLA-B27 in all patients suspected of axSpA (ASAS PFH OR, 2.6; 95% CI, 1.7–3.9; PFH of AS OR, 6.5; 95% CI, 3.5–12.1). When these patients were stratified according to ethnicity and degree of family relationship, positive associations were found between an ASAS PFH and HLA-B27 carriership in patients with a self-reported white (OR, 2.3; 95% CI, 1.4–3.9) or Asian ethnicity (OR, 3.1; 95% CI, 1.6–5.8) and with a PFH in first-degree relatives (OR, 2.9; 95% CI, 1.8–4.5), but not in second-degree relatives (OR, 1.7; 95% CI, 0.7–3.8) (Table 2). A PFH of AS was positively associated with

HLA-B27 carriership in all subgroups (white OR, 7.1; 95% CI, 2.9–17.1; Asian OR, 5.7; 95% CI, 2.5–13.2; first-degree relatives OR, 7.8; 95% CI, 3.8–16.0; second-degree relatives OR, 3.7; 95% CI, 1.2–11.6). A PFH of AAU, ReA, IBD, or psoriasis was not positively associated with HLA-B27 carriership in patients suspected of axSpA, regardless of the degree of family relationship or ethnicity (Table 2). In the multivariable analysis, similar results were found (data not shown).

Discussion

In patients suspected of axSpA in the worldwide ASAS cohort, a PFH of AS was the predominant PFH subtype and was associated, independently of other PFH subtypes, with HLA-B27 carriership, regardless of self-reported ethnicity or degree of family relationship. No positive associations were found between a PFH of AAU, ReA, IBD, or psoriasis and HLA-B27 carriership. However, it should be noted that in patients with CBP suspected of axSpA, a PFH of AAU, ReA, and IBD was less common than a PFH of AS, which is in line with previous studies. Somewhat stronger associations were found for patients with white ethnicity and for patients with a PFH in first-degree relatives. Nonetheless, a PFH of AS was strongly associated with HLA-B27 carriership in both white and Asian patients and in both first- and second-degree relatives.

Our study is in line with the study of Ez-Zaitouni et al. in two European cohorts because they reported that a PFH of AS is associated with HLA-B27 carriership, but a PFH of ReA, IBD, or psoriasis was not [14]. In this study, a PFH of ReA, IBD, and AAU was also less common than a PHF of AS. However, in contrast to our findings, Ez-Zaitouni et al. [14] also found that a PFH of AAU contributed to the identification of axSpA because this was associated with HLA-B27 carriership in patients with CBP. In our study, a PFH of AAU was rarely reported (1%), as compared with 5–6% in the study of Ez-Zaitouni et al., which may limit detecting a possible association with HLA-B27 carriership owing to sample size. We have no proper explanation why a PFH of AAU was less common in our study. It may be attributed to differences in ethnicity (European cohorts vs. worldwide cohort in our study). However, the frequency of a PFH of AAU was similarly low in white and Asian patients in our cohort (0.7% vs. 0.5%). Moreover, the frequency of AAU in patients suspected of axSpA was similar in our cohort (9% overall; 10% in white and 6% in Asian patients) as compared with 8% in the study by Ez-Zaitouni et al.

In a general practice setting or other low SpA prevalence settings, a PFH of AS could be used for identifying HLA-B27-positive patients among patients suspected of axSpA. The RADAR study showed that HLA-B27 is a good referral tool for identifying patients with axSpA, because HLA-B27 has a higher sensitivity than an ASAS PFH [17]. Therefore, it is recommended that a PFH of AS should be used as a criterion for referral to secondary care only when HLA-B27 testing is not feasible.

The current study investigated patients with axial symptoms (i.e., patients with CBP suspected of axSpA) of the ASAS cohort, and therefore it is important to emphasize that the results are not applicable to patients with predominantly peripheral symptoms. In patients with predominantly peripheral symptoms, a PFH of, for example, psoriasis could be important and relevant for identifying patients with an increased risk of pSpA [15].

An important strength of this study is that the ASAS study is a worldwide cohort, which enabled us to investigate different self-reported ethnicities. Another strength is the availability of extensive information on family history, which allowed us to investigate the role of first- and second-degree relatives for each manifestation of a PFH. A major limitation is the self-reported family history by patients. This could lead either to an underestimation if a patient forgets or is unaware that a relative has an SpA-related disease or to an overestimation if a patient is confused or mistaken in the type of disease of a relative. Nevertheless, in a clinical setting, the physician usually has to depend on patient-reported family history. Another limitation is the small percentage of patients with self-reported ethnicity other than being white or Asian. Only 5% of the patients reported to be Hispanic/Latino, black, mixed, Turkish, East Indian, or unknown ethnicity. Therefore, the results are applicable only to white or Asian populations, which corresponds to the largest population with axSpA worldwide [18]. Preferably, future research into the value of a PFH for identifying HLA-B27 carriership should be conducted in patients with other ethnicities. In this study, we focused on the use of a PFH of SpA for identifying patients with CBP who are at an increased risk of HLA-B27 carriership, but we did not investigate the potential added value of a PFH in diagnosing patients with axSpA. We are currently analyzing data from three independent axSpA cohorts to address this issue.

Conclusions

Our data, in combination with data from two European cohorts, show that a PFH of AS and possibly also a PFH of AAU, regardless of ethnicity (white or Asian) or degree of family relationship, is valuable for identifying patients with CBP who could be HLA-B27-positive and consequently have an increased risk of axSpA.

Abbreviations

AAU: Acute anterior uveitis; AS: Ankylosing spondylitis; ASAS: Assessment of SpondyloArthritis international Society; axSpA: Axial spondyloarthritis; CBP: Chronic back pain; CRP: C-reactive protein; ESR: Erythrocyte sedimentation rate; FDR: First-degree relative; HLA-B27: Human leukocyte antigen B27; IBD: Inflammatory bowel disease; IBP: Inflammatory back pain; MRI: Magnetic resonance imaging; NSAID: Nonsteroidal anti-inflammatory drug; PFH: Positive family history; pSpA: Peripheral spondyloarthritis;

ReA: Reactive arthritis; SDR: Second-degree relative; SI: Sacroiliac joints; SpA: Spondyloarthritis

Authors' contributions

MvL, DvdH, and FvG were responsible for the study conception and design. RL, JS, MR, and DvdH were responsible for acquisition of the data. MvL, DvdH, and FvG participated in interpretation and analysis of the data. MvL drafted and wrote the manuscript. MvL, AS, RL, JS, MR, DvdH, and FvG were involved in critically revising the manuscript for important intellectual content. All authors read and approved the final manuscript.

Consent for publication

Not applicable.

Competing interests

The authors declare that they have no competing interests.

Author details

[1]Department of Rheumatology, Leiden University Medical Center, P.O. Box 9600, 2300 RC Leiden, the Netherlands. [2]NOVA Medical School, Universidade Nova de Lisboa, Lisbon, Portugal. [3]Department of Rheumatology, Amsterdam Rheumatology & Immunology Center, Amsterdam, the Netherlands. [4]Department of Rheumatology, Zuyderland Hospital, Heerlen, the Netherlands. [5]Department of Rheumatology, Charité Campus Benjamin Franklin, Berlin, Germany. [6]German Rheumatism Research Centre, Berlin, Germany. [7]Department of Internal Medicine and Rheumatology, Klinikum Bielefeld Rosenhöhe, Bielefeld, Germany.

References

1. Sieper J, Poddubnyy D. Axial spondyloarthritis. Lancet. 2017;390(10089):73–84.
2. Brown MA, Kennedy LG, MacGregor AJ, Darke C, Duncan E, Shatford JL, Taylor A, Calin A, Wordsworth P. Susceptibility to ankylosing spondylitis in twins: the role of genes, HLA, and the environment. Arthritis Rheum. 1997; 40(10):1823–8.
3. Mathieu A, Paladini F, Vacca A, Cauli A, Fiorillo MT, Sorrentino R. The interplay between the geographic distribution of HLA-B27 alleles and their role in infectious and autoimmune diseases: a unifying hypothesis. Autoimmun Rev. 2009;8(5):420–5.
4. Bedendo A, Glorioso S, Venturi Pasini C, Fabiano F, Casara D, Cavallo A, Todesco S. A family study of ankylosing spondylitis. Rheumatol Int. 1984;5(1):29–32.
5. van der Linden SM, Valkenburg HA, de Jongh BM, Cats A. The risk of developing ankylosing spondylitis in HLA-B27 positive individuals: a comparison of relatives of spondylitis patients with the general population. Arthritis Rheum. 1984;27(3):241–9.
6. Brown MA, Laval SH, Brophy S, Calin A. Recurrence risk modelling of the genetic susceptibility to ankylosing spondylitis. Ann Rheum Dis. 2000;59(11):883–6.
7. Kim HW, Choe HR, Lee SB, Chang WI, Chae HJ, Moon JY, Kang J, Lee S, Song YW, Lee EY. Phenotype difference between familial and sporadic ankylosing spondylitis in Korean patients. J Korean Med Sci. 2014;29(6):782–7.
8. Geirsson AJ, Kristjansson K, Gudbjornsson B. A strong familiality of ankylosing spondylitis through several generations. Ann Rheum Dis. 2010;69(7):1346–8.
9. Amor B, Dougados M, Mijiyawa M. Criteria of the classification of spondylarthropathies [in French]. Rev Rhum Mal Osteoartic. 1990;57(2):85–9.
10. Dougados M, van der Linden S, Juhlin R, Huitfeldt B, Amor B, Calin A, Cats A, Dijkmans B, Olivieri I, Pasero G, et al. The European Spondylarthropathy study group preliminary criteria for the classification of spondylarthropathy. Arthritis Rheum. 1991;34(10):1218–27.
11. Rudwaleit M, van der Heijde D, Landewé R, Listing J, Akkoc N, Brandt J, Braun J, Chou CT, Collantes-Estevez E, Dougados M, et al. The development of Assessment of SpondyloArthritis international Society classification criteria for axial spondyloarthritis (part II): validation and final selection. Ann Rheum Dis. 2009;68(6):777–83.
12. Poddubnyy D, van Tubergen A, Landewé R, Sieper J, van der Heijde D, Assessment of SpondyloArthritis international Society (ASAS). Development of an ASAS-endorsed recommendation for the early referral of patients with a suspicion of axial spondyloarthritis. Ann Rheum Dis. 2015;74(8):1483–7.
13. Abawi O, van den Berg R, van der Heijde D, van Gaalen FA. Evaluation of multiple referral strategies for axial spondyloarthritis in the SPondyloArthritis Caught Early (SPACE) cohort. RMD Open. 2017;3(1):e000389.
14. Ez-Zaitouni Z, Hilkens A, Gossec L, Berg IJ, Landewé R, Ramonda R, Dougados M, van der Heijde D, van Gaalen F. Is the current ASAS expert definition of a positive family history useful in identifying axial spondyloarthritis? Results from the SPACE and DESIR cohorts. Arthritis Res Ther. 2017;19(1):118.
15. Rudwaleit M, van der Heijde D, Landewé R, Akkoc N, Brandt J, Chou CT, Dougados M, Huang F, Gu J, Kirazli Y, et al. The Assessment of SpondyloArthritis international Society classification criteria for peripheral spondyloarthritis and for spondyloarthritis in general. Ann Rheum Dis. 2011; 70(1):25–31.
16. Sepriano A, Landewé R, van der Heijde D, Sieper J, Akkoc N, Brandt J, Braun J, Collantes-Estevez E, Dougados M, Fitzgerald O, et al. Predictive validity of the ASAS classification criteria for axial and peripheral spondyloarthritis after follow-up in the ASAS cohort: a final analysis. Ann Rheum Dis. 2016;75(6):1034–42.
17. Sieper J, Srinivasan S, Zamani O, Mielants H, Choquette D, Pavelka K, Loft AG, Géher P, Danda D, Reitblat T, et al. Comparison of two referral strategies for diagnosis of axial spondyloarthritis: the Recognising and Diagnosing Ankylosing spondylitis Reliably (RADAR) study. Ann Rheum Dis. 2013;72(10):1621–7.
18. Dean LE, Jones GT, MacDonald AG, Downham C, Sturrock RD, Macfarlane GJ. Global prevalence of ankylosing spondylitis. Rheumatology (Oxford). 2014; 53(4):650–7.

18

CYLD suppression enhances the pro-inflammatory effects and hyperproliferation of rheumatoid arthritis fibroblast-like synoviocytes by enhancing NF-κB activation

Le-meng Zhang[1†], Jing-Jing Zhou[1,2*†] (iD) and Chun-lei Luo[3]

Abstract

Background: Rheumatoid arthritis fibroblast-like synoviocytes (RA-FLSs) actively drive joint inflammation and degradation by producing inflammatory cytokines and matrix-degrading molecules, making them key factors in the pathogenesis of RA. Cylindromatosis (CYLD) is a tumor suppressor that downregulates nuclear factor kappa-light-chain-enhancer of activated B cells (NF-κB) activation by deubiquitinating NF-κB essential modulator and tumor necrosis factor receptor-associated factors 2 and 6. In this study, we aimed to determine CYLD expression in the synovium of patients with RA, analyze its correlation with NF-κB activation and clinical disease activity, further investigate CYLD expression in RA-FLSs, and explore CYLD's roles and mechanisms in the pro-inflammatory effects, proliferation, apoptosis, and cell cycles of RA-FLSs.

Methods: We obtained synovia from 50 patients with active RA and 20 with osteoarthritis (OA) and then cultured FLSs from the samples. We determined CYLD expression in the synovia of RA patients and in FLSs via reverse transcription polymerase chain reaction (RT-PCR). CYLD was depleted by lentiviral CYLD short hairpin ribonucleic acid. We used RT-PCR and enzyme-linked immunosorbent assay to analyze the expression of pro-inflammatory cytokines, matrix metalloproteinases (MMPs), and receptor activator of nuclear factor kappa-B ligand (RANKL). We detected cell proliferation using Cell Counting Kit-8 and examined cell apoptosis and cell cycle using flow cytometry.

(Continued on next page)

* Correspondence: shamanhua1986@163.com
†Le-meng Zhang and Jing-Jing Zhou contributed equally to this work.
[1]Thoracic Medicine Department, Hunan Cancer Hospital, Changsha 410013, People's Republic of China
[2]Department of Rheumatology, Navy General Hospital, Beijing 100048, People's Republic of China
Full list of author information is available at the end of the article

(Continued from previous page)

Results: We obtained the following results:

1. In synovia from patients with RA, CYLD expression was significantly downregulated while NF-κB expression was distinctly upregulated, compared with synovia from patients with OA. Thus, there is a significant inverse correlation between CYLD and NF-κB in synovia affected by RA.
2. CYLD expression significantly decreased in RA-FLSs compared with OA-FLSs.
3. CYLD suppression enhanced the production of pro-inflammatory cytokines, MMPs, and RANKL by activating NF-κB in RA-FLSs.
4. CYLD suppression enhanced proliferation, reduced apoptosis, and increased cell division of RA-FLSs and aggravated the activity of NF-κB in RA-FLSs.

Conclusions: Via its regulation of NF-κB activation, CYLD may be involved in the pathogenesis of synovial inflammation in RA as well as in the pro-inflammatory effects and hyperproliferation of RA-FLSs. CYLD may therefore provide a potential target for the treatment of RA.

Keywords: Rheumatoid arthritis (RA), Cylindromatosis (CYLD), Fibroblast-like synoviocyte (FLS), Nuclear factor κ-light-chain-enhancer of activated B cells (NF-κB), Pro-inflammatory cytokines, Hyperproliferation

Background

Rheumatoid arthritis (RA) is a systemic and chronic inflammatory disease characterized by synovial hyperplasia formation, which mediates cartilage and bone destruction [1].The pathogenesis of RA is extraordinarily complicated and involves various kinds of cells, such as fibroblast-like synoviocytes (FLSs), T cells, B cells, monocytes/macrophages, and osteoclasts [2]. It has been indicated that each cell type plays distinct, complex, and interrelated roles in the development of RA [3]. In RA, the synovial lining thickness at the border of the joint cavity increases to 10–15 cell layers, compared with 1–3 cell layers in normal individuals [4, 5]. Prior studies have demonstrated that FLSs are the predominant cell type in the terminal layer of the hyperplastic synovium and at the sites of invasion in adjacent cartilage and bone joints, and that they vigorously contribute to the initiation and early perpetuation of RA [4, 6].

FLSs in RA, also known as synovial fibroblasts or type B synoviocytes, occur early after onset with visible erosion at cartilage–bone junctions [7]. FLS activation involves multiple factors, including Toll-like receptor (TLR) activation, inflammatory factors, matrix degradation products, and epigenetic modifications [8]. Activated RA-FLSs are highly able to recruit, retain, and activate both cells of the immune system and resident joint cells through hyperproduction of a broad array of pro-inflammatory cytokines, matrix metalloproteinases (MMPs), and chemokines, leading to the initiation and maintenance of chronic inflammation and progressive joint destruction [9]. The pro-inflammatory cytokine tumor necrosis factor alpha (TNF-α) is regarded as one of the most central cytokines that significantly triggers inflammation and joint destruction, which is confirmed by the clinical efficacy of TNF-α-blocking agents [10].

TNF-α, interleukin-1β (IL-1β), interleukin-6 (IL-6), and interleukin-8 (IL-8), the most important cytokines, can obviously aggravate inflammatory reactions and increase the influx of additional pro-inflammatory cells into the synovium to sustain regulatory feedback loops and induce production of MMPs, cathepsins, and aggrecanases [11, 12]. The synovium is the main source of MMPs and cathepsins in RA, and in situ hybridization studies have localized collagenase messenger ribonucleic acid (mRNA) nearly exclusively to RA-FLSs [13]. Activated MMPs can significantly drive the degradation of the extracellular matrix (ECM) and facilitate cartilage and bone erosion, while inhibition of MMPs can greatly alleviate the invasiveness of RA-FLSs into cartilage [14–16]. RA-FLSs also influence bone destruction via modulation of osteoclastogenesis by secreting receptor activator of nuclear factor kappa-light-chain-enhancer of activated B cells (NF-κB) ligand (RANKL) [17]. Denosumab, a human monoclonal antibody that specifically binds RANKL, has been effective for the treatment of RA-associated bone loss [18, 19]. In addition, synovial hyperplasia in RA appears to be caused at least in part by the impairment of apoptosis in RA-FLSs and synovial macrophages, while deficient apoptosis has been shown to prolong RA-FLS survival by increasing the production of anti-apoptotic molecules like B-cell lymphoma 2 (Bcl-2), sentrin-1 (SUMO-1), and Fas-associated death domain-like interleukin-1- converting enzyme inhibitory protein (FLIP) [19, 20].

Cylindromatosis (CYLD) was initially identified as a tumor suppressor that is mutated in patients with familial cylindromatosis, a genetic condition that predisposes patients for the development of skin appendage tumors (cylindroma) [21]. CYLD is a key adaptor that regulates various signaling pathways to modulate diverse physiological processes, ranging from immune response and inflammation to cell cycle progression, spermatogenesis, and osteoclastogenesis [22]. Emerging evidence suggests that CYLD primarily downregulates NF-κB signaling by deubiquitinating NF-κB essential modulator (NEMO) and several upstream regulators like TNF receptor-associated factors 2 and 6 (TRAF2 and TRAF6) and TGF-β-activated kinase 1 (Tak1) [23–25]. The family of NF-κB transcription factors plays a large role in mediating the expression of large numbers of genes during the inflammatory response. Many previous in vitro and in vivo studies on the contribution of components of NF-κB signaling pathways to the pathogenesis of RA have shown that NF-κB plays prominent roles in inflammation, cartilage degradation, cell proliferation, angiogenesis, and pannus formation [26]. Until now, however, the role and the underlying mechanism of CYLD in local inflammation and joint destruction in RA have been poorly elucidated. Therefore, in this study, we determined CYLD expression in synovia from patients with RA and analyzed its correlation with NF-κB activation or clinical disease activity. Then we investigated CYLD expression in RA-FLSs and explored its roles and mechanisms in pro-inflammatory effects, proliferation, apoptosis, and cell cycles of RA-FLSs.

Methods

Patients

We recruited 50 Chinese patients with RA who fulfilled the 1987 revised criteria of the American College of Rheumatology (ACR) for RA [27] or the 2010 ACR/ European League Against Rheumatism (EULAR) classification criteria for RA [28] from the Department of Rheumatology and Orthopedics. All RA patients had a Disease Activity Score 28-joint assessment (DAS28) ≥ 3.0 (active disease). We obtained the names of 20 patients with osteoarthritis (OA) who fulfilled established clinical criteria as "less-inflamed" disease controls from the Department of Rheumatology and Orthopedics [29, 30]. This study was conducted in compliance with the Helsinki Declaration, and the protocol was approved by the Ethics Committee of Navy General Hospital, Beijing, China. All patients gave written informed consent.

Disease assessments

Clinical data of all patients with RA were collected at baseline, including tender joint count of 28 joints (28TJC), swollen joint count of 28 joints (28SJC), patient and provider global assessment of disease activity (PtGA and PrGA, respectively), pain visual analog scale (pain VAS), Chinese-language version of Stanford Health Assessment Questionnaire (HAQ) [31], erythrocyte sedimentation rate (ESR), C-reactive protein (CRP), rheumatoid factor (RF), and anti-cyclic citrullinated peptide antibody (ACPA). We assessed disease activity with

DAS28 using 4 variables, including CRP (DAS28 [4]-CRP) [32].

Synovial tissue collection

We collected the synovium from patients with RA via biopsy with a closed Parker Pearson needle [33]. We obtained at least six pieces of synovial tissue per patient to minimize sampling error [34]. The synovia were obtained from the knees of OA patients by closed-needle biopsy, arthroplasty, or arthroscopy. We fixed all samples in 10% neutral formalin and embedded them in paraffin. Sections (5 μm) were cut serially and mounted on adhesive glass slides. The sealed slides were stored at – 20 °C until staining.

Immunohistochemistry (IHC)

We stained serial sections of synovial tissues with hematoxylin and eosin (H&E) and a three-step immunoperoxidase method for IHC. Sections were incubated with CYLD (Abcam, Cambridge, MA, USA) at 1/100 dilution overnight at 4 °C after deparaffinization and retrieval, then with EnVision mouse or rabbit conjugate (Dako/Agilent, Santa Clara, CA, USA) for 30 min at 37 °C. We used 3,3′-diaminobenzidine (DAB)-positive substrate for the color reaction, and we counterstained sections with hematoxylin. We used nonspecific isotype immunoglobulin G (IgG) as a negative control. We determined the percentage of CYLD-positive staining cells in the lining layers and sublining area by manually observing five different fields at × 400 magnification.

Fibroblast-like synoviocyte (FLS) culture

We isolated FLSs from the synovial tissues using the modified tissue culture method [35], shredded fresh synovial tissues into small pieces, and digested them in type I collagenase (Sigma-Aldrich, St. Louis, MO, USA) for 2 h at 37 °C. The cells were cultured with complete Dulbecco's modified Eagle's medium–Ham's F-12 (DMEM/ F12; Gibco Life Technologies, Shanghai, China) containing 100 g/ml streptomycin, 100 units/ml penicillin, and 20% fetal bovine serum (FBS; Gibco Life Technologies, Australia) in a humidified 5% CO_2 incubator. Our in vitro study used FLSs from passages 3–5.

Immunofluorescence (IF) staining of FLSs

After fixation and permeabilization, we blocked the FLSs with 5% bovine serum albumin (BSA), then incubated the cells in phosphate-buffered saline (PBS) containing rabbit anti-human polyclonal antibody to CYLD (Abcam, USA) or normal rabbit IgG (control) overnight at 4 °C. The secondary antibody (red) was Alexa Fluor 633 conjugated goat anti-rabbit IgG (Invitrogen, Carlsbad, CA, USA), used at a 1:1000 dilution for 1 h at 37 °C. We used 4,′6-diamindino-2-phenylindole (DAPI;

Sigma-Aldrich) to stain the cell nuclei (blue) at a concentration of 1.43 µM for 3 min and mounted ProLong Gold Antifade Reagent (P36934; Invitrogen) to the coverslips. Images were examined and analyzed with a 160 Zeiss LSM 510 confocal microscope (Carl Zeiss AG, Jena, Germany).

Lentivirus infection in RA-FLSs

We performed gene silencing with lentiviral short hairpin RNA (shRNA). The sh-CYLD targeting sequence was GCCCAATACCAATGGAAGTAT. We cloned shRNA into pLKO.1 (gv248) lentiviral vectors, added culture supernatants containing shRNA to RA-FLSs in the presence of polybrene, and selected the cells using 1 µg/ml puromycin after 24 h. Stable cell lines were verified by reverse transcription polymerase chain reaction (RT-PCR) and Western blot.

Reverse transcription polymerase chain reaction (RT-PCR)

We isolated total RNA from the synovium or cells using RNAiso Plus (Takara Bio, Inc., Kusatsu, Japan) per the manufacturer's instructions and synthesized complementary DNA (cDNA) samples using a reverse transcription kit (PrimeScript RT Master Mix; Takara Bio). We amplified the cDNA using specific oligonucleotide primers (Table 1). We performed quantitative real-time PCR (RT-qPCR) using SYBR Premix Ex Taq (Tli RNase H Plus;

Table 1 Primers for reverse transcription-polymerase chain reaction (RT-PCR)

β-actin	Sense: 5′-GGACTTCGA GCAAGAGATGG-3′
	Antisense: 5′-TGTGTTGGCGTACAGGTCTTTG-3′
NF-κB	Sense: 5′-ATGTGGAGATCATTGAGCAGC-3′
	Antisense: 5′-CCTGGTCCTGTGTAGCCATT-3′
CYLD	Sense: 5′-ACGCCACAATCTTCATCACACT-3′
	Antisense: 5′-AGGTCGTGGTCAAGGTTTCACT-3′
TNF-α	Sense: 5′-GCTAAGAGGGAGAGAAGCAACTACA-3′
	Antisense: 5′-GAAGAGGCTGAGGAACAAGCA-3′
IL-6	Sense: 5′-CTGCGCAGCTTTAAGGAGTTC-3′
	Antisense: 5′-CAATCTGAGGTGCCCATGCTA-3′
IL-1β	Sense: 5′-CCAGCTACGAATCTCCGACC-3′
	Antisense: 5′-CATGGCCACAACAACTGACG-3′
IL-8	Ssense: 5′-GTGCAGAGGGTTGTGGAGAAGTTT-3′
	Antisense: 5′-TCACTGGCATCTTCACTGATTCTTG-3′
MMP-1	Ssense: 5′- AAAATTACACGCCAGATTTGCC-3′
	Antisense: 5′- GGTGTGACATTACTCCAGAGTTG-3′
MMP-3	Sense: 5′- TTTCCAGGGATTGACTCAAAGA-3′
	Antisense: 5′- AAGTGCCCATATTGTGCCTTC-3′
RANKL	Sense: 5′-ACCAGCATCAAAATCCCAAG-3′
	Antisense: 5′-CCCCAAAGTATGTTGCATCC-3′

Takara Bio). The reactions were initiated with denaturation of cDNA templates at 95 °C for 30 s, 95 °C for 5 s, and 60 °C for 30 s, then amplification for 40–50 cycles. We ran samples in triplicate in a Roche LightCycler 480 sequence detection system (Roche, Basel, Switzerland) per the manufacturer's instructions. All primers used in this study were synthesized by Invitrogen Genetech Co. Ltd. (Shanghai, China). As a control for sample loading, we performed PCR amplification of the housekeeping gene *β-actin* for each sample. We normalized and quantified PCR signals by comparing the cycle threshold value of the gene in question, in triplicate, with *β-actin*. Each bar represents mean ± standard deviation (SD) of three independent experiments was showed in Figs. 3 and 4.

Western blot analysis

After transfection, we separated cytoplasmic protein from nuclear protein using NE-PER nuclear and cytoplasmic extraction reagents (Thermo Scientific–Pierce, Rockford, IL, USA). We measured protein concentrations by bicinchoninic acid (BCA) protein assay (Pierce, Rockford, IL, USA). Protein (50 µg) was loaded onto 12% gradient sodium dodecyl sulfate- polyacrylamide gel electrophoresis (SDS-PAGE) gel under denaturing conditions and electrotransferred to nitrocellulose membranes. We blocked the blots with 5% milk in Tris-buffered saline-Tween (TBST) for 1 h at room temperature, then probed them with antibodies against CYLD (Abcam), p-nuclear factor of κ-light polypeptide gene enhancer in B-cells inhibitor-α (IκBα), T-IκBα, p-NF-κB p65 (Ser536), and NF-κB p65 (all CST (Cell Signaling Technology, Inc), USA; all 1:1000), glyceraldehyde 3-phosphate dehydrogenase (GAPDH; CST; 1:1000) and Histone H3 (CST; 1:2000) at 4 °C overnight. After washing them with TBST, we incubated the membranes with horseradish peroxidase (HRP)-conjugated secondary antibody (EarthOx Life Sciences, Millbrae, CA, USA) at 1:5000 dilution for 1 h at room temperature. We visualized immunoreactive bands by enhanced chemiluminescence (ECL; Amersham Pharmacia Biotech, Little Chalfont, UK) reaction. We conducted densitometric analyses on protein bands using a scanning imager, ImageQuant TL software (GE Healthcare Life Sciences) and the G:BOX Gel & Blot Imaging Series (Syngene, Cambridge, UK) and normalized the bands against the intensity of Histone H3 or GAPDH, expressing it as a fold change relative to untreated controls. Each blot is representative of at least three similar independent experiments.

Enzyme-linked immunosorbent assay (ELISA)

We used ELISA (R&D Systems, Minneapolis, MN, USA) per the manufacturer's instructions to detect the amounts of TNF-α, IL-1β, IL-6, MMP-1, MMP-3, and RANKL in the culture supernatants of the stably transduced RA-FLSs. Briefly, we added the culture supernatant mixed with assay buffer to wells coated with anti-TNF-α, IL-1β, IL-6, MMP-1, MMP-3, and RANKL antibody at 37 °C for 60 min. We then added HRP-conjugated anti-human TNF-α, IL-1β, IL-6, MMP-1, MMP-3, and RANKL monoclonal antibody and incubated at 37 °C for 2 h, followed by incubation with colorimetric (tetramethylbenzidine) solution for another 10 min. After that, we measured relative absorbance, and three independent experiments were performed for each condition.

Cell proliferation assay

We seeded stably transduced RA-FLSs at a density of 5000 cells/well of each group in 96-well microtiter plates, then pre-incubated them in a humidified atmosphere with 5% CO_2 at 37 °C. We added 10 μl of Cell Counting Kit-8 (CCK-8; Dojindo Molecular Technologies, Inc., Kyushu, Japan) solution to each well and incubated the RA-FLSs at 37 °C for 2 h at various time points (0, 24, 48, and 72 h after initial seeding). We used a microplate reader to detect absorbance at wavelength 450 nm (450 optical density [OD]). All experiments were conducted in triplicate.

Apoptosis detection assay and cell cycle analysis by flow cytometry (FCM)

To study the effects of CYLD on RA-FLS apoptosis, we used sodium nitroprusside (SNP; Sigma-Aldrich) to induce apoptosis of stably transduced RA-FLSs. We measured apoptosis by detecting allophycocyanin (APC)-conjugated annexin-V and 7-aminoactinomycin D (7-AAD) using FCM (BD Biosciences Pharmingen, San Diego, CA, USA). For cell cycle analysis, we fixed and permeabilized the RA-FLSs with cold ethanol overnight, then treated them with propidium iodide (PI) and RNA enzyme (RNase) before subjecting them to fluorescence-activated cell sorting (FACS) analysis. We determined cell cycle distribution and quantification using FCM and CellQuest software (BD Biosciences, Mountain View, CA, USA). Each condition was repeated independently three times.

Statistical analysis

We performed statistical analysis using SPSS for Windows statistical software version 13.0 (SPSS Inc., Chicago, IL, USA). Data are presented as mean ± standard deviation (SD) of three independent experiments. We used one-way analysis of variance (ANOVA) to compare data among groups and Bonferroni's test for post hoc comparison. To assess the correlation between synovial expression of CYLD and NF-κB and that between CYLD expression in RA-FLSs and histological or clinical parameters, we used Spearman's rank-order correlation. A P value < 0.05 was considered statistically significant.

Results

Characteristics of the study patients

Table 2 shows baseline demographic and clinical characteristics of all RA patients. Age and gender did not differ between patients with RA and those with OA. Thirty-eight of the RA patients were female and 12 were male. The mean age was 60 (range 49–64) years. The mean disease duration was 38 (range 14–110) months. Of the RA patients, 92% (46/50) had positive RF, while 82% (41/50) were positive for ACPA. All RA patients had DAS28 [4]-CRP values > 3.0. The mean DAS28 [4]-CRP score was 5.02 (range 3.0–6.8). Among the patients with RA, 54% (27/50) had never been treated with corticosteroids or disease-modifying anti-rheumatic drugs (DMARDs). Most of them had taken only Chinese herbals and/or painkillers to relieve arthralgia. A total of 16% (8/50) had taken corticosteroids alone before being referred to our hospital. A total of 30% (15/50) accepted one or more DMARDs, including methotrexate, leflunomide, sulfasalazine, hydroxychloroquine, or etanercept.

Synovial CYLD and NF-κB expression in RA and OA

The following results were obtained by RT-PCR analysis of synovia from 50 RA patients and 20 OA patients. Figure 1a shows that CYLD mRNA expression in synovia from RA patients was significantly decreased compared with that in synovia from OA controls (0.59 ± 1.81 vs.

Table 2 Baseline demographic and clinical features of RA patients in the study

Characteristic	RA patients ($n = 50$)
Demographic	
Age, years, median (IQR)	60 (49~ 64)
Female, n (%)	38 (76)
Disease status	
Disease duration, months, median (IQR)	38 (14–110)
ESR (mm/h), median (IQR)	80 (54~ 105)
CRP (mg/dl), median (IQR)	4.37 (1.82~ 6.75)
Rheumatoid factor-positive, n (%)	46 (92)
ACPA-positive, n (%)	41 (82)
DAS28, median (IQR)	5.02 (3.0~ 6.8)
Previous medications, n (%)	
Corticosteroids	19 (38)
Methotrexate	20 (40)
Leflunomide	6 (12)
Sulfasalazine	2 (4)
Hydroxychloroquine	7 (14)
Etanercept	5 (10)

RA rheumatoid arthritis, *IQR* interquartile range, *ESR*, erythrocyte sedimentation rate, *CRP*, C-reactive protein, *ACPA*, anti-cyclic citrullinated peptide antibody, *DAS28*, Disease Activity Score 28-joint assessment, *n*, number of patients, *SD*, standard deviation

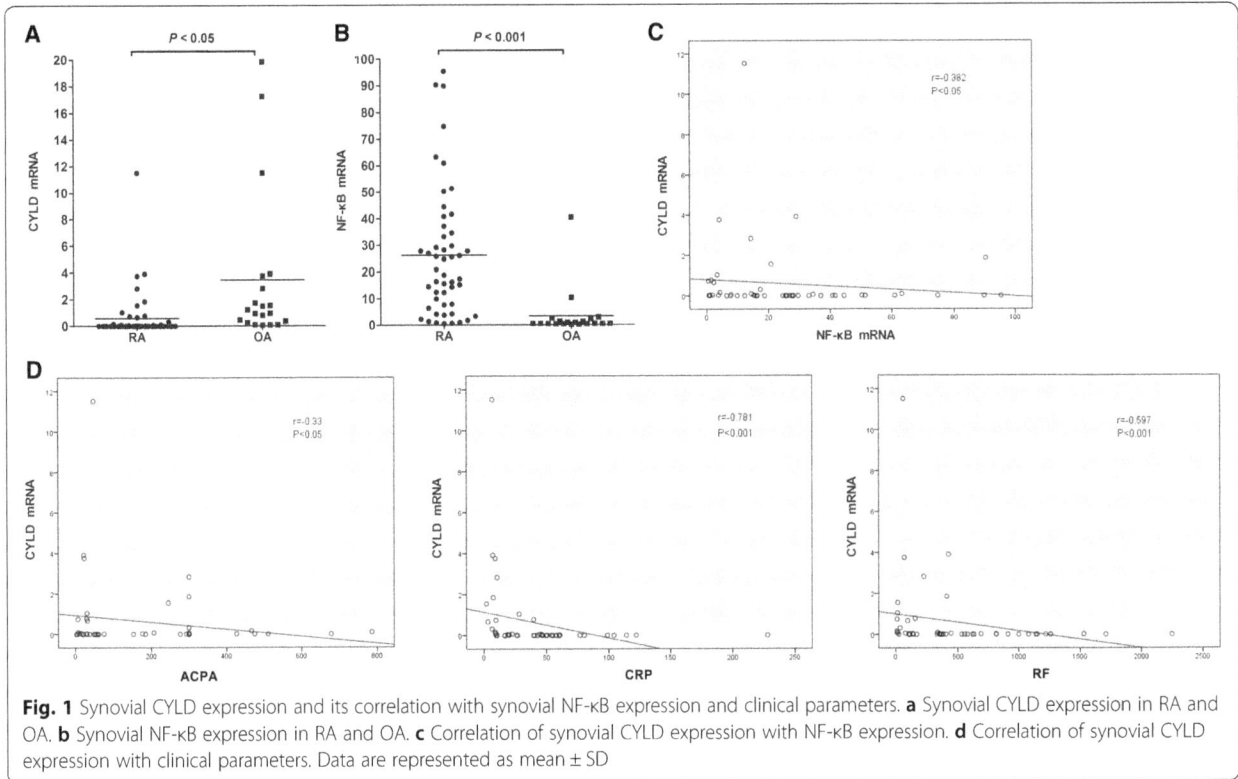

Fig. 1 Synovial CYLD expression and its correlation with synovial NF-κB expression and clinical parameters. **a** Synovial CYLD expression in RA and OA. **b** Synovial NF-κB expression in RA and OA. **c** Correlation of synovial CYLD expression with NF-κB expression. **d** Correlation of synovial CYLD expression with clinical parameters. Data are represented as mean ± SD

3.46 ± 5.77; $P < 0.05$). Figure 1b indicates that NF-κB mRNA expression in synovia from RA patients was obviously increased compared with that in synovia from OA controls (26.17 ± 24.36 vs. 3.42 ± 9.00; $P < 0.001$).

Correlation of synovial CYLD expression with NF-κB expression

To find the association between CYLD and NF-κB, we examined the correlation between CYLD and NF-κβ mRNA expression in synovia from RA patients. Using Spearman's test, we found a significant inverse correlation between CYLD and NF-κβ mRNA expression in synovia from RA patients (Fig. 1c; $r = -0.382$, $P < 0.01$).

Correlation of synovial CYLD expression with clinical parameters

Spearman's test showed conspicuous correlations between synovial CYLD mRNA expression and ACPA, CRP and RF (Fig. 1d; $r = -0.330$, $P < 0.05$; $r = -0.781$, $P < 0.001$; $r = -0.597$, $P < 0.001$, respectively). There was no significant correlation between CYLD mRNA and 28TJC, 28SJC, PtGA, PrGA, HAQ, ESR, Simple or Clinical Disease Activity Index (SDAI and CDAI, respectively) or DAS28 (all $P > 0.05$).

Expression of CYLD in RA-FLSs

We observed CYLD expression in the lining and sublining layer of synovium from RA patients, finding intense staining in the endochylema as well as the nuclei of lining cells (both macrophage-like synoviocytes and FLSs) and sublining inflammatory cells (mostly in lymphocytes and plasma cells; Fig. 2A). To further investigate whether CYLD expression was aberrant in FLSs, we determined CYLD expression in 25 RA-FLSs and 15 OA-FLSs. Via RT-PCR we found that expression of CYLD mRNA in RA-FLSs was significantly lower than in OA-FLS controls (Fig. 2B; 0.41 ± 0.43 vs. 1.23 ± 0.84; $P < 0.01$), and via IF staining we also found that expression of CYLD in RA-FLSs was obviously lower than in OA-FLSs (Fig. 2C).

shRNA transfection suppressed CYLD expression in RA-FLSs

To investigate whether the constitutive expression of CYLD in RA-FLSs could be decreased by lentiviral CYLD shRNA (sh-CYLD), we transfected RA-FLSs with sh-CYLD or lentiviral vector (sh-GFP). RT-PCR showed that expression of CYLD in mRNA levels was remarkably downregulated in RA-FLSs transfected with sh-CYLD, compared with those transfected with sh-GFP (Fig. 3a; 0.20 ± 0.04 vs. 1.00 ± 0.00; $P < 0.01$). Western

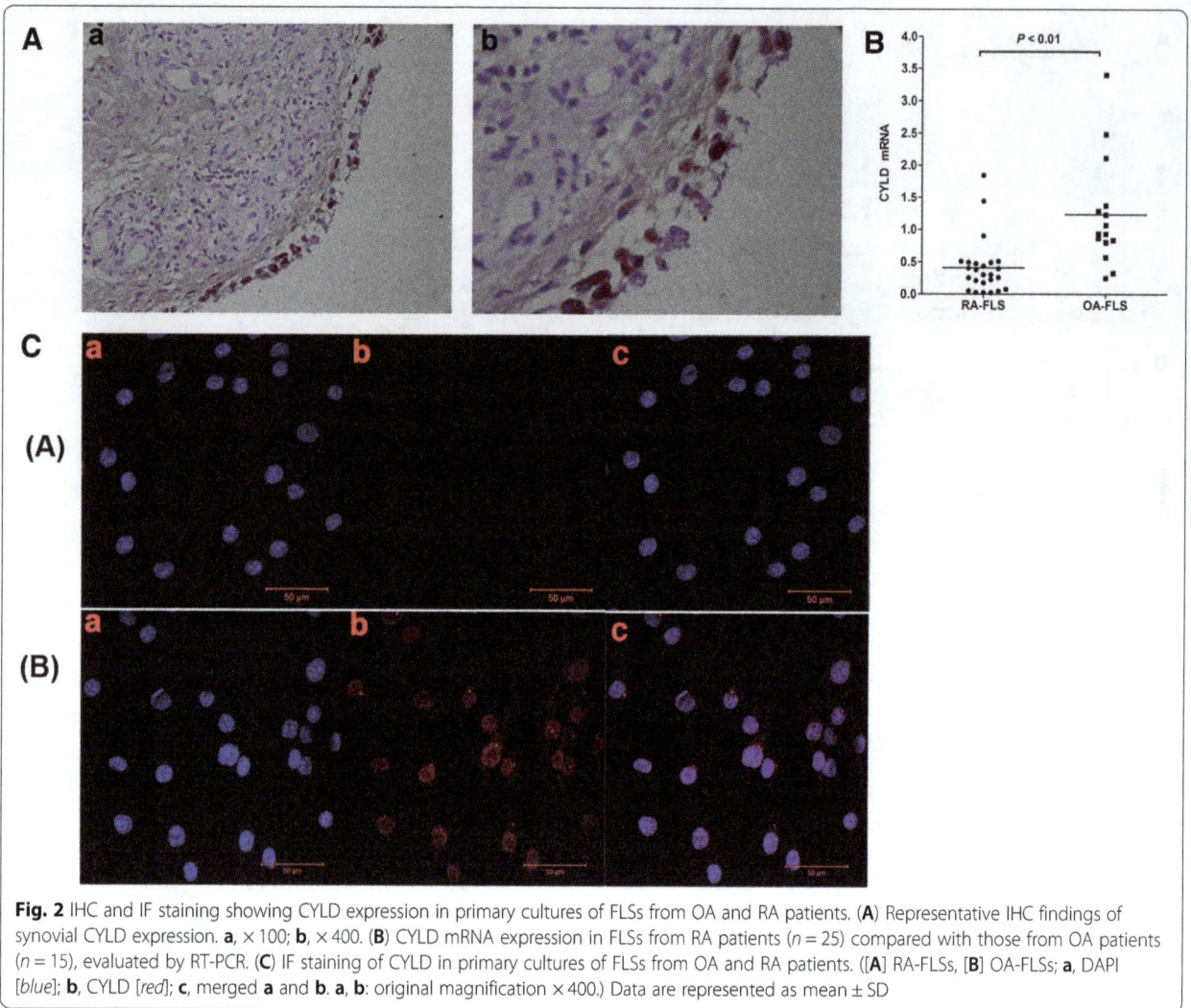

Fig. 2 IHC and IF staining showing CYLD expression in primary cultures of FLSs from OA and RA patients. (**A**) Representative IHC findings of synovial CYLD expression. **a**, × 100; **b**, × 400. (**B**) CYLD mRNA expression in FLSs from RA patients (n = 25) compared with those from OA patients (n = 15), evaluated by RT-PCR. (**C**) IF staining of CYLD in primary cultures of FLSs from OA and RA patients. ([**A**] RA-FLSs, [**B**] OA-FLSs; **a**, DAPI [blue]; **b**, CYLD [red]; **c**, merged **a** and **b**. **a**, **b**: original magnification × 400.) Data are represented as mean ± SD

blot indicated similar results for protein levels (Fig. 3b; 0.21 ± 0.03 vs. 1.00 ± 0.00; P < 0.01).

CYLD knockdown enhanced the pro-inflammatory effects of RA-FLSs

To further determine the role CYLD plays in the pro-inflammatory effects of RA-FLSs, we compared pro-inflammatory cytokine production in CYLD-knockdown RA-FLSs with that in RA-FLSs infected with sh-GFP. After sh-CYLD transfection, not only was mRNA expression of pro-inflammatory cytokines such as TNF-α, IL-1β, IL-6, and IL-8 strengthened, but that of MMP-1, MMP-3, RANKL, and NF-κB was also obviously enhanced compared with sh-GFP transfection (Fig. 4a). Similarly, protein levels of TNF-α, IL-1β, IL-6, IL-8, MMP-1, MMP-3, and RANKL in the cell culture supernatants of sh-CYLD-transfected RA-FLSs were markedly higher than those in supernatants of sh-GFP-transfected RA-FLSs (Fig. 4b).

CYLD knockdown enhanced RA-FLS proliferation

CCK-8 test results showed increased RA-FLS proliferation in sh-CYLD transfection groups compared with sh-GFP transfection groups (Fig. 5A). FCM analyses of annexin-V, APCA, and PI revealed that lentivirus-mediated inhibition of CYLD significantly prevented early and total apoptosis (LR and TR, respectively) but not late apoptosis (UR) when compared with the sh-GFP groups (Fig. 5B; LR 4.98 ± 0.94 vs. 7.15 ± 0.10, P = 0.016; UR 1.65 ± 1.14 vs. 3.51 ± 1.19, P = 0.122; TR 6.63 ± 0.21 vs. 10.67 ± 1.28, P = 0.029). The data also showed that CYLD knockdown markedly mitigated LR and TR but not UR in the presence of SNP, compared with the sh-GFP groups (Fig. 5B; LR 14.95 ± 0.71 vs. 35.30 ± 6.20, P = 0.005; UR 5.22 ± 0.78 vs. 8.80 ± 3.74, P = 0.236; TR 20.17 ± 1.41 vs. 44.10 ± 6.80, P = 0.004). The percentage of cells in G0/G1 phase was significantly decreased in sh-CYLD-transfected RA-FLSs compared with the sh-GFP groups (Fig. 5C; 51.80 ± 0.83 vs. 84.15 ± 1.18; P = 0.000). Conversely, the percentage of cells in S-phase

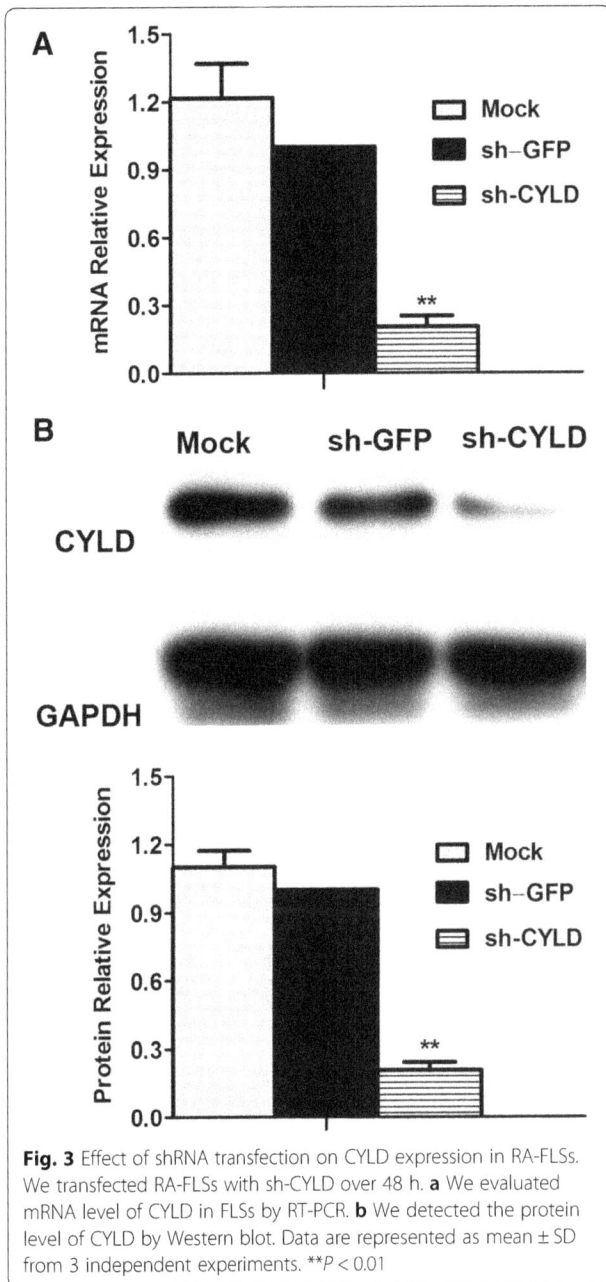

Fig. 3 Effect of shRNA transfection on CYLD expression in RA-FLSs. We transfected RA-FLSs with sh-CYLD over 48 h. **a** We evaluated mRNA level of CYLD in FLSs by RT-PCR. **b** We detected the protein level of CYLD by Western blot. Data are represented as mean ± SD from 3 independent experiments. **$P < 0.01$

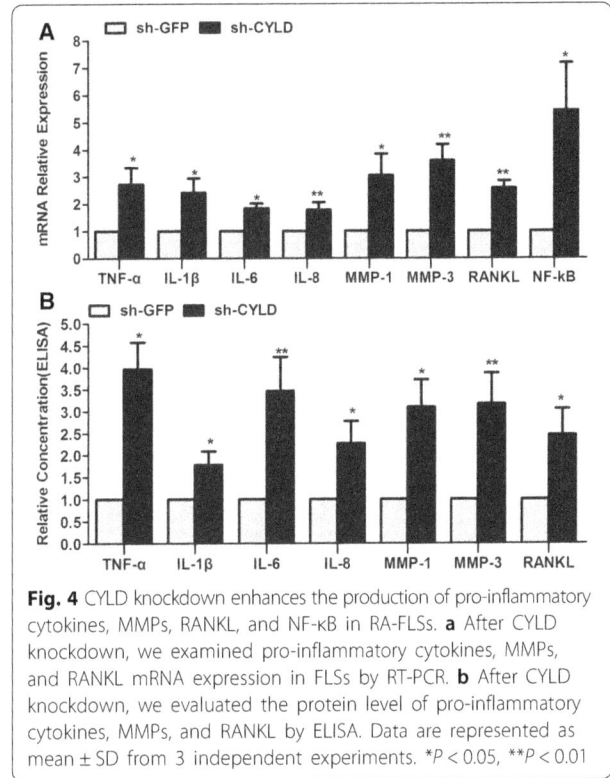

Fig. 4 CYLD knockdown enhances the production of pro-inflammatory cytokines, MMPs, RANKL, and NF-κB in RA-FLSs. **a** After CYLD knockdown, we examined pro-inflammatory cytokines, MMPs, and RANKL mRNA expression in FLSs by RT-PCR. **b** After CYLD knockdown, we evaluated the protein level of pro-inflammatory cytokines, MMPs, and RANKL by ELISA. Data are represented as mean ± SD from 3 independent experiments. *$P < 0.05$, **$P < 0.01$

was apparently enhanced in sh-CYLD-transfected RA-FLSs compared with the sh-GFP groups (Fig. 5C; 40.83 ± 2.92 vs. 12.10 ± 1.02; $P = 0.000$). Annexin-V assay results showed that the percentage of cells in G2/M phase was not significantly different between the sh-CYLD and the sh-GFP transfection groups (Fig. 5C; 7.38 ± 2.26 vs. 3.75 ± 0.51; $P = 0.053$).

CYLD knockdown aggravated NF-κB and IκBα activation in RA-FLSs

To explore the mechanism of CYLD on induction of pro-inflammatory cytokines, production of MMPs and RANKL, increased RA-FLS proliferation, decreased apoptosis, and

cell cycle, we measured upstream NF-κB signaling by RT-PCR and Western blot. We showed that CYLD knockdown visibly aggravated NF-KB activity in RA-FLSs nuclei and IκBα in RA-FLSs cytoplasm and obviously decreased the level of total IκBα in RA-FLS cytoplasm (Fig. 6a), but not the total of NF-κB in RA-FLSs (Figs. 4a and 6b).

Discussion

CYLD was initially reported as a tumor suppressor with deubiquitinating enzyme activity that is mutated in familial cylindromatosis. It suppresses the activation of NF-κB, which plays central roles in inflammation, immune responses, carcinogenesis, protection against apoptosis, and promotion of cell proliferation [21]. Our current study showed that CYLD expression in synovia from RA patients was significantly downregulated compared with that in synovia from OA patients. Conversely, NF-κB expression was distinctly upregulated in the RA synovium compared with the OA synovium. This result is consistent with that of a past study which found that NF-κB activation is higher in RA than in OA [36]. In addition, we found a significant inverse correlation between CYLD and NF-κB in the RA synovium, suggesting that NF-κB activation is suppressed when CYLD function is normal, but that it tends to be enhanced in the absence of functional CYLD. Moreover, synovial CYLD expression correlates significantly with ACPA, CRP, and RF. Above all, our results support the possibility that

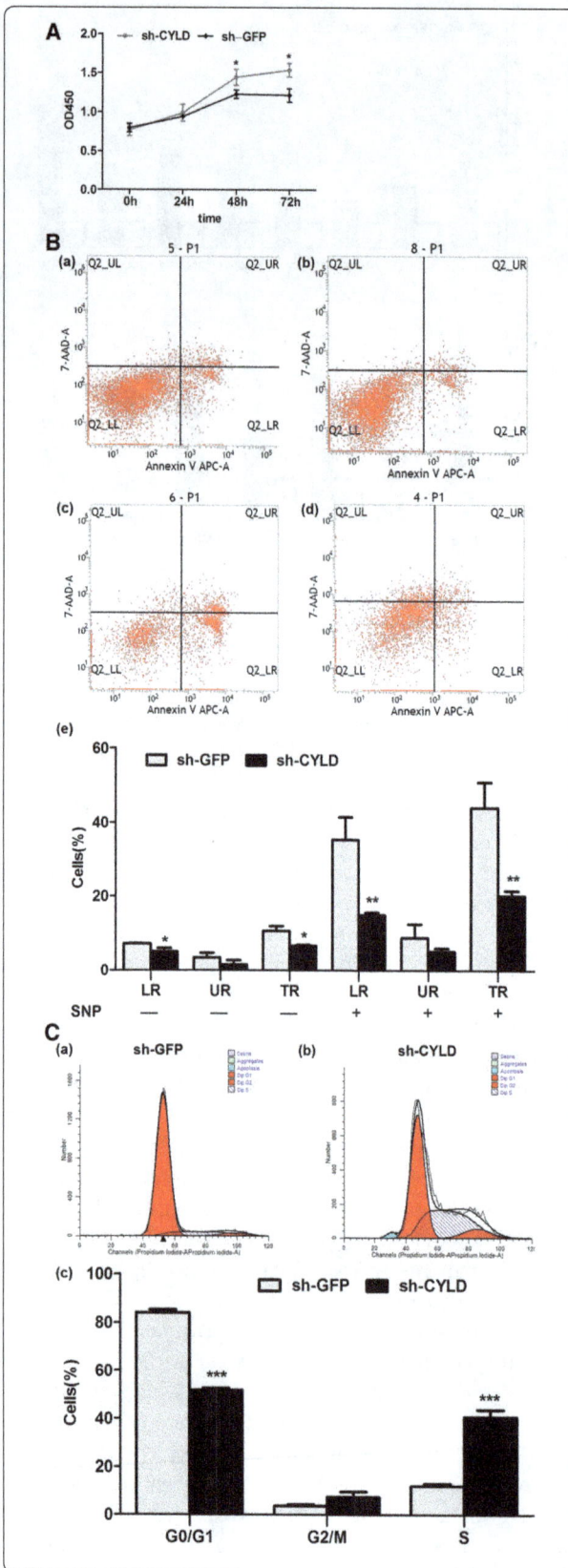

Fig. 5 Effects of CYLD on cell proliferation, apoptosis, and cell cycle in RA-FLSs. We transfected RA-FLSs with sh-CYLD or sh-GFP. (**A**) CCK-8 test showed increased RA-FLSs proliferation in the sh-CYLD transfection group compared with the sh-GFP transfection group. (**B**) FCM analysis demonstrating the effect of CYLD suppression on cell apoptosis. (**C**) FCM analysis demonstrating the effect of CYLD suppression on cell cycle progression. Data are represented as mean $\pm$ SD from 3 independent experiments. $*P < 0.05$, $**P < 0.01$, $***P < 0.001$

NF-κB activation accompanied by loss of CYLD may be a crucial step in the development and progression of RA. Thus, we postulated that functional relevant loss of CYLD expression may contribute to RA development and progression and may provide a new target for therapeutic strategies.

RA is a chronic inflammatory disease characterized by persistent inflammation of the diarthrodial joints with synovial hyperplasia and progressive joint destruction. In

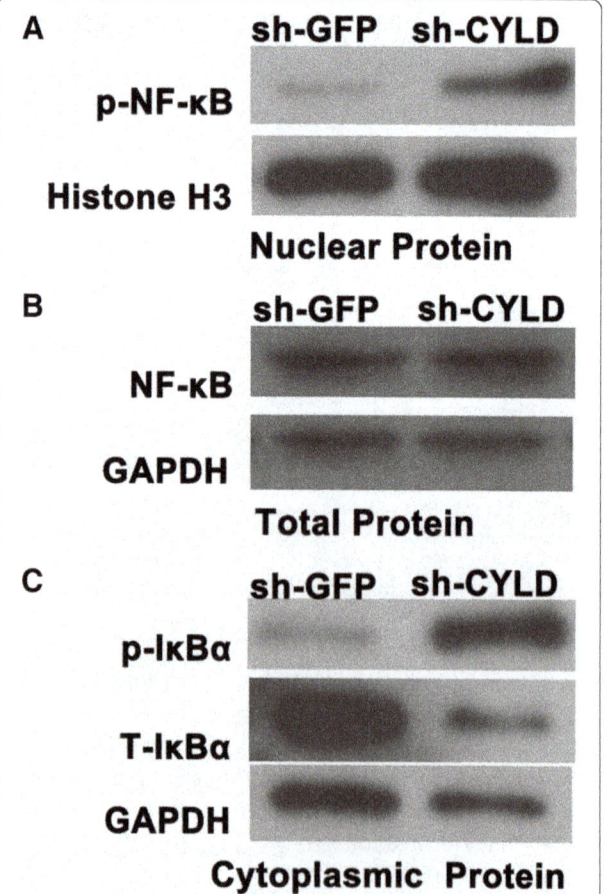

Fig. 6 Effects of CYLD on NF-κB and IκBα activation in RA-FLSs. **a** After CYLD knockdown, we detected the protein level of NF-κB in RA-FLSs nuclei by Western blot. **b** After CYLD knockdown, we detected the protein level of NF-κB in RA-FLSs by Western blot. **c** After CYLD knockdown, we examined the protein level of p-IκBα and T-IκBα in RA-FLSs cytoplasm by Western blot

the terminal layer of the hyperplastic rheumatoid synovium, FLSs are the dominant cell types. Similar to tumor cells, they can be expanded in cell culture over several passages and escape contact inhibition to invade and degrade the adjacent cartilage and bone [37]. Activated RA-FLSs can be detected early after RA onset by visible erosions at cartilage–bone junctions [7].There, RA-FLSs can be activated by (among other things) inflammatory factors, TLR activation, matrix degradation products, and epigenetic modifications [8]. Recent studies have revealed that at an initial stage of synovial activation, TLRs are the key recognition structures of innate immune stimuli, such as microbial components, endogenous ligands, liberated cellular RNA, and DNA fragments from necrotic cells within the synovial fluid [38, 39]. TLRs are stimulated by their respective ligands; they dimerize and recruit downstream adaptor molecules, which propagate signals that converge at NF-κB through the TRAF6, TRAF3, and IL-1- and IL-1R-associated kinase 1/4 (IRAK1/4) complex and induce the production cytokines such as TNF-α, IL-1β, and IL-6 [40]. In addition, RA-FLS activation is not only the response to active inflammation within the synovium and the presence of inflammatory cells but constitutes an intrinsic feature of RA-FLSs. This inflammation-independent activation has been elegantly confirmed by studies in which human RA-FLSs implanted into a severe combined immunodeficient (SCID) mouse model of RA attached to and invaded co-implanted healthy human cartilage without cells of the immune system [41]. In addition, Murphy Roths Large mice with or without lymphoproliferation (MRL – lpr/lpr mice) can spontaneously develop RA-like arthritis, indicating that synovial cell proliferation and invasion into joint structures occur even before inflammatory cells migrate into the synovium [42]. Hence, RA-FLSs potentially contribute to the initiation and early progression of RA and are thus key factors in the pathogenesis of RA. Therefore, targeting the aggressive, joint-destructive, and pro-inflammatory properties of RA-FLSs is a recent approach to RA treatment.

Activated NF-κB plays a central role in regulating the expression of numerous genes during the inflammatory response, which is the fundamental process of RA. Generally, NF-κB is present in the cytoplasm as a heterodimeric complex composed of the p50 and p65 subunits, which are associated with inhibitory κB proteins (IκBs) [43]. NF-κB activation typically occurs following specific serine/threonine kinase IκB kinase (IKK) signalosome activation, leading to the phosphorylation and subsequent dispatch of IκBs to the proteasome of protein degradation [44]. IκB degradation enables NF-κB to translocate to the nucleus, stimulating the transcription of specific genes. The IKK complex consists of at least three subunits, including the kinases IKK-α and IKK-β

and the associated regulatory subunit IKK-γ [44]. It has been demonstrated that NF-κB and IKK are abundant in RA-FLSs [26, 36]. NF-κB activation can robustly induce pro-inflammatory cytokines, MMPs, and RANKL production in RA-FLSs, which enhances the inflammatory cycle and contributes to joint erosion in RA [45, 46]. NF-κB has been shown to mediate fibronectin fragment-induced chondrocyte activation and to increase pro-inflammatory cytokines, chemokines, MMPs such as IL-6 and IL-8, and methyl-accepting chemotaxis protein-1 (MCP-1), growth-related oncogenes a, b, and g (*GRO-α*, *GRO-b*, and *GRO-g*, respectively), and MMP-13 production in human articular chondrocytes [47, 48]. TNF-α and IL-1β can strongly promote NF-κB activation and enhance the production of IL-6, IL-8, intercellular adhesion molecule 1 (ICAM-1), and collagenase in RA-FLSs [49]. TNF-α, IL-1β, and IL-6 are prominent pro-inflammatory cytokines in the inflammatory cascade of RA and have been widely studied as therapeutic interventions [5, 50].

Numerous studies in vitro and in vivo have validated that CYLD mediates NF-κB activation by deubiquitinating TRAF2, TRAF6, and NEMO, making it an important regulator in the adaptive immune response. However, the expression and exact roles of CYLD in the pro-inflammatory effects of RA-FLSs are unknown. We observed CYLD expression in the lining and sublining layers of RA synovium, with intense staining found in the endochylema as well as the nuclei of lining cells (both macrophage-like synoviocytes and FLSs) and sublining of inflammatory cells, implying that CYLD was expressed in RA-FLSs. Its expression in primarily cultured RA-FLSs was significantly lower than that in OA-FLSs. Our experiments also further demonstrated that suppression of CYLD by sh-CYLD enhanced mRNA expression and the secretion of pro-inflammatory cytokines in RA-FLSs, including TNF-α, IL-1β, IL-6, and IL-8; aggravated the activity of NF-κB in RA-FLS nuclei and IκBα in RA-FLS cytoplasm; and decreased the level of total IκBα in RA-FLS cytoplasm. This suggests that downregulated CYLD plays a conspicuous role in the pro-inflammatory effects of RA-FLSs via NF-κB signaling.

In joints with early-stage RA, activated RA-FLSs attach to and overgrow the articular cartilage surface, then invade and destroy cartilage and induce bone resorption via secretion of MMPs, cathepsins, and inflammatory cytokines and regulation of monocyte-to-osteoclast differentiation [51, 52]. MMPs include collagenases (MMP-1, MMP-8, and MMP-13), gelatinases (MMP-2, MMP-9), stromelysins (MMP-3, MMP-7, MMP-10, MMP-11, and MMP-12), and membrane-type (MT) MMPs (MT1-MMP, MT2-MMP, MT3-MMP, and MT4-MMP). In situ hybridization studies have validated that lining cells are the major source of MMP-1 and MMP-3 in the synovium, especially RA-FLSs [53, 54]. MMP-1 cleaves collagens I, II, VII, and X, while inhibition of MMP-1 synthesis significantly reduces the cartilage invasiveness of FLSs in the SCID mouse model for RA [55]. MMP-3 can degrade cartilage proteoglycans and type IX collagen and activate other pro-MMPs, including pro-MMP-1 and pro-MMP-9 [56]. In addition, osteoclasts are the major course of local and systemic abnormalities of bone remodeling, including bone erosion and both focal and systemic osteoporosis [57]. RANKL is one of the key molecules for osteoclastic differentiation and activity that have been found to be strongly expressed at sites of bone erosion in RA synovium, especially in RA-FLSs [58]. Studies performed in human RA-FLSs have indicated that IL-1β mediates the production of MMP-1 and MMP-3 by regulating NF-κB activation [59]. Inhibition of NF-κB and Jun N-terminal kinase (JNK) activation significantly decreases production of pro-inflammatory cytokines (TNF-α, IL-1β, IL-6, and IL-8) and MMPs (MMP-1 and MMP-3) in RA-FLSs [60]. It has also been reported that NF-κB suppression obviously reduces RANKL expression in human RA-FLSs and in FLSs from mice with adjuvant-induced arthritis (AA) [61, 62]. As CYLD plays a pivotal role in regulating NF-κB activation, it is not clear whether it is involved in the synthesis of MMP-1, MMP-3, and RANKL in RA-FLSs. We showed that CYLD inhibition in RA-FLSs apparently enhanced MMP-1, MMP-3, and RANKL production and NF-κB activity, implying that CYLD participated in mediating RA-FLS-induced cartilage and bone destruction via NF-κB signaling.

In the pathology of RA, it is widely acknowledged that the progressive destruction of articular cartilage relies on the evolution of hyperplastic synovial tissue, while hyperplasia in FLSs depends on dysregulated proliferation and apoptosis [63]. Thus, promoting RA-FLS apoptosis and reducing RA-FLS proliferation are new treatment strategies for RA. It has been reported that CYLD attenuates NF-κB signaling by removing lysine63 (Lys63)-linked polyubiquitin chains from TRAF2 or TRAF6, leading to programmed cell death [64]. Previous studies have also revealed that CYLD suppression leads to decreased apoptosis and increased proliferation by activating NF-κB [23, 65]. In the present study, we found that CYLD inhibition distinctly enhanced proliferation, reduced apoptosis, and increased the cell division of RA-FLSs and aggravated the activity of NF-κB in these cells, suggesting that CYLD is involved in RA-FLS hyperproliferation in RA. However, a recent report indicated that the loss of CYLD in mouse keratinocytes enhances cell proliferation by increasing the nuclear activity of Bcl-30-associated NF-κB p50 and p52 subunits, rather than by increasing classical p65/p50 NF-κB action. This

implies that the mechanism of CYLD-mediated NF-κB inhibition may vary by cell type [65].

Conclusions

In summary, downregulated CYLD may be involved in the pathogenesis of inflammation in the RA synovium by regulating classical NF-κB activation, as well as in the pro-inflammatory effects and hyperproliferation of RA-FLSs. Thus, CYLD may provide a potential target for the treatment of RA. However, the precise mechanism of interaction between CYLD and NF-κB in RA-FLSs remains unclear and requires further exploration. In addition, our study showed that CYLD is expressed not only in RA-FLSs but also in inflammatory cells, such as lymphocytes, and in plasma cells. Further studies are needed to investigate the expression and role of CYLD in regard to the pro-inflammatory effects, proliferation, apoptosis, and cell cycles of these cells.

Abbreviations
28SJC: Swollen joint count of 28 joints; 28TJC: Tender joint count of 28 joints; 7-AAD: 7-aminoactinomycin D; AA: Adjuvant-induced arthritis; ACPA: Anti-cyclic citrullinated peptide antibody; ACR: American College of Rheumatology; ANOVA: Aanalysis of variance; BCA: Bicinchoninic acid; Bcl-2: B-cell lymphoma 2; BSA: Bovine serum albumin; CCK-8: Cell Counting Kit-8; CDAI: Clinical Disease Activity Index; cDNA: Complementary deoxyribonucleic acid; CRP: C-reactive protein; CYLD: Cylindromatosis; DAB: 3,3'-Diaminobenzidine; DAPI: 4,'6-diamindino-2-phenylindole; DAS28 [4]-CRP: DAS28 with 4 variables, including CRP; DAS28: Disease Activity Score 28-joint assessment; DMARDs: Disease-modifying anti-rheumatic drugs; DMEM/F12: Dulbecco's modified Eagle's medium–Ham's F-12; ECL: Enhanced chemiluminescence; ECM: Extracellular matrix; ELISA: Enzyme-linked immunosorbent assay; ESR: Erythrocyte sedimentation rate; EULAR: European League Against Rheumatism; FACS: Fluorescence-activated cell sorting; FBS: Fetal bovine serum; FCM: Flow cytometry; FLIP: Fas-associated death domain-like interleukin-1-converting enzyme inhibitory protein; FLS: Fibroblast-like synoviocyte; GAPDH: Glyceraldehyde 3-phosphate dehydrogenase; GRO-a: Growth-related oncogene-alpha; H&E: Hematoxylin and eosin; HAQ: Chinese-language version of Stanford Health Assessment Questionnaire; HRP: Horseradish peroxidase; ICAM-1: Intercellular adhesion molecule 1; IgG: Immunoglobulin G; IKK: IκB kinase; IL-1β: Interleukin-1 beta; IL-6: Interleukin-6; IL-8: Interleukin-8; IRAK1/4: IL-1- and IL-1R-associated kinase 1/4; IκB: Inhibitory κB protein; IκBα: Nuclear factor of κ-light polypeptide gene enhancer in B-cells inhibitor-α; LR: Early apoptosis; Lys63: Lysine63; MCP-1: Methyl-accepting chemotaxis protein; MMP: Matrix metalloproteinase; MRL – lpr/lpr mice: Murphy Roths Large mice with or without lymphoproliferation; mRNA: Messenger ribonucleic acid; MT: Membrane type; n: Number of patients; NEMO: NF-κB essential modulator; NF-κB: Nuclear factor κ-light-chain-enhancer of activated B cells; OA: Osteoarthritis; OD: Optical density; Pain VAS: Pain visual analog scale; PBS: Phosphate-buffered saline; PI: Propidium iodide; PrGA: Provider global assessment of disease activity; PtGA: Patient global assessment of disease activity; RA: Rheumatoid arthritis; RANKL: receptor activator of nuclear factor kappa-B ligand; RF: Rheumatoid factor; RNase: Ribonuclease; RT-PCR: Reverse transcription polymerase chain reaction; RT-qPCR: Quantitative reverse transcription polymerase chain reaction; SCID: Severe combined immunodeficiency; SD: Standard deviation; SDAI: Simple Disease Activity Index; SDS-PAGE: Sodium dodecyl sulfate-polyacrylamide gel electrophoresis; sh-CYLD: Lentiviral CYLD shRNA; sh-GFP: Lentiviral vector; shRNA: Short hairpin ribonucleic acid; SNP: Sodium nitroprusside; SUMO-1: Sentrin-1; Tak1: TGF-β-activated kinase 1; TBST: Tris-buffered saline-Tween; TLR: Toll-like receptor; TNF-α: Tumor necrosis factor alpha; TR: Total apoptosis; TRAF2: TNF receptor-associated factor 2; TRAF6: TNF receptor-associated factor 6; UR: Late apoptosis

Acknowledgements
We wish to thank all the patients and the staff members of the medical staff for their cooperation.

Funding
This work was mainly supported by a grant from the National Natural Science Foundation of China (No. 81401631).

Authors' contributions
JJZ and LMZ participated in study development and collection of patient samples, performed experiments, and actively wrote the first draft of the manuscript. CLL actively participated in all aspects of this process. All authors read and approved the final manuscript.

Consent for publication
All participants have approved publication of the data in this manuscript.

Competing interests
The authors declare that they have no competing interests.

Author details
[1]Thoracic Medicine Department, Hunan Cancer Hospital, Changsha 410013, People's Republic of China. [2]Department of Rheumatology, Navy General Hospital, Beijing 100048, People's Republic of China. [3]Department of Nephrology, Ningbo First Hospital, Ningbo 3150102, People's Republic of China.

References
1. Malemud CJ. Intracellular signaling pathways in rheumatoid arthritis. J Clin Cell Immunol. 2013;4:160.
2. Wang Q, Ma Y, Liu D, Zhang L, Wei W. The roles of B cells and their interactions with fibroblast-like synoviocytes in the pathogenesis of rheumatoid arthritis. Int Arch Allergy Immunol. 2011;155(3):205–11.
3. Karsdal MA, Woodworth T, Henriksen K, Maksymowych WP, Genant H, Vergnaud P, Christiansen C, Schubert T, Qvist P, Schett G, et al. Biochemical markers of ongoing joint damage in rheumatoid arthritis—current and future applications, limitations and opportunities. Arthritis Res Ther. 2011; 13(2):215.
4. Muller-Ladner U, Ospelt C, Gay S, Distler O, Pap T. Cells of the synovium in rheumatoid arthritis. Synovial fibroblasts. Arthritis Res Ther. 2007;9(6):223.
5. Perlman H, Pope RM. The synovial lining micromass system: toward rheumatoid arthritis in a dish? Arthritis Rheum. 2010;62(3):643–6.
6. Fan W, Zhou ZY, Huang XF, Bao CD, Du F. Deoxycytidine kinase promotes the migration and invasion of fibroblast-like synoviocytes from rheumatoid arthritis patients. Int J Clin Exp Pathol. 2013;6(12):2733–44.
7. Noss EH, Brenner MB. The role and therapeutic implications of fibroblast-like synoviocytes in inflammation and cartilage erosion in rheumatoid arthritis. Immunol Rev. 2008;223:252–70.
8. Neumann E, Lefevre S, Zimmermann B, Gay S, Muller-Ladner U. Rheumatoid arthritis progression mediated by activated synovial fibroblasts. Trends Mol Med. 2010;16(10):458–68.
9. Lefevre S, Meier FM, Neumann E, Muller-Ladner U. Role of synovial fibroblasts in rheumatoid arthritis. Curr Pharm Des. 2015;21(2):130–41.
10. Hoff M, Kvien TK, Kalvesten J, Elden A, Kavanaugh A, Haugeberg G. Adalimumab reduces hand bone loss in rheumatoid arthritis independent

11. of clinical response: subanalysis of the PREMIER study. BMC Musculoskelet Disord. 2011;12:54.
11. Kasama T, Isozaki T, Takahashi R, Miwa Y. Clinical effects of tocilizumab on cytokines and immunological factors in patients with rheumatoid arthritis. Int Immunopharmacol. 2016;35:301–6.
12. Alam J, Jantan I, Bukhari SNA. Rheumatoid arthritis: recent advances on its etiology, role of cytokines and pharmacotherapy. Biomed Pharmacother. 2017;92:615–33.
13. Ahn JK, Huang B, Bae EK, Park EJ, Hwang JW, Lee J, Koh EM, Cha HS. The role of alpha-defensin-1 and related signal transduction mechanisms in the production of IL-6, IL-8 and MMPs in rheumatoid fibroblast-like synoviocytes. Rheumatology (Oxford). 2013;52(8):1368–76.
14. Itoh Y. Metalloproteinases: potential therapeutic targets for rheumatoid arthritis. Endocr Metab Immune Disord Drug Targets. 2015;15(3):216–22.
15. Araki Y, Mimura T. Matrix metalloproteinase gene activation resulting from disordered epigenetic mechanisms in rheumatoid arthritis. Int J Mol Sci. 2017;18(5):905.
16. Miller MC, Manning HB, Jain A, Troeberg L, Dudhia J, Essex D, Sandison A, Seiki M, Nanchahal J, Nagase H, et al. Membrane type 1 matrix metalloproteinase is a crucial promoter of synovial invasion in human rheumatoid arthritis. Arthritis Rheum. 2009;60(3):686–97.
17. Pusey MF. Anomalous weak values are proofs of contextuality. Phys Rev Lett. 2014;113(20):200401.
18. Cummings SR, San Martin J, McClung MR, Siris ES, Eastell R, Reid IR, Delmas P, Zoog HB, Austin M, Wang A, et al. Denosumab for prevention of fractures in postmenopausal women with osteoporosis. N Engl J Med. 2009;361(8):756–65.
19. Cohen SB, Dore RK, Lane NE, Ory PA, Peterfy CG, Sharp JT, van der Heijde D, Zhou L, Tsuji W, Newmark R. Denosumab treatment effects on structural damage, bone mineral density, and bone turnover in rheumatoid arthritis: a twelve-month, multicenter, randomized, double-blind, placebo-controlled, phase II clinical trial. Arthritis Rheum. 2008;58(5):1299–309.
20. Ha JE, Choi YE, Jang J, Yoon CH, Kim HY, Bae YS. FLIP and MAPK play crucial roles in the MLN51-mediated hyperproliferation of fibroblast-like synoviocytes in the pathogenesis of rheumatoid arthritis. FEBS J. 2008; 275(14):3546–55.
21. Bignell GR, Warren W, Seal S, Takahashi M, Rapley E, Barfoot R, Green H, Brown C, Biggs PJ, Lakhani SR, et al. Identification of the familial cylindromatosis tumour-suppressor gene. Nat Genet. 2000;25(2):160–5.
22. Sun SC. CYLD: a tumor suppressor deubiquitinase regulating NF-kappaB activation and diverse biological processes. Cell Death Differ. 2010;17(1): 25–34.
23. Brummelkamp TR, Nijman SM, Dirac AM, Bernards R. Loss of the cylindromatosis tumour suppressor inhibits apoptosis by activating NF-kappaB. Nature. 2003;424(6950):797–801.
24. Kovalenko A, Chable-Bessia C, Cantarella G, Israel A, Wallach D, Courtois G. The tumour suppressor CYLD negatively regulates NF-kappaB signalling by deubiquitination. Nature. 2003;424(6950):801–5.
25. Trompouki E, Hatzivassiliou E, Tsichritzis T, Farmer H, Ashworth A, Mosialos G. CYLD is a deubiquitinating enzyme that negatively regulates NF-kappaB activation by TNFR family members. Nature. 2003;424(6950):793–6.
26. Romanblas J, Jimenez S. NF-κB as a potential therapeutic target in osteoarthritis and rheumatoid arthritis. Osteoarthr Cartil. 2006;14(9):839–48.
27. Arnett FC, Edworthy SM, Bloch DA, McShane DJ, Fries JF, Cooper NS, Healey LA, Kaplan SR, Liang MH, Luthra HS, et al. The American Rheumatism Association 1987 revised criteria for the classification of rheumatoid arthritis. Arthritis Rheum. 1988;31(3):315–24.
28. Aletaha D, Neogi T, Silman AJ, Funovits J, Felson DT, Bingham CO 3rd, Birnbaum NS, Burmester GR, Bykerk VP, Cohen MD, et al. Rheumatoid arthritis classification criteria: an American College of Rheumatology/ European League Against Rheumatism collaborative initiative. Arthritis Rheum. 2010;62(9):2569–81.
29. Pessler F, Ogdie A, Diaz-Torne C, Dai L, Yu X, Einhorn E, Gay S, Schumacher HR. Subintimal Ki-67 as a synovial tissue biomarker for inflammatory arthropathies. Ann Rheum Dis. 2008;67(2):162–7.
30. Pessler F, Dai L, Diaz-Torne C, Gomez-Vaquero C, Paessler ME, Zheng DH, Einhorn E, Range U, Scanzello C, Schumacher HR. The synovitis of "non-inflammatory" orthopaedic arthropathies: a quantitative histological and immunohistochemical analysis. Ann Rheum Dis. 2008;67(8):1184–7.
31. Koh ET, Seow A, Pong LY, Koh WH, Chan L, Howe HS, Lim TH, Low CK. Cross cultural adaptation and validation of the Chinese Health

Assessment Questionnaire for use in rheumatoid arthritis. J Rheumatol. 1998;25(9):1705–8.

32. Anderson J, Caplan L, Yazdany J, Robbins ML, Neogi T, Michaud K, Saag KG, O'Dell JR, Kazi S. Rheumatoid arthritis disease activity measures: American College of Rheumatology recommendations for use in clinical practice. Arthritis Care Res. 2012;64(5):640–7.

33. Singh JA, Arayssi T, Duray P, Schumacher HR. Immunohistochemistry of normal human knee synovium: a quantitative study. Ann Rheum Dis. 2004; 63(7):785–90.

34. Gerlag D, Tak PP. Synovial biopsy. Best Pract Res Clin Rheumatol. 2005;19(3):387–400.

35. Kawakami A, Nakashima T, Sakai H, Hida A, Urayama S, Yamasaki S, Nakamura H, Ida H, Ichinose Y, Aoyagi T, et al. Regulation of synovial cell apoptosis by proteasome inhibitor. Arthritis Rheum. 1999;42(11):2440–8.

36. Handel ML, McMorrow LB, Gravallese EM. Nuclear factor-kappa B in rheumatoid synovium. Localization of p50 and p65. Arthritis Rheum. 1995; 38(12):1762–70.

37. Qu Z, Garcia CH, O'Rourke LM, Planck SR, Kohli M, Rosenbaum JT. Local proliferation of fibroblast-like synoviocytes contributes to synovial hyperplasia. Results of proliferating cell nuclear antigen/cyclin, c-myc, and nucleolar organizer region staining. Arthritis Rheum. 1994;37(2):212–20.

38. Brentano F, Kyburz D, Schorr O, Gay R, Gay S. The role of Toll-like receptor signalling in the pathogenesis of arthritis. Cell Immunol. 2005;233(2):90–6.

39. Brentano F, Schorr O, Gay RE, Gay S, Kyburz D. RNA released from necrotic synovial fluid cells activates rheumatoid arthritis synovial fibroblasts via Toll-like receptor 3. Arthritis Rheum. 2005;52(9):2656–65.

40. Anwar MA, Basith S, Choi S. Negative regulatory approaches to the attenuation of Toll-like receptor signaling. Exp Mol Med. 2013;45:e11.

41. Muller-Ladner U, Kriegsmann J, Franklin BN, Matsumoto S, Geiler T, Gay RE, Gay S. Synovial fibroblasts of patients with rheumatoid arthritis attach to and invade normal human cartilage when engrafted into SCID mice. Am J Pathol. 1996;149(5):1607–15.

42. Gay S, Gay RE, Koopman WJ. Molecular and cellular mechanisms of joint destruction in rheumatoid arthritis: two cellular mechanisms explain joint destruction? Ann Rheum Dis. 1993;52(Suppl 1):S39–47.

43. Lin TH, Pajarinen J, Lu L, Nabeshima A, Cordova LA, Yao Z, Goodman SB. NF-kappaB as a therapeutic target in inflammatory-associated bone diseases. Adv Protein Chem Struct Biol. 2017;107:117–54.

44. Llona-Minguez S, Baiget J, Mackay SP. Small-molecule inhibitors of IkappaB kinase (IKK) and IKK-related kinases. Pharmaceutical Patent Analyst. 2013; 2(4):481–98.

45. Huber LC. Synovial fibroblasts: key players in rheumatoid arthritis. Rheumatology. 2006;45(6):669–75.

46. Kim KW, Kim HR, Park JY, Park JS, Oh HJ, Woo YJ, Park MK, Cho ML, Lee SH. Interleukin-22 promotes osteoclastogenesis in rheumatoid arthritis through induction of RANKL in human synovial fibroblasts. Arthritis Rheum. 2012; 64(4):1015–23.

47. Pulai JI, Chen H, Im HJ, Kumar S, Hanning C, Hegde PS, Loeser RF. NF-kappa B mediates the stimulation of cytokine and chemokine expression by human articular chondrocytes in response to fibronectin fragments. J Immunol. 2005;174(9):5781–8.

48. Forsyth CB, Cole A, Murphy G, Bienias JL, Im HJ, Loeser RF Jr. Increased matrix metalloproteinase-13 production with aging by human articular chondrocytes in response to catabolic stimuli. J Gerontol A Biol Sci Med Sci. 2005;60(9):1118–24.

49. Aupperle K, Bennett B, Han Z, Boyle D, Manning A, Firestein G. NF-kappa B regulation by I kappa B kinase-2 in rheumatoid arthritis synoviocytes. J Immunol (Baltimore, Md : 1950). 2001;166(4):2705–11.

50. Canete JD, Hernandez MV, Sanmarti R. Safety profile of biological therapies for treating rheumatoid arthritis. Expert Opin Biol Ther. 2017;17(9):1089–103.

51. Muller-Ladner U, Gay S. MMPs and rheumatoid synovial fibroblasts: Siamese twins in joint destruction? Ann Rheum Dis. 2002;61(11):957–9.

52. Takayanagi H, Iizuka H, Juji T, Nakagawa T, Yamamoto A, Miyazaki T, Koshihara Y, Oda H, Nakamura K, Tanaka S. Involvement of receptor activator of nuclear factor kappaB ligand/osteoclast differentiation factor in osteoclastogenesis from synoviocytes in rheumatoid arthritis. Arthritis Rheum. 2000;43(2):259–69.

53. Okada Y, Takeuchi N, Tomita K, Nakanishi I, Nagase H. Immunolocalization of matrix metalloproteinase 3 (stromelysin) in rheumatoid synovioblasts (B cells): correlation with rheumatoid arthritis. Ann Rheum Dis. 1989;48(8):645–53.

54. Okada Y, Gonoji Y, Nakanishi I, Nagase H, Hayakawa T. Immunohistochemical demonstration of collagenase and tissue inhibitor of metalloproteinases (TIMP) in synovial lining cells of rheumatoid synovium. Virchows Archiv B, Cell Pathol Incl Mol Pathol. 1990;59(5):305–12.

55. Rutkauskaite E, Zacharias W, Schedel J, Muller-Ladner U, Mawrin C, Seemayer CA, Alexander D, Gay RE, Aicher WK, Michel BA, et al. Ribozymes that inhibit the production of matrix metalloproteinase 1 reduce the invasiveness of rheumatoid arthritis synovial fibroblasts. Arthritis Rheum. 2004;50(5):1448–56.

56. Ogata Y, Enghild JJ, Nagase H. Matrix metalloproteinase 3 (stromelysin) activates the precursor for the human matrix metalloproteinase 9. J Biol Chem. 1992;267(6):3581–4.

57. Schett G, Hayer S, Zwerina J, Redlich K, Smolen JS. Mechanisms of disease: the link between RANKL and arthritic bone disease. Nat Clin Pract Rheumatol. 2005;1(1):47–54.

58. Lee HY, Jeon HS, Song EK, Han MK, Park SI, Lee SI, Yun HJ, Kim JR, Kim JS, Lee YC, et al. CD40 ligation of rheumatoid synovial fibroblasts regulates RANKL-mediated osteoclastogenesis: evidence of NF-kappaB-dependent, CD40-mediated bone destruction in rheumatoid arthritis. Arthritis Rheum. 2006;54(6):1747–58.

59. Lee YR, Lee JH, Noh EM, Kim EK, Song MY, Jung WS, Park SJ, Kim JS, Park JW, Kwon KB, et al. Guggulsterone blocks IL-1beta-mediated inflammatory responses by suppressing NF-kappaB activation in fibroblast-like synoviocytes. Life Sci. 2008;82(23–24):1203–9.

60. Li N, Xu Q, Liu Q, Pan D, Jiang Y, Liu M, Liu X, Lin C. Leonurine attenuates fibroblast-like synoviocyte-mediated synovial inflammation and joint destruction in rheumatoid arthritis. Rheumatology. 2017;56(8):1417–27.

61. Lee EJ, So MW, Hong S, Kim YG, Yoo B, Lee CK. Interleukin-33 acts as a transcriptional repressor and extracellular cytokine in fibroblast-like synoviocytes in patients with rheumatoid arthritis. Cytokine. 2016;77:35–43.

62. Gao QF, Zhang XH, Yuan FL, Zhao MD, Li X. Recombinant human endostatin inhibits TNF-alpha-induced receptor activator of NF-kappaB ligand expression in fibroblast-like synoviocytes in mice with adjuvant arthritis. Cell Biol Int. 2016;40(12):1340–8.

63. Firestein GS. Invasive fibroblast-like synoviocytes in rheumatoid arthritis. Passive responders or transformed aggressors? Arthritis Rheum. 1996; 39(11):1781–90.

64. Weissman AM. Themes and variations on ubiquitylation. Nat Rev Mol Cell Biol. 2001;2(3):169–78.

65. Massoumi R, Chmielarska K, Hennecke K, Pfeifer A, Fassler R. Cyld inhibits tumor cell proliferation by blocking Bcl-3-dependent NF-kappaB signaling. Cell. 2006;125(4):665–77.

19

Serum biomarker for diagnostic evaluation of pulmonary arterial hypertension in systemic sclerosis

Lisa M. Rice[1*], Julio C. Mantero[1], Eric A. Stratton[1], Rod Warburton[2], Kari Roberts[2], Nicholas Hill[2], Robert W. Simms[1], Robyn Domsic[3], Harrison W. Farber[1] and Robert Layfatis[3]

Abstract

Background: Systemic sclerosis-associated pulmonary arterial hypertension (SSc-PAH) is one of the leading causes of death in SSc. Identification of a serum-based proteomic diagnostic biomarker for SSc-PAH would allow for rapid non-invasive screening and could positively impact patient survival. Identification and validation of novel proteins could potentially facilitate the identification of SSc-PAH, and might also point to important protein mediators in pathogenesis.

Methods: Thirteen treatment-naïve SSc-PAH patients had serum collected at time of diagnosis and were used as the discovery cohort for the protein-expression biomarker. Two proteins, Midkine and Follistatin-like 3 (FSTL3) were then validated by enzyme-linked immunosorbent assays. Midkine and FSTL3 were tested in combination to identify SSc-PAH and were validated in two independent cohorts of SSc-PAH ($n = 23$, $n = 11$).

Results: Eighty-two proteins were found to be differentially regulated in SSc-PAH sera. Two proteins (Midkine and FSTL3) were also shown to be elevated in publicly available data and their expression was evaluated in independent cohorts. In the validation cohorts, the combination of Midkine and FSTL3 had an area under the receiver operating characteristic curve (AUC) of 0.85 and 0.92 with respective corresponding measures of sensitivity of 76% and 91%, and specificity measures of 76% and 80%.

Conclusions: These findings indicate that there is a clear delineation between overall protein expression in sera from SSc patients and those with SSc-PAH. The combination of Midkine and FSTL3 can serve as an SSc-PAH biomarker and are potential drug targets for this rare disease population.

Keywords: Classification, Proteomic, Scleroderma, Biomarkers, Pulmonary arterial hypertension

Background

Cardiopulmonary involvement is the most common cause of morbidity and mortality in patients with systemic sclerosis (SSc). Twelve percent of SSc patients will develop SSc-associated pulmonary arterial hypertension (SSc-PAH); these patients have an estimated 50% 3-year survival [1]. Early and accurate diagnosis of PAH is clinically challenging and relies on right heart catheterization (RHC). RHC is invasive, is not suitable for screening, and so is typically performed only on patients with a high index of suspicion

based on echocardiogram and other criteria that are neither highly sensitive nor specific [2–4].

Earlier diagnosis and treatment with PAH-specific therapeutics is associated with better outcomes in patients with SSc-PAH [5, 6]. Thus, identification of a diagnostic biomarker that would allow for rapid non-invasive screening could positively impact patient survival, supplement current screening methods, and potentially reduce the need for diagnostic RHC.

Transthoracic echocardiography is the most widely accepted screening tool for the diagnosis of SSc-PAH. Echocardiographically estimated systolic PAP (sPAP) correlates reasonably ($r = 0.83$) with RHC [7], though it has potential limitations including an ~ 45% false positive rate [8–10]. Echocardiogram has also been studied

---

* Correspondence: lisarice@bu.edu
[1]Boston University School of Medicine, E5 Arthritis Center, 72 E Concord Street, Boston, MA 0211, USA
Full list of author information is available at the end of the article

in combination with other measures. PAH biomarkers such as brain natriuretic peptide (BNP) and the N-terminal fragment of pro-BNP (NT-proBNP) have similar diagnostic accuracy as the echocardiogram [11]. Natriuretic peptide levels of have been shown to correlate with hemodynamic measurements, predict disease prognosis and mortality among those with PAH [12]. They are also generally specific for SSc-PAH, but lack sensitivity [13]. As such, other potential biomarkers, such as osteopontin, pentraxin 3, C-reactive protein (CRP), interleukin (IL)1, IL8 and tumor necrosis factor alpha (TNFα) have been investigated as diagnostic tools. In preliminary studies, some have appeared superior to both BNP and NT-proBNP [14–17]. However, these findings are tempered by the fact that they are single studies and have yet to be validated.

The clinical use of gene expression for classifying different biological disease states is well established [18]. We have previously described SSc-PAH associated gene-expression patterns in peripheral blood mononuclear cells (PBMCs) that highlight IFN-regulation and monocyte/macrophage activation in disease pathogenesis [17, 19]. Thus, we hypothesized that wide-scale proteomic studies of serum might identify a diagnostic biomarker of SSc-PAH. This hypothesis was further supported by our previous small proteomic study, in which we identified 17 cytokines associated with SSc-PAH [17].

In the present study, we utilized a proteomic technology to identify novel proteins specific to the diagnosis of SSc-PAH. We show that in combination, Follistatin-like 3 (FSTL3) and Midkine (MDK) are highly diagnostic for SSc-PAH, and have validated these biomarkers in two independent cohorts. These results suggest that serum assays in patients with PAH could be dramatically improved with identification of these serum biomarkers and, thus, aid in the earlier diagnosis of SSc-PAH.

Methods

Patient selection

Institutional review boards at Boston University, University of Pittsburgh, and Tufts University approved the collection of all serum samples and clinical data. Written informed consent was obtained from all patients before sample collection. Diagnosis of PAH was made by RHC: mean pulmonary artery pressure (mPAP) of ≥ 25 mmHg, a pulmonary capillary wedge pressure of ≤ 15 mmHg, and a pulmonary vascular resistance of ≥ 3 Wood units [20]. Diagnosis of SSc was made by a rheumatologist and date of disease onset is recorded as date of first non-Raynaud's symptom. There are two subcategories of SSc, limited cutaneous systemic sclerosis (lcSSc) and diffuse cutaneous

systemic sclerosis (dcSSc). This distinction is based on extent and location of skin disease. The majority of patients included in this study were lcSSc patients with limited skin disease, any exceptions are noted in the detailed description of each patient cohort included. All samples in the discovery cohort ($n = 13$) were collected at Boston University. Patients had limited skin disease (lcSSc) and were PAH treatment-naïve. Sera were collected at time of diagnostic RHC and were analyzed by SOMAscan (SomaLogic Boulder, CO, USA), which allowed for the capability to examine 1129 proteins simultaneously. Sixteen subjects with lcSSc and no clinical evidence of PAH (medical records were reviewed by a clinical expert in the field, forced vital capacity [FVC] > 70%, negative RHC, or no record of an abnormal finding on an echocardiograph) or interstitial lung disease (ILD), diagnosed by high-resolution CT scans (HRCTs), served as controls. Protein data were analyzed for differences in lcSSc-PAH patients (Wilcoxon signed-rank test). Analytes for further study were selected based on the q values (false discovery rates [FDR] < 0.1). These parsed analytes were clustered and visualized using the R environment for statistical computing (version 3.2.1). The clustering was unsupervised and used Spearman's correlation and average linkage. Identification of pathways linked to the differentially expressed proteins was performed using Qiagen's Ingenuity Pathway Analysis (IPA, Qiagen, Redwood City, CA, USA). Subjects in validation cohorts diagnosed with ILD based on HRCTs were included when measured FVC was > 70%. The discovery cohort was from Boston University, and the validation cohort one was from both Tufts University as well as Boston University and validation cohort two was from University of Pittsburgh.

Subjects enrolled with signed informed written consent by the institutional review board of Boston University also included patients with dcSSc, as well as lcSSc subjects showing evidence of ILD (confirmed by HRCT) and healthy controls. Sera from these subjects were also analyzed by SOMAScan, after collection into a serum separator tube, allowed to clot, aliquoted, and stored at –80 °C.

ELISA validations and statistical analysis

Concentrations of candidate proteins were measured in duplicate using commercial ELISA kits for FSTL3 (DFLRG0: R&D Systems, Minneapolis, MN, USA), or for MDK (ab193761: Abcam, Cambridge, MA, USA).

Putative biomarker protein concentrations were log2-transformed to better approximate a normal distribution and obtain reliable odds ratio (OR) estimates [21]. Wilcoxon signed-rank test were used to test the difference in SSc analyte concentrations from lcSSc-PAH. Models of discreet variables were developed using logistic regression and multiple logistic regression. Sensitivity and specificity of discrete variables were assessed using receiver operating characteristic (ROC) curves, plotting the sensitivity on the y-axis and 1-specificity on the x-axis. The area under the curve (AUC) of a ROC was computed to provide a global measure of performance and for comparing biomarker performance, with AUC of 0.90–.1 considered excellent, 0.80–0.90 considered good, 0.7–0.8 considered fair, 0.6–0.7 considered poor, 0.5–0.06 considered without value. Youden's J statistic was used to calculate the best threshold level of the biomarker that gives equal weight to sensitivity and specificity [22].

Publicly available gene expression data were downloaded from GEO: http://www.ncbi.nlm.nih.gov/geo/. The data included five data sets with relevant SSc subpopulations. The first data set was derived from the peripheral blood mononuclear cells (PBMCs) of lcSSc subjects with ($n = 15$) and without ($n = 21$) PAH. The data set was downloaded from GEO accession number GSE19617 [17]. A second data set from the PBMCs of PAH subjects including a systemic sclerosis subset. The data was downloaded from GEO accession number GSE33463 [23]. lcSSc subjects were with ($n = 37$) and without ($n = 19$) PAH. The third data set was derived from PBMCs of patients with SSc-PAH ($n = 10$) and SSc without ($n = 10$). The data set was downloaded with the GEO accession number GSE22356 [24]. The second type of data was derived from lung tissue from transplant subjects, there were $n = 6$ Ssc subjects with PAH and $n = 9$ subjects with normal lungs. The data set was downloaded with the GEO accession number GSE48149 [25]. The third type of data was derived from skin tissue of SSc subjects ($n = 61$) and healthy controls ($n = 36$). The data set

Table 1 Clinical characteristics

Baseline demographics	Discovery cohort		Validation cohort 1		Validation cohort 2	
	lcSSc-PAH	lcSSc-no PAH	lcSSc-PAH	lcSSc-no PAH	lcSSc-PAH	lcSSc-no PAH
Age (year)	$n = 13$	$n = 16$	$n = 23$	$n = 12$	$n = 11$	$n = 18$
Mean (SD)	65 (7.4)	50 (14)	66 (8.6)	54 (17.8)	66 (9.4)	62 (8.5)
Median (range)	65 (56–81)	57 (25–70)	64 (52–85)	52 (26–76)	66 (52–81)	63 (46–79)
Sex						
Female, % (n)	92% (12)	87.5% (14)	83% (19)	92% (11)	100% (11)	83% (15)
Male,% (n)	8% (1)	12.5% (2)	17% (4)	8% (1)	0% (0)	17% (3)
mPAP (mmHg)						
Mean (SD)	46 (9.1)	–	42 (12.3)	–	40 (10.8)	–
Median (range)	45 (34–68)	–	43 (26–69)	–	42 (25–54)	–
mPCWP (mmHg)						
Mean (SD)	10 (2.7)	–	10 (4.3)	–	10 (3.2)	–
Median (range)	11 (4–14)	–	11 (1–15)	–	9 (5–15)	–
PVR (Woods units)						
Mean (SD)	9 (4.9)	–	8 (5.3)	–	8 (4.1)[a]	–
Median (range)	8 (5–24)	–	6 (3–27)	–	7 (3–13)[a]	–
ILD (Dx by HRCT)						
Positive, % (n)	7% (1)	–	13% (3)	–	0% (0)	–
Negative, % (n)	83% (12)	–	87% (20)	–	100% (11)	–
Treatment						
Treated, % (n)	0% (0)	–	48% (11)	≈	100% (11)	–
Untreated, % (n)	100% (13)	–	52% (12)	–	0% (0)	–
BNP (pg/mL)						
Mean (SD)	261 (313)	–	411 (494)	–	–	–
Median (range)	140 (42–1054)	–	148 (12–1630)	–	–	–
Date of sample						
At time of RHC, % (n)	100% (13)	–	91% (21)	–	36% (4)	–

[a]Missing values

BNP, brain natriuretic peptide; lcSSc-PAH, limited cutaneous systemic sclerosis pulmonary arterial hypertension; ILD, interstitial lung disease; mPAP, mean pulmonary artery pressure; mPCWP, mean pulmonary capillary wedge pressure; PVR, pulmonary vascular resistance; RHC, right heart catheterization

was downloaded with the GEO accession number GSE58095 [26].

Results

Pathway analysis of protein expression

SOMAScan protein expression was evaluated in sera from 13 subjects with lcSSc-PAH and 16 subjects with lcSSc and no clinical evidence of PAH (Table 1). Detailed hemodynamic data are found in Additional file 1: Table S1.

Eighty-two proteins were found to be differentially regulated in lcSSc-PAH patients compared to lcSSc controls (FDR q ≤ 0.1, summarized in Additional file 2: Table S2. Of the 82 proteins that were significantly different between comparing subjects with lcSSc-PAH to lcSSc-no PAH 32 were increased and 50 decreased. Analytes meeting these criteria were analyzed by unsupervised clustering for both proteins and subjects. lcSSc-PAH and lcSSc controls clustered independently (Fig. 1). An unfiltered clustering

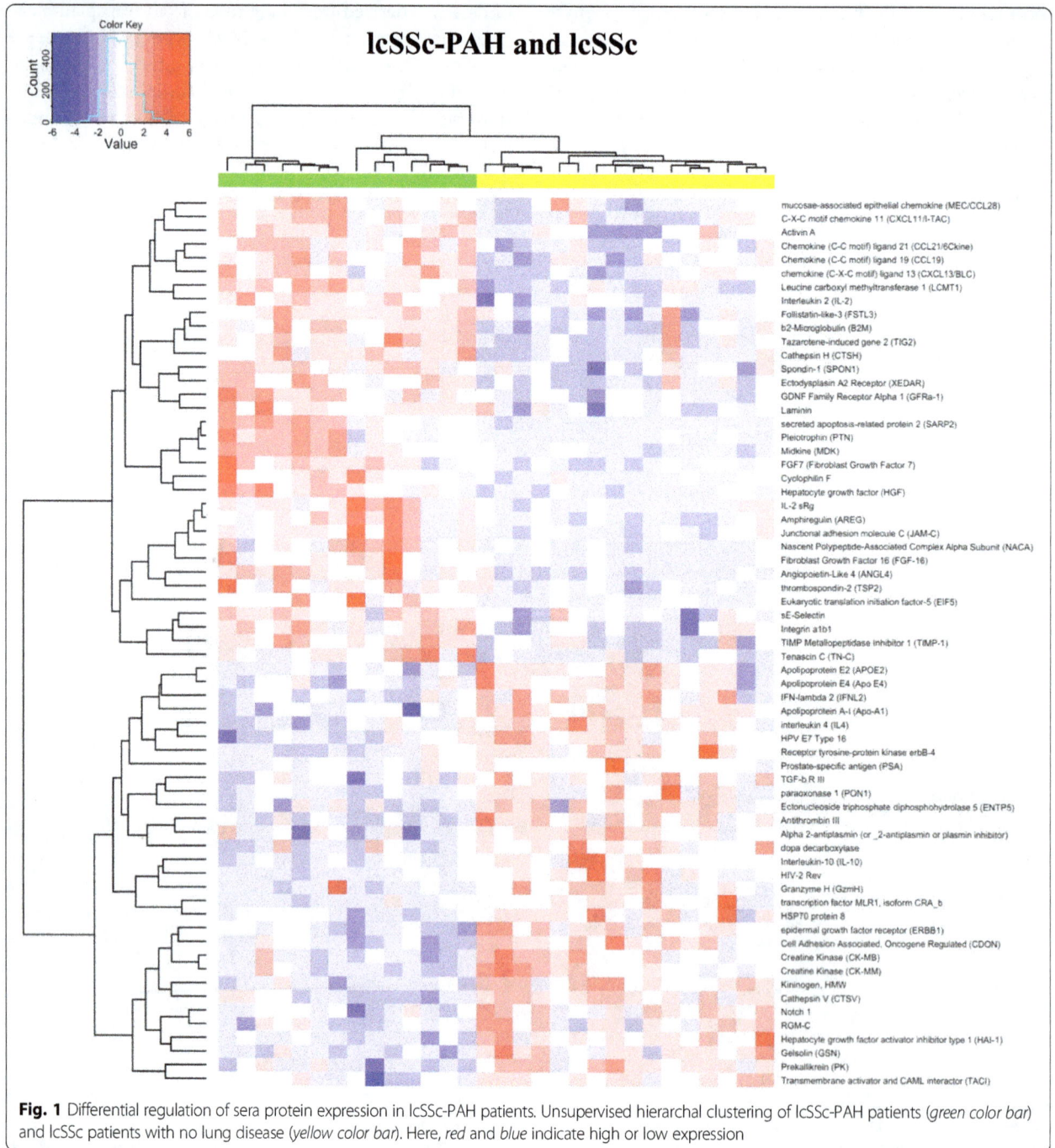

Fig. 1 Differential regulation of sera protein expression in lcSSc-PAH patients. Unsupervised hierarchal clustering of lcSSc-PAH patients (*green color bar*) and lcSSc patients with no lung disease (*yellow color bar*). Here, *red* and *blue* indicate high or low expression

diagram of all the measured proteins was also examined. The presence of PAH was the dominant signal in the serum proteome, as all the lcSSc-PAH cases clustered together without any structured stratification of groups (Additional file 3: Figure S1).

We mined publicly available data to identify which proteins of the 82 had been previously observed as differentially regulated in skin and lung tissue or PBMCs of SSc-PAH patients (Additional file 4: Table S3). The search yielded 16 proteins with corresponding differential expression by either fold change, absolute value log2 fold-change > 1 or adjusted *p* value ≤ 0.1 (*p* value was adjusted by Benjamini-Hochberg). About half of the identified proteins were related to the extracellular matrix including SFRP1, TNC, and TIMP1. Some immune markers were also seen

as differentially regulated across data sets including complement decay-accelerating factor (CD55), CD36, CD27, and CCL19 [17, 24]. MDK was the only protein previously observed to also be differentially regulated at the mRNA level in lung tissue [25].

The 82 proteins that were differentially regulated between lcSSc-PAH and lcSSc-no PAH controls were explored in greater depth by pathway analysis. There was a cluster of chemokine signaling molecules activated including CCL19, CXCL13, CXCL11, CCL28, and CCL21, as well as several transforming growth factor beta (TGF-β) regulated molecules including FSTL3 and Spondin-1. Using IPA several activated upstream regulators were identified within the data, including a strong interferon gamma (IFN-γ) signature (Fig. 2).

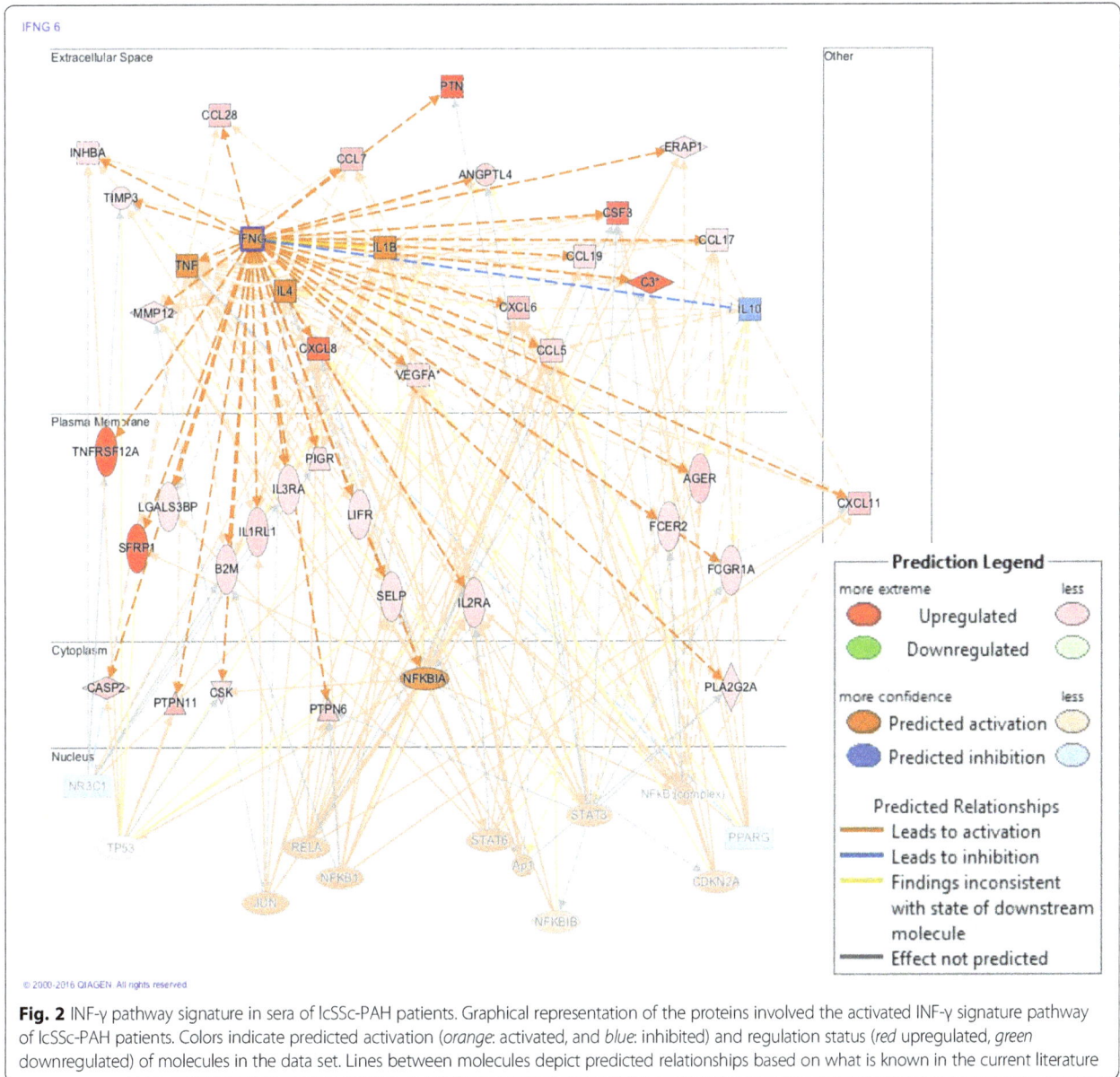

Fig. 2 INF-γ pathway signature in sera of lcSSc-PAH patients. Graphical representation of the proteins involved the activated INF-γ signature pathway of lcSSc-PAH patients. Colors indicate predicted activation (*orange*: activated, and *blue*: inhibited) and regulation status (*red* upregulated, *green* downregulated) of molecules in the data set. Lines between molecules depict predicted relationships based on what is known in the current literature

Putative biomarker selection and validation

Five of the proteins upregulated in lcSSc-PAH sera (FSTL3, Spondin-1, junctional adhesion molecule C (JAM-C), CCL28, and MDK) were investigated further for their individual ability to discriminate between subjects with lcSSc-PAH and lcSSc-no PAH in silico (logistic regression) based on biological relevance, their presence in different clusters and average fold change > 2 (Additional file 5: Figure S2). FSTL3 and MDK had nearly equal areas under the curve (AUC: 0.90 and 0.89). However, FSTL3 performed better then MDK when high sensitivity was required, and MDK performed better then FSTL3 when high specificity was required. Additionally, MDK and FSTL3 did not correlate with each other or with BNP (Additional file 6: Figure S3). This suggested that in combination these proteins would give additional information to the currently measured BNP. These proteins were investigated in combination using a generalized linear model. MDK and FSTL3 were also examined in other clinical subgroups of systemic sclerosis and were shown to be specifically upregulated compared to dcSSc, lcSSc-ILD (diagnosed by HRCT) (Fig. 3), healthy controls were included for reference.

The ability to discriminate between lcSSc subjects with and without PAH using Midkine and FSTL3 was confirmed by enzyme-linked immunosorbent assay (ELISA) on the patients originally analyzed by SOMAscan. Both proteins were elevated in subjects with SSc-PAH compared to those without PAH, and when modeled together using multiple logistic regression showed an increase in discriminatory power (Additional file 7: Figure S4).

Sera from two validation cohorts were then used to test the discrimination of Midkine and FSTL3 for lcSSc-PAH. Clinical characteristics in the validation cohorts were similar but not identical to the test cohort (Table 1, Additional file 1: Table S1 and Additional file 7: Table S4). In the validation cohorts not all samples were collected on the day of diagnostic RHC; as such, some patients were being treated for PAH. Additionally, some patients had other pulmonary complications, such as ILD. Yet, both cohorts demonstrated a consistent and significant increase ($p < 0.01$) in both FSTL3 and MDK protein concentrations in SSc-PAH patients compared to lcSSc-no PAH (Fig. 4). Logistic and multiple logistic models were created based on protein concentrations (Fig. 5). In the discovery cohort, the biomarker had an area under the ROC curve (AUC) of 0.94 (95% confidence interval (CI) 81 to 95), a sensitivity of 99%, and a specificity of 99%. In the first validation cohort, the biomarker had an AUC of 85% (95% CI 67 to 94), a sensitivity of 76%, and a specificity of 76%. In the second validation cohort, the biomarker had an AUC of 92% (95% CI 77 to 95), a sensitivity of 91%, and a specificity of 80%.

The discovery cohort was comprised of all untreated patients and one subject with ILD, while the second validation cohort was comprised of all treated patients with no subjects with ILD (Table 1, Additional file 1: Table S1, and Additional file 8: Table S4). However, the

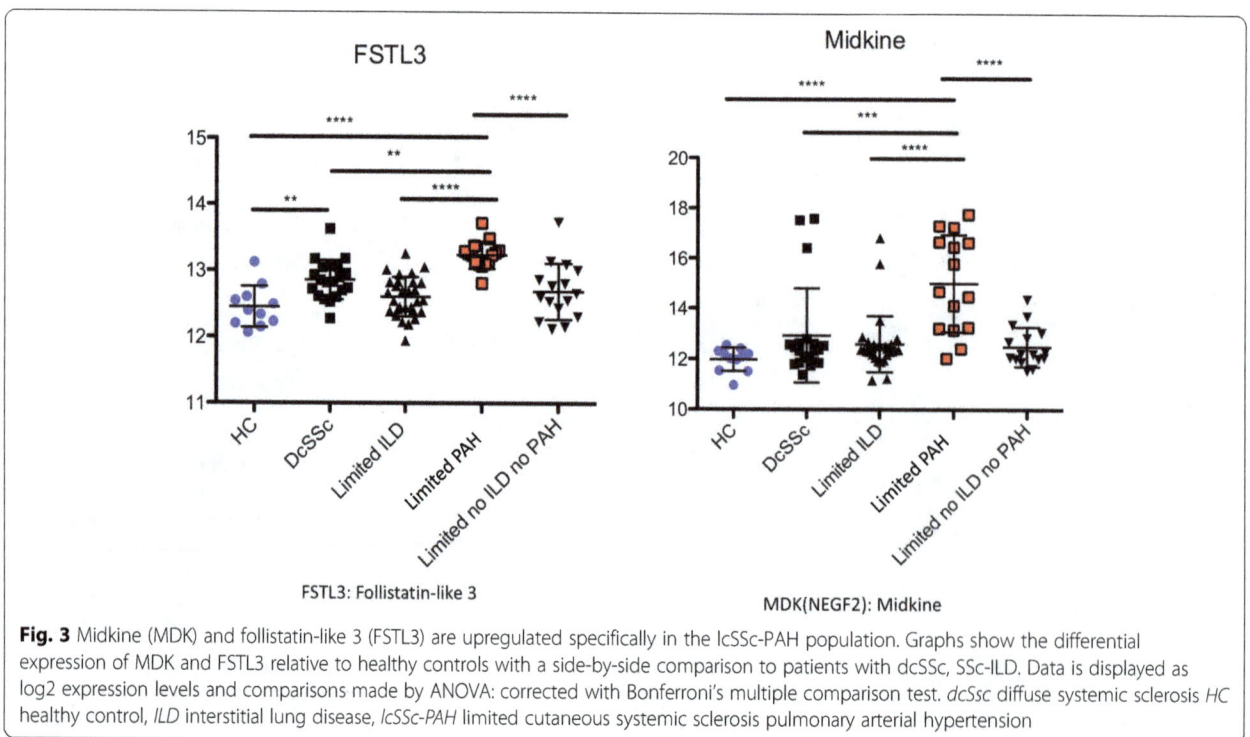

FSTL3: Follistatin-like 3

MDK(NEGF2): Midkine

Fig. 3 Midkine (MDK) and follistatin-like 3 (FSTL3) are upregulated specifically in the lcSSc-PAH population. Graphs show the differential expression of MDK and FSTL3 relative to healthy controls with a side-by-side comparison to patients with dcSSc, SSc-ILD. Data is displayed as log2 expression levels and comparisons made by ANOVA: corrected with Bonferroni's multiple comparison test. *dcSsc* diffuse systemic sclerosis *HC* healthy control, *ILD* interstitial lung disease, *lcSSc-PAH* limited cutaneous systemic sclerosis pulmonary arterial hypertension

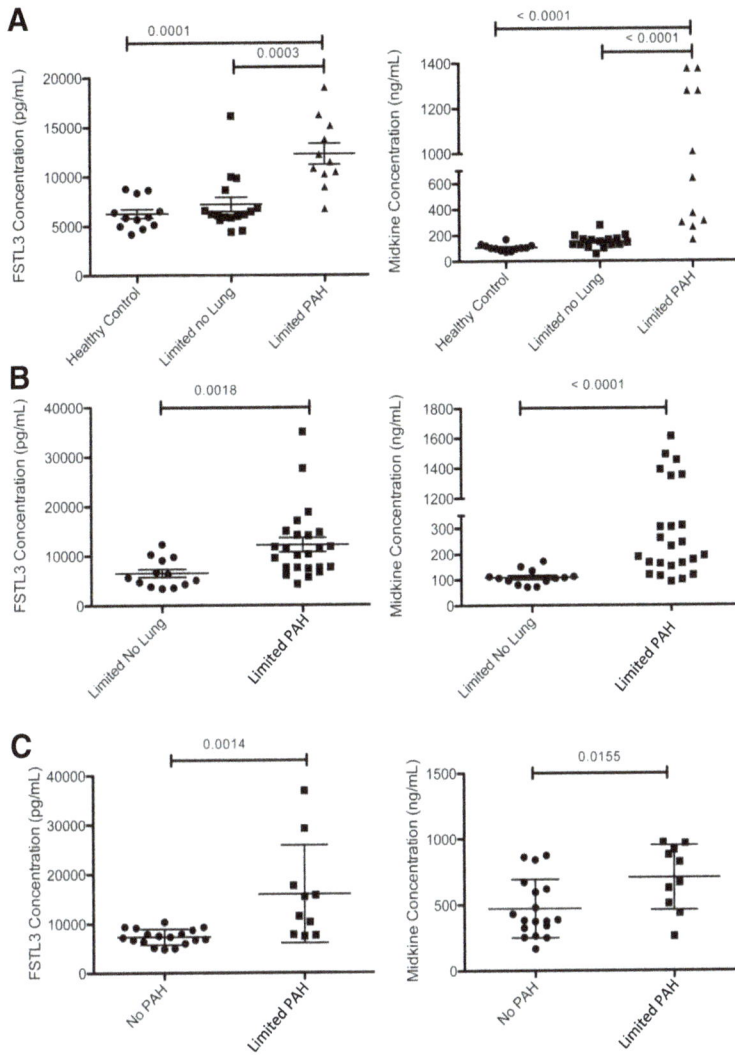

Fig. 4 ELISA validation cohort data. Graphs show differences (Wilcoxon signed-rank test) of lcSSc-PAH Follistatin-like 3 (FSTL3), and Midkine (MDK) protein concentrations as compared to SSc patients with no lung disease in the test cohort (A) as well as two independent validation cohorts (B and C). *PAH* pulmonary arterial hypertension

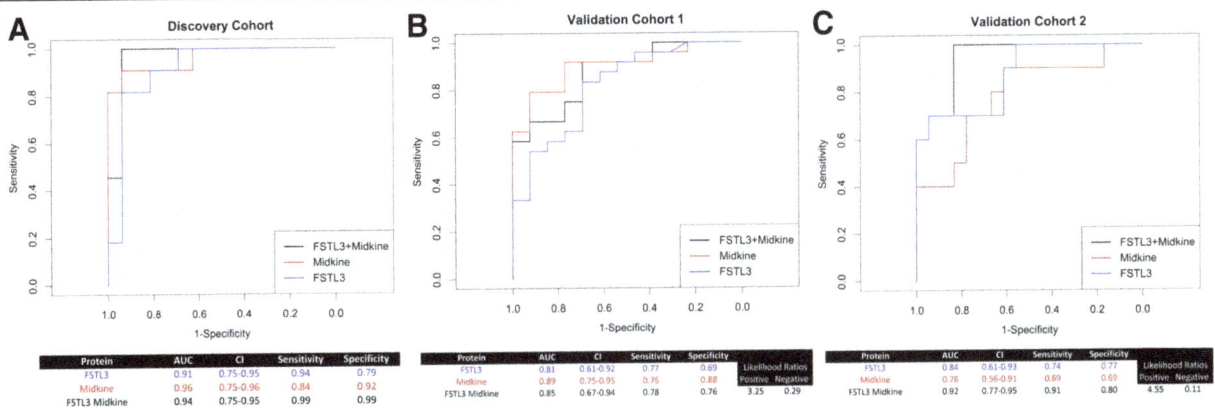

Fig. 5 Receiver operator characteristic curves of ELISA data. Graphs show differences Receiver operator characteristic curves of lcSSc-PAH follistatin-like 3 (FSTL3), and Midkine (MDK) protein concentrations as well as the two in combination as compared to lcSSc patients with no lung disease in the test cohort (A) as well as two independent validation cohorts (B and C)

first validation cohort had a mix of treated ($n = 11$) and untreated ($n = 12$) subjects as well as a mix of subjects with ($n = 3$) and without ($n = 20$) ILD (Table 1, Additional file 8: Table S4). After excluding subjects with ILD and patients treated for PAH, FSTL3 and MDK remained elevated ($p < 0.05$) in SSc-PAH patients compared to lcSSc-no PAH (Additional file 9: Figure S5). However, exclusion of these patients did not increase the parameters of the ROCs, with the AUC including all the patients remaining the highest at 85% (Additional file 9: Figure S5).

Discussion

Investigation into the circulating proteome of lcSSc-PAH allowed for the identification of multiple putative biomarkers. Our results show a circulating serum protein pattern that is associated with lcSSc-PAH compared to lcSSc-no PAH, thus identifying a potential serum proteomic biomarker for use in the diagnostic evaluation of lcSSc-PAH. In sum, we demonstrated that the combination of FSTL3 and MDK are highly associated with lcSSc-PAH.

Our results show that 82 circulating serum proteins are associated with lcSSc-PAH compared to lcSSc-no PAH; this data set allowed us a unique opportunity to examine potential upstream regulators of these proteins. Within those 82 differentially regulated proteins, there were a number of activated chemokines, CCL19, CXCL13, and CCL21, which are implicated in tertiary lymphoid structures [27]. In addition, many of the up-regulated proteins are regulated by INF-γ, thus confirming previously published gene-expression patterns that observed INF regulation in PBMCs of SSc-PAH [19].

From these 82 differentially regulated proteins, we showed that the combination of FSTL3 and MDK are highly associated for SSc-PAH in the independent cohorts, with an average sensitivity of 84% and an average specificity of 79%. These findings are plausible pathophysiologically. FSTL3, a TGF-β regulated protein, inhibits the protective actions of activin A on cardiac myocytes. We also previously observed that FSTL3 is elevated, compared to healthy controls, in the sera, PBMCs, and skin of patients with dcSSc [28]. The growth factor, MDK, has been implicated in the pathogenesis of hypertension, kidney disease, and lung fibrosis [29–31].

The lack of effect of various treatments in the validation data sets on biomarker performance suggests that this is a robust diagnostic biomarker. Also, that the roles of these biomarkers are upstream from the pathophysiologic processes affected by vasodilators, the most commonly available therapeutics. Additionally, some patients had radiographic evidence of ILD as well as SSc-PAH. The effect of ILD and PAH treatment was tested in a small subset of patients in validation cohort one. Including patients with ILD also bestowed no additional benefit to the diagnostic capabilities of FSTL3 and MDK.

Some samples were not collected at the time of diagnostic RHC (Table 1 and Additional file 9: Table S4) and thus the relationship between biomarker and clinical disease is less certain in these cases. In spite of this, there was still a significant increase in MDK and FSTL3 among patients with SSc-PAH. Of particular interest are those patients whose sera was collected prior to PAH diagnosis suggesting that these biomarkers might be elevated before PAH is clinically suspected. There has not been investigation of MDK or FSTL3 in other subset of SSc patients who might have increased concentrations of those specific proteins, such as patients with cardiac involvement or renal disease.

Conclusions

In sum, we have identified serum proteins that are strongly associated with SSc-PAH. Further investigation of these and other proteins has the potential to improve the diagnosis, care, and outcomes in this clinically challenging PAH subset.

Abbreviations

AUC: Area under the receiver operating characteristic curve; BNP: Brain natriuretic peptide; dcSSc: Diffuse systemic sclerosis; FDR: False discovery rate; FSTL3: Follistatin-like 3; FVC: Forced vital capacity; HRCT: High-resolution CT scan; ILD: Interstitial lung disease; INF-γ: Interferon gamma; lcSSc: Limited cutaneous systemic sclerosis; MDK: Midkine; mPAP: Mean pulmonary artery pressure; NT-proBNP: N-terminal fragment of pro-BNP; PBMC: Peripheral blood mononuclear cell; RHC: Right heart catheterization; ROC: Receiver operating characteristic curve; sPAP: Systolic PAP; SSc: Systemic sclerosis; SSc-PAH: Systemic sclerosis-associated pulmonary arterial hypertension; TNF-β: Transforming growth factor beta

Funding

This work was supported by National Institutes of Health, National Institute of Arthritis Musculoskeletal and Skin Disease grants; Scleroderma Core Centers (5P30AR061271), Scleroderma Center of Research Translation (1P50AR060780) and 2R01AR051089 to RL.

Authors' contributions

LMR and JCM contributed to interpretation, design, analysis, and acquisition. RL and HF contributed to conception, interpretation, and acquisition. ES, RW, KR, NH, RS, and RD contributed to acquisition. All authors participated in writing, reading, and approving the final manuscript.

Consent for publication

The manuscript does not contain any individual person's data in any form.

Competing interests

The authors declare that they have no competing interests.

Author details

[1]Boston University School of Medicine, E5 Arthritis Center, 72 E Concord Street, Boston, MA 0211, USA. [2]Tufts University, Boston, MA, USA. [3]University of Pittsburgh Medical Center, Pittsburgh, PA, USA.

References

1. Chaisson NF, Hassoun PM. Systemic sclerosis-associated pulmonary arterial hypertension. Chest. 2013;144(4):1346–56. https://doi.org/10.1378/chest.12-2396. published Online First: Epub Date
2. Chung L, Domsic RT, Lingala B, et al. Survival and predictors of mortality in systemic sclerosis-associated pulmonary arterial hypertension: outcomes from the pulmonary hypertension assessment and recognition of outcomes in scleroderma registry. Arthritis Care Res (Hoboken). 66(3):489–95. https://doi.org/10.1002/acr.22121. published Online First: Epub Date
3. Foris V, Kovacs G, Tscherner M, et al. Biomarkers in pulmonary hypertension: what do we know? Chest. 2013;144(1):274–83. https://doi.org/10.1378/chest.12-1246. published Online First: Epub Date
4. Hao Y, Thakkar V, Stevens W, et al. A comparison of the predictive accuracy of three screening models for pulmonary arterial hypertension in systemic sclerosis. Arthritis Res. Ther. 2015;17:7. https://doi.org/10.1186/s13075-015-0517-5. published Online First: Epub Date
5. Proudman SM, Stevens WM, Sahhar J, et al. Pulmonary arterial hypertension in systemic sclerosis: the need for early detection and treatment. Intern. Med. J. 2007;37(7):485–94. https://doi.org/10.1111/j.1445-5994.2007.01370.x. published Online First: Epub Date
6. Task Force for D, Treatment of Pulmonary Hypertension of European Society of C, European Respiratory S, et al. Guidelines for the diagnosis and treatment of pulmonary hypertension. Eur. Respir. J. 2009;34(6):1219–63. https://doi.org/10.1183/09031936.00139009. published Online First: Epub Date
7. Denton CP, Cailes JB, Phillips GD, et al. Comparison of Doppler echocardiography and right heart catheterization to assess pulmonary hypertension in systemic sclerosis. Br J Rheumatol. 1997;36(2):239–43.
8. Fisher MR, Forfia PR, Chamera E, et al. Accuracy of Doppler echocardiography in the hemodynamic assessment of pulmonary hypertension. Am. J. Respir. Crit. Care Med. 2009;179(7):615–21. https://doi.org/10.1164/rccm.200811-1691OC. published Online First: Epub Date
9. Badesch DB, Champion HC, Sanchez MA, et al. Diagnosis and assessment of pulmonary arterial hypertension. J. Am. Coll. Cardiol. 2009;54(1 Suppl):S55–66. https://doi.org/10.1016/j.jacc.2009.04.011. published Online First: Epub Date
10. McGoon M, Gutterman D, Steen V, et al. Screening, early detection, and diagnosis of pulmonary arterial hypertension: ACCP evidence-based clinical practice guidelines. Chest. 2004;126(1 Suppl):14S–34S. https://doi.org/10.1378/chest.126.1_suppl.14S. published Online First: Epub Date
11. Cavagna L, Caporali R, Klersy C, et al. Comparison of brain natriuretic peptide (BNP) and NT-proBNP in screening for pulmonary arterial hypertension in patients with systemic sclerosis. J. Rheumatol. 2010;37(10):2064–70. https://doi.org/10.3899/jrheum.090997. published Online First: Epub Date
12. Mathai SC, Bueso M, Hummers LK, et al. Disproportionate elevation of N-terminal pro-brain natriuretic peptide in scleroderma-related pulmonary hypertension. Eur Respir J. 2010;35(1):95–104. https://doi.org/10.1183/09031936.00074309. published Online First: Epub Date
13. Williams MH, Das C, Handler CE, et al. Systemic sclerosis associated pulmonary hypertension: improved survival in the current era. Heart. 2006;92(7):926–32. https://doi.org/10.1136/hrt.2005.069484. published Online First: Epub Date
14. Lorenzen JM, Nickel N, Kramer R, et al. Osteopontin in patients with idiopathic pulmonary hypertension. Chest. 2011;139(5):1010–7. https://doi.org/10.1378/chest.10-1146. published Online First: Epub Date
15. Malhotra R, Paskin-Flerlage S, Zamanian RT, et al. Circulating angiogenic modulatory factors predict survival and functional class in pulmonary arterial hypertension. Pulm Circ. 2013;3(2):369–80. https://doi.org/10.4103/2045-8932.110445. published Online First: Epub Date
16. Tamura Y, Ono T, Kuwana M, et al. Human pentraxin 3 (PTX3) as a novel biomarker for the diagnosis of pulmonary arterial hypertension. PLoS One. 2012;7(9):e45834. https://doi.org/10.1371/journal.pone.0045834. published Online First: Epub Date
17. Pendergrass SA, Hayes E, Farina G, et al. Limited systemic sclerosis patients with pulmonary arterial hypertension show biomarkers of inflammation and vascular injury. PLoS One. 2010;5(8):e12106. https://doi.org/10.1371/journal.pone.0012106. published Online First: Epub Date
18. Golub TR, Slonim DK, Tamayo P, et al. Molecular classification of cancer: class discovery and class prediction by gene expression monitoring. Science. 1999;286(5439):531–7.
19. Christmann RB, Hayes E, Pendergrass S, et al. Interferon and alternative activation of monocyte/macrophages in systemic sclerosis-associated pulmonary arterial hypertension. Arthritis Rheum. 2011;63(6):1718–28. https://doi.org/10.1002/art.30318. published Online First: Epub Date
20. Simonneau G, Gatzoulis MA, Adatia I, et al. Updated clinical classification of pulmonary hypertension. J. Am. Coll. Cardiol. 2013;62(25 Suppl):D34–41. https://doi.org/10.1016/j.jacc.2013.10.029. published Online First: Epub Date
21. Grund B, Sabin C. Analysis of biomarker data: logs, odds ratios, and receiver operating characteristic curves. Curr Opin HIV AIDS. 2010;5(6):473–9. https://doi.org/10.1097/COH.0b013e32833ed742. published Online First: Epub Date
22. Schisterman EF, Perkins NJ, Liu A, et al. Optimal cut-point and its corresponding Youden index to discriminate individuals using pooled blood samples. Epidemiology. 2005;16(1):73–81.
23. Cheadle C, Berger AE, Mathai SC, et al. Erythroid-specific transcriptional changes in PBMCs from pulmonary hypertension patients. PLoS One. 2012;7(4):e34951. https://doi.org/10.1371/journal.pone.0034951. published Online First: Epub Date
24. Risbano MG, Meadows CA, Coldren CD, et al. Altered immune phenotype in peripheral blood cells of patients with scleroderma-associated pulmonary hypertension. Clin. Transl. Sci. 2010;3(5):210–8. https://doi.org/10.1111/j.1752-8062.2010.00218.x. published Online First: Epub Date
25. Hsu ESH, Jordan RM, Lyons-Weiler J, Pilewski JM, Feghali-Bostwick CA. Lung tissues in patients with systemic sclerosis have gene expression patterns unique to pulmonary fibrosis and pulmonary hypertension. Arthritis Rheum. 2011;63(3):783–94.
26. Assassi S, Swindell WR, Wu M, et al. Dissecting the heterogeneity of skin gene expression patterns in systemic sclerosis. Arthritis Rheumatol. 2015;67(11):3016–26. https://doi.org/10.1002/art.39289. published Online First: Epub Date
27. Ruddle NH. Lymphatic vessels and tertiary lymphoid organs. J. Clin. Invest. 2014;124(3):953–9. https://doi.org/10.1172/JCI71611. published Online First: Epub Date
28. Rice LM, Mantero JC, Stifano G, et al. A Proteome-Derived Longitudinal Pharmacodynamic Biomarker for Diffuse Systemic Sclerosis Skin. J. Invest. Dermatol. 2017;137(1):62–70. https://doi.org/10.1016/j.jid.2016.08.027. published Online First: Epub Date
29. Cohen S, Shachar I. Midkine as a regulator of B cell survival in health and disease. Br. J. Pharmacol. 2014;171(4):888–95. https://doi.org/10.1111/bph.12419. published Online First: Epub Date
30. Sato W, Sato Y. Midkine in nephrogenesis, hypertension and kidney diseases. Br. J. Pharmacol. 2014;171(4):879–87. https://doi.org/10.1111/bph.12418. published Online First: Epub Date
31. Zhang R, Pan Y, Fanelli V, et al. Mechanical Stress and the Induction of Lung Fibrosis via the Midkine Signaling Pathway. Am. J. Respir. Crit. Care Med. 2015;192(3):315–23. https://doi.org/10.1164/rccm.201412-2326OC. published Online First: Epub Date

20

Tofacitinib inhibits granulocyte–macrophage colony-stimulating factor-induced NLRP3 inflammasome activation in human neutrophils

Makiko Yashiro Furuya[1], Tomoyuki Asano[1], Yuya Sumichika[1], Shuzo Sato[1], Hiroko Kobayashi[1], Hiroshi Watanabe[1], Eiji Suzuki[2], Hideko Kozuru[3], Hiroshi Yatsuhashi[3], Tomohiro Koga[4], Hiromasa Ohira[5], Hideharu Sekine[6], Atsushi Kawakami[4] and Kiyoshi Migita[1*]

Abstract

Background: Granulocyte–macrophage colony-stimulating factor (GM-CSF) has emerged as a crucial cytokine that activates myeloid cells to initiate tissue inflammation. However, the molecular actions of GM-CSF against innate immunity are still poorly characterized. Here, we investigated the *in vitro* effects of GM-CSF on the activation of human myeloid lineages, neutrophils, and the underlying intracellular signaling mechanism, including inflammasome activation.

Methods: Human neutrophils were stimulated with GM-CSF in the presence or absence of tofacitinib. The cellular supernatants were analyzed for interleukin-1 beta (IL-1β) and caspase-1 by enzyme-linked immunosorbent assay (ELISA) methods. Pro-IL-1β mRNA expressions in human neutrophils were analyzed by real-time polymerase chain reaction. Protein phosphorylation of neutrophils was assessed by Western blot using phospho-specific antibodies.

Results: Stimulation with GM-CSF alone, but not tumor necrosis factor-alpha, was shown to increase the release of IL-1β and cleaved caspase-1 (p20) from human neutrophils. Tofacitinib, which inhibits GM-CSF–induced Janus kinase 2 (Jak2)-mediated signal transduction, completely abrogated GM-CSF–induced IL-1β and caspase-1 (p20) secretion from neutrophils. GM-CSF stimulation also induced pro-IL-1β mRNA expression in neutrophils and induced NLR family pyrin domain-containing 3 (NLRP3) protein expression. Although tofacitinib pretreatment marginally inhibited GM-CSF–induced pro-IL-1β mRNA expression, tofacitinib completely abrogated NLRP3 protein expression in neutrophils.

Conclusions: These results indicate that GM-CSF signaling induces NLRP3 expression and subsequent IL-1β production by affecting neutrophils, which may cause the activation of innate immunity. Therefore, GM-CSF is a key regulator of the NLRP3 inflammasome and IL-1β production by activating innate immune cells. This process can be blocked by tofacitinib, which interferes with JAK/STAT signaling pathways.

Keywords: Granulocyte–macrophage colony-stimulating factor, Inflammasome, Interleukin-1 beta, Janus kinase, Neutrophils, NLR family pyrin domain-containing 3, Tofacitinib

* Correspondence: migita@fmu.ac.jp
[1]Department of Rheumatology, Fukushima Medical University School of Medicine, 1 Hikarigaoka, Fukushima, Fukushima 960-1295, Japan
Full list of author information is available at the end of the article

Background

Granulocyte–macrophage colony-stimulating factor (GM-CSF) is a hematopoietic growth factor that stimulates the proliferation of granulocytes and macrophages from bone marrow precursor cells [1]. Recent studies suggest that GM-CSF has many pro-inflammatory functions and plays an important role in the development of autoimmune and inflammatory diseases [2]. For example, GM-CSF plays a central role in the pathogenesis of rheumatoid arthritis (RA) by activating the differentiation and survival of macrophages and neutrophils in the rheumatoid synovium [3]. Moreover, a case report showed that the administration of GM-CSF exacerbated RA [4]. Conversely, therapies targeting GM-CSF have been demonstrated to be effective against patients with active RA [5]. These findings suggest that GM-CSF can prime monocyte/macrophage activation and inflammatory cytokine production, leading to a pro-inflammatory network loop that is maintained in rheumatoid synovitis [6].

GM-CSF has also been implicated in the progression of arthritis in mice expressing a transgene encoding human interleukin-1 alpha (IL-1α) [7], indicating a possible link between IL-1 and GM-CSF in inflammatory arthritis. IL-1β is a key cytokine involved in the regulation of immune responses as well as several inflammatory disorders [8]. The secretion of IL-1β, in contrast to that of other inflammatory cytokines, is a tightly controlled two-step process involving the induction of pro-IL-1β and its processing into mature IL-1β by caspase-1, in which NLR family pyrin domain-containing 3 (NLRP3) inflammasome activation plays a critical role [9]. Recent investigations suggest that GM-CSF can act as an enhancer of inflammasome-dependent IL-1β secretion in response to stimuli such as monosodium urate [10]. The GM-CSF receptor is expressed on myeloid cells, including neutrophils. It is a heterodimer of an α-subunit that binds a common β-subunit (c β) [11]. This c β subunit constitutively associates with Janus kinase 2 (JAK2) and undergoes tyrosine phosphorylation prior to the initiation of signaling [12]. Signal transducer and activation of transcription (STAT) is recruited into the cytoplasmic domain of cytokine receptors and is phosphorylated by receptor-associated JAK family kinases [13, 14].

The function of the JAK/STAT signaling pathway in neutrophils and its relationship with IL-1β production are poorly understood. Therefore, this study examined the role of GM-CSF in the cytokine network by determining its effect against neutrophils. We also determined whether an alternation of signal transduction by a JAK inhibitor could regulate the secretion of IL-1β. We report that GM-CSF directly induces IL-1β secretion from neutrophils by activating the NLRP3 inflammasome.

Methods

Reagents

Recombinant human GM-CSF and tumor necrosis factor-alpha (TNF-α) were purchased from PeproTech (Rocky Hill, NJ, USA). Anti-β-actin antibodies were purchased from Santa Cruz Biotechnology Inc. (Dallas, TX, USA). Anti-NLRP3 antibody was purchased from Merck Millipore (Billerica, MA, USA). Human IL-1β and caspase-1 (p20) enzyme-linked immunosorbent assay (ELISA) kits were purchased from R&D Systems (Minneapolis, MN, USA). Human IL-18 ELISA kits were purchased from MBL (Nagoya, Japan). Phospho-specific antibodies against JAK-1 (Tyr1022/1023), JAK-2 (Tyr1007/1008), STAT-5 (Tyr701), and STAT-3 (Tyr705) were purchased from Cell Signaling Technology (Beverly, MA, USA). Phospho-specific antibody against JAK3 (Tyr980) was purchased from Santa Cruz Biotechnology (Santa Cruz, CA, USA). Anti-phospho-1κB-α (Ser32), anti-phospho-NF-κB p65 (Ser536), anti-IκBα, and anti-NF-κB antibodies were purchased from Cell Signaling Technology (Danvers, MA, USA). Anti-phospho-specific Asc (Tyr-144) antibody was purchased from ECM Biosciences (Versailles, KY, USA). Anti-caspase-1 antibody (14F468) was purchased from Novus Biologics (Littleton, CO, USA). Tofacitinib was purchased from Sigma-Aldrich (Tokyo, Japan).

Neutrophil isolation

Venous peripheral blood was collected from healthy volunteers. Written informed consent for blood donation was obtained from each individual. The blood was layered on a Polymorphprep TM (Axis-Shield, Oslo, Norway) cushion and cells were isolated in accordance with the protocol of the manufacturer. Briefly, neutrophils were isolated on the basis of density, washed once in 0.5 N RPMI-1640 to restore osmolality, and then washed once more in RPMI-1640. Using this procedure, we obtained higher purity of $CD13^+$ neutrophils. The cells were subsequently diluted in complete medium consisting of RPMI-1640.

ELISA and Western blot analysis

Neutrophils $(2 \times 10^6/mL)$ were seeded in 24-well plates containing RPMI1640 supplemented with 10% heat-inactivated fetal bovine serum and stimulated with TNF-α or GM-CSF. Cell-free supernatants were collected by centrifugation at $400g$ for 5 min and assayed for IL-1β or caspase-1 (p20) using ELISA kits. Caspase-1 p20 detection was carried out by using a commercially available ELISA kit (Quntikine human caspase-1 p20, R&D Systems) in which monoclonal antibody specific to the p20 subunit of caspase-1 was pre-coated onto a microplate as captured antibody and bounded caspase-1 are detected by another p20-specific polyclonal antibody.

Reverse transcription–polymerase chain reaction

Total RNA was extracted from neutrophils by using the RNeasy total RNA isolation protocol (Qiagen, Crawley, UK) in accordance with the protocol of the manufacturer. First-strand cDNA was synthesized from 1 μg of total cellular RNA by using an RNA polymerase chain reaction kit (Takara Bio Inc., Otsu, Japan) with random primers. Thereafter, cDNA was amplified by using specific primers respectively. The amplification of the IL-1β transcripts was also accomplished on a Light Cycler (Roche Diagnostics, Mannheim, Germany) by using specific primers. The housekeeping gene fragment of glyceraldehydes-3-phosphates dehydrogenase (GAPDH) was used for verification of equal loading.

Cell lysis and Western blotting

Freshly isolated neutrophils were stimulated with GM-CSF (50 ng/mL) for the times indicated in the figure legends, and the cells were washed by ice-cold phosphate-buffered saline and lysed with RIPA Buffer (Sigma-Aldrich) supplemented with 1.0 mM sodium orthovanadate, 10 μg/mL aprotinin, and 10 μg/mL leupeptin for 20 min at 4 °C. After 5 min on ice, the cell lysates were centrifuged at 10,000g for 10 min at 4 °C. After centrifugation, cellular lysates (30 μg) were also subjected to 12% SDS-PAGE followed by Western blot with antibodies against human NLRP3 or β-actin with an ECL Western blotting kit (Amersham, Little Chalfont, UK). Only in the signal transduction analysis, cells were pretreated with tofacitinib for 30 min and then stimulated with GM-CSF. Western blot analysis using phospho-specific anti-JAK and STAT antibodies was performed with an ECL Western blotting kit (Amersham).

Statistical analysis

Differences between groups were examined for statistical significance by using the Student t test. P values of less than 0.05 were considered statistically significant.

Results

GM-CSF induces IL-1β secretion from human neutrophils

We investigated whether cytokine stimulation alone induces IL-1β secretion from human neutrophils. Neutrophils were stimulated with various amounts of TNF-α or GM-CSF, and the supernatants were analyzed for IL-1β by ELISA. The stimulation of human neutrophils with TNF-α alone did not induce IL-1β secretion, but a significant increase in IL-1β secretion occurred following stimulation with GM-CSF (Fig. 1). We also observed that GM-CSF–stimulated IL-1β secretion was completely abrogated by tofacitinib (Fig. 2). During NLRP3 inflammasome activation, a cleaved form of caspase-1 is released along with processed IL-1β [15]. Upon recruitment to an inflammasome complex, caspase-1 is

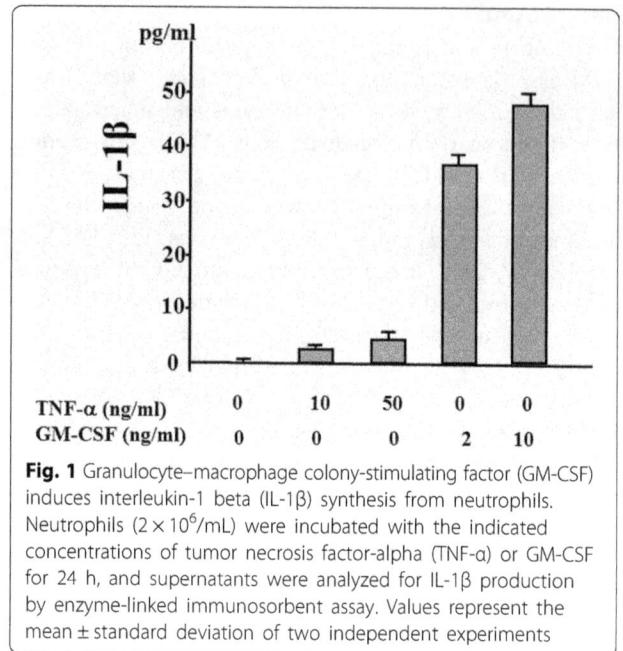

Fig. 1 Granulocyte–macrophage colony-stimulating factor (GM-CSF) induces interleukin-1 beta (IL-1β) synthesis from neutrophils. Neutrophils (2×10^6/mL) were incubated with the indicated concentrations of tumor necrosis factor-alpha (TNF-α) or GM-CSF for 24 h, and supernatants were analyzed for IL-1β production by enzyme-linked immunosorbent assay. Values represent the mean ± standard deviation of two independent experiments

activated and processed into mature caspase-1 formed of p10 and p20 subunits and these subunits have been shown to be secreted and be determined by measuring caspase-1 p20 in culture supernatant [15]. Therefore, we analyzed culture supernatants for the secretion of caspase-1 by using an ELISA specific for the cleaved form of caspase-1 (p20). We found that, consistent with IL-1β production, caspase-1 activation was induced in neutrophils stimulated with GM-CSF but not with

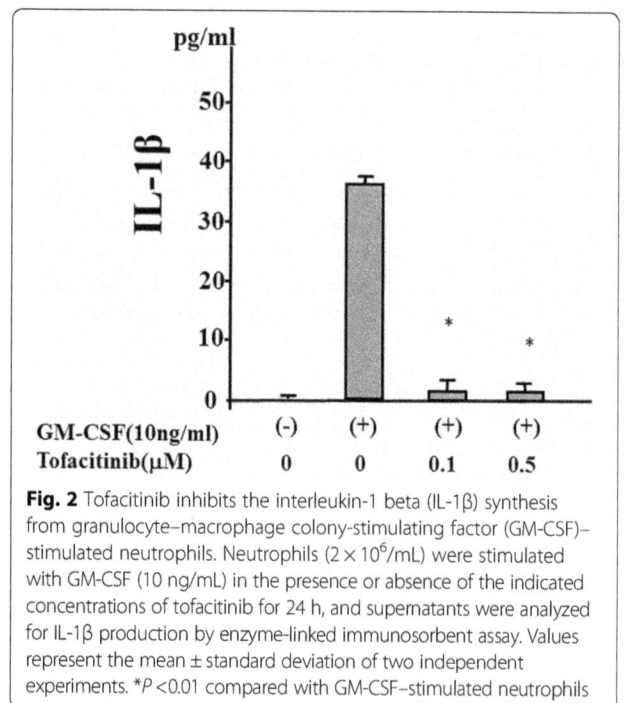

Fig. 2 Tofacitinib inhibits the interleukin-1 beta (IL-1β) synthesis from granulocyte–macrophage colony-stimulating factor (GM-CSF)–stimulated neutrophils. Neutrophils (2×10^6/mL) were stimulated with GM-CSF (10 ng/mL) in the presence or absence of the indicated concentrations of tofacitinib for 24 h, and supernatants were analyzed for IL-1β production by enzyme-linked immunosorbent assay. Values represent the mean ± standard deviation of two independent experiments. *$P < 0.01$ compared with GM-CSF–stimulated neutrophils

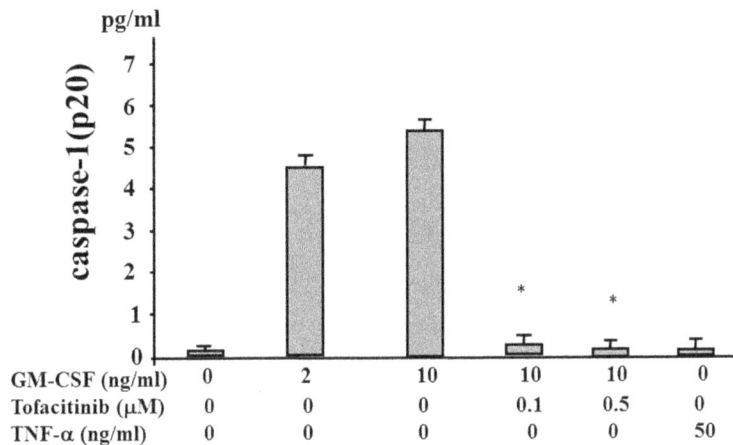

Fig. 3 Tofacitinib inhibits the caspase-1 (p20) release from granulocyte–macrophage colony-stimulating factor (GM-CSF)-stimulated neutrophils. Neutrophils (2×10^6/mL) were stimulated with GM-CSF (10 ng/mL) in the presence or absence of the indicated concentrations of tofacitinib for 24 h, and supernatants were analyzed for caspase-1 (p20) by enzyme-linked immunosorbent assay. Values represent the mean ± standard deviation of two independent experiments. *P <0.01 compared with GM-CSF–stimulated neutrophils. Abbreviation: *TNF-α* tumor necrosis factor-alpha

TNF-α. Tofacitinib inhibited the GM-CSF–induced increase in caspase-1 secretion from neutrophils (Fig. 3). We examined the expression of caspase-1 by using cellular lysates of GM-CSF–stimulated neutrophils. GM-CSF stimulation upregulated pro-caspase-1 expression as well as cleaved caspase-1 (p20) in neutrophils. Tofacitinib diminished this GM-CSF–induced cleaved form of caspase-1 (Fig. 4). The trypan blue dye exclusion test was performed to check cell viability of GM-CSF–treated neutrophils. However, there was no difference in cell viability assessed by trypan blue exclusion rates between untreated and GM-CSF-treated neutrophils (96.5 ± 4.1% versus 97.5 ± 2–3%, respectively).

Tofacitinib disrupts GM-CSF signaling in neutrophils

Because tofacitinib abrogates type 1 and type 2 cytokine receptor signaling by blocking JAK kinase, we next investigated whether JAK inhibition interferes with GM-CSF–mediated JAK/STAT signaling. To investigate the effects of tofacitinib on GM-CSF receptor signaling, freshly isolated neutrophils were pretreated with tofacitinib and stimulated with GM-CSF, and protein extracts were analyzed by immunoblotting with phospho-specific antibodies. We examined the phosphorylation status of JAK2 and two important downstream molecules of STAT3 and STAT5. As shown in Fig. 5, JAK2 and STAT3/5 were strongly phosphorylated after 10 min of stimulation with GM-CSF. By contrast, JAK1 or JAK3 phosphorylation was barely detected in GM-CSF–stimulated neutrophils under the same conditions (data not shown), whereas tofacitinib pretreatment (30 min) efficiently inhibited GM-CSF–induced phosphorylation of JAK2 and STAT3/5 (Fig. 6). These results indicate that tofacitinib interferes with the GM-CSF–induced STAT

signaling pathway downstream of JAK2. We also examined whether GM-CSF activates the NF-κB pathway in neutrophils. The phosphorylation of NF-κB and 1κB-α was induced in neutrophils by GM-CSF stimulation (Fig. 7). In this result, 1κB-α expression was marginally downregulated and this was probably due to the 1κB-α phosphorylation and subsequent degradation by GM-CSF stimulation. GM-CSF–induced JAK2/STAT3 activation and IL-1β production were compared between neutrophils isolated from healthy subjects and patients with RA. As shown in Fig. 8, GM-CSF stimulation induced JAK2/STAT3 phosphorylation in neutrophils isolated from healthy subjects and patients with RA. Similarly, GM-CSF stimulation induced IL-1β production from neutrophils but its induction did not differ

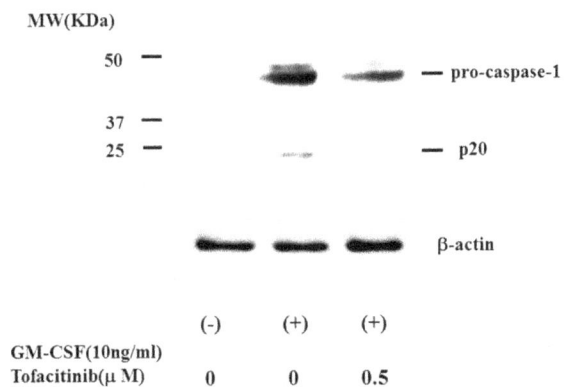

Fig. 4 Caspase-1 expressions in granulocyte–macrophage colony-stimulating factor (GM-CSF)-treated neutrophils. Neutrophils were treated with GM-CSF (10 ng/mL) in the presence or absence of tofacitinib for 12 h. Cellular lysates were analyzed by Western blotting by using anti-caspase-1 or anti-β-actin antibodies. Data are representative of two independent experiments. Abbreviation: *MW* molecular weight

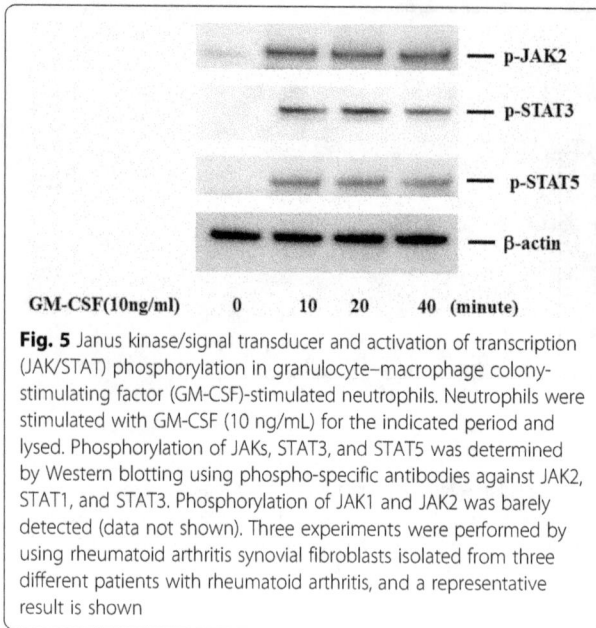

Fig. 5 Janus kinase/signal transducer and activation of transcription (JAK/STAT) phosphorylation in granulocyte–macrophage colony-stimulating factor (GM-CSF)-stimulated neutrophils. Neutrophils were stimulated with GM-CSF (10 ng/mL) for the indicated period and lysed. Phosphorylation of JAKs, STAT3, and STAT5 was determined by Western blotting using phospho-specific antibodies against JAK2, STAT1, and STAT3. Phosphorylation of JAK1 and JAK2 was barely detected (data not shown). Three experiments were performed by using rheumatoid arthritis synovial fibroblasts isolated from three different patients with rheumatoid arthritis, and a representative result is shown

significantly between healthy subjects and patients with RA (Fig. 9).

GM-CSF induces NLRP3 protein expression in neutrophils

We next examined whether tofacitinib modulates pro-IL-1β mRNA expression in GM-CSF–stimulated neutrophils. As shown in Fig. 10, GM-CSF is a potent inducer of pro-IL-1β mRNA expression in neutrophils, and tofacitinib could not completely prevent GM-CSF–induced pro-IL-1β mRNA expression Additional file 1. These findings were not consistent with observed IL-1β protein

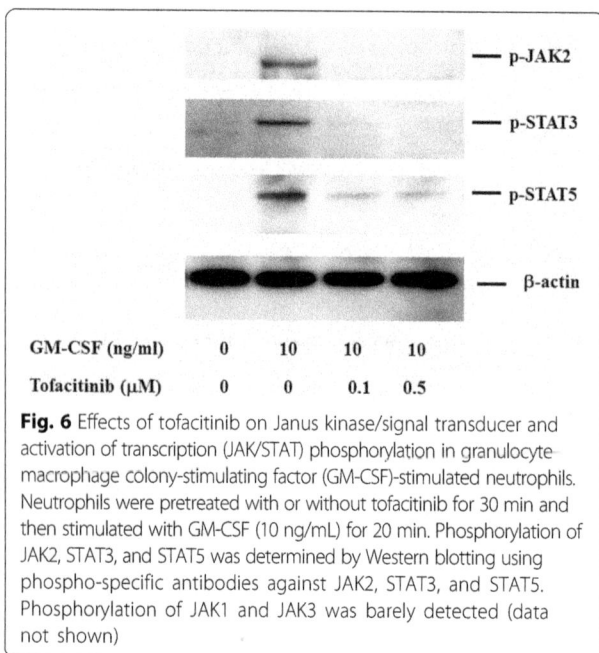

Fig. 6 Effects of tofacitinib on Janus kinase/signal transducer and activation of transcription (JAK/STAT) phosphorylation in granulocyte–macrophage colony-stimulating factor (GM-CSF)-stimulated neutrophils. Neutrophils were pretreated with or without tofacitinib for 30 min and then stimulated with GM-CSF (10 ng/mL) for 20 min. Phosphorylation of JAK2, STAT3, and STAT5 was determined by Western blotting using phospho-specific antibodies against JAK2, STAT3, and STAT5. Phosphorylation of JAK1 and JAK3 was barely detected (data not shown)

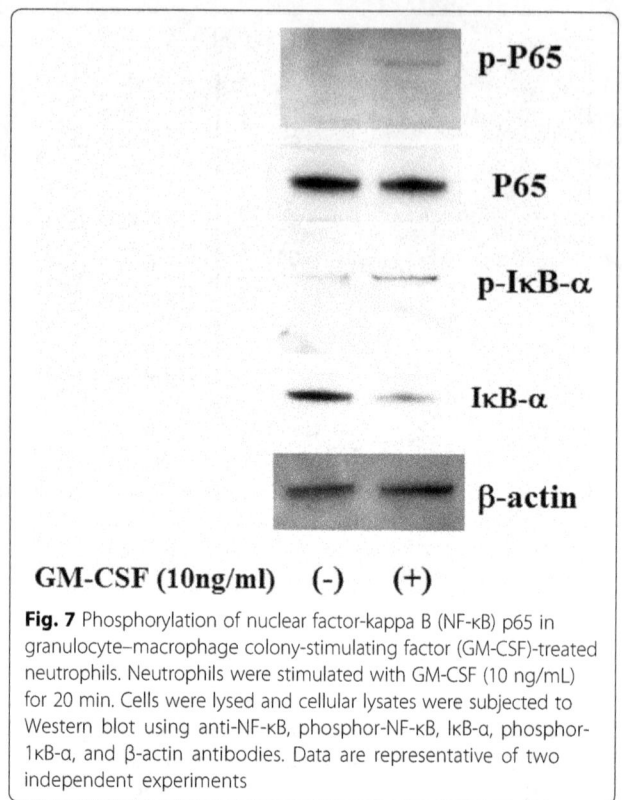

Fig. 7 Phosphorylation of nuclear factor-kappa B (NF-κB) p65 in granulocyte–macrophage colony-stimulating factor (GM-CSF)-treated neutrophils. Neutrophils were stimulated with GM-CSF (10 ng/mL) for 20 min. Cells were lysed and cellular lysates were subjected to Western blot using anti-NF-κB, phosphor-NF-κB, IκB-α, phosphor-1κB-α, and β-actin antibodies. Data are representative of two independent experiments

levels, which showed that tofacitinib completely blocked GM-CSF–induced IL-1β secretion from neutrophils.

Given the inhibitory effects of tofacitinib on GM-CSF–mediated caspase-1 activation and IL-1β production, we considered the possibility that this JAK inhibitor would also affect NLRP3 inflammasome expression in neutrophils. We therefore investigated the protein expression of NLRP3 in GM-CSF–stimulated neutrophils. Little NLRP3 expression was detected in untreated human neutrophils, whereas GM-CSF stimulation enhanced NLRP3 protein expression and this was inhibited by tofacitinib (Fig. 11). Phosphorylation of Tyr-144 residue of apoptosis-associated speck-like protein containing CARD (ASC) was critical for speck formation and caspase-1 activation during NLRP3 inflammasome activation [16]. We examined whether GM-CSF stimulation induces ASC phosphorylation in neutrophils. The result revealed that ASC could be phosphorylated in response to GM-CSF and tofacitinib diminished this ASC phosphorylation in neutrophils (Fig. 12).

Discussion

GM-CSF is a well-known hematopoietic factor but its function exceeds that of a simple growth factor [17]. GM-CSF modulates key aspects of both innate and adaptive immunity and plays an important role in the communication between pathogenic auto-reactive T helper (Th) cells and members of the myeloid lineages [18]. In experimental autoimmune encephalitis, the production of GM-CSF by

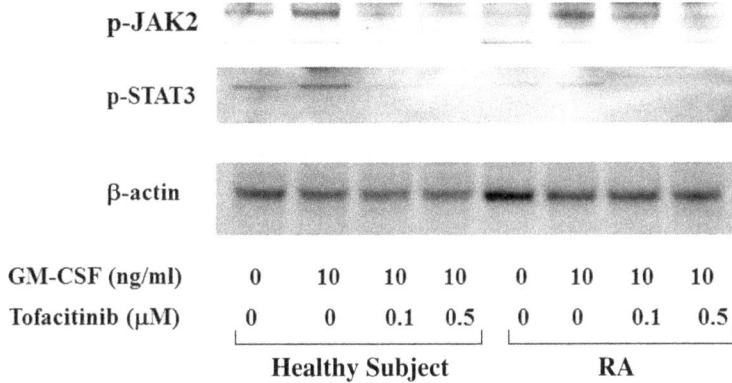

Fig. 8 Janus kinase 2/signal transducer and activation of transcription 3 (JAK2/STAT3) phosphorylation in granulocyte–macrophage colony-stimulating factor (GM-CSF)-stimulated neutrophils. Neutrophils from a healthy subject and a patient with rheumatoid arthritis (RA) were pretreated with tofacitinib for 30 min and then stimulated with GM-CSF (10 ng/mL) for 20 min. Cellular lysates were subjected to Western blot using anti-phospho JAK2 or anti-phospho STAT3 antibodies. Data are representative of three independent experiments

CD4[+] T cells is required to induce encephalitis [19], while GM-CSF secreted by RA synovial CD4[+] T cells promotes the differentiation of inflammatory dendritic cells [20]. The success of blocking the GM-CSF receptor in RA therapy suggests that neutralizing the GM-CSF axis could be a useful therapeutic strategy in RA [21].

Activated neutrophils possess many of the molecular properties of macrophages as drivers of inflammatory processes, and several drugs used to treat RA can target neutrophil functions [22]. In this study, we investigated the biological effects of GM-CSF against neutrophils as a major cell of the myeloid lineage. We describe the novel finding

that GM-CSF induces inflammasome-dependent IL-1β secretion in human neutrophils. In fact, unlike TNF-α stimulation, GM-CSF stimulation resulted in marked IL-1β secretion and enhanced IL-1β gene expression in neutrophils without the need for a priming signal. Our data strongly suggest that GM-CSF upregulates IL-1β gene expression at the transcriptional as well as the post-translational level in human neutrophils. Furthermore, GM-CSF stimulation was shown to induce the secretion of caspase-1 (p20) in parallel with the upregulation of NLRP3 protein expression in neutrophils. This increased NLRP3 protein expression likely contributes to the heightened IL-1β production following GM-CSF stimulation.

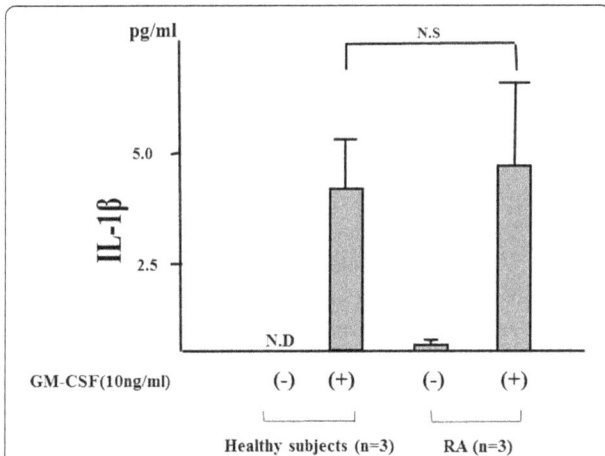

Fig. 9 Interleukin-1 beta (IL-1β) secretions from neutrophils isolated from healthy subjects and patients with rheumatoid arthritis (RA). Neutrophils (1×10^6/mL) derived from patients with RA ($n = 3$) or healthy subjects ($n = 3$) were incubated with or without granulocyte–macrophage colony-stimulating factor (GM-CSF) (10 ng/mL) for 24 h. IL-1β levels in supernatants of neutrophils stimulated with GM-CSF (10 ng/mL) were assessed by enzyme-linked immunosorbent assay. Values were represented as mean ± standard deviation. Abbreviations: *ND* not determined, *NS* not significant

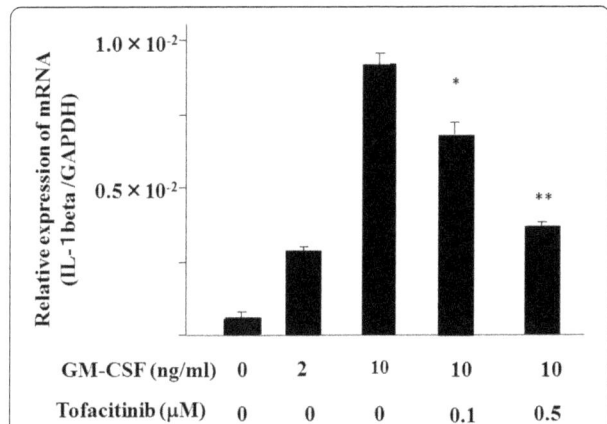

Fig. 10 Granulocyte–macrophage colony-stimulating factor (GM-CSF) induces the transcription of pro-interleukin-1 beta (pro-IL-1β) in human neutrophils. Neutrophils were stimulated with GM-CSF (10 ng/mL) in the presence or absence of tofacitinib for 8 h. The cells were harvested and analyzed for pro-IL-1β and glyceraldehydes-3-phosphates dehydrogenase (GAPDH) mRNA levels by real-time polymerase chain reaction. Values represent the mean ± standard deviation of two independent experiments. *$P < 0.01$ compared with GM-CSF–stimulated neutrophils. **$P < 0.001$ compared with GM-CSF–stimulated neutrophils

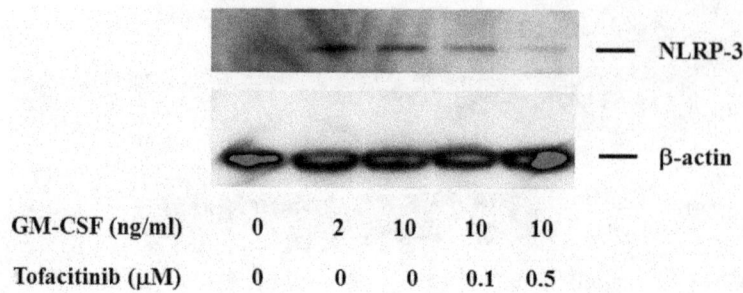

Fig. 11 NLR family pyrin domain-containing 3 (NLRP3) expression in neutrophils. Neutrophils were stimulated with granulocyte–macrophage colony-stimulating factor (GM-CSF) in the presence or absence of the indicated concentrations of tofacitinib for 24 h. Cellular lysates were analyzed by Western blot using anti-NLRP3 or anti-β-actin antibodies. Three experiments were performed by using different neutrophils, and a representative result is shown

Type 1 and type 2 cytokine receptors lack intrinsic enzymatic activity and associate with a family of cytoplasmic protein tyrosine kinases known as JAKs [23]. Upon cytokine-induced activation, JAKs phosphorylate the cytoplasmic tail of the receptors, leading to the recruitment of STATs, which are also phosphorylated by JAKs [23]. Activated STATs dimerize, translocate to the nucleus, and regulate the expression of target genes [14]. In this study, we demonstrated that tofacitinib, an inhibitor of the JAK family, interferes with JAK2-dependent GM-CSF–driven signaling. It has previously been demonstrated that JAK2 is important in the signal transduction cascade of GM-CSF signaling [13]. Tofacitinib demonstrated selectivity for JAK1 and JAK3 over JAK2 in a whole blood assay in which JAK2 was in its native conformation [24, 25]. Although it is unclear how tofacitinib might spare JAK2 in experiments with isolated JAK kinases, our data clearly showed that tofacitinib efficiently blocked GM-CSF–induced JAK2 phosphorylation in human neutrophils. Tofacitinib was first designed as a JAK3-specific inhibitor, but recent studies suggest that it could be a pan-JAK inhibitor [26].

Our data confirm that neutrophils respond to GM-CSF, which activates JAK2 and the downstream STAT3/STAT5 pathway, resulting in NLRP3 protein expression and IL-1β secretion. Neutrophils are thought to be essential in the pathogenesis of rheumatoid synovitis [27]. Our data suggest that GM-CSF–driven neutrophils play a non-redundant role during the T cell–mediated inflammatory process by polarizing the innate immune activation, including inflammasome activation and IL-1β induction as demonstrated in neutrophils previously [28]. Our data showed that GM-CSF sustains the expression of NLRP3 in neutrophils. Given that NLRP3 expression is known to activate innate immune cells [29], a functional NLRP3 inflammasome resulting in IL-1β induction within the synovium would be expected to contribute to rheumatoid synovitis. Our observations highlight the role of IL-1β by arthrogenic Th cells in the inflamed synovium. Therapeutic interventions targeting GM-CSF during rheumatoid inflammation are likely to restrict not only activated T cells producing GM-CSF but also GM-CSF–responding neutrophils and subsequent IL-1β secretion. This study provides evidence for how GM-CSF impacts on rheumatoid synovitis and which cell type requires a GM-CSF signaling event to mediate inflammation. Pathogenic T cells are the most abundant cellular infiltrates in the rheumatoid synovium and thus cause rheumatoid inflammation [30]. Our data suggest that JAK inhibitors have the potential to block multiple cytokine pathways, including the GM-CSF–mediated autoinflammatory cascade.

There was a limitation in our study. We measured the p20 subunit of caspase-1 in culture supernatants by using caspase-1 p20-specific ELISA. However, Western blot or enzymatic assay should be required to demonstrate the bioactive p20 subunit of caspase-1.

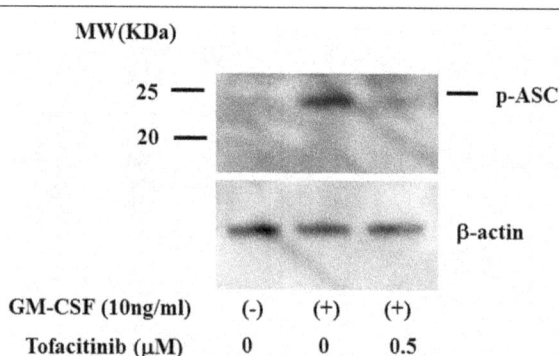

Fig. 12 Apoptosis-associated speck-like protein containing CARD (ASC) phosphorylation in granulocyte–macrophage colony-stimulating factor (GM-CSF)-treated neutrophils. Neutrophils were incubated with GM-CSF (10 ng/mL) in the presence or absence of tofacitinib for 8 h. Cellular lysates were subjected to Western blot using anti-phospho-ASC (Tyr-144) or anti-β-actin antibodies. Data are representative of two independent experiments. Abbreviation: *MW* molecular weight

Conclusion

We have shown that GM-CSF is a strong inducer of IL-1β by activating the inflammasome in neutrophils.

Our results indicate that GM-CSF signaling controls the pathogenic expression of IL-1β in neutrophils, which may cause innate cell activation, inflammation, and cartilage damage in RA. Therefore, GM-CSF emerges as a communicator between pathogenic lymphocytes and neutrophils through activating the NLRP3 inflammasome.

Abbreviations
ASC: Apoptosis-associated speck-like protein containing CARD; ELISA: Enzyme-linked immunosorbent assay; GM-CSF: Granulocyte–macrophage colony-stimulating factor; IL: Interleukin; JAK: Janus kinase; NF-κB: Nuclear factor-kappa B; NLRP3: NLR family pyrin domain-containing 3; RA: Rheumatoid arthritis; STAT: Signal transduction and activator of transcription; Th: T helper; TNF-α: Tumor necrosis factor-alpha

Funding
The study was supported by the Practical Research Project for Rare/ Intractable Diseases from the Japan Agency for Medical Research and Development (AMED).

Authors' contributions
MF, TA, YS, SS, HKob, HW, ES, and KM carried out the molecular biochemical studies, participated in the sequence alignment, and drafted the manuscript. HKoz and HY carried out the genetic assays. TK, HO, HS, AK, and KM participated in the sequence alignment and drafted the manuscript. TK and KM participated in the design of the study and performed the statistical analysis. All authors read and approved the final manuscript.

Consent for publication
Not applicable.

Competing interests
KM has received research grants from Chugai, Pfizer, and AbbVie. The other authors declare that they have no competing interests.

Author details
[1]Department of Rheumatology, Fukushima Medical University School of Medicine, 1 Hikarigaoka, Fukushima, Fukushima 960-1295, Japan. [2]Department of Rheumatology, Ohta Nishinouchi General Hospital Foundation, 2-5-20 Nishinouchi, Koriyama, Fukushima 963-8558, Japan. [3]Clinical Research Center, NHO Nagasaki Medical Center, Kubara 2-1001-1 Omura, Nagasaki 856-8562, Japan. [4]Department of Immunology and Rheumatology, Unit of Translational Medicine, Graduate School of Biomedical Sciences, Nagasaki University, Sakamoto1-7-1, Nagasaki 852-8501, Japan. [5]Department of Gastroenterology, Fukushima Medical University School of Medicine, 1 Hikarigaoka, Fukushima, Fukushima 960-1295, Japan. [6]Department of Immunology, Fukushima Medical University School of Medicine, 1 Hikarigaoka, Fukushima, Fukushima 960-1295, Japan.

References
1. Conti L, Gessani S. GM-CSF in the generation of dendritic cells from human blood monocyte precursors: recent advances. Immunobiology. 2008;213(9–10):859–70.
2. Becher B, Tugues S, Greter M. GM-CSF: from growth factor to central mediator of tissue inflammation. Immunity. 2016;45(5):963–73.
3. Cornish AL, Campbell IK, McKenzie BS, Chatfield S, Wicks IP. G-CSF and GM-CSF as therapeutic targets in rheumatoid arthritis. Nat Rev Rheumatol. 2009;5(10):554–9.
4. de Vries EG, Willemse PH, Biesma B, Stern AC, Limburg PC, Vellenga E. Flare-up of rheumatoid arthritis during GM-CSF treatment after chemotherapy. Lancet. 1991;338(8765):517–8.
5. Avci AB, Feist E, Burmester GR. Targeting GM-CSF in rheumatoid arthritis. Clin Exp Rheumatol. 2016;34(4 Suppl 98):39–44.
6. Shiomi A, Usui T. Pivotal roles of GM-CSF in autoimmunity and inflammation. Mediat Inflamm. 2015;2015:568543.
7. Yang YH, Hamilton JA. Dependence of interleukin-1-induced arthritis on granulocyte-macrophage colony-stimulating factor. Arthritis Rheum. 2001;44(1):111–9.
8. Dinarello CA, van der Meer JW. Treating inflammation by blocking interleukin-1 in humans. Semin Immunol. 2013;25(6):469–84.
9. Leemans JC, Cassel SL, Sutterwala FS. Sensing damage by the NLRP3 inflammasome. Immunol Rev. 2011;243(1):152–62.
10. Shaw OM, Steiger S, Liu X, Hamilton JA, Harper JL. Brief report: granulocyte-macrophage colony-stimulating factor drives monosodium urate monohydrate crystal-induced inflammatory macrophage differentiation and NLRP3 inflammasome up-regulation in an in vivo mouse model. Arthritis Rheumatol. 2014;66(9):2423–8.
11. Hercus TR, Thomas D, Guthridge MA, Ekert PG, King-Scott J, Parker MW, et al. The granulocyte-macrophage colony-stimulating factor receptor: linking its structure to cell signaling and its role in disease. Blood. 2009; 114(7):1289–98.
12. Watanabe S, Itoh T, Arai K. Roles of JAK kinases in human GM-CSF receptor signal transduction. J Allergy Clin Immunol. 1996;98(6 Pt 2):S183–91.
13. Al-Shami A, Mahanna W, Naccache PH. Granulocyte-macrophage colony-stimulating factor-activated signaling pathways in human neutrophils. Selective activation of Jak2, Stat3, and Stat5b. J Biol Chem. 1998;273(2):1058–63.
14. Darnell JE Jr. STATs and gene regulation. Science. 1997;277(5332):1630–5.
15. Shamaa OR, Mitra S, Gavrilin MA, Wewers MD. Monocyte Caspase-1 is released in a stable, active high molecular weight complex distinct from the unstable cell lysate-activated Caspase-1. PLoS One. 2015;10:e0142203.
16. Hara H, Tsuchiya K, Kawamura I, Fang R, Hernandez-Cuellar E, Shen Y, et al. Phosphorylation of the adaptor ASC acts as a molecular switch that controls the formation of speck-like aggregates and inflammasome activity. Nat Immunol. 2013;12:1247–55.
17. Fleetwood AJ, Cook AD, Hamilton JA. Functions of granulocyte-macrophage colony-stimulating factor. Crit Rev Immunol. 2005;25(5):405–28.
18. Belardelli F, Ferrantini M. Cytokines as a link between innate and adaptive antitumor immunity. Trends Immunol. 2002;23(4):201–8.
19. Croxford AL, Lanzinger M, Hartmann FJ, et al. The cytokine GM-CSF drives the inflammatory signature of CCR2+ monocytes and licenses autoimmunity. Immunity. 2015;43(3):502–14.
20. Reynolds G, Gibbon JR, Pratt AG, Wood MJ, Coady D, Raftery G, et al. Synovial CD4+ T-cell-derived GM-CSF supports the differentiation of an inflammatory dendritic cell population in rheumatoid arthritis. Ann Rheum Dis. 2016;75(5):899–907.
21. Wicks IP, Roberts AW. Targeting GM-CSF in inflammatory diseases. Nat Rev Rheumatol. 2016;12(1):37–48.
22. Pillinger MH, Abramson SB. The neutrophil in rheumatoid arthritis. Rheum Dis Clin N Am. 1995;21(3):691–714.
23. Schwartz DM, Bonelli M, Gadina M, O'Shea JJ. Type I/II cytokines, JAKs, and new strategies for treating autoimmune diseases. Nat Rev Rheumatol. 2016;12(1):25.
24. Vijayakrishnan L, Venkataramanan R, Gulati P. Treating inflammation with the Janus kinase inhibitor CP-690,550. Trends Pharmacol Sci. 2011;32(1):25–34.
25. Flanagan ME, Blumenkopf TA, Brissette WH, Brown MF, Casavant JM, Shang-Poa C, et al. Discovery of CP-690,550: a potent and selective Janus kinase (JAK) inhibitor for the treatment of autoimmune diseases and organ transplant rejection. J Med Chem. 2010;53(24):8468–84.
26. Baker KF, Isaacs JD. Novel therapies for immune-mediated inflammatory diseases: What can we learn from their use in rheumatoid arthritis, spondyloarthritis, systemic lupus erythematosus, psoriasis, Crohn's disease and ulcerative colitis? Ann Rheum Dis. 2018;77(2):175–87.
27. Kaplan MJ. Role of neutrophils in systemic autoimmune diseases. Arthritis Res Ther. 2013;15(5):219.
28. Mankan AK, Dau T, Jenne D, Hornung V. The NLRP3/ASC/Caspase-1 axis regulates IL-1β processing in neutrophils. Eur J Immunol. 2012;42(3):710–5.
29. Franchi L, Muñoz-Planillo R, Núñez G. Sensing and reacting to microbes through the inflammasomes. Nat Immunol. 2012;13(4):325–32.
30. Miossec P. Dynamic interactions between T cells and dendritic cells and their derived cytokines/chemokines in the rheumatoid synovium. Arthritis Res Ther. 2008;10(Suppl 1):S2.

21

Blocking CD248 molecules in perivascular stromal cells of patients with systemic sclerosis strongly inhibits their differentiation toward myofibroblasts and proliferation: a new potential target for antifibrotic therapy

Paola Di Benedetto[1]* ![ORCID], Vasiliki Liakouli[1], Piero Ruscitti[1], Onorina Berardicurti[1], Francesco Carubbi[1], Noemi Panzera[1], Salvatore Di Bartolomeo[1], Giuliana Guggino[2], Francesco Ciccia[2], Giovanni Triolo[2], Paola Cipriani[1] and Roberto Giacomelli[1]

Abstract

Background: Fibrosis may be considered the hallmark of systemic sclerosis (SSc), the end stage triggered by different pathological events. Transforming growth factor-β (TGF-β) and platelet-derived growth factor BB (PDGF-BB) are profibrotic molecules modulating myofibroblast differentiation and proliferation, respectively. There is evidence linking CD248 with these two molecules, both highly expressed in patients with SSc, and suggesting that CD248 may be a therapeutic target for several diseases. The aim of this work was to evaluate the expression of CD248 in SSc skin and its ability to modulate SSc fibrotic process.

Methods: After ethical approval was obtained, skin biopsies were collected from 20 patients with SSc and 10 healthy control subjects (HC). CD248 expression was investigated in the skin, as well as in bone marrow mesenchymal stem cells (MSCs) treated with TGF-β or PDGF-BB, by immunofluorescence, qRT-PCR, and Western blotting. Finally, in SSc-MSCs, the CD248 gene was silenced by siRNA.

Results: Increased expression of CD248 was found in endothelial cells and perivascular stromal cells of SSc skin. In SSc-MSCs, the levels of CD248 and α-smooth muscle actin expression were significantly higher than in HC-MSCs. In both SSc- and HC-MSCs, PDGF-BB induced increased expression of *Ki-67* when compared with untreated cells but was unable to modulate CD248 levels. After CD248 silencing, both TGF-β and PDGF-BB signaling were inhibited in SSc-MSCs.

Conclusions: CD248 overexpression may play an important role in the fibrotic process by modulating the molecular target, leading to perivascular cells differentiation toward myofibroblasts and interfering with its expression, and thus might open a new therapeutic strategy to inhibit myofibroblast generation during SSc.

Keywords: Systemic sclerosis, CD248, Fibrosis

* Correspondence: paola.dibenedetto1@univaq.it
[1]Department of Biotechnological and Applied Clinical Sciences, Rheumatology Unit, School of Medicine, University of L'Aquila, Delta 6 Building, Via dell'Ospedale, 67100 L'Aquila, Italy
Full list of author information is available at the end of the article

Background

CD248 (also known as *endosialin* or *tumor endothelial marker 1*) is a transmembrane receptor whose known ligands are fibronectin and type I/IV collagen. It is widely expressed on mesenchymal cells during embryonic life and is required for proliferation and migration of pericytes and fibroblasts [1]. Although CD248 expression is dramatically reduced during adult life, it may be upregulated during specific conditions such as malignancy, inflammation, and fibrosis [2–4]. It is well known that CD248 is expressed on the surface of cells of mesenchymal origin, including tumor-associated pericytes and activated fibroblasts, which are thought to play a key role in the development of tumor neovascular networks and stromal interaction [1]. The interruption of endosialin function, with antibody blockade or genetic knockouts, negatively affects tumor growth and angiogenesis in numerous cancer types [5–7]. Furthermore, in the experimental model of kidney fibrosis after unilateral ureteral obstruction (UUO), CD248$^{-/-}$ mice display downregulation of myofibroblast proliferation, thus decreasing the kidney fibrosis [8]. These biologic effects, in cancer and in reparative response, may be related to the ability of CD248 to modulate many signaling pathways involved in both cancer development and tissue repair, including platelet-derived growth factor BB (PDGF-BB), transforming growth factor-β (TGF-β), and Notch receptor protein [9]. Under normal conditions, pericytes that expressed high levels of CD248 were able to proliferate, responding to PDGF-BB stimulation [9], and higher expression of CD248 is required for imparting fibroblast sensitivity to the effects of TGF-β [10].

Owing to its multifunctional activities modulating innate immunity, cell proliferation, and vascular homeostasis [9, 11], CD248 may be considered a potential therapeutic target for several diseases [12], and currently, the results of a first-in-human, open-label, phase I study recruiting patients with extracranial solid tumors who failed standard chemotherapy and were treated with a biologic therapy targeting CD248 have been published, confirming the therapy's safety and a positive impact on different cancers [13].

Systemic sclerosis (SSc) is a connective tissue disease of unknown etiology with multiorgan involvement and heterogeneous clinical manifestations. The hallmark of early SSc is endothelial involvement, whereas later stages are characterized by an excessive accumulation of extracellular matrix (ECM), resulting in extended fibrosis in skin and internal organs [14, 15]. In the last few years, it has been clarified that endothelial cells (ECs) and pericytes, after injury, may differentiate toward myofibroblasts, which are committed to producing increased amounts of collagen [16–18], and this process has been proposed as a key pathogenic mechanism in SSc.

Several polypeptide mediators are involved in fibrosis during SSc, such as TGF-β and PDGF-BB. The latter is a potent pro-proliferative signal for mesenchyme-derived cells, including myofibroblasts [19, 20], whereas TGF-β primarily promotes myofibroblast activation, α-smooth muscle actin (α-SMA) expression, and collagen deposition [16, 21–26]. Interestingly, CD248 modulates both these pathways because of CD248 is required for imparting fibroblast sensitivity to the effects of TGF-β [9] and is crucial for optimal migratory response of activated fibroblasts to PDGF-BB [19].

The goal of this work is to investigate the expression of CD248 in skin perivascular stromal cells from patients with SSc and its ability in mediating pericyte differentiation toward myofibroblasts. Although the role of CD248 in the pathogenesis of SSc has not yet been established, its potential role in controlling vessel regression and fibrosis makes this molecule a potential therapeutic target in a clinical setting, different from cancer, and in which an effective therapeutic approach to prevent fibrosis is still an important unmet need.

Methods

Patients, control subjects, and skin biopsies

Full-thickness biopsy samples measuring 2×0.5 cm isolated from excisional biopsy were obtained from clinically involved skin of one-third of the distal forearm of patients with diffuse SSc according to the classification of LeRoy and colleagues [27]. All patients fulfilled the 2013 classification criteria for SSc [28]. Skin with a modified Rodnan skin score [29] ≥ 1 was considered to be clinically involved.

To be sure that 50% of our patients were in a very early phase of SSc, considering that the term *early* currently refers to an undifferentiated connective tissue disease at higher risk of developing into scleroderma, as suggested by the pivotal study of Koening et al. [30], more than to a time frame from the beginning of the disease, we further divided our patients into two subsets: patients fulfilling the classification criteria in less than 1 year from the onset of Raynaud's phenomenon (early-onset subset [EOS], $n = 10$) and all the others (long-standing subset [LSS], $n = 10$). Skin samples from the same region of ten age- and sex-matched healthy control subjects (HC) who underwent a surgical treatment for trauma were used for comparison. All patients with SSc underwent a 20-day washout from any immunosuppressive treatment and 1 month from intravenous prostanoids before skin biopsy was performed. During this period, only proton pump inhibitors and clebopride were allowed. Patients who could not undergo therapeutic washout owing to severe organ complications were not enrolled in the study. Biopsies were taken after informed consent was obtained, and the study was approved by our local ethics committee (ASL Avezzano Sulmona L'Aquila, protocol number 015408/17). Demographic and clinical characteristics of the patients are shown in Table 1. Each biopsy sample was divided into specimens for immunofluorescence (IF) and qRT-PCR. For IF, the specimens were fixed in 10% buffered formalin, dehydrated in graded alcohol series, and embedded in paraffin. Specimens used for qRT-PCR analyses were immediately immersed in liquid nitrogen and stored at − 80 °C until use.

Immunofluorescence

The IF analysis was performed on paraffin sections (thickness 3 μm) using a conjugated anti-CD248 antibody (Novus Biologicals, Littleton, CO, USA). Antigen retrieval was carried out using Dako Target Retrieval solution (Agilent Technologies, Santa Clara, CA, USA). Vasculature pericytes were highlighted using a Cy3-conjugated anti-α-SMA antibody (Sigma-Aldrich, St. Louis, MO, USA) and EC using unconjugated anti–von Willebrand factor (vWF) antibody (Dako, Glostrup, Denmark). The immunoreaction was revealed using secondary antibody

(Alexa Fluor; Life Technologies, Carlsbad, CA, USA). Cell nuclei were visualized using 4′,6-diamidino-2-phenylindole. Fluorescence was analyzed using a BX53 fluorescence microscope (Olympus, Center Valley, PA, USA). The intensity of fluorescence was measured using ImageJ software (National Institutes of Health, Bethesda, MD, USA).

Isolation, culture, and immunophenotyping of mesenchymal stem cells

After approval was provided by the local ethics committee (ASL Avezzano Sulmona L'Aquila) and written informed consent was obtained from patients, bone marrow was obtained by aspiration from the posterior superior iliac crest from the patients enrolled in the study. Samples of mesenchymal stem cells (MSC) from bone marrow donors were used as a control. MSC were obtained and expanded from both the subsets of five EOS and five LSS patients, as previously described [25]. Third-passage MSC were analyzed for the surface expression of MSC antigens (CD45, CD73, CD90, CD34, CD79a, PDGF receptor-β) and pericyte markers (α-SMA, SM22α, NG2, desmin, RGS5) by flow

Table 1 Clinical and demographic features of the 20 patients with diffuse systemic sclerosis

Sex/age (yr)	Disease duration at skin biopsy (yr from RP)	mRSS/score at skin biopsy	Autoantibodies	ILD	PAH	SRC	RP	DU
95% F	50% EOS 50% LSS		100% ANA/Scl70	25% ILD	15% PAH;	0% SCR	100% RP	30% DU
F/45	< 1	10/2	ANA/Scl-70	No	No	No	Yes	No
F/22	< 1	13/1	ANA/Scl-70	No	No	No	Yes	Yes
F/31	< 1	08/2	ANA/Scl-70	No	No	No	Yes	No
F/38	< 1	09/2	ANA/Scl-70	No	Yes	No	Yes	Yes
M/20	< 1	11/1	ANA/Scl-70	No	No	No	Yes	No
F/40	< 1	10/2	ANA/Scl-70	No	No	No	Yes	No
F/31	< 1	10/1	ANA/Scl-70	No	No	No	Yes	No
F/21	< 1	09/1	ANA/Scl-70	No	No	No	Yes	No
F/31	< 1	14/1	ANA/Scl-70	No	No	No	Yes	No
F/42	< 1	16/2	ANA/Scl-70	Yes	No	No	Yes	No
F/45	4	17/2	ANA/Scl-70	No	No	No	Yes	No
F/21	5	15/1	ANA/Scl-70	No	No	No	Yes	No
F/30	6	18/2	ANA/Scl-70	No	Yes	No	Yes	Yes
F/33	4	13/2	ANA/Scl-70	Yes	No	No	Yes	No
F/34	4	12/1	ANA/Scl-70	No	No	No	Yes	Yes
F/40	4	10/2	ANA/Scl-70	Yes	Yes	No	Yes	No
M/26	6	10/2	ANA/Scl-70	Yes	No	No	Yes	Yes
F/21	4	11/1	ANA/Scl-70	No	No	No	Yes	No
F/30	3	12/2	ANA/Scl-70	Yes	No	No	Yes	Yes
F/33	4	12/1	ANA/Scl-70	No	No	No	Yes	No

Abbreviations: EOS Early-onset subset, *LSS* Long-standing subset, *RP* Raynaud's phenomenon, *mRSS* Modified Rodnan skin score (maximum possible score 51), *ILD* Interstitial lung disease, *ANA* Antinuclear antibodies, *Scl-70* Antitopoisomerase, *PAH* Pulmonary arterial hypertension, *SRC* Scleroderma renal crisis, *DU* Digital ulcers
The internal organ involvement is referred to the time of biopsies

cytometry (FACScan; BD Biosciences, San Jose, CA, USA) as previously described [25] (data not shown).

MSC response to PDGF-BB and TGF-β

To establish the optimal concentration of PDGF-BB and TGF-β molecules, in our system, a dose-response curve was created, using P3 cells of one HC and one patient and evaluating the Ki-67 and α-SMA messenger RNA (mRNA) expression. Each experiment was performed in triplicate (data not shown). Both SSc-MSC and HC-MSC were cultured for 7 days in 1% FBS medium supplemented with selected doses of 10 ng/ml PDGF-BB (R&D Systems, Minneapolis, MN, USA) and 10 ng/ml TGF-β (R&D Systems). We used the TGF-β1 isoform. Media were changed every 2 days.

Small interfering RNA assay

To silence CD248 expression, SSc-MSC were transfected with Silencer Select CD248 small interfering RNA (siRNA; Life Technologies) [31] or with Silencer Select nontargeting scrambled (scr) siRNA (Life Technologies) using Lipofectamine™ 2000 reagent (Life Technologies). The CD248 gene was identified to be transcribed from a 2557-bp single-exon gene [32, 33].

Transfection was performed according to the manufacturer's instructions. Briefly, MSC were plated at 1×10^4 cells/cm^2 24 h prior to transfection. Cultures were incubated for 24 h with 30 pmol of siRNA in 2 ml of Opti-MEM (Life Technologies). After incubation, plates were washed, and cells were allowed to recover in growth conditions (1% FBS) supplemented with TGF-β (10 ng/ml) and PDGF-BB (10 ng/ml).

Western blot analysis

MSC, derived from two EOS and two LSS patients, were pelleted and lysed in lysis buffer (radioimmunoprecipitation assay buffer; Cell Signaling Technology, Danvers, MA, USA) for 30 min and cleared by centrifugation. The protein concentration was calculated by using a bicinchoninic acid protein assay kit (EuroClone, Pero, Italy). Proteins (40 μg) were separated by SDS-PAGE and transferred to nitrocellulose membranes. After blocking in 10% nonfat milk in Tris-buffered saline/1% Tween 20 and incubated with the primary antibodies α-SMA (Santa Cruz Biotechnology, Dallas, TX, USA) and CD248 (Novus Biologicals), horseradish peroxidase-conjugated secondary antibodies (Cell Signaling Technology) were appropriately used. The detection was performed using long-lasting chemiluminescent substrate (EuroClone). All the signals were quantified by normalizing to the β-actin signal (Santa Cruz Biotechnology). Immunoreactive bands were acquired using a ChemiDoc imaging system with Image Lab software (Bio-Rad Laboratories, Hercules, CA, USA) and quantified with densitometry using ImageJ software.

qRT-PCR analysis

Total RNA was extracted from MSC and whole biopsy using NucleoSpin RNA (Macherey-Nagel, Düren, Germany) and reverse-transcribed into complementary DNA (cDNA) with the High Capacity cDNA Reverse Transcription Kit (Applied Biosystems, Foster City, CA, USA). The qRT-PCR was run in triplicate. *Ki-67* and *GAPDH* gene expression were assessed using commercial TaqMan gene expression assay (Hs01032443_m1; Hs02 758991_g1, respectively). *α-SMA*, *CD248*, and *β-actin* expression was performed by using SYBR Green kits (Applied Biosystems). Primers were designed on the basis of reported sequences in the National Center for Biotechnology Information PrimerBank [β-actin: 5′-CCTGGC ACCCAGCACAAT-3′ (forward) and 5′-AGTACTCCG TGTGGATCGGC-3′ (reverse); α-SMA: 5′-CGGTGCT GTCTCTCTATGCC-3′ (forward) and 5′-CGCTCAGTC AGGATCTTCA-3′ (reverse); CD248: 5′-AGTGTTATT GTAGCGAGGGACA-3′ (forward) and 5′-CCTCTGGG AAGCTCGGTCTA-3′ (reverse)]. Results were analyzed after 45 cycles of amplification using the ABI 7500 Fast Real Time PCR System (Applied Biosystems).

Statistical analysis

Prism 5.0 software (GraphPad Software, La Jolla, CA, USA) was used for statistical analyses. Results are expressed as median (range). Owing to the nonparametric distribution of our data, the Mann-Whitney U test was used as appropriate for analyses. Statistical significance was expressed by a p value < 0.05.

Results

CD248 expression in skin SSc

Our results show that CD248 is overexpressed in SSc skin, and specifically in both EC and perivascular cells, when compared with HC skin, as observed in Fig. 1. Consistent with these findings, in whole SSc skin biopsies, CD248 mRNA expression was significantly increased when compared with HC skin, as assessed by qRT-PCR. Furthermore, in LSS skin, the CD248 mRNA expression was significantly increased when compared with EOS skin (Fig. 1g).

Interestingly, we observed that CD248 expression was not limited only to the cells of blood vessels; also other cells, proximal to microvessels, showed an increased expression of this marker (Fig. 1a–d, arrowheads). To better understand our findings, we performed different staining to identify the possible lineage of these cells, and as shown in Fig. 2, these cells surrounding the vascular trees coexpressed the CD90 marker, which is highly expressed in undifferentiated MSC [34]. Of interest, these CD90$^+$/CD248$^+$ cells were significantly increased in SSc skin when compared with HC skin (Fig. 2). Finally, the number of these CD90$^+$/CD248$^+$ cells

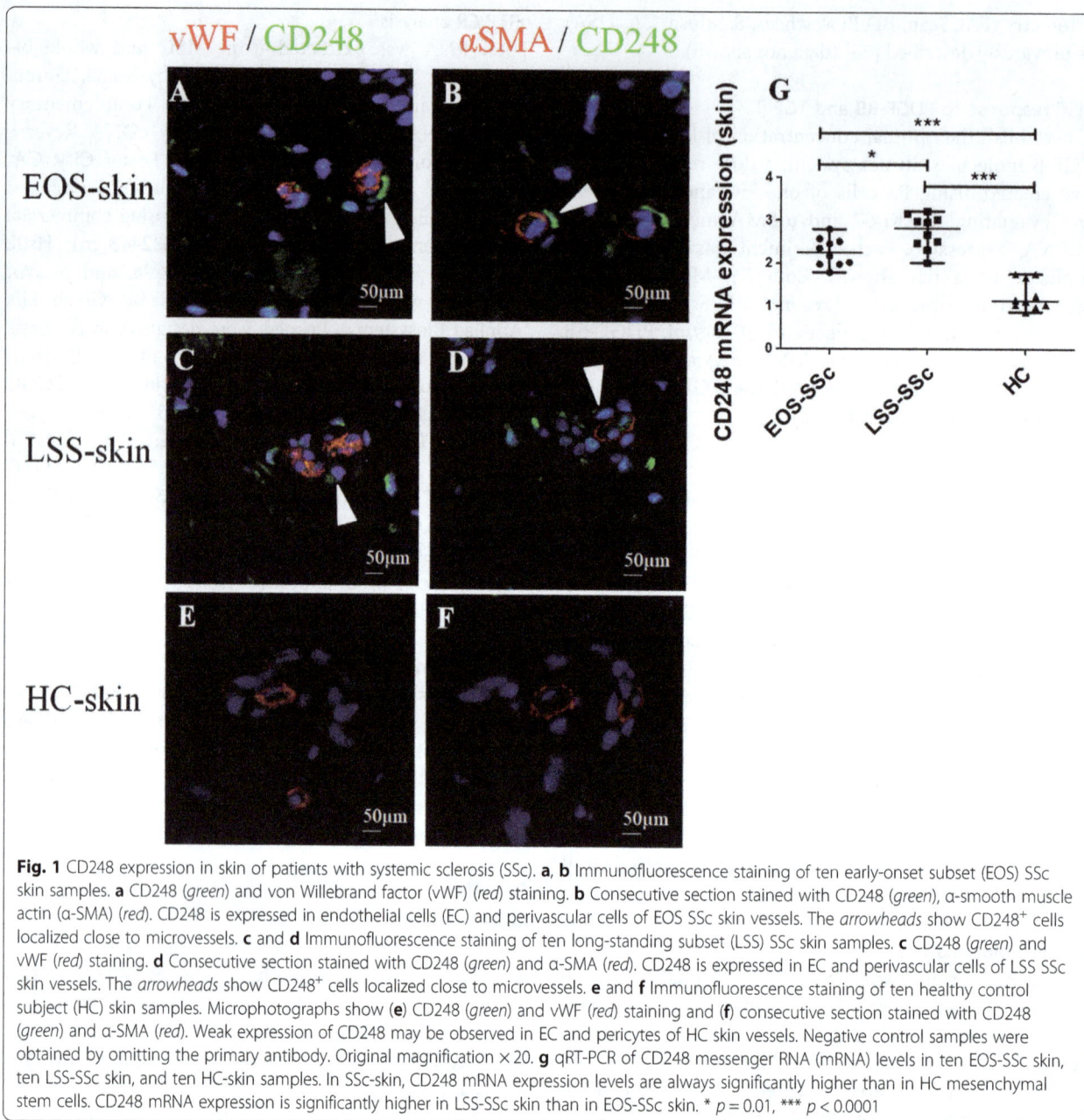

Fig. 1 CD248 expression in skin of patients with systemic sclerosis (SSc). **a, b** Immunofluorescence staining of ten early-onset subset (EOS) SSc skin samples. **a** CD248 (*green*) and von Willebrand factor (vWF) (*red*) staining. **b** Consecutive section stained with CD248 (*green*), α-smooth muscle actin (α-SMA) (*red*). CD248 is expressed in endothelial cells (EC) and perivascular cells of EOS SSc skin vessels. The *arrowheads* show CD248+ cells localized close to microvessels. **c** and **d** Immunofluorescence staining of ten long-standing subset (LSS) SSc skin samples. **c** CD248 (*green*) and vWF (*red*) staining. **d** Consecutive section stained with CD248 (*green*) and α-SMA (*red*). CD248 is expressed in EC and perivascular cells of LSS SSc skin vessels. The *arrowheads* show CD248+ cells localized close to microvessels. **e** and **f** Immunofluorescence staining of ten healthy control subject (HC) skin samples. Microphotographs show (**e**) CD248 (*green*) and vWF (*red*) staining and (**f**) consecutive section stained with CD248 (*green*) and α-SMA (*red*). Weak expression of CD248 may be observed in EC and pericytes of HC skin vessels. Negative control samples were obtained by omitting the primary antibody. Original magnification × 20. **g** qRT-PCR of CD248 messenger RNA (mRNA) levels in ten EOS-SSc skin, ten LSS-SSc skin, and ten HC-skin samples. In SSc-skin, CD248 mRNA expression levels are always significantly higher than in HC mesenchymal stem cells. CD248 mRNA expression is significantly higher in LSS-SSc skin than in EOS-SSc skin. * $p = 0.01$, *** $p < 0.0001$

was significantly higher in LSS SSc skin (Fig. 2c and d) than in EOS SSc skin (Fig. 2a and b).

TGF-β and PDGF-BB effects on CD248 expression in MSC

We investigated the functional role of CD248 in vitro in the perivascular differentiation toward myofibroblasts, by using MSC, a validated surrogate of perivascular cells [26]. Figure 3a shows that in SSc-MSC, CD248 mRNA expression levels were significantly higher than in HC-MSC [CD248 mRNA levels in untreated [UT] SSc-MSC 1.32 (1.25–1.50) vs UT HC-MSC 0.96 (0.73–1.17); $p < 0.0001$]. Furthermore, in SSc-MSC, TGF-β induced a significant decrease of CD248 mRNA expression levels when compared with UT SSc-MSC [CD248 mRNA levels in TGF-β SSc-MSC 0.74 (0.54–0.94) vs UT SSc-MSC 1.32 (1.25–1.50); $p < 0.0001$]. In HC-MSC, the TGF-β treatment induced a significant reduction of CD248 mRNA expression levels when compared with UT cells [CD248 mRNA levels in TGF-β HC-MSC 0.07 (0.03–0.15) vs UT HC-MSC 0.96 (0.73–1.17); $p < 0.0001$], although in SSc-MSC, the levels of CD248 expression were always significantly higher than in HC-MSC. On the contrary, no CD248 mRNA modulation was observed by using PDGF-BB, in both SSc- and HC-MSC [CD248 mRNA levels in PDGF-BB SSc-MSC 1.69 (1.24–1.85) vs UT SSc-MSC 1.32 (1.25–1.50); $p = $ ns; CD248 mRNA levels in

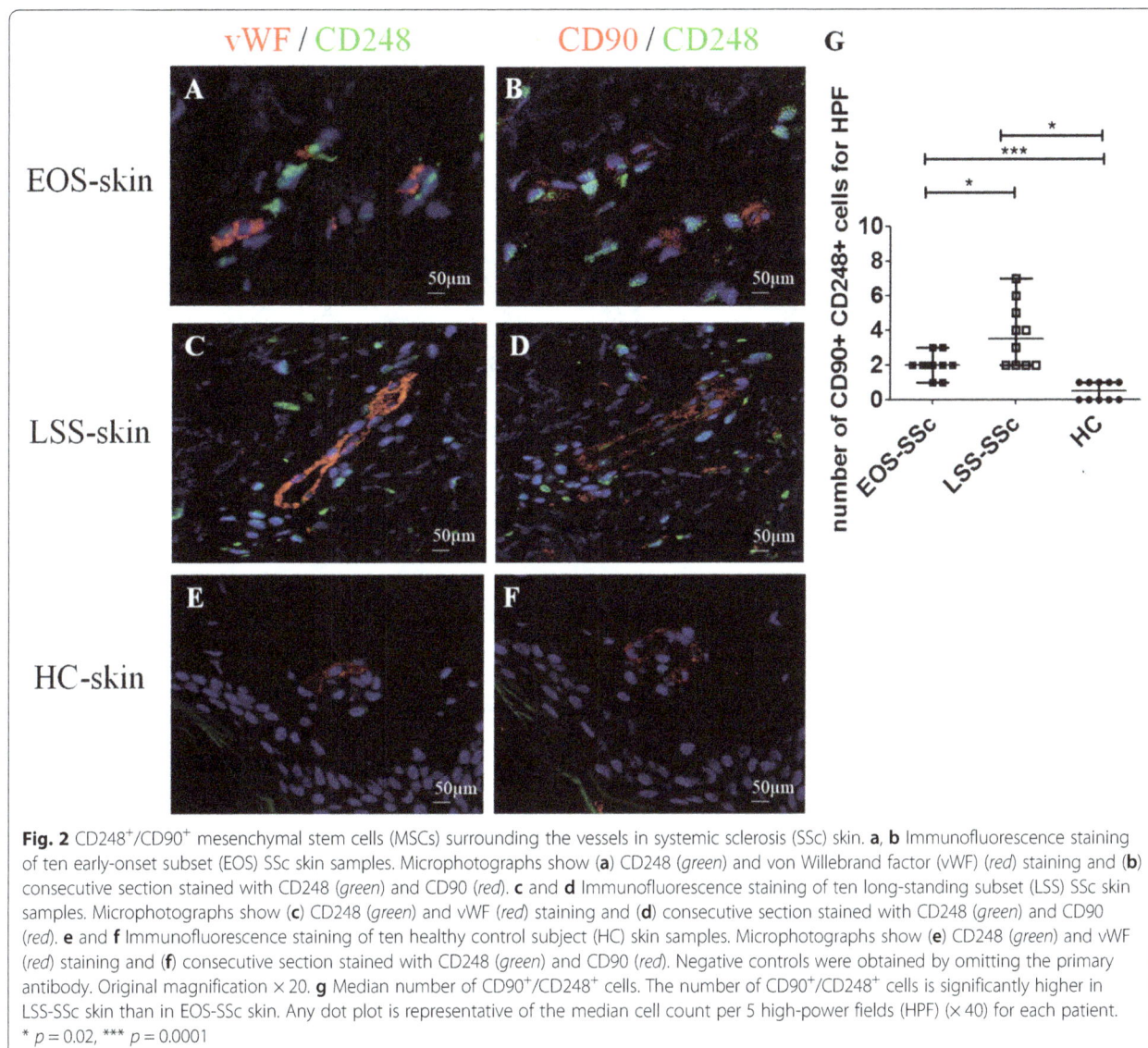

Fig. 2 CD248[+]/CD90[+] mesenchymal stem cells (MSCs) surrounding the vessels in systemic sclerosis (SSc) skin. **a**, **b** Immunofluorescence staining of ten early-onset subset (EOS) SSc skin samples. Microphotographs show (**a**) CD248 (*green*) and von Willebrand factor (vWF) (*red*) staining and (**b**) consecutive section stained with CD248 (*green*) and CD90 (*red*). **c** and **d** Immunofluorescence staining of ten long-standing subset (LSS) SSc skin samples. Microphotographs show (**c**) CD248 (*green*) and vWF (*red*) staining and (**d**) consecutive section stained with CD248 (*green*) and CD90 (*red*). **e** and **f** Immunofluorescence staining of ten healthy control subject (HC) skin samples. Microphotographs show (**e**) CD248 (*green*) and vWF (*red*) staining and (**f**) consecutive section stained with CD248 (*green*) and CD90 (*red*). Negative controls were obtained by omitting the primary antibody. Original magnification × 20. **g** Median number of CD90[+]/CD248[+] cells. The number of CD90[+]/CD248[+] cells is significantly higher in LSS-SSc skin than in EOS-SSc skin. Any dot plot is representative of the median cell count per 5 high-power fields (HPF) (× 40) for each patient. * $p = 0.02$, *** $p = 0.0001$

PDGF-BB HC-MSC 0.85 (0.72–1.0) vs UT HC-MSC 0.96 (0.73–1.17); p = n.s.].

TGF-β induces an increase of α-SMA in MSC

TGF-β treatment induced a significant increase of α-SMA mRNA expression in both SSc- and HC-MSC when compared with UT cells [α-SMA mRNA levels in TGF-β SSc-MSC 11.90 (9.36–15.87) vs UT SSc-MSC 7.53 (6.94–7.94); $p < 0.0001$; α-SMA mRNA levels in TGF-β HC-MSC 1.66 (1.14–2.48) vs UT HC-MSC 1.05 (0.84–1.18); $p < 0.0001$]. On the contrary, PDGF-BB treatment induced a significant decrease of α-SMA when compared with UT cells, in both HC- and SSc-MSC [α-SMA mRNA levels in PDGF-BB SSc-MSC 1.84 (1.52–2.01) vs UT SSc-MSC 7.53 (6.94–7.94); $p < 0.0001$; α-SMA mRNA levels in PDGF-BB HC-MSC 0.54 (0.24–0.70) vs UT HC-MSC 1.05 (0.84–1.18); $p < 0.0001$] (Fig.

3b). Western blot analysis confirmed the results of gene expression (Fig. 3d).

TGF-β and PDGF-BB effects on cell proliferation in MSC

To assess the proliferative ability of our cells, we performed qRT-PCR for Ki-67 gene expression, a molecule considered to be associated with active proliferation. We observed that TGF-β treatment induced a significant decrease of Ki-67 in both SSc- and HC-MSC; on the contrary, PDGF-BB induced a significant increase of Ki-67 when compared with UT cells in both SSc- and HC-MSC [Ki-67 mRNA levels in TGF-β SSc-MSC 0.0066 (0.0013–0.016) vs UT SSc-MSC 0.16 (0.08–0.23); $p < 0.0001$; Ki-67 mRNA levels in TGF-β HC-MSC 0.64 (0.54–0.84) vs UT HC-MSC 1.04 (0.85–1.26); $p < 0.0001$; Ki-67 mRNA levels in PDGF-BB SSc-MSC 0.63 (0.52–0.81) vs UT SSc-MSC 0.16 (0.08–

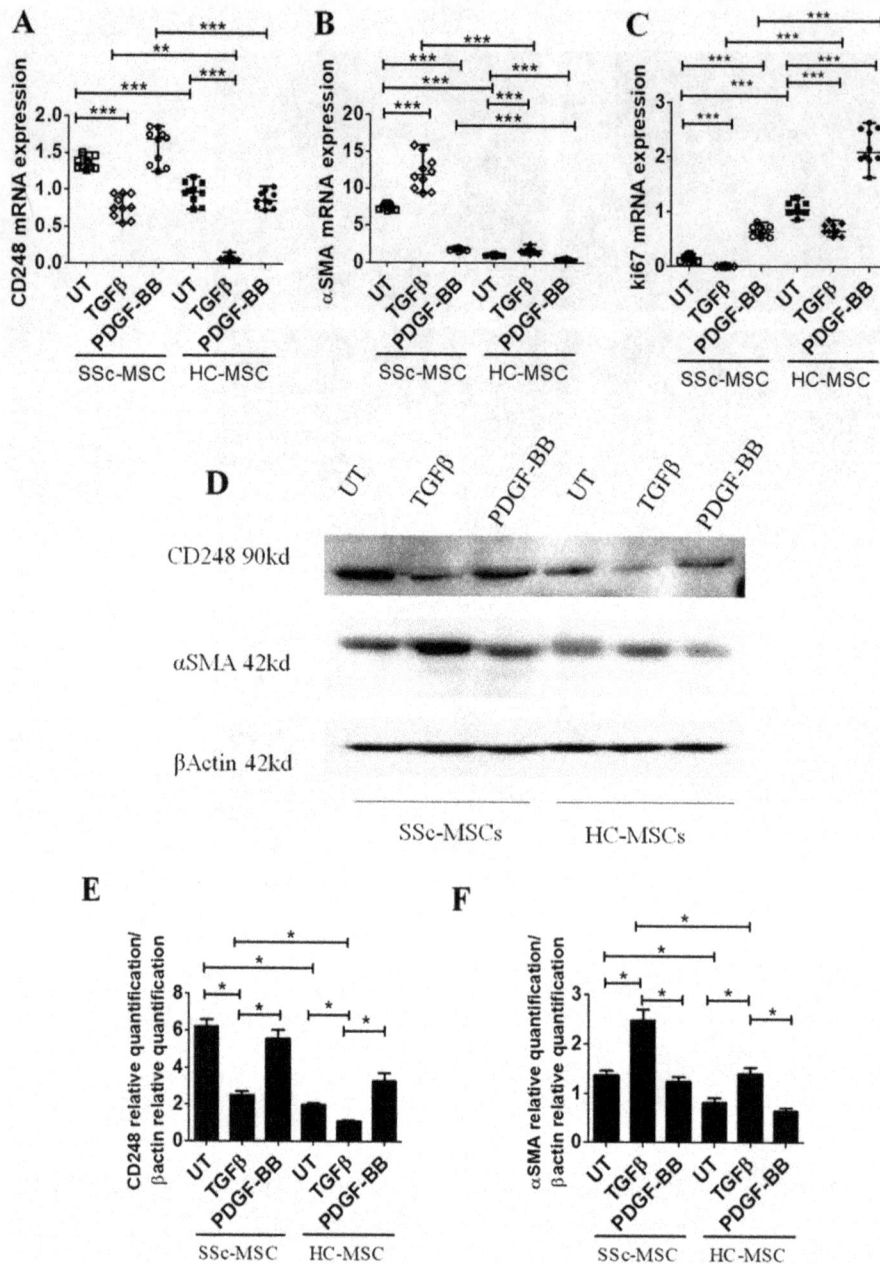

Fig. 3 Transforming growth factor (TGF)-β and platelet-derived growth factor (PDGF)-BB effects on CD248, α-smooth muscle actin (α-SMA), and Ki-67 expression in systemic sclerosis (SSc) mesenchymal stem cells (MSCs). **a** qRT-PCR of CD248 messenger RNA (mRNA) levels in ten SSc-MSC (five early-onset subset [EOS] and five long-standing subset [LSS]) and ten healthy control subject (HC) MSC samples. In SSc-MSCs, CD248 mRNA expression levels are always significantly higher than in HC-MSCs. **b** qRT-PCR of α-SMA mRNA levels in ten SSc-MSCs (five EOS and five LSS) and ten HC-MSCs. In SSc-MSCs, the α-SMA mRNA levels are always significantly higher than in HC-MSCs. In both SSc- and HC-MSCs, TGF-β treatment induces a significant increase of α-SMA mRNA expression compared with untreated (UT) cells. On the contrary, PDGF-BB treatment induces a significant decrease of α-SMA compared with UT cells in both HC- and SSc-MSCs. **c** qRT-PCR of Ki-67 mRNA levels in ten SSc-MSCs (five EOS and five LSS) and ten HC-MSCs. In both SSc- and HC-MSCs, TGF-β treatment induces a significant decrease of Ki-67; on the contrary, PDGF-BB induces a significant increase of Ki-67 when compared with UT cells in both SSc- and HC-MSCs. The TGF-β isoform used is TGF-β1. Any single dot in the figure represents the median of triplicate experiments for each patient ** $p = 0.0002$, *** $p = 0.0001$. **d** Western blot analyses performed in four SSc-MSCs (two EOS and two LSS) and four HC SSc-MSCs confirmed the results observed by qRT-PCR analyses. Pictures are representative of all experiments. **e** and **f** Densitometric analysis of (**e**) CD248 protein bands and (**f**) α-SMA protein bands. The values were expressed as protein relative quantification/β-actin relative quantification. * $p = 0.02$

Blocking CD248 molecules in perivascular stromal cells of patients with systemic sclerosis strongly inhibits...

217

0.23); $p < 0.0001$; Ki-67 mRNA levels in PDGF-BB HC-MSC 2.08 (1.63–2.63) vs UT HC-MSC 1.04 (0.85–1.26); $p < 0.0001$] (Fig. 3c).

CD248 silencing interferes with PDGF-BB and TGF-β signaling in SSc-MSC

To address the role of CD248 in this cytokine network, we inactivated CD248 gene product in SSc-MSC by transfecting these cells with CD248-siRNA or scr-siRNA. CD248-siRNA efficiently knocked down CD248 molecules in SSc-MSC (> 71%), and, after silencing, TGF-β was unable to modulate the CD248 expression (Fig. 4a). Figure 4b shows that in CD248 silenced MSC, TGF-β stimulation did not induce α-SMA mRNA upregulation. Furthermore, in the same cells, PDGF-BB was unable to induce an increased expression of Ki-67 gene levels when compared with scr-siRNA-treated MSC (Fig. 4c).

Western blot analysis confirmed the results of gene expression (Fig. 4d).

Discussion

This report is the first, to the best of our knowledge, indicating that CD248, first identified as a tumor vascular endothelial antigen [35] and considered a key molecule of myofibroblast generation, is deeply involved in TGF-β and PDGF-BB signaling transduction during the fibrosis associated with SSc and that its inhibition strongly interferes with the profibrotic pathways of these two cytokines. Recently, CD248 has been considered as a marker of stromal fibroblasts, pericyte subsets, and human MSC [36, 37], and in the experimental model of fibrosis, after UUO, a significant upregulation of CD248 was observed [3]. On the contrary, CD248$^{-/-}$ mice were protected from renal fibrosis and capillary rarefaction, probably

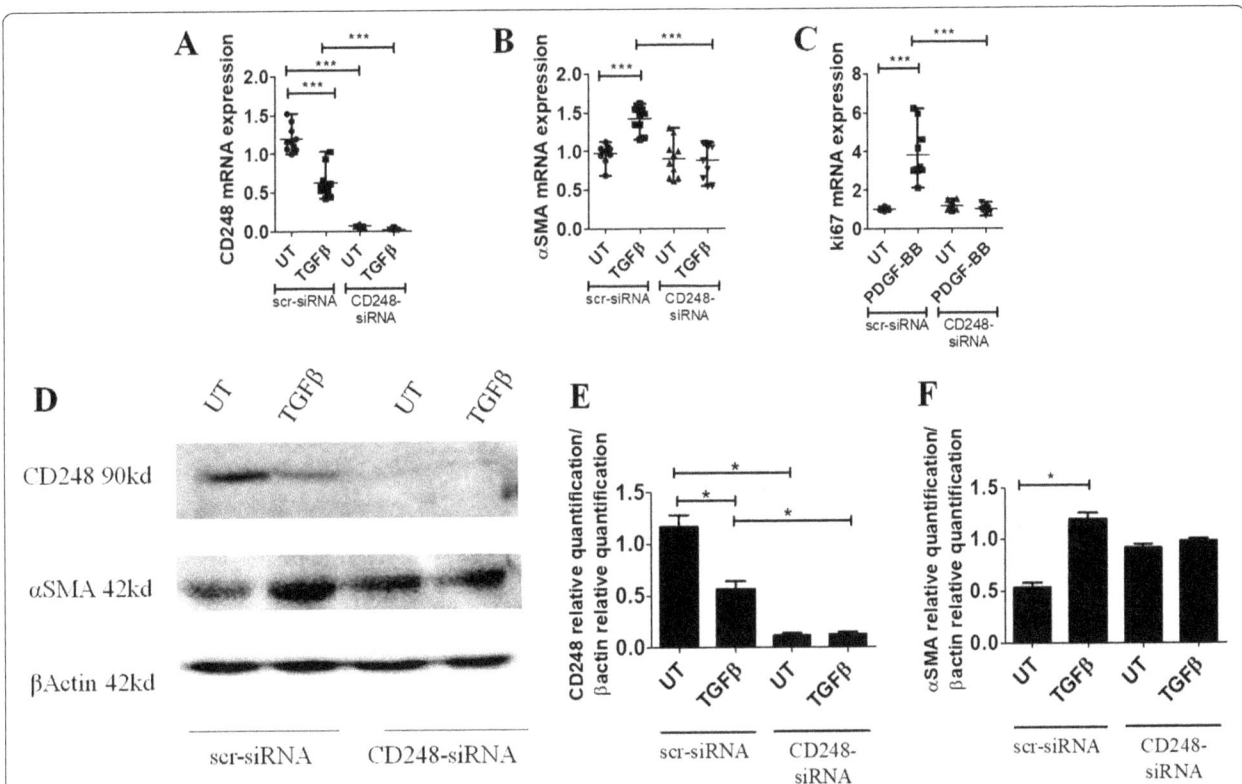

Fig. 4 Systemic sclerosis (SSc) mesenchymal stem cells (MSCs) silenced by small interfering RNA (siRNA) CD248. **a** qRT-PCR of CD248 in ten SSc-MSCs (five early-onset subset [EOS] and five long-standing subset [LSS]) transfected with specific CD248-siRNA or scrambled (scr)-siRNA. Cells transfected with CD248-siRNA show a decreased expression of the CD248 gene compared with cells transfected with scr-siRNA. In SSc-MSCs treated with scr-siRNA, the transforming growth factor (TGF)-β stimulus induces a significant decrease of CD248 expression. On the contrary, in CD248-siRNA cells, TGF-β is unable to modulate CD248 mRNA expression. **b** qRT-PCR of α-SMA in ten SSc-MSCs (five EOS and five LSS) transfected with specific CD248-siRNA or scr-siRNA. In SSc-MSCs treated with scr-siRNA, the TGF-β stimulus induces a significant increase of α-SMA mRNA expression. On the contrary, in CD248-siRNA cells, TGF-β is unable to modulate α-SMA mRNA expression. **c** qRT-PCR of Ki-67 in ten SSc-MSCs (five EOS and five LSS) transfected with specific CD248-siRNA or scr-siRNA. In SSc-MSCs treated with scr-siRNA, the PDGF-BB stimulus induces a significant increase of Ki-67 mRNA expression. On the contrary, in CD248-siRNA cells, PDGF-BB is unable to modulate Ki-67 mRNA expression. The TGF-β isoform used is TGF-β1. Any single dot in the figure represents the median of triplicate experiments for each patient. *** $p = 0.0001$. **d** Western blot analyses performed in four SSc-MSCs (two EOS and two LSS) confirmed the results observed by qRT-PCR analyses. Pictures are representative of all experiments. **e** and **f** Densitometric analysis of (**e**) CD248 protein bands and (**f**) α-SMA protein bands. The values were expressed as protein relative quantification/β-actin relative quantification. * $p = 0.02$

inhibiting pericyte differentiation toward α-SMA⁺ interstitial myofibroblasts and preventing vascular instability and collagen production [3]. Furthermore, it has been reported that CD248 expressed on pericytes can promote EC apoptosis, probably impairing the cross-talk between EC integrins and vascular endothelial growth factor (VEGF) receptor 2, leading to the attenuation of VEGF signaling [38]. On these bases, CD248 may be considered a key target in those pathologic processes in which vascular damage and fibrosis are strongly joined in SSc.

In our present study, we chose to include in the patient cohort only patients affected by the Scl70⁺ diffuse form of the disease, because this subset rapidly progresses from vascular damage to fibrosis and may be considered a good "human model" to evaluate the link between vascular damage and fibrosis. In fact, it is well known that anti-Scl70 antibody is one of the typical autoimmune markers in SSc, occurring in 60.8% of cases of diffuse SSc and 23.4% of cases of limited SSc [39]. The presence of anti-Scl70 antibody is associated with severity of the disease, decreased survival [40], and evidence of pulmonary fibrosis [41]. We observed that CD248 was constitutively overexpressed on SSc cells derived from mesenchymal lineage. In SSc skin, we observed that CD248 was expressed on stromal fibroblasts and perivascular cells located in close proximity to the vessel, when compared with healthy skin, and the number of CD248⁺ cells significantly increased over time. Furthermore, in LSS-SSc biopsy, the CD248 mRNA expression of whole biopsy was significantly increased when compared with EOS-SSc. Of note, IF showed that the CD248⁺ cells coexpressed CD90, a molecule highly expressed in all the undifferentiated MSC [42, 43]. Currently, although we do not have a single cell marker capable of defining MSC, available literature suggests that CD90, which is highly expressed in all MSC, regardless of the source, may be considered a good marker to identify undifferentiated MSC [34]. The increased CD248 expression in perivascular cells of patients with SSc highly coexpressing the stem marker CD90 may suggest that in these MSC, both the profibrotic machinery and cells' differentiation toward myofibroblasts may be activated.

Furthermore, our results showed that increased CD248 expression may be observed also in EC of SSc skin biopsies. It has been reported that CD248 may be expressed by endothelial progenitor cells [44] and tumor EC, together with pericytes and tumor-associated fibroblasts, during active cancer angiogenesis [38, 45]. It has been proposed that CD248 expressed by EC may interact with ECM proteins as well as tumor stromal cells to promote vascular invasion and migration [46]; in fact, CD248 expression was induced in EC when cultured in Matrigel, suggesting that endosialin could be induced in

EC exposed to a complex extracellular environment [46]. In our setting, we hypothesize that SSc-EC may express CD248 as a compensatory mechanism to support angiogenesis in the context of a disease characterized by progressive desertification of vascular tree.

We investigated the functional role of CD248 in vitro in the perivascular differentiation toward myofibroblasts by using MSC, a validated surrogate of perivascular cells [26, 47]. Although the possible role of the CD248 molecule in SSc pathogenesis is largely unknown, it has been reported that this molecule is involved in the fibroproliferative process by modulating the PDGF-BB pathway [21] and collaborating with the TGF-β pathway to induce α-SMA expression [48]. In HC cells, TGF-β induced significantly decreased of CD248 when compared with UT cells. On the contrary, SSc-MSC displayed significantly higher CD248 expression than HC cells in both TGF-β-stimulated and unstimulated cultures. Recently, it has been shown that TGF-β strongly suppresses CD248 expression in healthy murine fibroblast cell lines; on the contrary, during cancer, where significantly higher CD248 levels are reported, mirroring what we observed in our cells, TGF-β failed to downregulate CD248 expression [49]. Although TGF-β is not a promoter of CD248 expression, CD248 may collaborate with TGF-β to induce α-SMA, possibly via downregulation of Notch3 [9, 12] and upregulation of interleukin 6 (IL6), C-C motif chemokine ligand 2 (CCL2), TGF-β1, and TGF-βR1 [48]. In fact, it has been reported that Notch3 may prevent the TGF-β1 induction of α-SMA, working as a molecular brake on smooth muscle gene transcription [50]. Furthermore, IL6, CCL2, TGF-β1, and TGF-βR1, activated by CD248, may strongly stimulate α-SMA [51]. Thus, we may hypothesize that CD248 overexpression in SSc-MSC may play its profibrotic role, exacerbating the TGF-β effects [52], by removing the Notch3 control and promoting α-SMA expression by its own downstream mediators. In fact, after silencing CD248, cells were unable to induce α-SMA expression after TGF-β stimulus, thus confirming the key role of CD248 in increasing the TGF-β effects in SSc-MSC.

To date, conflicting results have been reported in available literature concerning the expression of different smooth muscle genes during fibroblast proliferation and activation. Transcript levels of Sm22 are elevated in fibroblasts derived from mice lacking the cytoplasmic domain of CD248 [12], and CD248 knockdown did not affect the in vitro expression of α-SMA in normal human lung fibroblast [31]. On the contrary, in in vitro cultured human pericytes, the ability of TGF-β to induce α-SMA expression was lost in the CD248-specific siRNA-transfected primary human brain vascular pericytes, suggesting that α-SMA induction is CD248-dependent [53]. Furthermore, in an experimental model of liver fibrosis, the total liver mRNA of collagen and α-SMA was reduced in CD248-deficient mice compared with wild-type mice [19], and in a model of renal fibrosis, no increase of α-SMA molecule was observed in CD248-deficient mice [8]. These discrepancies may be partially explained by the different experimental models, the differences in cell manipulation, the intensity and quality of stimuli, and the different levels of efficacy in CD248 silencing.

To assess the contribution of CD248 in modulating the proliferative ability of SSc-MSC, we evaluated the expression of Ki-67 gene expression, which strongly correlates with cellular proliferation [19]. PDGF-BB induced a significant increase of Ki-67 levels when compared with UT cells in both HC- and SSc-MSC.

The role of CD248 in PDGF-BB signaling has been studied in human pericytes and hepatic stellate cells (HSC), commonly considered the precursors of septal myofibroblasts in liver fibrosis. PDGF-BB currently is considered one of the most potent HSC mitogens known, and it plays a key regulatory role in HSC proliferation during hepatic fibrogenesis [19]. It has been proposed that CD248 regulates the PDGF-BB pathway, thus controlling cell proliferation [54].

After CD248 silencing, we observed a strong inhibition of PDGF-BB-mediated cell proliferation, suggesting that this process is under CD248 control, thus decreasing the myofibroblast accumulation and confirming previous reports [23] in which primary renal fibroblasts isolated from CD248-knockout mice displays both decreased cell proliferation and reduced collagen secretion when compared with wild-type mice. Currently, it is still unclear how CD248 may modulate this proliferative signal: via the matrix-binding properties of CD248 and/or by the well-known ability of this molecule to potentiate PDGF-BB signaling. Recent studies in hepatic fibrosis, however, have provided evidence that HSC CD248$^{-/-}$ display normal levels of PDGF receptors, suggesting that the antiproliferative effect of CD248$^{-/-}$ HSCs is not mediated through the modulation of PDGF receptor expression [19].

Conclusions

Our study shows that SSc perivascular cells overexpress CD248, which is involved in SSc pericyte transition toward myofibroblasts, and CD248 silencing may prevent pericyte-to-myofibroblast transition, proliferation, vascular instability, and tissue fibrosis. Taken together, our data suggest that targeting CD248 expression may be considered a potential target in order to block tissue fibrosis and vascular desertification during SSc.

Abbreviations

CCL2: C-C motif chemokine ligand 2; cDNA: Complementary DNA; ECM: Extracellular matrix; EC: Endothelial cell(s); EOS: Early-onset subset; HC: Healthy control subject(s); HSC: Hepatic stellate cell(s); IF: Immunofluorescence; IL6: Interleukin 6; LSS: Long-standing subset; mRNA: Messenger RNA; MSC: Mesenchymal stem cell(s); PDGF-BB: Platelet-derived growth factor BB; RP: Raynaud's phenomenon; scr-siRNA: Nontargeting scrambled small interfering RNA; siRNA: Small interfering RNA; α-SMA: α-Smooth muscle actin; SSc: Systemic sclerosis; TGF-β: Transforming growth factor-β; UUO: Unilateral ureteral obstruction; VEGF: Vascular endothelial growth factor; vWF: Von Willebrand factor

Acknowledgements

The authors thank Federica Sensini and Anna Rita Lizzi for their technical assistance.

Authors' contributions

PDB was responsible for study conception and design, data interpretation, literature search, figure creation, manuscript writing, and paper revision and approval. VL was responsible for data collection, data interpretation, literature search, and paper revision and approval. PR was responsible for data collection, data interpretation, literature search, and paper revision and approval. OB was responsible for data collection, data interpretation, literature search, and paper revision and approval. FCa was responsible for data collection, data interpretation, literature search, and paper revision and approval. NP was responsible for data collection, data interpretation, literature search, and paper revision and approval. SDB was responsible for data collection, data interpretation, literature search, and paper revision and approval. FCi was responsible for data collection, data interpretation, literature search, and paper revision and approval. GG was responsible for data collection, data interpretation, literature search, and paper revision and approval. GT was responsible for data collection, data interpretation, literature search, and paper revision and approval. PC was responsible for study conception and design, data interpretation, manuscript writing, and paper revision and approval. RG was responsible for study conception and design, data interpretation, manuscript writing, and paper revision and approval. All authors gave final approval for submitting the manuscript for review and agree to be accountable for all aspects of the work.

Consent for publication

Not applicable.

Competing interests

The authors declare that they have no competing interests.

Author details

[1]Department of Biotechnological and Applied Clinical Sciences, Rheumatology Unit, School of Medicine, University of L'Aquila, Delta 6 Building, Via dell'Ospedale, 67100 L'Aquila, Italy. [2]Department of Internal Medicine, Division of Rheumatology, University of Palermo, Piazza delle Cliniche 2, 90127 Palermo, Italy.

References

1. Lax S, Hardie D, Wilson A, Douglas M, Anderson G, Huso D, et al. The pericyte and stromal marker CD248 (endosialin) is required for efficient lymph node expansion. Eur J Immunol. 2010;40:1884–9.
2. Bagley RG, Honma N, Weber W, Boutin P, Rouleau C, Shankara S, et al. Endosialin/TEM1/CD248 is a pericyte marker of embryonic and tumor neovascularisation. Microvasc Res. 2008;76:180–8.

3. Smith SW, Eardley KS, Croft A, Nwosu J, Howie AJ, Cockwell P, et al. CD248+ stromal cells are associated with progressive chronic kidney disease. Kidney Int. 2011;80:199–207.

4. Maia M, de Vriese A, Janssens T, Moons M, van Landuyt K, Tavernier J, et al. CD248 and its cytoplasmic domain: a therapeutic target for arthritis. Arthritis Rheum. 2010;62:3595–606.

5. Rettig WJ, Garin-Chesa P, Healey JH, Su SL, Jaffe EA, Old LJ. Identification of endosialin, a cell surface glycoprotein of vascular endothelial cells in human cancer. Proc Natl Acad Sci U S A. 1992;89:10832–6.

6. Rouleau C, Curiel M, Weber W, Smale R, Kurtzberg L, Mascarello J, et al. Endosialin protein expression and therapeutic target potential in human solid tumors: sarcoma versus carcinoma. Clin Cancer Res. 2008;14:7223–36.

7. Brady J, Neal J, Sadakar N, Gasque P. Human endosialin (tumor endothelial marker 1) is abundantly expressed in highly malignant and invasive brain tumors. J Neuropathol Exp Neurol. 2004;63:2374–83.

8. Smith SW, Croft AP, Morris HL, Naylor AJ, Huso DL, Isacke CM, Savage CO, Buckley CD. Genetic deletion of the stromal cell marker CD248 (endosialin) protects against the development of renal fibrosis. Nephron. 2015;131:265–77.

9. Chang-Panesso M, Humphreys BD. CD248/endosialin: a novel pericyte target in renal fibrosis. Nephron. 2015;131:262–4.

10. Maia M, DeVriese A, Janssens T, Moons M, Lories RJ, Tavernier J, et al. CD248 facilitates tumor growth via its cytoplasmic domain. BMC Cancer. 2011;11:162.

11. Teicher BA. Newer vascular targets: endosialin (review). Int J Oncol. 2007;30: 305–12.

12. Valdez Y, Maia M, Conway EM. CD248: reviewing its role in health and disease. Curr Drug Targets. 2012;13:432–9.

13. Diaz LA, Coughlin CM, Weil SC, Fishel J, Gounder MM, Lawrence S, et al. A first-in-human phase I study of MORAb-004, a monoclonal antibody to endosialin in patients with advanced solid tumors. Clin Cancer Res. 2015;21: 1281–8.

14. Denton CP, Black CM, Abraham DJ. Mechanisms and consequences of fibrosis in systemic sclerosis. Nat Clin Pract Rheumatol. 2006;2:134–44.

15. Gabrielli A, Avvedimento EV, Krieg T. Scleroderma. N Engl J Med. 2009;360: 1989–2003.

16. Cipriani P, Di Benedetto P, Ruscitti P, Capece D, Zazzeroni F, Liakouli V, et al. The endothelial-mesenchymal transition in SSc is induced by the synergistic effect of ET-1 and TGF-β and may be blocked by macitentan, a new dual ET-1 receptor antagonist. J Rheumatol. 2015;42:1808–16.

17. Cipriani P, Di Benedetto P, Ruscitti P, Campese AF, Liakouli V, Carubbi F, et al. Impaired endothelium-mesenchymal stem cells cross-talk in systemic sclerosis: a link between vascular and fibrotic features. Arthritis Res Ther. 2014;16:442.

18. Jimenez SA. Role of endothelial to mesenchymal transition in the pathogenesis of the vascular alterations in systemic sclerosis. ISRN Rheumatol. 2013;23:835948.

19. Wilhelm A, Aldridge V, Haldar D, Naylor AJ, Weston CJ, Hedegaard D, et al. CD248/endosialin critically regulates hepatic stellate cell proliferation during chronic liver injury via a PDGF-regulated mechanism. Gut. 2016;65:1175–85.

20. Cipriani P, Di Benedetto P, Dietrich H, Ruscitti P, Liakouli V, Carubbi F, Pantano I, Berardicurti O, Sgonc R, Giacomelli R. Searching for a good model for systemic sclerosis: the molecular profile and vascular changes occurring in UCD-200 chickens strongly resemble the early phase of human systemic sclerosis. Arch Med Sci. 2016;12:828–43.

21. Jiménez SA, Castro SV, Piera-Velázquez S. Role of growth factors in the pathogenesis of tissue fibrosis in systemic sclerosis. Curr Rheumatol Rev. 2010;6:283–94.

22. Sacchetti C, Bai Y, Stanford SM, Di Benedetto P, Cipriani P, Santelli E, et al. PTP4A1 promotes TGFβ signaling and fibrosis in systemic sclerosis. Nat Commun. 2017;8(1):1060.

23. Cipriani P, Di Benedetto P, Liakouli V, Del Papa B, Di Padova M, Di Ianni M, Marrelli A, Alesse E, Giacomelli R. Mesenchymal stem cells (MSCs) from scleroderma patients (SSc) preserve their immunomodulatory properties although senescent and normally induce T regulatory cells (Tregs) with a functional phenotype: implications for cellular-based therapy. Clin Exp Immunol. 2013;173:195–206.

24. Cipriani P, Marrelli A, Liakouli V, Di Benedetto P, Giacomelli R. Cellular players in angiogenesis during the course of systemic sclerosis. Autoimmun Rev. 2011;10:641–6.

25. Cipriani P, Di Benedetto P, Ruscitti P, Liakouli V, Berardicurti O, Carubbi F, et al. Perivascular cells in diffuse cutaneous systemic sclerosis overexpress

26. Cipriani P, Marrelli A, Di Benedetto P, Liakouli V, Carubbi F, Ruscitti P, et al. Scleroderma mesenchymal stem cells display a different phenotype from healthy controls; implications for regenerative medicine. Angiogenesis. 2013;16:595–607.

27. LeRoy EC, Black C, Fleischmajer R, Jablonska S, Krieg T, Medsger TA, et al. Scleroderma (systemic sclerosis): classification, subsets and pathogenesis. J Rheumatol. 1988;15:202–5.

28. van den Hoogen F, Khanna D, Fransen J, Johnson SR, Baron M, Tyndall A, et al. 2013 Classification criteria for systemic sclerosis: an American College of Rheumatology/European League Against Rheumatism collaborative initiative. Ann Rheum Dis. 2013;72:1747–55.

29. Kahaleh MB, Sultany GL, Smith EA, Huffstutter JE, Loadholt CB, Le Roy EC. A modified scleroderma skin scoring method. Clin Exp Rheumatol. 1986;4:367–9.

30. Koenig M, Joyal F, Fritzler MJ. Autoantibodies and microvascular damage are independent predictive factors for the progression of Raynaud's phenomenon to systemic sclerosis: a twenty-year prospective study of 586 patients, with validation of proposed criteria for early systemic sclerosis. Arthritis Rheum. 2008;58:3902–12.

31. Bartis D, Crowley LE, D'Souza VK, Borthwick L, Fisher AJ, Croft AP, et al. Role of CD248 as a potential severity marker in idiopathic pulmonary fibrosis. BMC Pulm Med. 2016;16:51.

32. Huang HP, Hong CL, Kao CY, Lin SW, Lin SR, Wu HL et al. Gene targeting and expression analysis of mouse Tem1/endosialin using a lacZ reporter. Gene Expr Patterns. 2011;11:316–26.

33. Christian S, Ahorn H, Koehler A, Eisenhaber F, Rodi HP, Garin-Chesa P, et al. Molecular cloning and characterization of endosialin, a C-type lectin-like cell surface receptor of tumor endothelium. J Biol Chem. 2001;276:7408–14.

34. Moraes DA, Sibov TT, Pavon LF, Alvim PQ, Bonadio RS, Da Silva JR, et al. A reduction in CD90 (THY-1) expression results in increased differentiation of mesenchymal stromal cells. Stem Cell Res Ther. 2016;7:97.

35. Christian S, Winkler R, Helfrich I, Boos AM, Besemfelder E, Schadendorf D, Augustin HG. Endosialin (Tem1) Is a Marker of Tumor-Associated Myofibroblasts and Tumor Vessel-Associated Mural Cells. Am J Pathol. 2008; 172(2):486–94.

36. MacFadyen JR, Haworth O, Roberston D, Hardie D, Webster MT, Morris HR, et al. Endosialin (TEM1, CD248) is a marker of stromal fibroblasts and is not selectively expressed on tumour endothelium. FEBS Lett. 2005;579:2569–75.

37. Bagley RG, Weber W, Rouleau C, Yao M, Honma N, Kataoka S, et al. Human mesenchymal stem cells from bone marrow express tumor endothelial and stromal markers. Int J Oncol. 2009;34:619–27.

38. Simonavicius N, Robertson D, Bax DA, Jones C, Huijbers IJ, Isacke CM. Endosialin (CD248) is a marker of tumor-associated pericytes in high-grade glioma. Mod Pathol. 2008;21:308–15.

39. Walker UA, Tyndall A, Czirják L, Denton C, Farge-Bancel D, Kowal-Bielecka O, et al. Clinical risk assessment of organ manifestations in systemic sclerosis: a report from the EULAR Scleroderma Trials and Research group database. Ann Rheum Dis. 2007;66:754–63.

40. Jacobsen S, Ullman S, Shen GQ, Wiik A, Halberg P. Influence of clinical features, serum antinuclear antibodies, and lung function on survival of patients with systemic sclerosis. J Rheumatol. 2001;28:2454–9.

41. Diot E, Giraudeau B, Diot P, Degenne D, Ritz L, Guilmot JL, et al. Is anti-topoisomerase I a serum marker of pulmonary involvement in systemic sclerosis? Chest. 1999;116:715–20.

42. Dominici M, Le Blanc K, Mueller I, Marini FC, Krause DS, Deans RJ, et al. Minimal criteria for defining multipotent mesenchymal stromal cells: the International Society for Cellular Therapy position statement. Cytotherapy. 2006;8:315–7.

43. Horwitz EM, Le Blanc K, Dominici M, Mueller I, Slaper-Cortenbach I, Marini FC, et al. Clarification of the nomenclature for MSC: the International Society for Cellular Therapy position statement. Cytotherapy. 2005;7:393–5.

44. Bagley RG, Rouleau C, St Martin T, Boutin P, Weber W, Ruzek M, et al. Human endothelial precursor cells express tumor endothelial marker 1/ endosialin/CD248. Mol Cancer Ther. 2008;7:2536–46.

45. Wesseling P, Schlingemann RO, Rietveld FJ, Link M, Burger PC, Ruiter DJ. Early and extensive contribution of pericytes/vascular smooth muscle cells to microvascular proliferation in glioblastoma multiforme: an immuno-light and immuno-electron microscopic study. J Neuropathol Exp Neurol. 1995;54:304–10.

46. Carson-Walter EB, Winans BN, Whiteman MC, Liu Y, Jarvela S, Haapasalo H, et al. Characterization of TEM1/endosialin in human and murine brain tumors. BMC Cancer. 2009;9:417.

47. Crisan M, Yap S, Casteilla L, Chen CW, Corselli M, Park TS, et al. A perivascular origin for mesenchymal stem cells in multiple human organs. Cell Stem Cell. 2008;3:301–13.

48. Kontsekova S, Polcicova K, Takacova M, Pastorekova S. Endosialin: molecular and functional links to tumor angiogenesis. Neoplasma. 2016;63:183–92.

49. Suresh Babu S, Valdez Y, Xu A, O'Byrne AM, Calvo F, Lei V, et al. TGFβ-mediated suppression of CD248 in non-cancer cells via canonical Smad-dependent signaling pathways is uncoupled in cancer cells. BMC Cancer. 2014;14:113.

50. Kennard S, Liu H, Lilly B. Transforming growth factor-β (TGF-1) down-regulates *Notch3* in fibroblasts to promote smooth muscle gene expression. J Biol Chem. 2008;283:1324–33.

51. Murray LA, Argentieri RL, Farrell FX, Bracht M, Sheng H, Whitaker B, et al. Hyper-responsiveness of IPF/UIP fibroblasts: interplay between TGFβ1, IL-13 and CCL2. Int J Biochem Cell Biol. 2008;40:2174–82.

52. Cipriani P, Di Benedetto P, Ruscitti P, Verzella D, Fischietti M, Zazzeroni F, et al. Macitentan inhibits the transforming growth factor-β profibrotic action, blocking the signaling mediated by the ETR/TβRI complex in systemic sclerosis dermal fibroblasts. Arthritis Res Ther. 2015;17:247.

53. Rybinski K, Imtiyaz HZ, Mittica B, Drozdowski B, Fulmer J, Furuuchi K, Fernando S, Henry M, Chao Q, Kline B, Albone E, Wustner J, Lin J, Nicolaides NC, Grasso L, Zhou Y. Targeting endosialin/CD248 through antibody-mediated internalization results in impaired pericyte maturation and dysfunctional tumor microvasculature. Oncotarget. 2015;22:25429–40.

54. Tomkowicz B, Rybinski K, Sebeck D, Sass P, Nicolaides NC, Grasso L, et al. Endosialin/TEM-1/CD248 regulates pericyte proliferation through PDGF receptor signaling. Cancer Biol Ther. 2010;9:908–15.

22

Factors associated with the achievement of biological disease-modifying antirheumatic drug-free remission in rheumatoid arthritis: the ANSWER cohort study

Motomu Hashimoto[1]*[ID], Moritoshi Furu[2], Wararu Yamamoto[1,3], Takanori Fujimura[4], Ryota Hara[4], Masaki Katayama[5], Akira Ohnishi[6], Kengo Akashi[6], Shuzo Yoshida[7], Koji Nagai[7], Yonsu Son[8], Hideki Amuro[8], Toru Hirano[9], Kosuke Ebina[10], Ryuji Uozumi[11], Hiromu Ito[1,2], Masao Tanaka[1], Koichiro Ohmura[12], Takao Fujii[13] and Tsuneyo Mimori[12]

Abstract

Background: Clinical remission can be maintained after the discontinuation of biological disease-modifying antirheumatic drugs (bDMARDs) in some patients with rheumatoid arthritis (RA) (bDMARD-free remission (BFR)). It is unknown which bDMARD is advantageous for achieving BFR or under which conditions BFR can be considered. This study aimed to determine the factors associated with BFR achievement in clinical practice.

Methods: Patients with RA were enrolled from a Japanese multicenter observational registry. Patients with RA who achieved clinical remission (Disease Activity Score 28—C-reactive protein < 2.3) at the time of bDMARD discontinuation were included. Serial disease activities and treatment changes were followed up. BFR was considered to have failed if the disease activity exceeded the remission cutoff value or if bDMARDs were restarted.

Results: Overall, 181 RA patients were included. BFR was maintained in 21.5% of patients at 1 year after bDMARD discontinuation. BFR was more successfully achieved after discontinuation of anti-tumor necrosis factor (TNF) monoclonal antibodies (TNFi(mAb)) (infliximab, adalimumab, and golimumab), followed by CTLA4-Ig (abatacept), soluble TNF receptor or Fab fragments against TNF fused with polyethylene glycol (etanercept and certolizumab), and anti-interleukin-6 receptor Ab (tocilizumab). After multivariate analysis, sustained remission (> 6 months), Boolean remission, no glucocorticoid use at the time of bDMARD discontinuation, and use of TNFi(mAb) or CTLA4-Ig remained as independent factors associated with BFR.

Conclusions: BFR can be achieved in some patients with RA after bDMARD discontinuation in clinical practice. Use of TNFi(mAb) or CTLA4-Ig, sustained remission, Boolean remission, and no glucocorticoid use at the time of bDMARD discontinuation are advantageous for achieving BFR.

Keywords: Rheumatoid arthritis, Biological disease-modifying antirheumatic drugs, Discontinuation, Tumor necrosis factor

* Correspondence: mohashim@kuhp.kyoto-u.ac.jp
[1]Department of Advanced Medicine for Rheumatic Diseases, Graduate School of Medicine, Kyoto University, 53 Kawahara-cho, Shogoin, Sakyo-ku, Kyoto 606-8507, Japan
Full list of author information is available at the end of the article

Background

Intensive treatment strategies utilizing biological disease-modifying antirheumatic drugs (bDMARDs) have revolutionized rheumatoid arthritis (RA) treatment. Remission or low disease activity is now a realistic goal for most patients. After achieving remission, it would be advantageous if remission could be maintained without using bDMARDs (bDMARDs-free remission (BFR)) because of the associated cost-effectiveness and prevention of adverse events. It would be of clinical importance to determine which bDMARD is advantageous for achieving BFR and in what conditions BFR could be successfully maintained in daily clinical practice [1].

Discontinuation of bDMARDs after remission has been attempted in previous studies, including prospective uncontrolled trials and randomized controlled trials (RCTs) [2–17]. For example, discontinuation of infliximab (IFX) was attempted in patients with established RA, and low disease activity was maintained in 43% of patients at 1 year after discontinuation in the RRR study [5]. Similarly, remission was maintained in 58% of patients with established RA at 6 months after discontinuation of adalimumab (ADA) in the HONOR study [8]. The remission maintenance rate after discontinuation of a soluble tumor necrosis factor (TNF) receptor, etanercept (ETN), was low (28%) compared to that in the ETN continuation group (50 mg/week; 59%) or the ETN reduction group (25 mg/week: 69%) at 1 year in the PRESERVE study [11, 12]. However, the ENCOURAGE study showed that 54% of patients maintained clinical remission after discontinuation of ETN [13]. Certolizumab pegol (CZP) (Fab fragments against TNF fused with polyethylene glycol) was discontinued after achieving remission in early RA patients, and 42% of patients remained in remission 1 year after discontinuation in the C-OPERA study [14]. Discontinuation of bDMARDs has also been attempted for non-TNF inhibitors. For example, abatacept (ABT) was withdrawn along with concomitant methotrexate (MTX) treatment after achieving remission, and "drug-free remission" was maintained in 15% of patients in the AVERT study [15]. "Drug-free remission" was also maintained after discontinuation of the anti-interleukin (IL)-6 receptor antibody tocilizumab (TCZ) in 9% of patients in the DREAM study [16] and 14% of patients in the ACT-RAY study [17], respectively, after 1 year.

However, the results of these clinical trials cannot be compared because each clinical trial was conducted under different conditions, with different patient backgrounds (early or established RA), study designs (prospective uncontrolled trials or RCTs), protocols (bDMARD free or drug free), and failure outcomes (remission, low disease activity, or restart of bDMARDs) [1, 18]. BFR achievability may vary depending on the type of bDMARDs, which have different modes of action (TNF inhibitors (TNFi),

CTLA4-Ig (ABT), and IL-6R inhibitors (IL-6Ri)). In addition to the typical classification of bDMARDs according to target molecules, TNFi can be classified into two groups: fully functional monoclonal antibodies with an immunoglobulin Fc portion (TNFi(mAb)), such as IFX, ADA, and golimumab (GLM); and soluble TNF absorption molecules (TNFi(R/P)), such as soluble TNF receptor (ETN) or Fab fragments against TNF fused with polyethylene glycol (CZP). It is possible that TNFi(mAb) (IFX, ADA, and GLM) might be more advantageous for achieving BFR than TNFi(R/P) (ETN and CZP) because anti-TNF monoclonal antibodies have higher cytotoxic activity against transmembrane TNF-expressing cells via complement-dependent and antibody-dependent cell-mediated cytotoxicity and inhibit granulomatous inflammation [19, 20]. However, this hypothesis cannot be tested by clinical trials that use totally different protocols. Therefore, the data from these clinical trials are not sufficient for determining how and when BFR can be successfully achieved in typical clinical practice.

Observational data from registries of patients in typical clinical practice could potentially contribute to answering these questions and providing real-world data that could be applied in daily clinical practice [21]. The Kansai Consortium for Well-being of Rheumatic Disease Patients (ANSWER) cohort was an observational multicenter registry of patients with RA in the Kansai district in Japan [22]. The data of patients at six universities (Kyoto University, Osaka University, Osaka Medical University, Kansai Medical University, Kobe University, and Nara Medial University) and associated hospitals were included. From 2011 to 2016, 4461 patients with RA were registered, and 52,654 serial disease activities were available from the database.

With the aforementioned in mind, the aim of this study was to determine which bDMARD is advantageous for achieving BFR and in what conditions BFR can be successfully achieved in typical clinical practice by utilizing the data from this multicenter observational cohort.

Methods

Study design and participants

We retrospectively analyzed the data for the ANSWER cohort from 2011 to 2016. Patients with RA fulfilled the 2010 ACR/European League Against Rheumatism (EULAR) criteria. In this study, we included all RA patients with Disease Activity Score 28—C-reactive protein (DAS28-CRP) < 2.3 (remission) at the time of bDMARD discontinuation to those with serial disease activity and treatment records that were fully available before and after bDMARD discontinuation. We used a DAS28-CRP remission cutoff value of 2.3, which has been validated in Japanese patients [23]. The study was approved by the ethics committee of Kyoto University (approval number R0357) as well as the ethics committees of all six institutions (Osaka University, Osaka Medical College, Kansai Medical University, Kobe University, Nara Medical University, and Osaka Red Cross Hospital). The study was conducted in accordance with the Declaration of Helsinki and written informed consent was obtained from all participants.

Treatments

In this study, the following bDMARDs were used: IFX, ADA, GLM, ETN, CZP, ABT, and TCZ. These were categorized into four groups based on their mode of action: TNFi(mAb) (IFX, ADA, and GLM); TNFi(R/P) (ETN and CZP); CTLA4-Ig (ABT); and anti-IL-6Ri antibodies (TCZ). Other bDMARDs such as rituximab or targeted synthetic DMARDs such as JAK inhibitors were not permitted for use in patients with RA in Japan during the study period. The reasons for the discontinuation of bDMARDs were remission, inefficiency, toxic adverse events, and nontoxic reasons [22]. The conventional synthetic DMARDs (csDMARDs) used in this study were MTX, sulfasalazine, bucillamine, tacrolimus, leflunomide, iguratimod, and gold compounds. The glucocorticoids used in this study were prednisolone, methylprednisolone, and betamethasone; these were converted into prednisolone-equivalent doses.

Outcomes

BFR failure was defined if DAS28-CRP exceeded 2.3 or if bDMARDs were restarted (including previous biologics or introduction of new bDMARDs). Changes in concomitant csDMARDs (including MTX) or glucocorticoids were not regarded as failures. If the disease activity record was not available for more than 6 months, then the case was regarded as censored at the date of the last disease activity record.

Statistical analysis

The Kaplan–Meier method was used to estimate the median time to BFR failure from bDMARD discontinuation. A Cox proportional hazard model was used to investigate the factors associated with BFR and to obtain hazard ratios (HRs) with 95% confidence intervals (CIs). The following variables were included in univariate analysis: age, sex, disease duration, type of bDMARD, disease duration, anti-cyclic citrullinated peptide (CCP) antibody and rheumatoid factor (RF) status, bDMARD status (naïve or switched), reason for bDMARD discontinuation (physician's intentional bDMARD discontinuation due to remission induction or not), remission maintenance period before bDMARD discontinuation, achievement of Boolean remission at the time of discontinuation, use and dosage of MTX at the time of bDMARD

discontinuation, and use and dosage of glucocorticoids at the time of bDMARD discontinuation. The variables included in the multivariate analysis were selected based on the results of the univariate analysis and clinical meaningfulness. Survival curves based on the Cox proportional hazard model were evaluated for patients in each category after adjustment for covariates using direct adjusted survival estimation [24]. Two-sided $p < 0.05$ was considered statistically significant. All statistical analyses were performed using SAS statistical software, version 9.4 (SAS Institute, Cary, NC, USA).

Results

Patient characteristics

From 2011 to 2016, bDMARDs were used for 1307 cases in the ANSWER cohort, and serial disease activity was available for 572 cases. Based on the inclusion criteria, 181 patients with disease activity under the DAS28-CRP remission cutoff value (< 2.3) at the time of bDMARD discontinuation were included in the study and serial disease activity and treatment changes were followed up after bDMARD discontinuation.

At the time of bDMARD discontinuation, the study participants were 49 years old on average and had a disease duration of 7.6 years (Table 1). The bDMARDs used in the patients were IFX ($n = 40$), ADA ($n = 25$), GLM ($n = 26$), ETN ($n = 22$), CZP ($n = 10$), ABT ($n = 12$), and TCZ ($n = 27$). In 65.2% of patients, bDMARDs were the first-ever bDMARDs used (bDMARD-naïve). In 18.8% of patients, bDMARDs were intentionally discontinued by physicians owing to remission induction. At the time of bDMARD discontinuation, 78.5% and 42.5% of patients received MTX and glucocorticoids, respectively. All patients were treated with some DMARDs after bDMARD discontinuation, and none of them achieved drug-free remission. Patients' baseline characteristics according to the different types of bDMARDs administered are presented in Table 1.

Maintenance of BFR

After bDMARD discontinuation, the BFR maintenance rates were 21.5% and 12.2% at 1 and 2 years, respectively, based on the Kaplan–Meier method. The median duration until BFR failure was 70 days (range 58–93 days). BFR failed because of disease activity flares and reinitiation of bDMARDs in 61.2% and 48.8% of patients, respectively.

Types of bDMARDs and maintenance of BFR

First, we analyzed the association between the types of bDMARDs and BFR maintenance. The BFR rates according to each bDMARD are shown in Additional file 1: Figure S1. Interestingly, among multiple TNF inhibitors, the BFR rate was clearly different between

Table 1 Patient demographics at the time of bDMARD discontinuation

Type of biologic	All	TNFi(mAb)	TNFi(R/P)	CTLA4-Ig	IL-6Ri	p value
	(N = 181)	(N = 95)	(N = 32)	(N = 17)	(N = 37)	
Age (years)	49.0 ± 16.7	50.8 ± 15.7	45.9 ± 17.5	49.4 ± 18.2	46.8 ± 18.3	0.42
Female sex, n (%)	144 (79.6)	77 (81.1)	27 (84.4)	12 (70.6)	28 (75.7)	0.62
Disease duration (years)	7.6 ± 9.2	5.3 ± 6.9	11.2 ± 11.5	8.0 ± 7.8	10.2 ± 11.3	< 0.01
Current smoking, n (%)	11 (11.1)	9 (17.3)	0 (0)	1 (9.1)	1 (4.2)	0.19
bDMARD-naïve, n (%)	118 (65.2)	76 (80.1)	18 (56.3)	11 (64.7)	18 (48.6)	< 0.01
Discontinuation due to remission, n (%)	34 (18.8)	25 (26.3)	4 (12.5)	3 (17.6)	2 (5.4)	0.03
Remission maintenance period (days)	130.6 ± 185.0	162.0 ± 211.0	125.3 ± 155.8	98.3 ± 140.2	69.5 ± 135.7	0.06
DAS28-CRP	1.6 ± 0.4	1.5 ± 0.39	1.7 ± 0.4	1.7 ± 0.4	1.7 ± 0.4	< 0.01
Boolean remission achieved, n (%)	61 (33.7)	34 (35.8)	18 (56.3)	1 (5.9)	8 (21.6)	< 0.01
MTX use, n (%)	142 (78.5)	70 (73.7)	29 (90.6)	10 (58.8)	33 (89.2)	0.01
MTX dose (mg/week)	7.1 ± 2.9	8.3 ± 3.0	7.5 ± 2.4	9.0 ± 3.6	7.5 ± 2.6	0.11
Glucocorticoid use, n (%)	77 (42.5)	40 (42.1)	8 (25.0)	12 (70.6)	17 (45.9)	0.02
Glucocorticoid dose (mg/day)	5.9 ± 9.5	7.4 ± 12.9	4.5 ± 3.6	4.9 ± 2.0	3.9 ± 2.2	0.44
ACPA positive, n (%)	125 (86.2)	68 (89.5)	26 (34.2)	8 (53.3)	26 (86.7)	0.54
RF positive, n (%)	114 (77.0)	57 (75.0)	15 (62.5)	13 (86.7)	29 (87.9)	0.04

Demographic and clinical characteristics at the time of bDMARD discontinuation summarized as means ± standard deviations for continuous data and as numbers (percentages) for categorical data. Analysis of variance and the chi-squared test were used to compare the clinical characteristics among different groups for continuous variables and categorical variables, respectively

bDMARD biological disease-modifying antirheumatic drug, *TNFi(mAb)* monoclonal antibodies against TNF (infliximab, adalimumab, and golimumab), *TNFi(R/P)* soluble TNF receptor or Fab fragments against TNF fused with polyethylene glycol (etanercept and certolizumab), *CTLA4-Ig* abatacept, *IL-6Ri* interleukin-6 receptor inhibitor (tocilizumab), *DAS28-CRP* Disease Activity Score 28—C-reactive protein, *MTX* methotrexate, *ACPA* anti-citrullinated protein antibodies, *RF* rheumatoid factor, *TNF* tumor necrosis factor

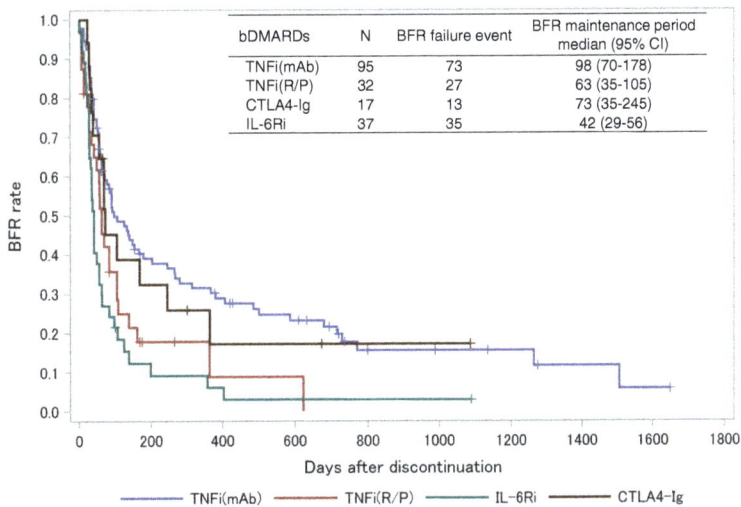

bDMARDs	N	BFR failure event	BFR maintenance period median (95% CI)
TNFi(mAb)	95	73	98 (70-178)
TNFi(R/P)	32	27	63 (35-105)
CTLA4-Ig	17	13	73 (35-245)
IL-6Ri	37	35	42 (29-56)

Fig. 1 Kaplan–Meier survival curve for maintaining bDMARD-free remission after discontinuation of different types of bDMARDs. *X* axis represents days after bDMARD discontinuation. *Y* axis represents rates of maintained BFR. BFR failure defined if DAS28-CRP exceeded 2.3 or if bDMARDs restarted. If disease activity not available for more than 6 months, patient was regarded as censored case at date of last disease activity record. Kaplan–Meier method used to estimate BFR maintenance time. bDMARD biological disease-modifying antirheumatic drug, BFR biological disease-modifying antirheumatic drug-free remission, TNFi(mAb) monoclonal antibodies against TNF (infliximab, adalimumab, and golimumab), TNFi(R/P) soluble TNF receptor or Fab fragments against TNF fused with polyethylene glycol (etanercept and certolizumab), CTLA4-Ig abatacept, IL-6Ri interleukin-6 receptor inhibitor (tocilizumab), CI confidence interval, TNF tumor necrosis factor

patients administered TNFi(mAb) (IFX, ADA, GLM) and those administered TNFi(R/P) (ETN and CZP) (Fig. 1). The longest median BFR maintenance period was after TNFi(mAb) administration, followed by CTLA4Ig, TNFi(R/P), and IL-6Ri (Table 2). TNFi(mAb) use was associated with a decreased risk of BFR failure compared with TNFi(R/P) and IL-6Ri use (Table 2). CTLA4-Ig use was associated with a decreased risk of BFR failure compared to IL-6Ri use (Table 2).

Because the patient backgrounds were different for those treated with different bDMARDs (Table 1), the BFR rate was compared only for the bDMARD-naïve patients (Additional file 2: Figure S2). Similar to the results in all patients, BFR was maintained the longest after withdrawal of TNFi(mAb), followed by CTLA4-Ig, TNFi(R/P), and IL-6Ri (Additional file 2: Figure S2). TNFi(mAb) use was consistently associated with a decreased risk of BFR failure compared with TNFi(R/P) use (Additional file 3: Table S1).

Clinical factors and achievement of BFR

We analyzed clinical factors that were associated with BFR maintenance (Table 2). Shorter disease duration (< 2 years) was associated with a decreased risk of BFR failure. Anti-CCP antibody and RF status or smoking status did not significantly affect BFR failure (Table 2). bDMARD-naïve patients were at a decreased risk for BFR failure compared to bDMARD-switched patients. bDMARD discontinuation due to remission was associated with a decreased risk of BFR failure.

If remission was continuously maintained for > 6 months before bDMARD discontinuation, patients achieved better BFR. Achievement of Boolean remission at the time of bDMARD discontinuation was also significantly associated with a decreased risk of BFR failure. The use and dosage of MTX at the time of bDMARD discontinuation were associated with a decreased risk of BFR failure, whereas glucocorticoid use at the time of discontinuation inversely increased the risk of BFR failure.

Table 2 Hazard ratios for bDMARD-free remission failure (univariate analysis)

Factor	HR (95% CI)	p value
Type of bDMARD		
TNFi(mAb)/TNFi(R/P)	0.56 (0.35–0.87)	0.01
TNFi(mAb)/CTLA4-Ig	0.87 (0.48–1.57)	0.65
TNFi(mAb)/IL-6Ri	0.42 (0.28–0.63)	< 0.01
CTLA4-Ig/TNFi(R/P)	0.64 (0.33–1.24)	0.19
CTLA4-Ig/IL-6Ri	0.48 (0.25–0.91)	0.03
TNFi(R/P)/IL-6Ri	0.75 (0.46–1.25)	0.27
Age (years)	1.00 (0.99–1.01)	0.88
Sex, female/male	0.79 (0.53–1.20)	0.26
Disease duration, < 2 years/≥ 2 years	0.63 (0.45–0.88)	0.01
Disease duration (years)	1.03 (1.01–1.05)	< 0.01
Smoking status, current/previous or never	0.62 (0.27–1.21)	0.17
Anti-CCP antibody, positive/negative	1.47 (0.84–2.81)	0.19
Rheumatoid factor, positive/negative	1.39 (0.91–2.21)	0.13
bDMARD-naïve, naïve/switch	0.56 (0.40–0.79)	< 0.01
Reason for discontinuation, remission/other reason	0.36 (0.22–0.58)	< 0.01
Boolean remission at the time of discontinuation, achieved/not achieved	0.42 (0.29–0.60)	< 0.01
Remission maintenance period before discontinuation, > 6 months/≥ 6 months	0.33 (0.22–0.50)	< 0.01
Methotrexate usage at the time of discontinuation, yes/no	0.65 (0.45–0.96)	0.03
Methotrexate dosage at the time of discontinuation (mg/week)	0.95 (0.92–0.99)	0.02
Glucocorticoid usage at the time of discontinuation, yes/no	2.03 (1.46–2.82)	< 0.01
Glucocorticoid dosage at the time of discontinuation (mg/day)	1.01 (0.98–1.02)	0.56

Patients classified based on types of bDMARDs, disease duration, anti-CCP or RF status, smoking status, bDMARD status (naïve or switched), reasons for bDMARD discontinuation, DAS28-CRP remission maintenance period before bDMARD discontinuation, achievement of Boolean remission at time of bDMARD discontinuation, and concomitant use of MTX or glucocorticoids at time of bDMARD discontinuation. HRs with 95% CIs obtained using Cox's proportional hazard model

bDMARD biological disease-modifying antirheumatic drug, *HR* hazard ratio, *CI* confidence interval, *TNFi(mAb)* monoclonal antibodies against TNF (infliximab, adalimumab, and golimumab), *TNFi(R/P)* soluble TNF receptor or Fab fragments against TNF fused with polyethylene glycol (etanercept and certolizumab), *CTLA4-Ig* abatacept, *IL-6Ri* interleukin-6 receptor inhibitor (tocilizumab), *DAS28-CRP* Disease Activity Score 28—C-reactive protein, *CCP* cyclic citrullinated peptide, *TNF* tumor necrosis factor, *RF* rheumatoid factor, *MTX* methotrexate

Multivariate analysis of factors associated with BFR maintenance

We performed a multivariate analysis of factors associated with BFR failure, including the types of bDMARDs and clinical factors selected based on the results of univariate analysis and clinical significance (Table 3). In addition, adjusted survival curves for different types of bDMARDs were constructed from the results of the multivariable Cox regression model (Fig. 2). After multivariate analysis, sustained remission (> 6 months) before bDMARD discontinuation, Boolean remission at the time of bDMARD discontinuation, and glucocorticoid-free medication at the time of bDMARD discontinuation remained as independent factors associated with a decreased risk of BFR failure. After adjustment, there was no significant difference in the BFR rate between pairs of bDMARDs, except for TNFi(mAb) and IL-6Ri. However, the adjusted survival curve revealed a clear difference between use of TNFi(mAb) or CTLA4-Ig and use of TNFi(R/P) or IL-6Ri (Fig. 2). Consistently, use of TNFi(mAb) or CTLA4-Ig was significantly associated with better survival for BFR compared with use of TNFi(R/P) or IL-6Ri (HR 0.64; 95% CI 0.42–0.96; p = 0.03), even after adjustment.

Discussion

In this study, we analyzed favorable conditions for BFR achievement after bDMARD discontinuation in typical clinical practice using a multicenter RA registry in Japan (the ANSWER cohort). We found the following: BFR was achieved in 21.5% of patients at 1 year after

bDMARD discontinuation in typical clinical practice; TNFi(mAb) or CTLA4-Ig was advantageous for achieving BFR compared with TNFi(R/P) or IL-6Ri; and sustained remission, Boolean remission, and glucocorticoid-free medication at the time of bDMARD discontinuation were important factors associated with a decreased risk of BFR failure. These findings will help decision-making in daily clinical practice when considering bDMARD discontinuation.

In this study, BFR was achieved in 21.5% of patients at 1 year after bDMARD discontinuation; the rate of BFR was lower than the rates reported in previous clinical trials [1, 3–6, 14]. The low BFR achievability in this study may be because of the stricter BFR protocol used (maintaining remission at every visit) or the diverse patient backgrounds encountered in daily clinical practice (longer disease duration, fewer bDMARD-naive patients, more patients with comorbidities, etc.). The results of this study suggest that maintaining BFR after bDMARD discontinuation is more difficult in typical clinical practice than has been reported by clinical trials.

The present results showed that TNFi(mAb) is more advantageous for achieving BFR than TNFi(R/P). This is the first study to show a substantial difference between TNFi(mAb) and TNFi(R/P) with respect to the achievability of BFR in the same observational cohort. TNFi(mAb) not only binds to soluble TNF-α but also to transmembrane TNF-α, the binding of which induces outside-to-inside signaling, leading to apoptosis of the pathogenic cells bearing transmembrane TNF-α [19]. Therefore, TNFi(mAb) but not TNFi(R/P) may not only neutralize soluble TNF but also inhibit the granuloma

Table 3 Hazard ratios for bDMARD-free remission failure (multivariate analysis)

Factor	HR (95% CI)	p value
Type of bDMARD		
TNFi(mAb)/TNFi(R/P)	0.67 (0.42–1.08)	0.10
TNFi(mAb)/CTLA4-Ig	1.04 (0.54–1.97)	0.91
TNFi(mAb)/IL-6Ri	0.63 (0.40–0.99)	0.05
CTLA4-Ig/TNFi(R/P)	0.65 (0.33–1.29)	0.22
CTLA4-Ig/IL-6Ri	0.61 (0.31–1.18)	0.14
TNFi(R/P)/IL-6Ri	0.93 (0.56–1.56)	0.79
Disease duration < 2 years /≥ 2 years	0.97 (0.65–1.44)	0.89
bDMARD-naïve, naïve/switch	0.85 (0.57–1.26)	0.42
Reason for discontinuation, remission/other reason	0.66 (0.38–1.14)	0.13
Boolean remission at the time of discontinuation, achieved/not achieved	0.63 (0.42–0.93)	0.02
Remission maintenance period before discontinuation, > 6 months/≥ 6 months	0.50 (0.32–0.78)	0.00
Methotrexate usage at the time of discontinuation, yes/no	1.10 (0.70–1.74)	0.67
Glucocorticoid usage at the time of discontinuation, yes/no	1.50 (1.05–2.15)	0.03

Cox's proportional hazard model used to determine factors associated with maintenance of bDMARD-free remission in multivariate analysis. Factors included in the analysis selected according to results of univariate analysis and clinical meaningfulness

bDMARD biological disease-modifying antirheumatic drug, *HR* hazard ratio, *CI* confidence interval, *TNFi(mAb)* monoclonal antibodies against TNF (infliximab, adalimumab, and golimumab), *TNFi(R/P)* soluble TNF receptor or Fab fragments against TNF fused with polyethylene glycol (etanercept and certolizumab), *CTLA4-Ig* abatacept, *IL-6Ri* interleukin-6 receptor inhibitor (tocilizumab), *TNF* tumor necrosis factor

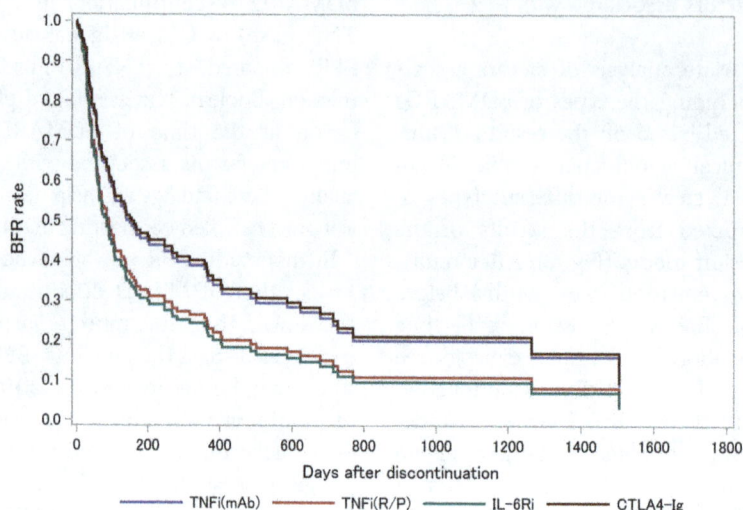

Fig. 2 Adjusted survival curve based on Cox proportional hazard model. *X* axis represents days after bDMARD discontinuation. *Y* axis represents rates of maintained BFR. Survival curves adjusted for covariates based on Cox proportional hazard model. BFR biological disease-modifying antirheumatic drug-free remission, TNFi(mAb) monoclonal antibodies against TNF (infliximab, adalimumab, and golimumab), TNFi(R/P) soluble TNF receptor or Fab fragments against TNF fused with polyethylene glycol (etanercept and certolizumab), CTLA4-Ig abatacept, IL-6Ri interleukin-6 receptor inhibitor (tocilizumab), TNF tumor necrosis factor

formation of TNF-expressing cells. The latter might create favorable conditions for successful BFR achievement after TNFi(mAb) discontinuation [19]. In addition, TNF-α inhibition might expand or restore the suppressive function of regulatory T (Treg) cells that are important for the maintenance of immunological tolerance [25–27]. Transmembrane TNF-α might be involved in this process because ADA but not ETN drives regulatory T-cell expansion via TNF-receptor 2 expressed by Treg cells [28].

CTLA4-Ig provided better survival for BFR, followed by TNFi(mAb) in the unadjusted model (Fig. 1), whereas it was almost equal to TNFi(mAb) in the adjusted model (Fig. 2). Since CTLA4-Ig targets CD4 T cells upstream of the pathological condition of RA, it might be easier to maintain a good condition even after discontinuation of bDMARDs. In fact, CTLA4-Ig reduces the number of follicular helper T cells and consequently reduces the number of switched memory B cells and autoantibodies, which may favor BFR achievement [29, 30].

It is known that IL-6 inhibition increases Treg and reduces effector T cells, which can create favorable conditions for immunological tolerance [30]. However, the BFR rate after IL-6Ri use was not as high as that associated with TNFi(mAb) or CTLA4-Ig use. Since the IL-6 signal is restored after discontinuation of TCZ, it is possible that a Treg-dominant condition might be reversed after withdrawal of IL-6Ri. Alternatively, DAS28-CRP remission might not be suited as the cutoff value considering BFR after TCZ therapy because TCZ masks CRP production and DAS28-CRP remission by TCZ can be overestimated.

Even using any bDMARDs, BFR can be achieved only in 21.5% of patients at 1 year after bDMARD discontinuation. This result suggests that immunological tolerance that could lead to long-lasting BFR has not yet been established after current bDMARD therapies, and there are still unmet needs for an RA "cure."

This study demonstrated that BFR can be successfully achieved after achieving sustained and strict remission at the time of bDMARD discontinuation (Table 3). This result is mostly consistent with previous recommendations and the consensus for bDMARD discontinuation [1]. The importance of minimal disease activity for > 6 months has been indicated in clinical trials [1]. The importance of achieving more stringent remission than DAS28 remission before withdrawing bDMARDs has been indicated by previous studies; for example, using a lower DAS28-CRP cutoff value or the absence of Doppler signals on an ultrasonogram [5, 8, 31]. This study showed that sustained and stringent remission at the time of bDMARD discontinuation is important for successfully achieving BFR, not only in clinical trials but also in real-world clinical practice.

This study also showed that no glucocorticoid use at the time of bDMARD discontinuation is important for achieving BFR. The importance of tapering the glucocorticoid dose before bDMARD discontinuation has been suggested in the EULAR recommendations, which state the following: "If a patient is in persistent remission after having tapered glucocorticoids, one can consider tapering bDMARDs" [32]. However, the clinical evidence supporting this recommendation is insufficient. The present study strongly suggests that the glucocorticoid dose should first

Factors associated with the achievement of biological disease-modifying antirheumatic drugfree remission...

229

be tapered when considering bDMARD discontinuation because the use of glucocorticoids at the time of bDMARD discontinuation was associated with failure of BFR in the real-world observational cohort (Table 3).

The present study has several limitations. First, the number of patients was small. Even including a multicenter cohort, serial disease activity at every visit was available only in limited cases. Therefore, the present results need to be confirmed by future studies including a larger number of participants. Second, due to the small number of study participants, all patients who met the inclusion and exclusion criteria were included regardless of the reasons for drug discontinuation. The reason for drug discontinuation may have affected the BFR survival time, although we adjusted for discontinuation due to remission in multivariate analysis. Third, since this study had a retrospective design and used an observational cohort from daily clinical practice, the unknown background factors (e.g., the use of csDMARDs other than MTX or disease status at the initiation of bDMARDs) may have affected the results. Finally, the radiographic progression of joint destruction was not evaluated in this study. Notably, bDMARDs have strong protective activity against bone destruction; therefore, radiographic destruction can be inhibited by bDMARD use, even though disease activity cannot be fully controlled [33, 34]. Future studies should address whether radiographic remission can be maintained if strict BFR is maintained after bDMARD discontinuation.

Conclusions

This study investigated the real-world conditions affecting BFR achievement in patients with RA. Although BFR is difficult to achieve in typical clinical practice, after strained and strict remission without glucocorticoid use, bDMARDs can be successfully withdrawn while retaining remission after discontinuation. Furthermore, TNFi(mAb) or CTLA4-Ig may be more advantageous for achieving BFR than TNFi(R/P) or IL-6Ri.

Abbreviations
ABT: Abatacept; ADA: Adalimumab; ANSWER: Kansai Consortium for Well-being of Rheumatic Disease Patients; bDMARD: Biological disease-modifying antirheumatic drug; BFR: bDMARD-free remission; CCP: Cyclic citrullinated peptide; CI: Confidence interval; csDMARD: Conventional synthetic DMARD; CZP: Certolizumab pegol; DAS28-CRP: Disease Activity Score 28—C-reactive protein; ETN: Etanercept; EULAR: European League Against Rheumatism; GLM: Golimumab; HR: Hazard ratio; IFX: Infliximab; IL: Interleukin; MTX: Methotrexate; RA: Rheumatoid arthritis; RCT: Randomized controlled trial; RF: Rheumatoid factor; TCZ: Tocilizumab; TNFi: TNF inhibitor; TNFi(mAb): Monoclonal antibodies against TNF; TNFi(R/P): Soluble TNF receptor or Fab fragments against TNF fused with polyethylene glycol

Acknowledgements
The authors thank all medical staff at all institutions participating in the ANSWER cohort study for providing data.

Authors' contributions
MH was responsible for conception and design. MF, WY, TF, RH, MK, AO, KA, SY, KN, YS, HA, TH, KE, HI, MT, KO, TF, and TM contributed to execution or analysis and interpretation of the data. MH and RU contributed to statistical analysis. MH prepared the manuscript. All authors read and approved the final manuscript.

Consent for publication
Not applicable.

Competing interests
MH and MT are affiliated with a department that is financially supported by four pharmaceutical companies (Mitsubishi-Tanabe, Chugai, Ayumi, and UCB Japan) and the city government (Nagahama City). MH received a research grant from Astellas. AO received a research grant from Eisai, Asahi-Kasei Pharma, and Mitsubishi-Tanabe. TH received a research grant and/or speaker fee from Astellas, Chugai, Eisai, Mitsubishi Tanabe, Abbvie, and Asahi-Kasei. MT received research grants from Astellas, Abbvie, Pfizer, and Taishotoyama. HI received a research grant and/or speaker fee from Bristol-Myers, Astellas, Asahi-Kasei, and Eli Lily. TF received a research grant and/or speaker fee from Pfizer Japan Inc., Ono Pharmaceutical Co., Ltd, Daiichi Sankyo Co., Ltd, Mitsubishi-Tanabe Pharma Corporation, Eisai Co., Ltd, AbbVie GK, and Astellas Pharma Inc. KO received a research grant and/or speaker fee from Abbvie, Astellas, Bristol-Myers Squibb, Eli Lily, Mitsubishi-Tanabe, Pfizer, and Takeda. TM received research grants from Acterion, Astellas, Asahi Kasei Pharma, Ayumi, Chugai, Daiichi Sankyo, Eisai, JB, Mitsubishi Tanabe, MSD, Nippon Shinyaku, Pfizer, Sanofi, and Takeda, and has participated in speakers' bureaus for Astellas, Bristol-Myers Squibb, Chugai, and Mitsubishi-Tanabe. The remaining authors have no financial conflicts of interest to disclose concerning this manuscript. The pharmaceutical companies had no role in the design of the study, the collection or analysis of the data, the writing of the manuscript, or the decision to submit the manuscript for publication.

Author details
[1]Department of Advanced Medicine for Rheumatic Diseases, Graduate School of Medicine, Kyoto University, 53 Kawahara-cho, Shogoin, Sakyo-ku, Kyoto 606-8507, Japan. [2]Department of Orthopedic Surgery, Graduate School of Medicine, Kyoto University, Kyoto, Japan. [3]Department of Health Information Management, Kurashiki Sweet Hospital, Kurashiki, Japan. [4]The Center for Rheumatic Diseases, Nara Medical University, Nara, Japan. [5]Department of Rheumatology, Osaka Red Cross Hospital, Osaka, Japan. [6]Department of Rheumatology and Clinical Immunology, Kobe University Graduate School of Medicine, Kobe, Japan. [7]Department of Internal Medicine (IV), Osaka Medical College, Osaka, Japan. [8]First Department of Internal Medicine, Kansai Medical University, Osaka, Japan. [9]Department of Respiratory Medicine, Allergy and Rheumatic Disease, Graduate School of Medicine, Osaka University, Osaka, Japan. [10]Department of Orthopaedic Surgery, Osaka University, Graduate School of Medicine, Osaka, Japan. [11]Department of Biomedical Statistics and Bioinformatics, Graduate School of Medicine, Kyoto University, Kyoto, Japan. [12]Department of Rheumatology and Clinical Immunology, Graduate School of Medicine, Kyoto University, Kyoto, Japan. [13]Department of Rheumatology and Clinical Immunology, Wakayama Medical University, Wakayama, Japan.

References
1. Schett G, Emery P, Tanaka Y, et al. Tapering biologic and conventional DMARD therapy in rheumatoid arthritis: current evidence and future directions. Ann Rheum Dis. 2016;75(8):1428–37.
2. Quinn MA, Conaghan PG, O'Connor PJ, et al. Very early treatment with infliximab in addition to methotrexate in early, poor-prognosis rheumatoid arthritis reduces magnetic resonance imaging evidence of synovitis and damage, with sustained benefit after infliximab withdrawal: results from a twelve-month randomized, double-blind, placebo-controlled trial. Arthritis Rheum. 2005;52(1):27–35.

3. van den Broek M, Klarenbeek NB, Dirven L, et al. Discontinuation of infliximab and potential predictors of persistent low disease activity in patients with early rheumatoid arthritis and disease activity score-steered therapy: subanalysis of the BeSt study. Ann Rheum Dis. 2011;70(8):1389–94.

4. Allaart CF, Lems WF, Huizinga TW. The BeSt way of withdrawing biologic agents. Clin Exp Rheumatol. 2013;31(4 Suppl 78):S14–8.

5. Tanaka Y, Takeuchi T, Mimori T, et al. Discontinuation of infliximab after attaining low disease activity in patients with rheumatoid arthritis: RRR (remission induction by Remicade in RA) study. Ann Rheum Dis. 2010;69(7):1286–91.

6. Ghiti Moghadam M, Vonkeman HE, Ten Klooster PM, et al. Stopping tumor necrosis factor inhibitor treatment in patients with established rheumatoid arthritis in remission or with stable low disease activity: a pragmatic multicenter, open-label randomized controlled trial. Arthritis Rheumatol. 2016;68(8):1810–7.

7. Harigai M, Takeuchi T, Tanaka Y, et al. Discontinuation of adalimumab treatment in rheumatoid arthritis patients after achieving low disease activity. Mod Rheumatol. 2012;22(6):814–22.

8. Tanaka Y, Hirata S, Kubo S, et al. Discontinuation of adalimumab after achieving remission in patients with established rheumatoid arthritis: 1-year outcome of the HONOR study. Ann Rheum Dis. 2015;74(2):389–95.

9. Tanaka Y, Yamanaka H, Ishiguro N, et al. Adalimumab discontinuation in patients with early rheumatoid arthritis who were initially treated with methotrexate alone or in combination with adalimumab: 1 year outcomes of the HOPEFUL-2 study. RMD Open. 2016;2(1):e000189.

10. Tanaka Y, Yamanaka H, Ishiguro N, et al. Low disease activity for up to 3 years after adalimumab discontinuation in patients with early rheumatoid arthritis: 2-year results of the HOPEFUL-3 study. Arthritis Res Ther. 2017;19(1):56.

11. Smolen JS, Nash P, Durez P, et al. Maintenance, reduction, or withdrawal of etanercept after treatment with etanercept and methotrexate in patients with moderate rheumatoid arthritis (PRESERVE): a randomised controlled trial. Lancet. 2013;381(9870):918–29.

12. Smolen JS, Szumski A, Koenig AS, et al. Predictors of remission with etanercept-methotrexate induction therapy and loss of remission with etanercept maintenance, reduction, or withdrawal in moderately active rheumatoid arthritis: results of the PRESERVE trial. Arthritis Res Ther. 2018;20(1):8.

13. Yamanaka H, Nagaoka S, Lee SK, et al. Discontinuation of etanercept after achievement of sustained remission in patients with rheumatoid arthritis who initially had moderate disease activity-results from the ENCOURAGE study, a prospective, international, multicenter randomized study. Mod Rheumatol. 2016;26(5):651–61.

14. Atsumi T, Tanaka Y, Yamamoto K, et al. Clinical benefit of 1-year certolizumab pegol (CZP) add-on therapy to methotrexate treatment in patients with early rheumatoid arthritis was observed following CZP discontinuation: 2-year results of the C-OPERA study, a phase III randomised trial. Ann Rheum Dis. 2017;76(8):1348–56.

15. Emery P, Burmester GR, Bykerk VP, et al. Evaluating drug-free remission with abatacept in early rheumatoid arthritis: results from the phase 3b, multicentre, randomised, active-controlled AVERT study of 24 months, with a 12-month, double-blind treatment period. Ann Rheum Dis. 2015;74(1):19–26.

16. Nishimoto N, Amano K, Hirabayashi Y, et al. Drug free REmission/low disease activity after cessation of tocilizumab (Actemra) monotherapy (DREAM) study. Mod Rheumatol. 2014;24(1):17–25.

17. Huizinga TW, Conaghan PG, Martin-Mola E, et al. Clinical and radiographic outcomes at 2 years and the effect of tocilizumab discontinuation following sustained remission in the second and third year of the ACT-RAY study. Ann Rheum Dis. 2015;74(1):35–43.

18. Yoshida K, Sung YK, Kavanaugh A, et al. Biologic discontinuation studies: a systematic review of methods. Ann Rheum Dis. 2014;73(3):595–9.

19. Horiuchi T, Mitoma H, Harashima S, et al. Transmembrane TNF-alpha: structure, function and interaction with anti-TNF agents. Rheumatology (Oxford). 2010;49(7):1215–28.

20. Mitoma H, Horiuchi T, Tsukamoto H, Ueda N. Molecular mechanisms of action of anti-TNF-alpha agents—comparison among therapeutic TNF-alpha antagonists. Cytokine. 2018;101:56–63.

21. Nikiphorou E, Buch MH, Hyrich KL. Biologics registers in RA: methodological aspects, current role and future applications. Nat Rev Rheumatol. 2017;13(8):503–10.

22. Ebina K, Hirao M, Takagi K, et al. Comparison of the effects of forefoot joint-preserving arthroplasty and resection-replacement arthroplasty on walking plantar pressure distribution and patient-based outcomes in patients with rheumatoid arthritis. PLoS One. 2017;12(8):e0183805.

23. Inoue E, Yamanaka H, Hara M, et al. Comparison of disease activity score (DAS)28-erythrocyte sedimentation rate and DAS28-C-reactive protein threshold values. Ann Rheum Dis. 2007;66(3):407–9.

24. Makuch RW. Adjusted survival curve estimation using covariates. J Chronic Dis. 1982;35(6):437–43.

25. Ehrenstein MR, Evans JG, Singh A, et al. Compromised function of regulatory T cells in rheumatoid arthritis and reversal by anti-TNFalpha therapy. J Exp Med. 2004;200(3):277–85.

26. Nadkarni S, Mauri C, Ehrenstein MR. Anti-TNF-alpha therapy induces a distinct regulatory T cell population in patients with rheumatoid arthritis via TGF-beta. J Exp Med. 2007;204(1):33–9.

27. Nie H, Zheng Y, Li R, et al. Phosphorylation of FOXP3 controls regulatory T cell function and is inhibited by TNF-alpha in rheumatoid arthritis. Nat Med. 2013;19(3):322–8.

28. Nguyen DX, Ehrenstein MR. Anti-TNF drives regulatory T cell expansion by paradoxically promoting membrane TNF-TNF-RII binding in rheumatoid arthritis. J Exp Med. 2016;213(7):1241–53.

29. Scarsi M, Paolini L, Ricotta D, et al. Abatacept reduces levels of switched memory B cells, autoantibodies, and immunoglobulins in patients with rheumatoid arthritis. J Rheumatol. 2014;41(4):666–72.

30. Nakayamada S, Kubo S, Yoshikawa M, Miyazaki Y, Yunoue N, Iwata S, Miyagawa I, Hirata S, Nakano K, Saito K, Tanaka Y. Differential effects of biological DMARDs on peripheral immune cell phenotypes in patients with rheumatoid arthritis. Rheumatology (Oxford). 2018;57(1):164–74.

31. Naredo E, Valor L, De la Torre I, et al. Predictive value of Doppler ultrasound-detected synovitis in relation to failed tapering of biologic therapy in patients with rheumatoid arthritis. Rheumatology (Oxford). 2015;54(8):1408–14.

32. Smolen JS, Landewe R, Bijlsma J, et al. EULAR recommendations for the management of rheumatoid arthritis with synthetic and biological disease-modifying antirheumatic drugs: 2016 update. Ann Rheum Dis. 2017;76(6):960–77.

33. Smolen JS, Han C, Bala M, et al. Evidence of radiographic benefit of treatment with infliximab plus methotrexate in rheumatoid arthritis patients who had no clinical improvement: a detailed subanalysis of data from the anti-tumor necrosis factor trial in rheumatoid arthritis with concomitant therapy study. Arthritis Rheum. 2005;52(4):1020–30.

34. Smolen JS, Avila JC, Aletaha D. Tocilizumab inhibits progression of joint damage in rheumatoid arthritis irrespective of its anti-inflammatory effects: disassociation of the link between inflammation and destruction. Ann Rheum Dis. 2012;71(5):687–93.

23

Polydatin effectively attenuates disease activity in lupus-prone mouse models by blocking ROS-mediated NET formation

Pan Liao[1,2†], Yi He[1,2†], Fangyuan Yang[1,2], Guihu Luo[1,2], Jian Zhuang[1,2], Zeqing Zhai[1,2], Lili Zhuang[1,2], Zhuomiao Lin[3], Jiehuang Zheng[3] and Erwei Sun[1,2*] (iD)

Abstract

Background: Neutrophil extracellular trap (NET) formation has been described to be closely involved in the pathogenesis of systemic lupus erythematosus (SLE). In this study, we aimed to investigate the effect of polydatin (PD) on NET formation and its effects on disease activity in lupus-prone mouse models.

Methods: In vitro, neutrophils from SLE patients and healthy people stimulated with phorbol 12-myristate 13-acetate (PMA) or phosphate-buffered saline (PBS) were treated with PD, and reactive oxygen species (ROS) production and NET formation examined. In vivo, pristane-induced lupus (PIL) mice were treated with vehicle, PD, mycophenolate mofetil (MMF) or cyclophosphamide (CYC) while MRL/*lpr* mice were treated with vehicle or PD. Proteinuria, serum autoantibodies, ROS production, NET formation and kidney histopathology were tested.

Results: Consistent with previous findings, blood neutrophils from SLE patients showed increased spontaneous NET formation. Both in vivo and in vitro, PD treatment significantly inhibited ROS production and NET release by neutrophils. In MRL/*lpr* mouse model, PD administration reduced the proteinuria, circulating autoantibody levels, and deposition of NETs and immune complex in the kidneys. In addition, PD treatment ameliorated lupus-like features in PIL mice as MMF or CYC did.

Conclusions: PD treatment inhibited ROS-mediated NET formation and ameliorated lupus manifestations in both PIL mice and MRL/*lpr* mice. These results highlight the involvement of NETosis in SLE pathogenesis and reveal that PD might be a potential therapeutic agent for SLE or other autoimmune diseases.

Keywords: Neutrophil extracellular trap, NETosis, Reactive oxygen species, Systemic lupus erythematosus, Polydatin

Introduction

Systemic lupus erythematosus (SLE) is a chronic progressive autoimmune disorder manifested by autoantibody overproduction and multi-organ involvement [1]. It is prominently prevalent in African, Asian, Hispanic and American patients [2] and mostly occurs in young women [3]. Over the past decades, most studies on SLE have focused on the dysregulation of adaptive immunity [4, 5]. Although abnormalities of B and T lymphocytes are considered to play central roles in the pathogenesis and development of SLE [6], the active role of the innate immune system in induction of autoimmune response in SLE is equally important. Neutrophils, the most abundant sensory and effector cells in the innate immune system, have attracted more attention in recent years [7].

NETosis is a specific form of cell death of neutrophils, during which the chromatin decondenses and is released into extracellular space with cytoplasmic proteins, forming neutrophil extracellular traps (NETs) [8]. Indeed, increased NET deposition has been found in the skin and kidneys of SLE patients [9]. Neutrophils from SLE patients have been shown to exhibit an increased propensity for NET formation [7, 10]. Owing to the presence of

* Correspondence: sunew@smu.edu.cn
†Pan Liao and Yi He contributed equally to this work.
[1]Department of Rheumatology and Immunology, The Third Affiliated Hospital, Southern Medical University, No. 183, Zhongshan Avenue West, Tianhe District, Guangzhou 510630, China
[2]Institute of Clinical Immunology, Academy of Orthopedics Guangdong Province, Guangzhou, China
Full list of author information is available at the end of the article

DNase1 inhibitors or anti-NET antibodies, most SLE patients show defective NET degradation. The impaired clearance of NETs has been reported to be closely associated with renal involvement [11]. In addition, NETs activate plasmacytoid dendritic cells and NLRP3 inflammasome in macrophage to release inflammatory cytokines including type I interferons, interleukin (IL)-1 and IL-18, further amplifying inflammatory and immune responses [12–14]. More importantly, many studies have indicated that NET formation causes tissue damage and vascular injury in patients with SLE [9, 15, 16]. Taken together, NETosis plays an important role in the pathogenesis and development of SLE. To date, efforts have been paid to examining the underlying molecular mechanisms of NETosis and found that ROS is necessary for NETosis [17]. A ROS scavenger, N-acetyl cysteine (NAC), has been reported to significantly prevent NET formation [18, 19]. In particular, spontaneous NETosis could also be inhibited by Mito TEMPO, a specific scavenger for mitochondrial ROS production [10].

Polydatin (PD) is an active stilbene compound extracted from a traditional Chinese herb (*Polygonum cuspidatum*). It has gained particular interest because of its strong anti-oxidative effects by blocking the generation of ROS [20, 21]. PD has just been accomplished a phase II clinical trial for irritable bowel syndrome (IBS) and identified to ameliorate IBS-related manifestations [22]. However, to our knowledge, no researches have examined whether PD inhibits the NET formation or has a therapeutic effect on SLE. Therefore, the purpose of this study was to investigate the potential effects of PD on NET formation and determine whether PD is effective in lupus-prone mouse models.

Materials and Methods
Mice
Female BALB/c mice (6–8-weeks) were obtained from Experimental Animal Center of Southern Medical University (Guangzhou, China). Female MRL/*lpr* mice (6–8-weeks old) were purchased from SLAC Laboratory Animal Company (Shanghai, China). All animals were maintained under specific pathogen-free conditions in the laboratory animal center of Southern Medical University (Guangzhou, China).

The protocols of animal experimentation were approved by the Ethics Committee of The Third Affiliated Hospital, Southern Medical University (No. L2017032).

Pristane-induced lupus (PIL) and MRL/*lpr* mouse models
PIL was induced by a single intraperitoneal injection of 500 μl pristane (Sigma-Aldrich, St. Louis, MO, USA) in female BALB/c mice at 6–to 8 weeks of age and followed over 26 weeks. Mouse 24-h urine was collected every 2 weeks, beginning when the mice were at the age of 12 weeks. Treatments started when proteinuria was evident in all Balb/c mice, and continued for another 16 weeks. In clinical practice, mycophenolate mofetil (MMF) and cyclophosphamide (CYC) are two common immunosuppressive drugs for lupus nephritis. Therefore, these two drugs were selected as positive controls. PIL mice were divided into four groups with nine mice in each group, named PIL model, PD, CYC and MMF groups respectively. In the PIL model group, mice received the same amount of vehicle solution (dehydrated alcohol-propylene glycol-Na2CO3-NaHCO3 buffer (pH 8.5)) for PD instead. Six normal mice were also treated with vehicle only as control. In PD group, mice were injected intraperitoneally with a dose of 45 mg/kg PD (a generous gift from Professor Ke-seng Zhao) every day, as reported previously [23, 24]. In CYC group, mice were administrated with CYC (1.8 mg/mouse, weekly, obtained from Baxter Oncology GmbH, Halle, Germany) by intraperitoneal injection. In MMF group, mice were treated with MMF (100 mg/kg, purchased from Huadong Pharmaceutical Co., Ltd, Hangzhou, China) by daily oral gavage [25, 26]. MRL/*lpr* mice were divided into two groups and then received PD (45 mg/kg) or an equal volume of vehicle by daily intraperitoneal injection for 8 weeks.

Isolation of neutrophils from human and mice
The human blood samples (5 ml each) were obtained from healthy donors and SLE subjects from The Third Affiliated Hospital, Southern Medical University. Human blood neutrophils were isolated by dextran sedimentation and centrifugation [27]. For the isolation of mouse neutrophils, femurs and tibias of mice were removed and bone marrow collected. The bone marrow-derived neutrophils were obtained using mouse bone marrow neutrophil cell isolation kit (TBD Sciences, Tianjin, China), following the manufacturer's instructions.

Cell viability assay
Human blood neutrophils were incubated in the absence or presence of various concentrations of PD (50, 75, 100, 125 and 150 μg/mL) and the cell viability tested by Cell Counting Kit (CCK-8) (Dojindo, Beijing, China) following the manufacturer's instructions.

ROS assessment
Neutrophils isolated from human blood or mouse bone marrow were incubated with 10 μM 2′,7′-dichlorodihydrofluorescein diacetate (DCFH-DA) (Sigma-Aldrich) in Roswell Park Memorial Institute-1640 (RPMI-1640) at 37 °C for 20 min. After three washes with RPMI-1640, neutrophils were transferred into a 96-well plate (1×10^6 cells/well in 200 μl). Then they were stimulated with 25 nM PMA (Sigma-Aldrich) for 30 mins (some cells

were pretreated with PD for 1 h), and the fluorescence intensity measured by SpectraMax M3 (Molecular Devices, San Jose, CA, USA) fluorescent plate reader at 485 nm (excitation)/520 nm (emission).

Quantification of NETs

To quantify spontaneous and phorbol 12-myristate 13-acetate (PMA)-induced NETs, neutrophils isolated from human blood (3×10^5 cells/well in 200 µl) were seeded into black, flat-bottomed, 96-well plates and cultured with phosphate-buffered saline (PBS) or 25 nM PMA in a humidified incubator at 37 °C with CO_2 (5%) for 4 h. Extracellular DNA was stained with the membrane-impermeable DNA-binding dye-SYTOX green (Thermo Fisher Scientific, Waltham, MA, USA). The plates were analyzed using SpectraMax M3 fluorescent plate reader (Molecular Devices) at excitation 485 nm and emission 520 nm. The spontaneous NET release by mouse bone marrow-derived neutrophils was measured similarly as NET formation tested in human blood neutrophils.

Immunofluorescence analysis of NET formation

Human blood neutrophils were pretreated with or without PD for 1 h. These prepared neutrophils were placed on cytospins and stimulated with 25 nM PMA or PBS for 4 h. Alternatively, bone marrow-derived neutrophils from PD-, solvent-, or saline-treated mice were directly placed on cytospins and cultured in the absence of serum for 4 h. And then all those neutrophils were fixed with 1 ml PBS/1% paraformaldehyde. After blocking with 5% fetal bovine serum, the cytospins were stained with rabbit anti-myeloperoxidase (MPO) antibody (Abcam, catalog ab208670, Cambridge, UK) in combination with a second Cy3-conjugated goat anti-rabbit immunoglobulin G (IgG) antibody (Servicebio, catalog GB21303, Boston, MA, USA). The DNA was visualized by 4′, 6′-diamidino-2-phenylindole (DAPI) (Thermo Fisher Scientific). After being mounted, specimens were analyzed using a fluorescence microscope.

Proteinuria detection

All mice were placed in metabolic cages for 24 h urine collection. The concentrations of proteinuria were detected by Bradford Protein Quantification Kit (Bioteke Corporation, Beijing, China). The following scale was used for assessment: 0 score = 0–30 mg/dl; 2 score = 100–300 mg/dl; 3 score = 300–2000 mg/dl; 4 score>2000 mg/dl.

Quantification of autoantibodies in serum

The serum levels of anti-dsDNA antibodies and anti-Sm antibodies were measured with enzyme-linked immunosorbent assay (ELISA) kits in accordance with the manufacturer's instructions (Cusabio Life Science Inc., Wuhan, China).

Flow cytometry analysis

To test the percentage of necrotic cells in peripheral blood-derived neutrophils from mice, heparinized blood samples were lysed with Lysing Buffer (BD Biosciences, San Jose, CA, USA) to eliminate erythrocytes. And then single-cell suspensions were stained with FITC-labeled Ly6G (BD Biosciences) and propidium iodide (BD Biosciences). Flow cytometry acquisition was performed with the FACSVerse™ (BD Biosciences) and the stained cells analyzed with flow cytometry software.

Assessment of histopathological changes and IgG deposition in kidneys

Kidney tissues were fixed with 10% formalin and embedded in paraffin for preparation. And then these paraffin-embedded sections were stained with hematoxylin and eosin (H&E). Histopathological changes in kidneys were reviewed by the pathologist who was blinded to the experimental information. Lupus disease activity was graded by the Austin score, as described previously [28].

For assessment of mouse IgG deposition in kidneys, frozen sections were analyzed. The frozen sections were blocked with 5% fetal bovine serum and then stained with Alexa Fluor 555-conjugated goat anti-mouse IgG (Abcam, catalog ab150114). Twenty-five glomeruli per kidney of mouse were examined by two observers in a blinded manner. Based on the mean intensity of fluorescence, the scores for IgG deposition were estimated on a scale of 0–3, according to previously described methods [29].

Assessment of NET formation in kidneys

Formalin-fixed and paraffin-embedded kidney sections were blocked with 5% fetal bovine serum, and then the MPO-stained with rabbit anti-myeloperoxidase antibody (Abcam, catalog ab208670) in combination with a second Cy3-conjugated goat anti-rabbit IgG (H + L) antibody (Servicebio, catalog GB21303). The chromatin was stained with DAPI (Thermo Fisher Scientific). Colocalization of myeloperoxidase and chromatin was recognized as NETs. Ten glomeruli per animal were analyzed for NET staining and the percentage of NET-stained glomeruli calculated.

Statistical analysis

Data are represented as the mean ± SD. According to data distribution, statistical analysis was performed by Student's t test, one-way analysis of variance or the non-parametric Wilcoxon rank-sum test. P values < 0.05 were considered significant differences. All data were analyzed by SPSS software (version 20.0) (IBM Corp., Armonk, NY, USA).

Results

SLE patients showed enhanced spontaneous NET formation

Previous studies have indicated that neutrophils from SLE patients exhibit high potential for spontaneous NET formation. Here, to test spontaneous NET formation, neutrophils were isolated from SLE patients and healthy controls (HCs), and then cultured in RPMI-1640 for 4 h. Indeed, we found that neutrophils from SLE patients spontaneously released higher levels of NETs than healthy control neutrophils (Fig. 1a and b).

PD significantly inhibited the PMA-induced NET formation by blocking ROS production

We first checked the cytotoxicity of PD on the neutrophils by CCK-8 assay and found that PD had no cytotoxic effect on neutrophils even at a concentration as high as 150 μg/ml (Fig. 1c). Based on this result in combination with other previous studies [25], we selected PD 100 μg/ml for the following vitro experiments.

Many studies have demonstrated that ROS overproduction plays a crucial role in NET formation. PMA is a strong inducer of NET formation dependent on ROS production. To identify whether PD could reduce intracellular ROS production, neutrophils were treated with PD for 1 h and then stimulated with PMA for 30 min. Treatment with PD significantly suppressed PMA-stimulated ROS generation (Fig. 1d).

Next, to investigate the effects of PD on NET formation, neutrophils were pretreated with PD for 1 h, followed by stimulation with PMA for 4 h. We found that PMA stimulation significantly increased NET formation by both SLE neutrophils and HC neutrophils, while PD treatment could markedly suppress the PMA-induced NET formation in both groups (Fig. 1e and f). Overall, these results indicated that PD treatment inhibited PMA-induced NET generation perhaps by blocking ROS production.

PD treatment alleviated lupus-like features in MRL/*lpr* mice

To date, increasing evidence has suggested that NETosis is closely associated with the pathogenesis and progression of SLE. In present study, we used two different lupus-prone mouse models to evaluate the effects of PD treatment on SLE development. MRL/*lpr* mice spontaneously develop severe lupus-like features characterized by multiple autoantibodies to nuclear antigens, proteinuria and glomerulonephritis. Here, we treated MRL/*lpr* mice with PD at the age of 12 weeks and continued PD treatment for another 8 weeks. Importantly, PD treatment resulted in a dramatic reduction in proteinuria at the 20 weeks of age (Fig. 2a). MRL/*lpr* mice showed high levels of circulating anti-dsDNA and anti-Sm antibodies, similarly PD treatment markedly reduced those autoantibody levels (Fig. 2b). In addition, kidney H&E staining

revealed that Austin scores of kidneys were significantly decreased in PD treated MRL/*lpr* mice (Fig. 2c). Moreover, less deposition of IgG was found in the kidneys of PD-treated mice (Fig. 2d). Particularly, abundant NETs (overlapping DNA and MPO staining) in the glomeruli were easily detected in vehicle-treated MRL/*lpr* mice, but rarely found in PD-treated MRL/*lpr* mice (Fig. 2e). Taken together, these findings suggested that PD treatment could alleviate lupus-like features in MRL/*lpr* mice and reduced the NET formation in the kidney tissue.

PD treatment also ameliorated lupus manifestations in PIL mice

Mycophenolate mofetil (MMF) and cyclophosphamide (CYC) are commonly accepted and effective treatments for lupus nephritis, so we chose these two drugs as positive controls to further investigate the effects of PD treatment on SLE mice. As expected, both MMF and CYC treatments could significantly reduce proteinuria levels, autoantibody levels and Austin activity scores (Fig. 3a, b and c). Similarly, we also found that PD treatment reduced lupus-associated manifestations in PIL mice and decreased NET deposition in the kidneys. However, there were no significant differences in proteinuria levels, autoantibody levels and Austin activity scores among PD, MMF and CYC groups. Compared with vehicle-treated PIL mice, proteinuria levels were significantly decreased in PD-treated PIL mice (Fig. 3a). Furthermore, dramatically decreased levels of serum anti-dsDNA and anti-Sm antibodies were also found in PD-treated PIL mice (Fig. 3b). Additionally, PD treatment markedly reduced the Austin scores and IgG deposition in kidneys (Fig. 3c and d). Finally, we also found that there was a significant decrease in NET formation in the glomeruli of PD-treated PIL mice (Fig. 3e).

Treatment of PIL mice with PD prevented spontaneous NET formation in vivo

Since PD treatment significantly reduced the NET deposition in kidneys of lupus-prone MRL/*lpr* mice, we further identified whether PD treatment could also inhibit NET formation by neutrophils from lupus-prone mice in vivo. Because NETosis is a form of cell death with membrane rupture, we analyzed the percentage of necrotic cells in peripheral blood-derived neutrophils with flow cytometry, illustrated by the percentage of Ly6G$^+$PI$^+$ cells. As shown in Fig. 4a, necrotic cells were notably decreased in neutrophils treated with PD. Then, we detected for spontaneous NET release by bone marrow-derived neutrophils. As expected, spontaneous NET formation was significantly increased by bone marrow-derived neutrophils from PIL mice, but was inhibited by PD treatment (Fig. 4b). In addition, PD

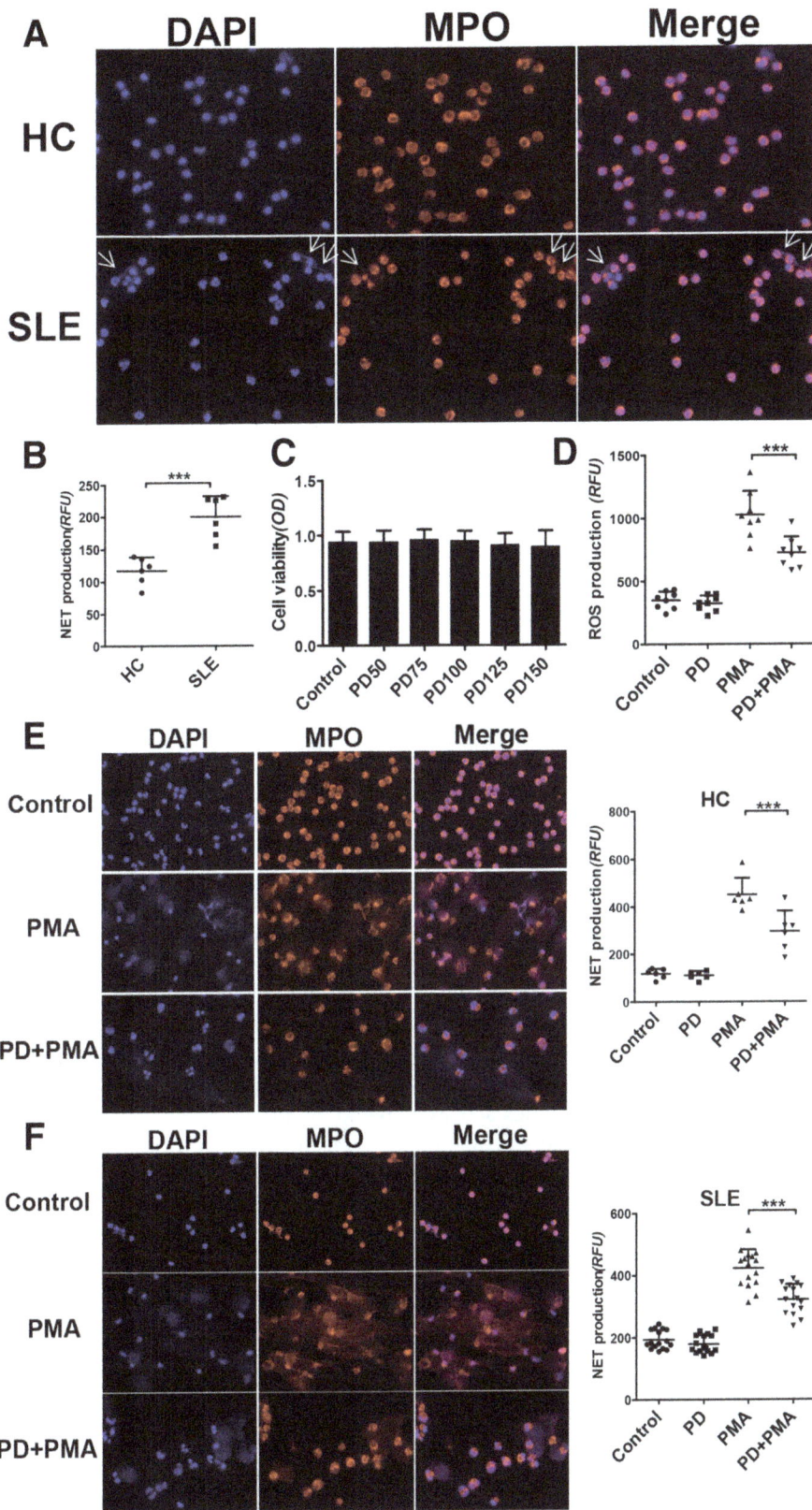

Fig. 1 (See legend on next page.)

Fig. 1 SLE patients displayed increased spontaneous NET formation and PD inhibited PMA-induced NET formation by blocking ROS production. **a** Neutrophils were isolated from peripheral blood of SLE patients and healthy controls (HC) and then incubated with RPMI-1640 for 4 h. Representative fluorescence microscopic images showing NETs that contained DNA (*blue*) and MPO (*red*) (×400). *White arrows* indicated NETs. **b** Neutrophils from SLE patients spontaneously released increased NETs. NET formation was quantified by SpectraMax M3 fluorescent plate reader. **c** Cell viability of PD-treated neutrophils. Cell viability of neutrophils was measured by CCK-8 assay after stimulation of PD (50, 75, 100, 125 and 150 µg/mL). **d** Neutrophils were isolated from SLE subjects and pretreated with PD for 1 h, followed by stimulation with PMA for 30 min. Cells were stained with DCFH-DA, and the fluorescence intensity was measured. **e–f** Neutrophils prepared from healthy controls (HC) and SLE patients, were treated with PD for 1 h and then exposed to PMA for 4 h. NET formation was quantified as described in Materials and Methods (*right*). Representative fluorescence microscopic images of NET formation from HC and SLE patients are shown (×400) on the left, respectively. For all experiments, data were shown as mean ± SD, *$p < 0.05$; **$p < 0.01$; ***$p < 0.001$. *DAPI* 4′, 6′-diamidino-2-phenylindole, *HC* healthy control, *MPO* myeloperoxidase, *NET* neutrophil extracellular trap, *PD* polydatin, *PMA* phorbol 12-myristate 13-acetate, *SLE* systemic lupus erythematosus

treatment effectively prevented the ROS production by bone marrow-derived neutrophils (Fig. 4c). Collectively, our findings demonstrated that PD treatment suppressed NET formation in pristane-induced lupus mice possibly by reducing ROS generation.

Discussion

Studies have demonstrated that NETosis plays a significant role in the pathogenesis and progression of SLE. NETosis is recognized as a specific cell death of neutrophils. Based on our prior studies [30, 31], we proposed a "cell death recognition model" for the immune system: consequence of immune responses depends on the ways of cell death. This "cell death" recognition model may well explain the role of NETosis in SLE pathogenesis. During the process of NETosis, intracellular components are released into extracellular space, leading to the presentation of autoantigens to host immune system and the release of damage-associated molecular patterns (DAMPs) that amplify inflammatory and immune responses. It is worth mentioning that peptidylarginine deiminase (PAD) inhibition limited lupus-related skin, renal and vascular damage by preventing NET formation in various lupus-prone mouse models [32, 33]. Moreover, a Janus kinase (JAK) inhibitor, tofacitinib, disrupted NET generation and displayed therapeutic capacity for lupus activity and lupus-related vascular damage [34]. Therefore, modulation of NETosis would be a potential therapeutic avenue for SLE. Consistent with previous studies, in this study we also identified that neutrophils from SLE patients were more prone to undergo NETosis, emphasizing the importance of blocking NETosis for SLE treatment.

During NETosis, ROS generated by nicotinamide adenine dinucleotide phosphate (NADPH)-oxidase mediates the activation of protein-arginine deiminase 4 (PAD4), resulting in decondensation of chromatin and the loss of the nuclear membrane [35]. Subsequently, the decondensed chromatin decorated with cytoplasmic and granule components are released to the extracellular space [35]. It has been shown that inhibiting intracellular or mitochondrial ROS production could effectively prevent NETosis [10, 19]. Thus, blocking ROS production

may be of importance for reducing NETosis and alleviating SLE disease activity.

Therefore, in this study, we investigated the effects of PD on ROS-mediated NET formation and further determined therapeutic effects of PD on lupus-prone mice. We first examined whether PD could reduce ROS production by neutrophils. It is well-known that PD exhibits powerful anti-oxidative properties by the inhibition of ROS release by various kinds of cells, such as umbilical vein endothelial cells [32], cardiomyocytes [36] and podocytes [37]. However, whether PD could suppress ROS production by immune cells, especially neutrophils, is still obscure. In this study, it was found that increased intracellular ROS production by human neutrophils was abrogated by PD treatment. Also, PD treatment markedly inhibited ROS production by bone marrow-derived neutrophils from PIL mice. These results demonstrated that PD could prevent ROS production by neutrophils and suggested that PD might inhibit NET formation through blocking ROS production.

Next, we demonstrated the suppressing effects of PD on NET formation. Importantly, we found that PD significantly reduced PMA-induced NET formation by SLE neutrophils and HC neutrophils in vitro. And we detected the percentage of Ly6G+PI+ cells in peripheral blood of PIL mice and found that PD treatment prevented neutrophils from necrosis, indirectly implying that NETosis was inhibited by PD treatment in vivo. More directly, PD treatment reduced spontaneous NET formation by bone marrow-derived neutrophils. To our knowledge, this is the first report that PD inhibits NET formation both in vivo and in vitro. Therefore, these findings combined with previous results indicate that PD exhibits inhibitory effects on NET formation by reducing ROS production and provide a new approach to modulation of NETosis for SLE treatment.

The combination of pristane-induced lupus model, an environmental factor-induced lupus mouse model, with MRL/*lpr* model, one of spontaneous murine lupus models, can best mimic human lupus, which is mostly affected by environment factors and genetic susceptibility [38]. Therefore, we used two lupus-prone models to

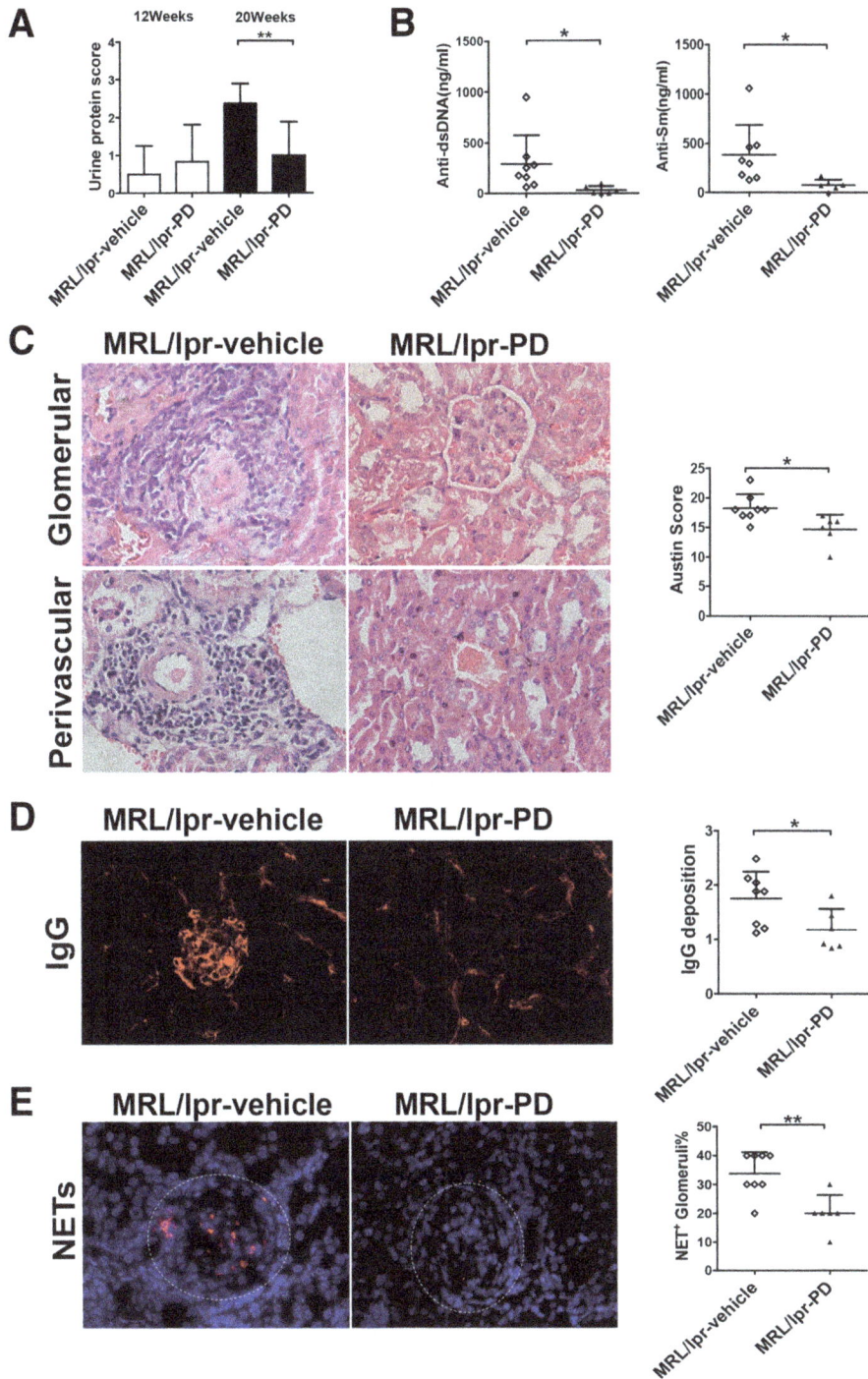

Fig. 2 PD markedly reduced autoantibody production, renal disease activity and NET deposition in MRL/*lpr* mouse model. MRL/*lpr* mice were treated with vehicle or with PD (45 mg/kg) by daily i.p. injection for 8 weeks. **a** The proteinuria concentrations were measured by Bradford Protein Quantification Kit and then the urine protein score assessed as described in Materials and Methods. **b** The levels of anti-dsDNA antibodies and anti-Sm antibodies were examined at the age of 20 weeks. **c** On the *left,* representative H&E staining of glomerular and renal vascular lesions in kidneys was shown (×400). On the *right,* Austin scores of kidneys were determined. **d** On the *left,* representative staining of IgG deposition (*red*) in glomeruli of kidneys was shown (×400). On the *right,* the average score of IgG deposition was calculated as described in Materials and Methods. **e** NET formation in kidneys was determined as colocalization of DNA (*blue*) and MPO (red). Representative fluorescent images were shown (×400) on the left. Ten glomeruli per animal were examined for NET staining and the percentage of NET-stained glomeruli per animal was calculated and shown on the right. NET$^+$ Glomeruli% = positive NET-stained glomeruli/total glomeruli per field. For all experiments, vehicle-treated MRL/*lpr* mice, $N = 8$; PD-treated MRL/*lpr* mice, $N = 6$; data were shown as mean ± SD, *$p < 0.05$; **$p < 0.01$; ***$p < 0.001$. *IgG* immunoglobulin G, *NET* neutrophil extracellular trap, *PD* polydatin

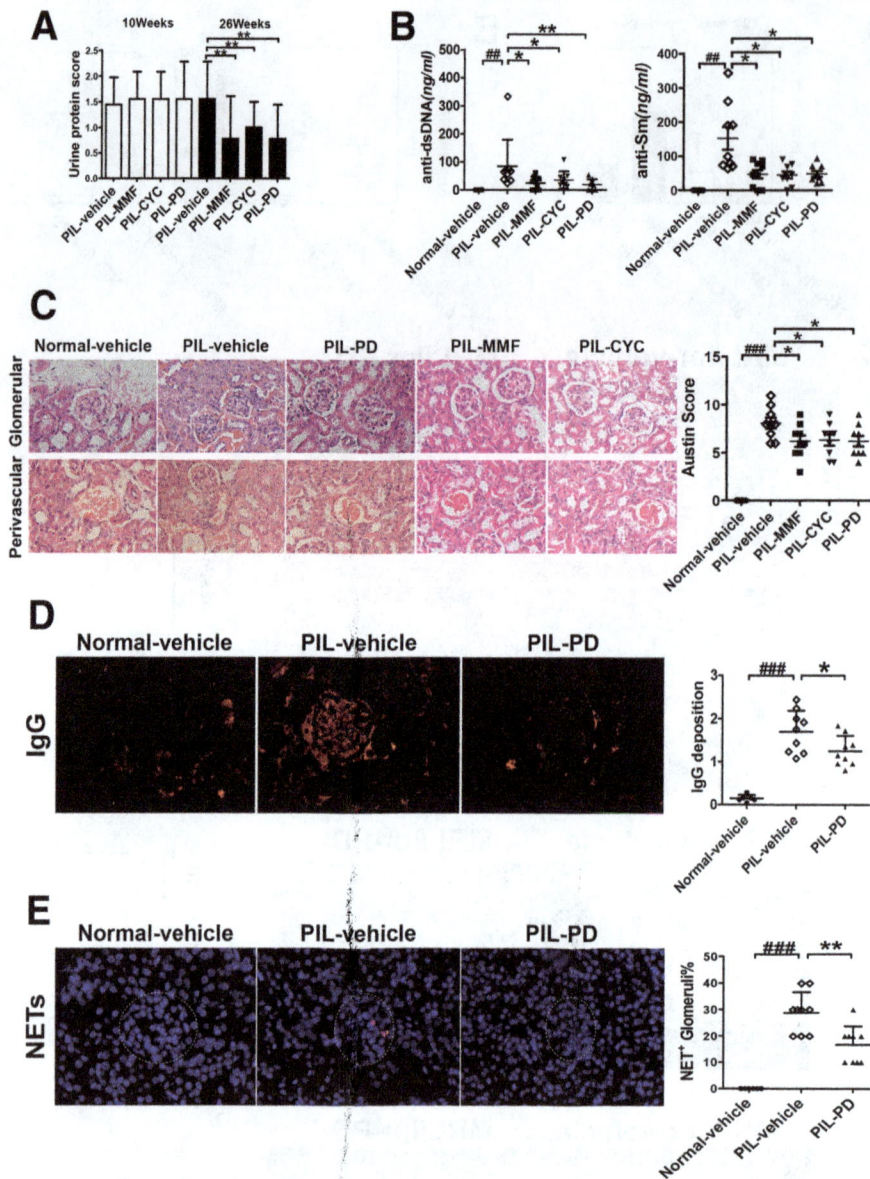

Fig. 3 PD ameliorated lupus manifestations and reduced NET deposition in the kidneys in PIL mouse model. PIL mice were treated with vehicle or with PD (45 mg/kg, daily), CYC (1.8 mg/mouse, weekly), MMF (100 mg/kg, daily) for 16 weeks. **a** The proteinuria was assessed as described in Materials and Methods. **b** The levels of anti-dsDNA antibodies and anti-Sm antibodies were examined by ELISA. **c** On the *left*, representative H&E staining of glomerular and renal vascular lesions in kidneys was shown (× 400). On the *right*, Austin scores of kidneys were shown. **d** On the *left*, the glomeruli were stained for IgG deposition and the representative staining images were shown (× 400). On the *right*, 25 glomeruli were analyzed and the average score was calculated for each kidney as described in Materials and Methods. **e** On the *left*, representative staining images of NET formation in kidneys were shown. Colocalization of DNA (*blue*) and MPO (*red*) in kidneys was consistent with NET formation (× 400). On the right, the percentage of NET-stained glomeruli per animal was determined. For all experiments, N = 6 for normal mice; $N = 9$ for each group of treated PIL mice; data were shown as Mean ± SD, *$p < 0.05$; **$p < 0.01$; ***$p < 0.001$. *CYC* cyclophosphamide, IgG immunoglobulin G, *MMF* mycophenolate mofetil, *PD* polydatin, *PIL* pristane-induced lupus

assess the effects of PD on SLE pathogenesis and development. As expected, we found that PD effectively ameliorated lupus-like features in MRL/*lpr* mice, showed by the reduction in levels of circulating anti-dsDNA and anti-Sm antibodies, and the improvement in pathology of kidneys. To better mimic the effect of drugs on the

development of human lupus clinically, we chose Balb/c mice that had developed proteinuria for further experiments. To our surprise, PD treatment exhibited the same capacity for ameliorating lupus-like features in PIL mice as traditional therapeutic agents targeting T and B lymphocytes (like MMF and CYC) did. Thus, these

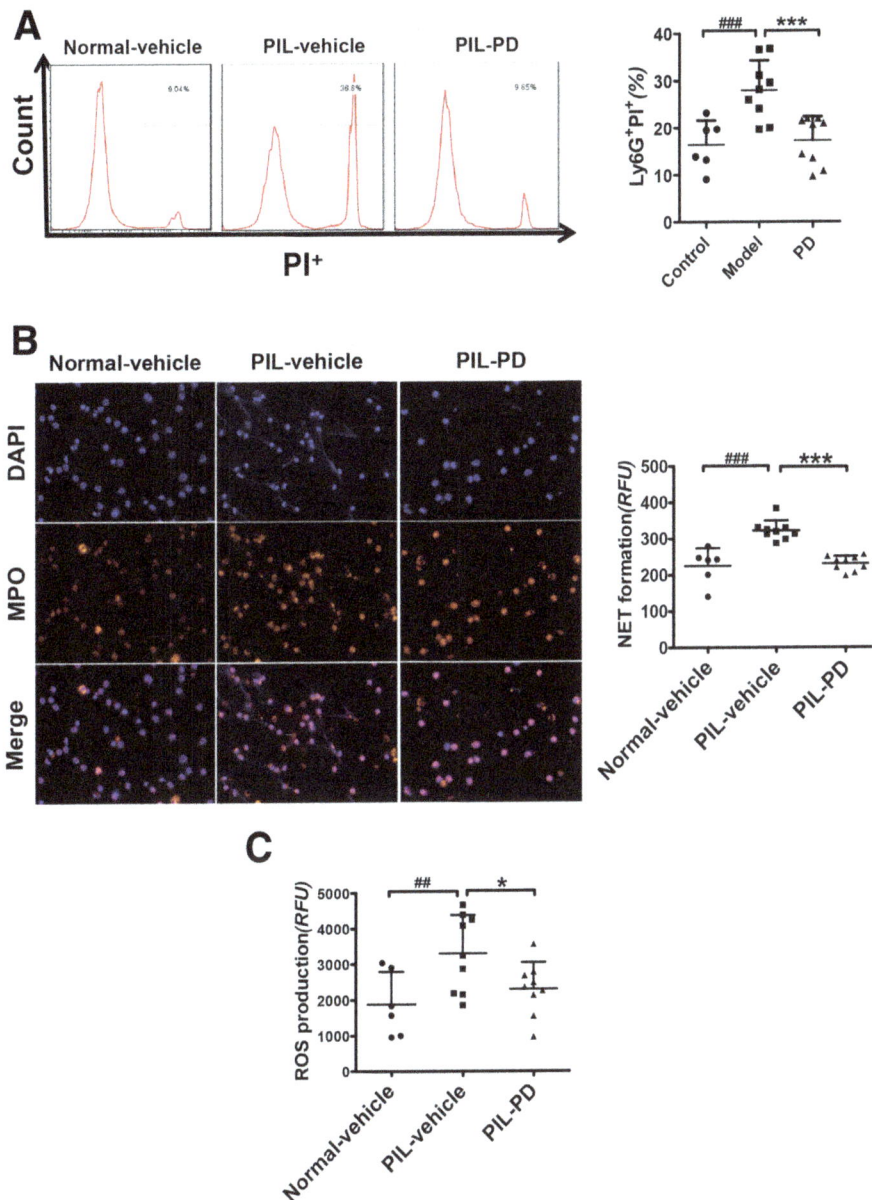

Fig. 4 In vivo, PD prevented spontaneous NET formation in pristane-induced lupus mice through inhibition of ROS. **a** After eliminating erythrocytes, the remaining cells from the mouse peripheral blood were incubated in RPMI-1640 with 5% fetal bovine serum. The percentage of Ly6G⁺PI⁺ cells in mouse peripheral blood was tested by flow cytometry. **b** Bone marrow-derived neutrophils from mice were cultured in the absence of serum for 4 h and then the spontaneous NET formation measured. **c** ROS production by the bone marrow-derived neutrophil was measured. For all experiments, data were represented as mean ± SD, $^{\#}p < 0.05$; $^{\#\#}p < 0.01$; $^{\#\#\#}p < 0.001$ were for comparisons between vehicle-treated PIL mouse model and vehicle-treated normal mice; $^{*}p < 0.05$; $^{**}p < 0.01$; $^{***}p < 0.001$ compared the vehicle and PD-treated PIL mice. *DAPI* 4′, 6′-diamidino-2-phenylindole, *MPO* myeloperoxidase, *NET* neutrophil extracellular trap, *PD* polydatin, *PIL* pristane-induced lupus

results confirmed that PD had high therapeutic effect for lupus-prone mice. For further revealing the mechanisms involved in the therapeutic effects of PD on SLE, we investigated whether PD treatment could prevent NET formation by neutrophils and decrease the deposition of NETs in kidneys in vivo. As a result, PD treatment significantly inhibited NET formation by bone marrow-derived neutrophils and reduced the deposition of NETs in

kidneys. All the above investigations demonstrated that PD effectively ameliorated lupus-like manifestations in lupus-prone mice perhaps via abrogating NET formation.

A previous study showed that PD treatment limited the symptoms of collagen-induced arthritis for its anti-oxidative and anti-inflammatory effects [26]. Some studies have identified increased levels of NETs in peripheral blood, synovial fluid and rheumatoid nodules of

Arthritis: A Growing Concern

RA patients, suggesting that NET formation may also be correlated with RA [39, 40]. Therefore, our results may provide evidence for an alternative mechanism of PD treatment for rheumatoid arthritis.

Conclusions

Our study clearly demonstrated that PD significantly blocked ROS-mediated NET formation and effectively attenuated many lupus-like manifestations in two lupus-prone mouse models. These results indicate that PD may have potential clinical values in treating SLE or other autoimmune diseases.

Abbreviations

CYC: Cyclophosphamide; DAMP: Damage-associated molecular pattern; DAPI: 4 6'-diamidino-2-phenylindole; DCFH-DA: 2',7'-Dichlorodihydrofluorescein diacetate; ELISA: Enzyme-linked immunosorbent assay; H&E: Hematoxylin and eosin; HC: Healthy controls; IBS: Irritable bowel syndrome; IgG: Immunoglobulin G; IL: Interleukin; JAK: Janus kinase; MMF: Mycophenolate mofetil; MPO: Myeloperoxidase; NAC: N-acetyl cysteine; NADPH: Nicotinamide adenine dinucleotide phosphate; NET: Neutrophil extracellular trap; PAD: Peptidylarginine deiminase; PBS: Phosphate-buffered saline; PD: Polydatin; PIL: Pristane-induced lupus; PMA: Phorbol 12-myristate 13-acetate; ROS: Reactive oxygen species; RPMI-1640: Roswell Park Memorial Institute 1640; SLE: Systemic lupus erythematosus

Acknowledgements

The authors would like to thank Professor Ke-seng Zhao from Guangdong Key Laboratory of Shock and Microcirculation Research of Southern Medical University for the gift of polydatin.

Funding

This work was supported by grants from National Natural Science Foundation of China (Grant Nos. 81501417, 81671623, 81873880, 81471613, 81601434) and Guangdong Project of Science and Technology (No. 2017A070713014).

Authors' contributions

PL carried out most of the experiments, participated in the analysis of data, and drafted the manuscript. YH participated in the design of the study, data analysis and interpretation, and drafted the manuscript. FYY participated in the animal experiments and performed the statistical analysis. GHL and JZ participated in the immunofluorescence assay and carried out the flow cytometry analysis. ZQZ participated in the collection of samples and clinical data. LLZ participated in assessment of histopathological changes and revising of the manuscript. JHZ and ZML participated in the animal experiments. EWS conceived the idea for the project, participated in its design and coordination, and modified the manuscript. All authors read and approved the final manuscript.

Consent for publication

Not applicable.

Competing interests

The authors declare that they have no competing interests.

Author details

[1]Department of Rheumatology and Immunology, The Third Affiliated Hospital, Southern Medical University, No. 183, Zhongshan Avenue West, Tianhe District, Guangzhou 510630, China. [2]Institute of Clinical Immunology, Academy of Orthopedics Guangdong Province, Guangzhou, China. [3]School of Pharmaceutical Science, Southern Medical University, Guangzhou, China.

References

1. Tsokos GC. Systemic lupus erythematosus. N Engl J Med. 2011;365(22):2110–21.
2. Carter EE, Barr SG, Clarke AE. The global burden of SLE: prevalence, health disparities and socioeconomic impact. Nat Rev Rheumatol. 2016;12(10):605–20.
3. McMurray RW, May W. Sex hormones and systemic lupus erythematosus: review and meta-analysis. Arthritis Rheum. 2003;48(8):2100–10.
4. Crispin JC, Kyttaris VC, Terhorst C, Tsokos GC. T cells as therapeutic targets in SLE. Nat Rev Rheumatol. 2010;6(6):317–25.
5. Dorner T, Jacobi AM, Lee J, Lipsky PE. Abnormalities of B cell subsets in patients with systemic lupus erythematosus. J Immunol Methods. 2011; 363(2):187–97.
6. Crispin JC, Liossis SN, Kis-Toth K, Lieberman LA, Kyttaris VC, Juang YT, Tsokos GC. Pathogenesis of human systemic lupus erythematosus: recent advances. Trends Mol Med. 2010;16(2):47–57.
7. Denny MF, Yalavarthi S, Zhao W, Thacker SG, Anderson M, Sandy AR, McCune WJ, Kaplan MJ. A distinct subset of proinflammatory neutrophils isolated from patients with systemic lupus erythematosus induces vascular damage and synthesizes type I IFNs. J Immunol. 2010;184(6):3284–97.
8. Yang H, Biermann MH, Brauner JM, Liu Y, Zhao Y, Herrmann M. New Insights into Neutrophil Extracellular Traps: Mechanisms of Formation and Role in Inflammation. Front Immunol. 2016;7:302.
9. Villanueva E, Yalavarthi S, Berthier CC, Hodgin JB, Khandpur R, Lin AM, Rubin CJ, Zhao W, Olsen SH, Klinker M, et al. Netting neutrophils induce endothelial damage, infiltrate tissues, and expose immunostimulatory molecules in systemic lupus erythematosus. J Immunol. 2011;187(1):538–52.
10. Lood C, Blanco LP, Purmalek MM, Carmona-Rivera C, De Ravin SS, Smith CK, Malech HL, Ledbetter JA, Elkon KB, Kaplan MJ. Neutrophil extracellular traps enriched in oxidized mitochondrial DNA are interferogenic and contribute to lupus-like disease. Nat Med. 2016;22(2):146–53.
11. Hakkim A, Furnrohr BG, Amann K, Laube B, Abed UA, Brinkmann V, Herrmann M, Voll RE, Zychlinsky A. Impairment of neutrophil extracellular trap degradation is associated with lupus nephritis. Proc Natl Acad Sci U S A. 2010; 107(21):9813–8.
12. Garcia-Romo GS, Caielli S, Vega B, Connolly J, Allantaz F, Xu Z, Punaro M, Baisch J, Guiducci C, Coffman RL, et al. Netting neutrophils are major inducers of type I IFN production in pediatric systemic lupus erythematosus. Sci Transl Med. 2011;3(73):20r–73r.
13. Lande R, Ganguly D, Facchinetti V, Frasca L, Conrad C, Gregorio J, Meller S, Chamilos G, Sebasigari R, Riccieri V, et al. Neutrophils activate plasmacytoid dendritic cells by releasing self-DNA-peptide complexes in systemic lupus erythematosus. Sci Transl Med. 2011;3(73):19r–73r.
14. Kahlenberg JM, Carmona-Rivera C, Smith CK, Kaplan MJ. Neutrophil extracellular trap-associated protein activation of the NLRP3 inflammasome is enhanced in lupus macrophages. J Immunol. 2013;190(3):1217–26.
15. Smith CK, Vivekanandan-Giri A, Tang C, Knight JS, Mathew A, Padilla RL, Gillespie BW, Carmona-Rivera C, Liu X, Subramanian V, et al. Neutrophil extracellular trap-derived enzymes oxidize high-density lipoprotein: an additional proatherogenic mechanism in systemic lupus erythematosus. Arthritis Rheum. 2014;66(9):2532–44.
16. Carmona-Rivera C, Zhao W, Yalavarthi S, Kaplan MJ. Neutrophil extracellular traps induce endothelial dysfunction in systemic lupus erythematosus through the activation of matrix metalloproteinase-2. Ann Rheum Dis. 2015;74(7):1417–24.
17. Pinegin B, Vorobjeva N, Pinegin V. Neutrophil extracellular traps and their role in the development of chronic inflammation and autoimmunity. Autoimmun Rev. 2015;14(7):633–40.
18. Patel S, Kumar S, Jyoti A, Srinag BS, Keshari RS, Saluja R, Verma A, Mitra K, Barthwal MK, Krishnamurthy H, et al. Nitric oxide donors release extracellular traps from human neutrophils by augmenting free radical generation. Nitric Oxide. 2010;22(3):226–34.

19. Lai ZW, Hanczko R, Bonilla E, Caza TN, Clair B, Bartos A, Miklossy G, Jimah J, Doherty E, Tily H, et al. N-acetylcysteine reduces disease activity by blocking mammalian target of rapamycin in T cells from systemic lupus erythematosus patients: a randomized, double-blind, placebo-controlled trial. Arthritis Rheum. 2012;64(9):2937–46.

20. Qiao H, Chen H, Dong Y, Ma H, Zhao G, Tang F, Li Z. Polydatin attenuates H2O2-induced oxidative stress via PKC pathway. Oxidative Med Cell Longev. 2016;2016:5139458.

21. Pang N, Chen T, Deng X, Chen N, Li R, Ren M, Li Y, Luo M, Hao H, Wu J, et al. Polydatin prevents methylglyoxal-induced apoptosis through reducing oxidative stress and improving mitochondrial function in human umbilical vein endothelial cells. Oxidative Med Cell Longev. 2017;2017:7180943.

22. Cremon C, Stanghellini V, Barbaro MR, Cogliandro RF, Bellacosa L, Santos J, Vicario M, Pigrau M, Alonso CC, Lobo B, et al. Randomised clinical trial: the analgesic properties of dietary supplementation with palmitoylethanolamide and polydatin in irritable bowel syndrome. Aliment Pharmacol Ther. 2017;45(7):909–22.

23. Jiang KF, Zhao G, Deng GZ, Wu HC, Yin NN, Chen XY, Qiu CW, Peng XL. Polydatin ameliorates Staphylococcus aureus-induced mastitis in mice via inhibiting TLR2-mediated activation of the p38 MAPK/NF-kappaB pathway. Acta Pharmacol Sin. 2017;38(2):211–22.

24. Li B, Wang XL. Effective treatment of polydatin weakens the symptoms of collagen-induced arthritis in mice through its anti-oxidative and anti-inflammatory effects and the activation of MMP-9. Mol Med Rep. 2016;14(6):5357–62.

25. Jonsson CA, Svensson L, Carlsten H. Beneficial effect of the inosine monophosphate dehydrogenase inhibitor mycophenolate mofetil on survival and severity of glomerulonephritis in systemic lupus erythematosus (SLE)-prone MRLlpr/lpr mice. Clin Exp Immunol. 1999;116(3):534–41.

26. Jonsson CA, Erlandsson M, Svensson L, Molne J, Carlsten H. Mycophenolate mofetil ameliorates perivascular T lymphocyte inflammation and reduces the double-negative T cell population in SLE-prone MRLlpr/lpr mice. Cell Immunol. 1999;197(2):136–44.

27. Caudrillier A, Kessenbrock K, Gilliss BM, Nguyen JX, Marques MB, Monestier M, Toy P, Werb Z, Looney MR. Platelets induce neutrophil extracellular traps in transfusion-related acute lung injury. J Clin Invest. 2012;122(7):2661–71.

28. Austin HR, Muenz LR, Joyce KM, Antonovych TT, Balow JE. Diffuse proliferative lupus nephritis: identification of specific pathologic features affecting renal outcome. Kidney Int. 1984;25(4):689–95.

29. Zhao J, Wang H, Dai C, Wang H, Zhang H, Huang Y, Wang S, Gaskin F, Yang N, Fu SM. P2X7 blockade attenuates murine lupus nephritis by inhibiting activation of the NLRP3/ASC/caspase 1 pathway. Arthritis Rheum. 2013;65(12):3176–85.

30. Sun E. Cell death recognition model for the immune system. Med Hypotheses. 2008;70(3):585–96.

31. Sun EW, Shi YF. Apoptosis: the quiet death silences the immune system. Pharmacol Ther. 2001;92(2–3):135–45.

32. Knight JS, Zhao W, Luo W, Subramanian V, O'Dell AA, Yalavarthi S, Hodgin JB, Eitzman DT, Thompson PR, Kaplan MJ. Peptidylarginine deiminase inhibition is immunomodulatory and vasculoprotective in murine lupus. J Clin Invest. 2013;123(7):2981–93.

33. Knight JS, Subramanian V, O'Dell AA, Yalavarthi S, Zhao W, Smith CK, Hodgin JB, Thompson PR, Kaplan MJ. Peptidylarginine deiminase inhibition disrupts NET formation and protects against kidney, skin and vascular disease in lupus-prone MRL/lpr mice. Ann Rheum Dis. 2015;74(12):2199–206.

34. Furumoto Y, Smith CK, Blanco L, Zhao W, Brooks SR, Thacker SG, Abdalrahman Z, Sciume G, Tsai WL, Trier AM, et al. Tofacitinib ameliorates murine lupus and its associated vascular dysfunction. Arthritis Rheum. 2017;69(1):148–60.

35. Jorch SK, Kubes P. An emerging role for neutrophil extracellular traps in noninfectious disease. Nat Med. 2017;23(3):279–87.

36. Ling Y, Chen G, Deng Y, Tang H, Ling L, Zhou X, Song X, Yang P, Liu Y, Li Z, et al. Polydatin post-treatment alleviates myocardial ischaemia/reperfusion injury by promoting autophagic flux. Clin Sci (Lond). 2016;130(18):1641–53.

37. Ni Z, Tao L, Xiaohui X, Zelin Z, Jiangang L, Zhao S, Weikang H, Hongchao X, Qiujing W, Xin L. Polydatin impairs mitochondria fitness and ameliorates podocyte injury by suppressing Drp1 expression. J Cell Physiol. 2017;232(10):2776–87.

38. Du Y, Sanam S, Kate K, Mohan C. Animal models of lupus and lupus nephritis. Curr Pharm Des. 2015;21(18):2320–49.

39. Khandpur R, Carmona-Rivera C, Vivekanandan-Giri A, Gizinski A, Yalavarthi S, Knight JS, Friday S, Li S, Patel RM, Subramanian V, et al. NETs are a source of citrullinated autoantigens and stimulate inflammatory responses in rheumatoid arthritis. Sci Transl Med. 2013;5(178):140r–78r.

40. Wang W, Peng W, Ning X. Increased levels of neutrophil extracellular trap remnants in the serum of patients with rheumatoid arthritis. Int J Rheum Dis. 2018;21(2):415–21.

24

E2F2 directly regulates the STAT1 and PI3K/AKT/NF-κB pathways to exacerbate the inflammatory phenotype in rheumatoid arthritis synovial fibroblasts and mouse embryonic fibroblasts

Shiguan Wang[1,2,3], Lin Wang[2,3,4], Changshun Wu[5], Shui Sun[5] and Ji-hong Pan[2,3,4*]

Abstract

Background: Expression of E2F transcription factor 2 (E2F2), a transcription factor related to the cell cycle, is abnormally high in rheumatoid arthritis synovial fibroblasts (RASFs). Deregulated expression of E2F2 leads to abnormal production of proinflammatory cytokines, such as interleukin (IL)-1α, IL-1β, and tumor necrosis factor (TNF)-α in RASFs. However, the underlying mechanism by which E2F2 regulates expression of IL-1α, IL-1β, and TNF-α has not been fully elucidated. This study aimed to elucidate this mechanism and confirm the pathological roles of E2F2 in rheumatoid arthritis (RA).

Methods: *E2f2* knockout (KO) and wild-type (WT) mice were injected with collagen to induce RA. Cytokine production was assessed by quantitative real-time polymerase chain reaction (qRT-PCR) and enzyme-linked immunosorbent assay (ELISA). Western blot and qRT-PCR were performed to evaluate the effect of E2F2 on signaling pathway activity. Chromatin immunoprecipitation (ChIP)-PCR and luciferase assays were used to detect the transcriptional activity of target genes of E2F2. Nuclear translocation of STAT1 and p65 were assayed by Western blot, co-immunoprecipitation (co-IP), and immunofluorescence experiments.

Results: The occurrence and severity of collagen-induced arthritis were decreased in *E2f2*-KO mice compared with WT mice. The expression of IL-1α, IL-1β, and TNF-α was also suppressed in mouse embryonic fibroblasts (MEFs) from *E2f2*-KO mice and RASFs with E2F2 knocked down. Mechanistically, we found that E2F2 can upregulate the expression of STAT1 and MyD88 through direct binding to their promoters, facilitate the formation of STAT1/MyD88 complexes, and consequently activate AKT. However, silencing STAT1/MyD88 or inactivating AKT significantly attenuated the induction of IL-1α, IL-1β, and TNF-α caused by the introduction of E2F2.

Conclusions: This study confirms the pathological role of E2F2 in RA and found that the E2F2-STAT1/MyD88-Akt axis is closely related with the inflammatory phenotype in RASFs.

Keywords: Cytokine, Inflammation, Rheumatoid arthritis, Synovial fibroblast, E2F2

* Correspondence: pjh933@sohu.com
[2]Shandong Medicinal Biotechnology Centre, Jingshi Road, Jinan 250000, Shandong, China
[3]Key Lab for Biotechnology Drugs of Ministry of Health, Jinan 250000, Shandong, China
Full list of author information is available at the end of the article

Background

Rheumatoid arthritis (RA) is a systemic autoimmune disease resulting in severe inflammation and morphological changes to skeletal tissues, including bone and joint damage. Cartilage degradation, synovial hyperplasia, fibroblast-like synoviocyte infiltration into cartilage and bone surfaces, and subchondral bone erosion are all pathological hallmarks of RA [1]. Accumulating evidence suggests that activated rheumatoid arthritis synovial fibroblasts (RASFs) play an important role in the pathogenesis of arthritic joint destruction [2, 3]. The process of arthritic joint destruction results in a marked secretion of inflammatory cytokines, including interleukin (IL)-1α, IL-1β, and tumor necrosis factor (TNF)-α, which are important in inducing adaptive immunity in RASFs [4]. In RA, excessive inflammatory molecules such as IL-1α, IL-1β, and TNF-α are secreted and subsequently mediate the destruction of cartilage and bone [5]. The identification of pathogenic genes regulating inflammation in the microenvironment of the inflamed joint is crucial to understand the pathogenesis of RA and may also provide new targets for diagnosis and treatment.

E2F transcription factor 2 (E2F2) encodes a periodic cycling molecule involved in transcription factor activity, sequence-specific DNA binding, and core promoter binding. Inhibition of E2F expression by an E2F decoy oligonucleotide inhibits the proliferation of synovial cells and prevents cartilage invasion [6]. A microarray study of peripheral blood mononuclear cells from RA patients found that a significant number of RA-associated genes contain E2F-binding motifs in their promoters, suggesting that E2F2 may play a role in RA pathogenesis [7–9].

In our previous microarray analysis, E2F2 was highly expressed in RA synovial tissue [10]. In RASFs, activated NF-κB can bind to the promoter region of E2F2, and activated E2F2 can bind to the promoter of IL-6 which, in turn, can promote the progression of arthritis [7]. Our recent data further showed that expression of E2F2 can promote upregulation of IL-1α, IL-1β, and TNF-α, although the mechanism underlying this function remains to be discovered. In the present study, RASFs and a gene knockout (KO) mouse model were used to investigate the signaling pathways involved in the pathogenic role of E2F2 in RA.

Methods

Cell acquisition and arthritis models

Synovial tissues were collected during knee joint replacement surgery from patients with RA (n = 14; five males, nine females, aged 35 to 75 years old, mean age 55 years). All patients fulfilled the 1987 American College of Rheumatology revised criteria for RA diagnosis. Written informed consent was obtained from each patient, and all samples were rendered anonymous. The Ethical Committee of the Shandong Academy of Medicinal Sciences approved this study (approval number 2014–2019).

E2F2 knockout mice

Twenty transgenic founder (F0) $E2f2^{+/-}$ mice (C57Bl6:12 9Sv background, 11 females, 9 males) from The Jackson Laboratory (JAX, Bar Harbor, Maine, USA) were identified using polymerase chain reaction (PCR) with genomic DNA. Female and male transgenic F0 mice were mated to produce the F1 generation. Tail clips were dissected from F1 mice at postnatal day 12 and subjected to PCR to determine $E2f2$ expression. Eight-week-old male and female mice ($E2f2^{+/-}$) were mated to obtain $E2f2^{-/-}$ and wild-type (WT) mice. These mice were maintained on a normal light/dark cycle in cages with microisolator lids, and genotyped by standard PCR [11, 12]. All procedures were approved by the Animal Care and Use Committee of the Shandong Academy of Medical Sciences.

Collagen-induced arthritis (CIA) model

CIA is a well-established mouse model for human RA [13]. Arthritic mice develop swollen joints, chronic inflammation, and joint destruction. CIA was induced by injecting a type II collagen at 2 mg/mL (Chondrex, Washington, USA) and complete Freud's adjuvant (Sigma-Aldrich, Mannheim, Germany) 1:1 emulsion (200 μL) at the base of the tail in 10-week-old male WT and $E2f2^{-/-}$ mice. A type II collagen and incomplete Freud's adjuvant (Sigma-Aldrich) 1:1 emulsion was injected (200 μL) at the base of the tail in 14-week-old mice. Mice were monitored once per day for symptoms of arthritis.

Mouse embryonic fibroblast (MEF) cell culture

$E2f2^{-/-}$ and wild-type MEFs were obtained from $E2f2^{+/-}$ maternal embryos at 13.5 days gestation as previously described [12]. The extracted MEFs were cultured in Dulbecco's modified Eagle's medium (DMEM) high glucose medium containing 10% serum and 1% penicillin/streptomycin.

Stimulation assays

Primary RASFs were isolated and cultured as described previously [14], and cells were used between passages 3 and 7. We screened many commonly used inflammatory stimulators including IL-1β, TNF-α, interferon (IFN)α, lipopolysaccharide (LPS), and IL-6 to stimulate RASF and MEFs, but we found LPS to be the most efficient. RASFs were plated in 24-well plates (3–5 × 10⁵ cells/well) and stimulated for 12 h with LPS (from *Escherichia coli* J5; Sigma, St Louis, MO, USA). The dilution buffer, phosphate-buffered saline (PBS), was applied as a control. Activation of PI3K/AKT pathways was blocked using LY294002 (Calbiochem, MCE, New Jersey, USA) and NF-κB inhibitor PDTC (M4005, Abmole Bioscience, Hong Kong, China).

Luciferase reporter gene assay

HEK239T cells (2×10^4 cells/well; 96-well plate) were seeded in triplicate in 24-well plates and transfected with 80 ng/well STAT1 and MyD88 luciferase reporter plasmids using Lipofectamine 2000, as described by the manufacturer (Invitrogen, Carlsbad, CA, USA). The reporter gene plasmids used were: pGL4.10-STAT1 promoter-WT; pGL4.10-STAT1 promoter-mutant (mut); pcDNA3.1(+)-E2F2; pRL-CMV (control) and pGL4.10-MyD88 promoter-WT; pcDNA3.1(+)-E2F2; and pRL-CMV (control). All plasmids were constructed by Obio (Obio, Shanghai, China). In all cases, 40 ng/well of phRL-TK reporter gene activity was measured using the Dual Luciferase Assay system (Promega, Madison, Wisconsin, USA). Data are expressed as the mean fold induction ± SEM relative to control levels from a minimum of three separate experiments.

Small interfering RNA (siRNA) and adenovirus transfection in RASFs and MEFs

RASFs (2×10^5 cells in 100-mm diameter dishes or 8×10^4 cells in six-well plates) were transiently transfected with siRNA targeting E2F2 (SI00375410, Qiagen, Hilden, Germany) or negative control siRNA (1,027,281, Qiagen) using HiPerFect transfection reagent (Qiagen) following the manufacturer's instructions, and all experiments were performed 24 h after transfection. The specific siRNAs targeting STAT1 were designed and synthesized by RuiboBio (RuiboBio, Guangzhou, China), and the most effective single siRNA was used for further experiments as follows: STAT1 (homo): CCTACGAACATGACCCTAT; STAT1 (mus): CTGTGATGTTAGATAAACA; MyD88 (homo): CCATCAAGTACAAGGCAAT. RASFs (2×10^5 cells in 100-mm diameter dishes or 8×10^4 cells in six-well plates) were infected by E2F2 and STAT1 adenovirus (2×10^5 pfu/mL) or empty adenovirus (ViGeneBiosciences, JiNan, China) using ADV-HR (ViGeneBiosciences) following the manufacturer's instructions. MEFs (2×10^5 cells in 100-mm diameter dishes or 8×10^4 cells in six-well plates) were infected by STAT1 adenovirus (2×10^5 pfu/mL) or empty adenovirus (Obio, Shanghai, China) using ADV-HR (Obio) following the manufacturer's instructions.

Enzyme-linked immunosorbent assay (ELISA)

Cells were cultured and stimulated as described above, and supernatants were collected at 12 h. The release of IL-1α, IL-1β, and TNF-α was analyzed by ELISA (Multi-Sciences, Hang Zhou, China) according to the manufacturer's instructions. Serum was extracted from fresh blood in 20-week-old mice. After centrifugation to remove particulates, the release of IL-1α, IL-1β, and

TNF-α was analyzed by ELISA (MultiSciences) according to the manufacturer's instructions.

Western blot

Whole cell lysates were separated by sodium dodecyl sulfate-polyacrylamide gel electrophoresis (SDS-PAGE) and transferred onto a 0.45-μm Immobilon-P transfer membrane (Merck Millipore, Darmstadt, Germany). They then underwent immunoblotting with the following specific primary antibodies overnight at 4 °C: anti-E2F2 (1:1000, Millipore), anti-STAT1 (1:1000, CST, Boston, MA, USA), anti-AKT (1:1000, CST), phospho-AKT (1:1000, CST), phospho-p65 NF-κB (1:1000, Affinity, Cincinnati, OH, USA) or p65 NF-κB (1:1000, Affinity), and anti-MyD88 (1:1000, Affinity). After washing with TBST, the membrane was incubated with each corresponding secondary antibody for 1 h at 37 °C. Detection was performed using an ECL Plus detection system (Thermo Scientific, Pittsburgh, PA, USA).

Co-immunoprecipitation (co-IP) assays

Immunoprecipitation was carried out to assess the interaction between STAT1 and MyD88. After harvesting the RASFs and MEFs, the supernatants were incubated overnight at 4 °C with rabbit anti-STAT1 (1:200, CST) and then protein A/G-Sepharose beads (Beyotime, Suzhou, China) conjugated to STAT1. The samples were then electrophoresed through gradient SDS-polyacrylamide gels and transferred to membranes that were probed with mouse anti-STAT1 (1:1000, Proteintech, Wuhan, China). Following incubation with horseradish peroxidase-conjugated secondary antibodies (458, MBL, Tokyo, Japan) the blots were developed using an ECL Plus detection system (Thermo Scientific).

RNA extraction and quantitative real-time PCR (qRT-PCR)

Total RNA was extracted from cultured cells and human tissues using TRIzol Reagent (Invitrogen) according to the manufacturer's protocol. RNA was reverse-transcribed using a ReverTra Ace qPCR RT Kit (Toyobo, Tokyo, Japan). qRT-PCR was conducted using a Light-Cycler 480 (Roche, Basel, Switzerland) with the following protocol: denaturation at 95 °C for 10 min, 40 cycles of denaturation at 95 °C for 10 s, annealing at 60 °C for 1 min, and extension at 72 °C for 1 s. The forward and reverse primers are shown in Table 1. All primers were synthesized by BGI (Beijing, China). Each sample was analyzed in triplicate. The $2^{-\triangle\triangle Ct}$ method of relative quantification was used to calculate changes in the expression of target genes.

Chromatin immunoprecipitation (ChIP)-PCR

RASFs and MEFs were treated with LPS for 12 h and then fixed with 1% formaldehyde for 10 min at room

Table 1 Primers used for real-time polymerase chain reaction

Primer name	Primer base sequence (5′ to 3′)
GAPDH (homo)	Forward: CACCATCT TCCAGGAGC; Reverse: AGTGGACTCCACGACGTA
GAPDH (mus)	Forward: AAAGGGTCATCATCTCCG; Reverse: CAATCTTGAGTGAGTTGTCATATTTC
E2F2 (homo)	Forward: CCTTGGA GGCTACTGACAGC; Reverse: CCACAGGTAGTCGTCCTGGT
E2F2 (mus)	Forward: TGTTTCCCTGGGAGGATTATT; Reverse: TTTGGGACAGTGGGTGTTTA
STAT1 (homo)	Forward: TACACCTACGAACATGACCC; Reverse: TGAAGGTGCGGTCCCATAA
STAT1 (mus)	Forward: TGGGAAGTATTATTCCAGACCAAA; Reverse: AGTCTTGATGTATCCAGTTCG
MyD88 (homo)	Forward: CTGGCCTCTGCGCATATTC;Reverse: CTCCCTGCTCACATCATTAC
MyD88 (mus)	Forward: TGCCAGCGAGCTAATTG;Reverse: CACATTCCTTGCTCTGTAGATA
AKT1 (homo)	Forward: GGCGTGGTCATGTACGA; Reverse: TTCTCATGGTCCTGGTTGTAG
AKT1 (mus)	Forward: GGACGGGCACATCAAGATAA; Reverse: CCGCAGAATGTCTTCATAG
AKT2 (homo)	Forward: TACACCTACGAACATGACCC; Reverse: TGAAGGTGCGGTCCCATAA
AKT2 (mus)	Forward: TTCAGAAGTGGACACAAGGT; Reverse: GGGTCCAGGCTGTCATATC
IL-1α (homo)	Forward: CGTCAGGCAGAAGTTTGTCA; Reverse: TTAGAGTCGTCTCCTCCCGA
IL-1α (mus)	Forward: ATCACAGGTAGTGAGACCGA; Reverse: AGCTGATGTGAAGTAGTTCTTAG
IL-1β (homo)	Forward: CTAAAGTATGGGCTGGACTG; Reverse: AGCTTCAATGAAAGACCTCA
IL-1β (mus)	Forward: CAAGGAGAACCAAGCAACGA; Reverse: TTTCATTACACAGGACAGGTATAGA
TNF-α (homo)	Forward: TGTCTACTGAACTTCGGGGT; Reverse: TCACAGAGCAATGACTCCAA
TNF-α (mus)	Forward: AGGTTCTCTTCAAGGGACAA; Reverse: GACTTTCTCCTGGTATGAGATAG

IL interleukin, *TNF* tumor necrosis factor

temperature. DNA was broken into 200–1000 bp fragments using a sonicator (10^6 cells in 200 μL volume, ultrasound 10 s, stop 10 s, repeated seven times). Chromatin was immunoprecipitated with immunoglobulin (Ig)G (Sigma) and anti-E2F2 (Millipore). The association of E2F2 with STAT1 and MyD88 was measured by RT-PCR (predenaturation at 95 °C for 5 min, followed by 95 °C for 30 s, 65 °C for 30 s, and 72 °C for 30 s, 35 cycles) using immunoprecipitated chromatin from RASFs with the following primers: STAT1: 5′- TGCATAGGGCTCAGGCA -3′ (forward) and 5′- CCCTTAGCCTCTTTCTGTTC -3′ (reverse) and 5′- TGAGGTAGGTAGGCCCTT -3′ (forward) and 5′-TCTTAGGGTGAACTCGGCA -3′ (reverse); MyD88: 5′- CTAAATACTTCCGAGACGCC -3′ (forward) and 5′- CAGTTAGAGAGCTTGTCACAC -3′ (reverse).

Immunofluorescence microscopy

MEFs and RASFs were grown in 48-well plates with LPS stimulation for 12 h. Preconditioned cells were washed three times with PBS slowly for 3 min each and then fixed with 4% paraformaldehyde for 10 min, washed three times with PBS (3 min each) and then treated with 5% bovine serum albumin (BSA) for 1 h. Cells were then incubated with monoclonal anti-MyD88 (1:100) and polyclonal anti-STAT1 (1:100) antibodies overnight at 4 °C. After three rinses, FITC- and TRITC-conjugated secondary antibodies were used to visualize the proteins by fluorescence microscopy (Olympus Corporation, FV3000, Tokyo, Japan). The nuclei were stained with 4′,6′-diamidino-2-phenylinndole (DAPI).

Histological analysis

Paws were fixed for 24 h in 10% buffered formalin and decalcified in 15% ethylenediaminetetraacetic acid (EDTA). The paws were then embedded in paraffin, and serial 5-μm sagittal sections were cut and stained with hematoxylin and eosin (H&E). Sections were also stained with Safranin O-Fast Green to determine the depletion of proteoglycans.

Statistical analysis

Statistical analysis was performed using the GraphPad Prism 5 software package (La Jolla, CA, USA). Results were considered statistically significant at $P < 0.05$. The results are expressed as mean ± SEM of five different experiments. The data were analyzed by two-way analysis of variance (ANOVA) followed by Bonferroni's multiple comparison test. The statistical significance of differences in the central tendencies were designated as $*P < 0.05$, $**P < 0.01$, and $***P < 0.001$.

Results

Amelioration of the CIA inflammatory phenotype in *E2f2* KO mice

We previously found that E2F2 expression is significantly upregulated in the RA synovium. To determine the role of E2F2 in RA pathogenesis, *E2f2* KO mice were constructed. WT and *E2f2*$^{-/-}$ mice were immunized by a collagen adjuvant mixture. Among *E2f2*$^{-/-}$ mice, 8% (1/12) showed obvious swelling 20 days after the second immunization, and 25% (3/12) showed obvious swelling 50 days after the second immunization. Among WT mice, 58% (7/12) showed obvious swelling 20 days after the second immunization, and 83% (10/12) showed obvious swelling 50 days after the second immunization (Fig. 1a). Meanwhile, the severity of arthritis in WT mice 20 days after the second immunization was significantly higher than in *E2f2*$^{-/-}$ mice (Fig. 1b). Edema and erythema/redness in the paws of WT mice was more obvious than in *E2f2*$^{-/-}$ mice at 50 days after the second immunization (Fig. 1c). An immunochemistry assay showed that joint destruction and inflammatory

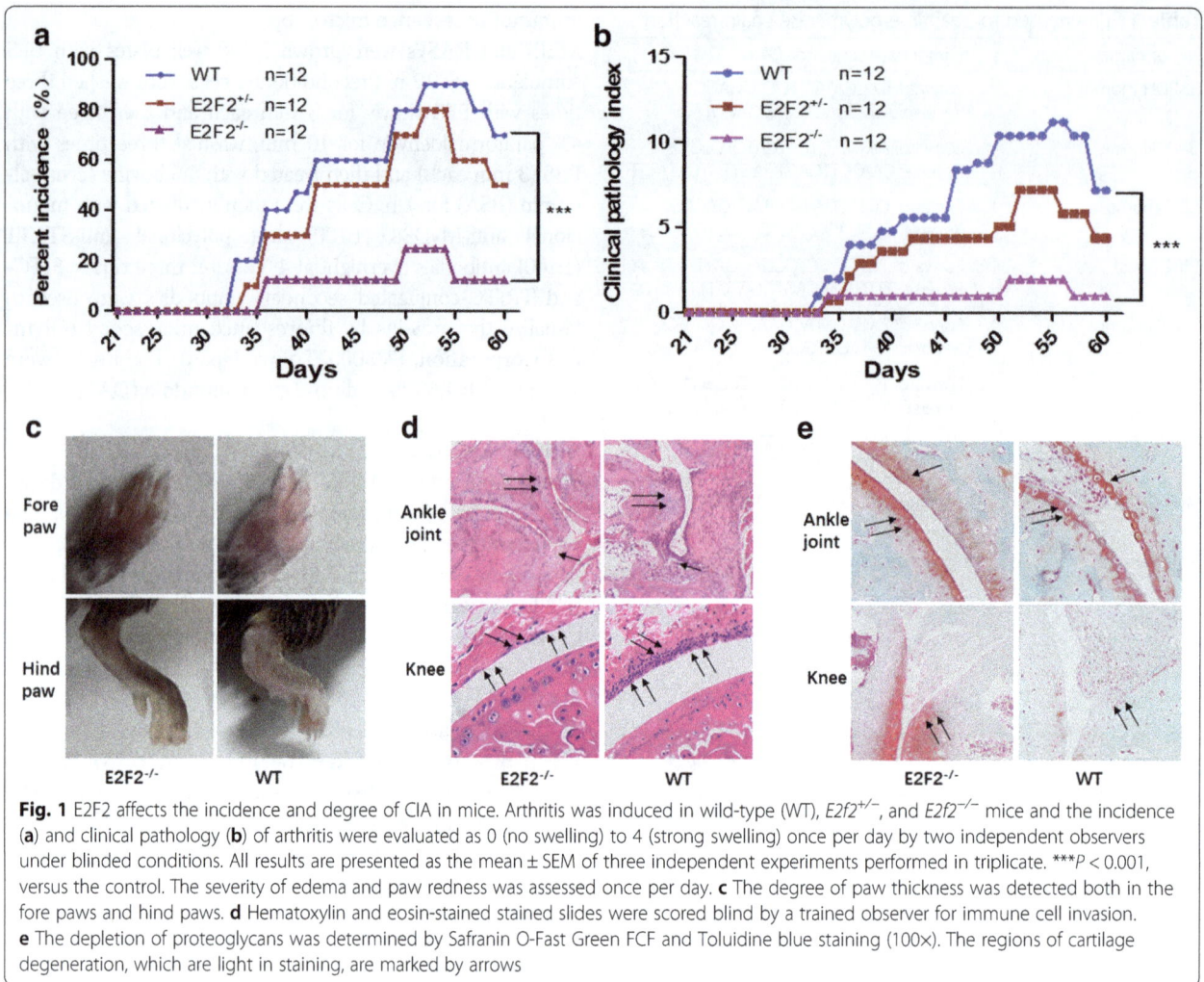

Fig. 1 E2F2 affects the incidence and degree of CIA in mice. Arthritis was induced in wild-type (WT), *E2f2*+/−, and *E2f2*−/− mice and the incidence (**a**) and clinical pathology (**b**) of arthritis were evaluated as 0 (no swelling) to 4 (strong swelling) once per day by two independent observers under blinded conditions. All results are presented as the mean ± SEM of three independent experiments performed in triplicate. ***P < 0.001, versus the control. The severity of edema and paw redness was assessed once per day. **c** The degree of paw thickness was detected both in the fore paws and hind paws. **d** Hematoxylin and eosin-stained stained slides were scored blind by a trained observer for immune cell invasion. **e** The depletion of proteoglycans was determined by Safranin O-Fast Green FCF and Toluidine blue staining (100×). The regions of cartilage degeneration, which are light in staining, are marked by arrows

accumulation were significantly decreased in *E2f2*−/− mice (Fig. 1d). Next, cartilage degradation was assessed by Safranin O-Fast Green staining, a method for detecting depletion of cartilage. Cartilage loss was significantly decreased in the knee joints of *E2f2*−/− mice (Fig. 1e).

Reduced expression of IL-1α, IL-1β, and TNF-α in E2F2−/− MEFs

Inflammatory factors (IL-1α, IL-1β, and TNF-α) play an important role in the progression of RA, and we previously found that siRNAs targeting E2F2 can inhibit the expression of inflammatory cytokines in RASFs [7]. To further verify this result, WT and *E2f2*−/− MEFs were obtained from *E2f2*+/− mice and stimulated with LPS for 12 h. qRT-PCR showed that *E2f2* KO significantly inhibited the expression of IL-1α (Fig. 2a), IL-1β (Fig. 2b), and TNF-α (Fig. 2c). ELISA results also confirmed that secretion of IL-1α (Fig. 2d), IL-1β (Fig. 2e), and TNF-α (Fig. 2f) was inhibited in *E2f2* KO MEFs. Secreted IL-1α, IL-1β, and TNF-α was significantly reduced in the blood

of the *E2f2*−/− CIA model compared with WT models 60 days after the second immunization (Fig. 2g).

E2F2 regulates expression of STAT1 and activation of AKT

We further investigated the molecular mechanism by which E2F2 regulates inflammatory cytokines in RA. Control RASFs and their corresponding E2F2 knockdown RASFs from three different RA patients were harvested. RNA-seq was performed to screen target genes downstream of E2F2. Differentially expressed genes following siRNA knockdown of E2F2 were identified (Fig. 3a). qRT-PCR was performed for in-vitro verification. Using KEGG pathway analysis, we found that E2F2 had an obvious effect on two pathways, STAT1 and PI3K/AKT/NF-κB (Fig. 3b). We confirmed this effect using qRT-PCR and Western blot in RASFs and MEFs, and found that E2F2 can affect the phosphorylation activity of AKT but had no significant effect on the expression of AKT1 and AKT2 (Fig. 3c–f).

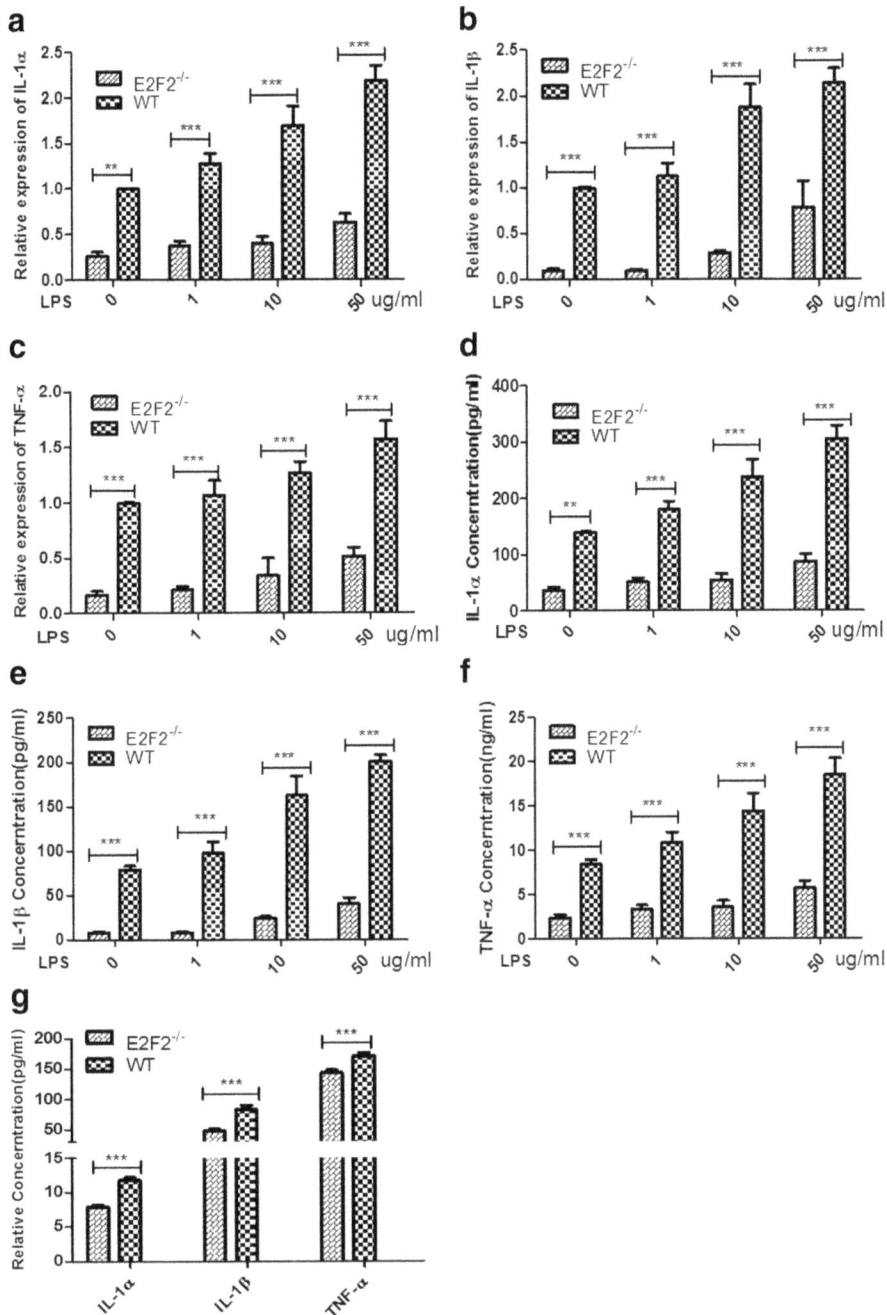

Fig. 2 E2F2 is required for production of inflammatory factors in MEFs. MEFs were treated with different concentrations of lipopolysaccharide (LPS) for 12 h. Expression and dose-dependent effects of interleukin (IL)-1α (**a**), IL-1β (**b**), and tumor necrosis factor (TNF)-α (**c**) were detected by qRT-PCR. **$P < 0.01$, ***$P < 0.001$, versus vehicle control. Dose-dependent effects of secreted IL-1α (**d**), IL-1β (**e**), and TNF-α (**f**) were detected by ELISA. **$P < 0.01$, ***$P < 0.001$, versus vehicle control. IL-1α, IL-1β, and TNF-α in serum of $E2f2^{-/-}$ and wild-type (WT) mice were measured by ELISA (**g**). **$P < 0.01$, ***$P < 0.001$, versus WT

E2F2 regulates IL-1α, IL-1β, and TNF-α expression by activating the STAT1 pathway in RASFs and MEFs

Under LPS stimulation, activated STAT1 proteins can translocate to the cell nucleus and induce transcription of target genes, which may regulate downstream cytokine (IL-1α, IL-1β, TNF-α) production and inflammatory cell infiltration [15, 16]. STAT1, IRF8, and SPI1 can form a complex that binds to the promoter region of IL-1β and promotes its transcription [15]. To test whether E2F2 can directly regulate the expression of STAT1, RASFs were

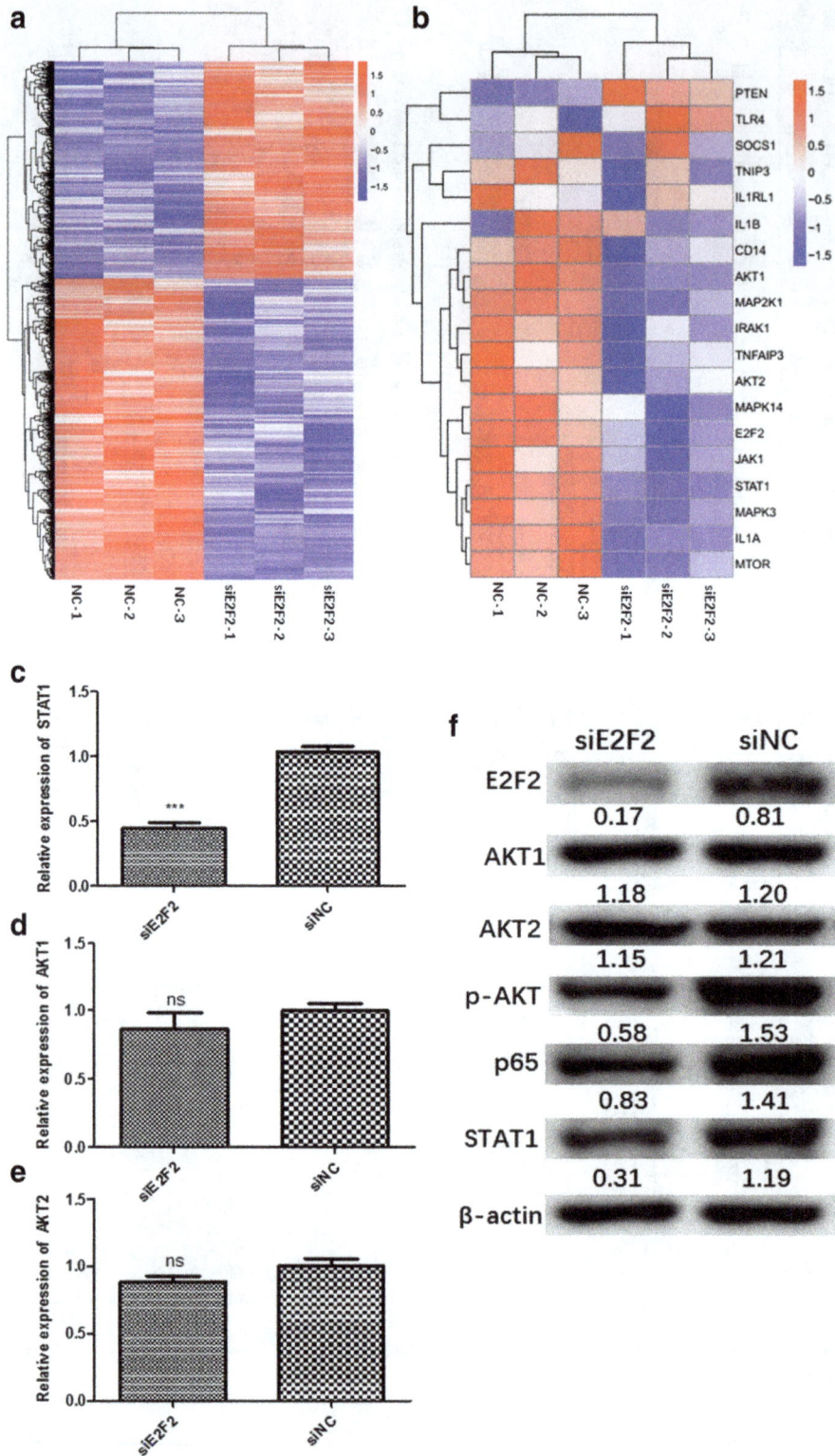

Fig. 3 (See legend on next page.)

(See figure on previous page.)
Fig. 3 E2F2 participates in RA inflammation through STAT1 and PI3K/AKT/NF-κB pathways. RNA-seq was performed to screen target genes downstream of E2F2 in RASFs. **a,b** Heat maps indicate the most differentially expressed genes in RASFs with E2F2 knocked-down. Colored bands represent the change in gene expression: red, downregulation; blue, upregulation. **c–e** In-vitro verification of genes related to inflammation in RA was performed using qRT-PCR. mRNA levels of STAT1 (**c**), AKT1 (**d**), and AKT2 (**e**). **f** Western blot was performed to test inhibitory effects of siE2F2 on expression of E2F2, STAT1, AKT1, AKT2, p-AKT, and the p65 subunit of NF-κB. All results are presented as the mean ± SEM of three independent experiments performed in triplicate. NC knockdown scramble control, si small interfering

transfected with adenovirus-E2F2 to overexpress E2F2 or siE2F2 to suppress E2F2 expression with or without LPS (10 μg/mL). qRT-PCR and Western blot showed that E2F2 can significantly regulate STAT1 at both the mRNA (Fig. 4a) and protein (Fig. 4c) level. Similarly, mRNA

(Fig. 4b) and protein (Fig. 4d) levels of STAT1 in WT MEFs were significantly lower than in *E2f2*⁻/⁻ MEFs with or without LPS (1 μg/mL).

To further explore the mechanism by which E2F2 regulates STAT1, we found two binding sites of E2F2 on the

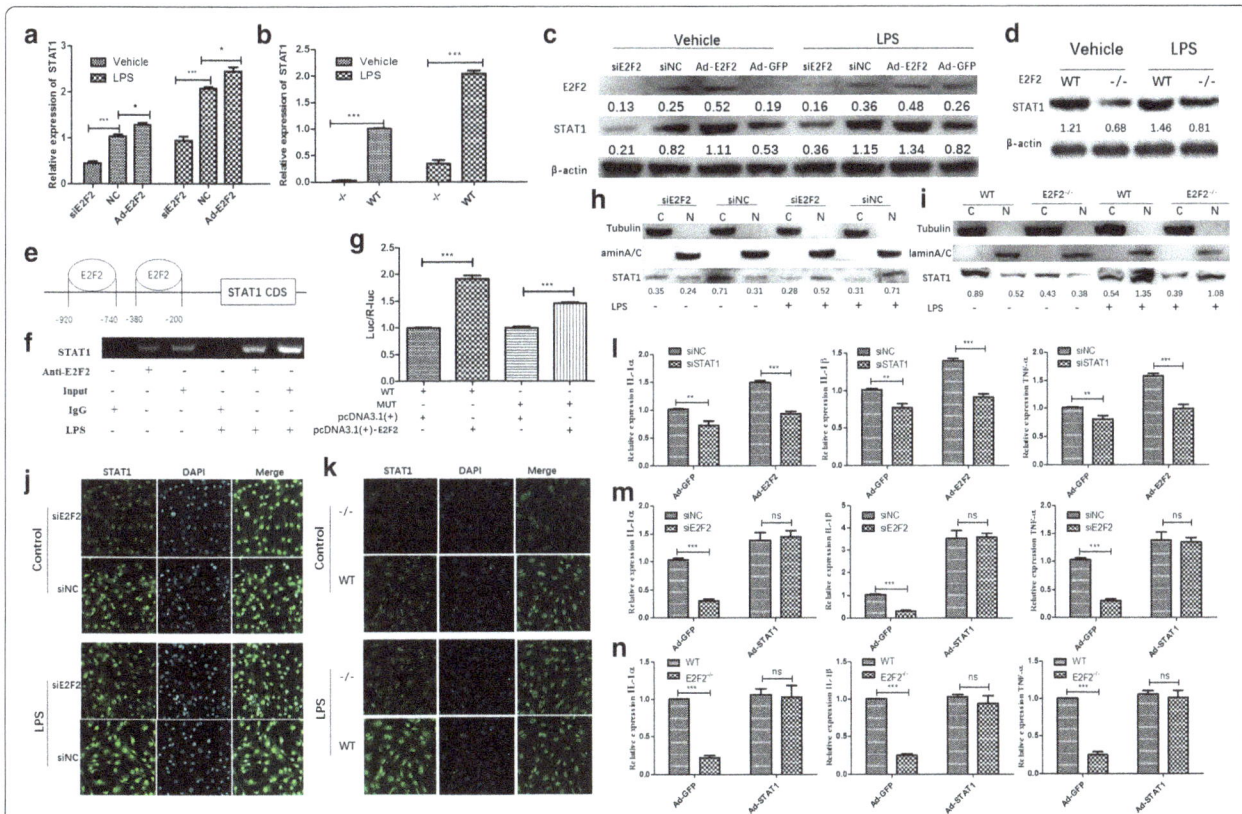

Fig. 4 STAT1 mediates E2F2 regulation of interleukin (IL)-1α, IL-1β, and tumor necrosis factor (TNF)-α expression. **a–d** Effect of E2F2 on STAT1. E2F2 was overexpressed by adenovirus infection or inhibited by small interfering RNA (siRNA) with or without lipopolysaccharide (LPS; 10 μg/mL). qRT-PCR (**a,b**) and Western blot (**c,d**) were performed to detect expression of STAT1. **e** Schematic representation of STAT1 promoters, primers for the ChIP assay, and the E2F2 binding motif in the STAT1 promoter. ChIP (**f**) and luciferase (Luc) reporter assays (**g**) were performed to show that E2F2 was recruited to the *STAT1* gene promoter in RASFs in the presence of LPS. Nuclear and cytoplasmic proteins were fractionally extracted from E2F2 knocked-down RASFs (**h**) and *E2f2*⁻/⁻ MEFs (**i**). Effects of E2F2 on nuclear translocation of STAT1 were determined by Western blot. (Lamin A/C as a reference for nuclear extraction (N); Tubulin as a reference for cytoplasmic extraction (C).) Effect of E2F2 on nuclear translocation of STAT1 was observed using confocal fluorescence microscopy both in E2F2-silenced RASFs (**j**) and *E2f2*⁻/⁻ MEFs (**k**). STAT1 (green) was detected using anti-STAT1 antibody. Nuclei were stained with DAPI (blue). **l** In E2F2-overexpressing RASFs, IL-1α, IL-1β, and TNF-α were analyzed by qRT-PCR after silencing STAT1 in the presence of LPS stimulation (10 μg/mL). **m** In STAT1-overexpressing RASFs, IL-1α, IL-1β, and TNF-α were analyzed by qRT-PCR after silencing E2F2 in the presence of LPS stimulation (10 μg/mL). **n** In *E2f2*⁻/⁻ MEFs, expression of IL-1α, IL-1β, and TNF-α was detected using qRT-PCR after STAT1 overexpression in the presence of LPS stimulation (10 μg/mL). The results shown are means ± SEM of three independent experiments performed in triplicate. *P < 0.05, **P < 0.01, ***P < 0.001, versus the control. Ad-GFP adenovirus encoding green fluorescent protein, NC knockdown scramble control, ns not significant, siE2F2 small interfering RNA knockdown of E2F2, WT wild-type

(See figure on previous page.)
Fig. 5 MyD88 mediates regulation of the PI3K/AKT/NF-κB pathway by E2F2. **a,b** E2F2 can regulate expression of PI3K/AKT/NF-κB. E2F2-silenced RASFs and *E2f2*$^{-/-}$ MEFs were cultured with or without lipopolysaccharide (LPS). Western blot was performed to detect phosphorylation of AKT and NF-κB P65 both in E2F2-silenced RASFs (**a**) and *E2f2*$^{-/-}$ MEFs (**b**). **c,d** Effect of E2F2 on translocation of p65. E2F2 knocked-down RASFs (**c**) and *E2f2*$^{-/-}$ MEFs (**d**) were cultured under LPS stimulation (10 μg/mL) for 12 h; nuclear and cytoplasmic proteins were extracted separately and then Western blot was performed (Lamin A/C as a reference for nuclear extraction (N); Tubulin as a reference for cytoplasmic extraction (C).) **e,f** Effects of E2F2 on p65 nuclear translocation both in RASFs (Fig. 4e) and MEFs (Fig. 4f) observed using confocal fluorescence microscopy. **g–j** E2F2-silenced RASFs and *E2f2*$^{-/-}$ MEFs were cultured with or without LPS. qRT-PCR (**g,h**) and Western blot (**i,j**) were performed to detect the effect of E2F2 on MyD88. **k** Schematic representation of the MyD88 promoter, primers for the ChIP assay, and the E2F2 binding motif in the MyD88 promoter. **l,m** E2F2 was recruited to the *MyD88* gene promoter in RASFs in the presence of LPS. ChIP (**l**) and luciferase (Luc) reporter assay (**m**) were performed in RASFs and MEFs in the presence or absence of LPS (10 μg/mL). **n** MyD88 mediated the effect of E2F2 on PI3K/AKT/NF-κB pathways. Western blot showed that knockdown of MyD88 could significantly inhibit the phosphorylation of AKT and P65 in the presence or absence of E2F2 overexpression. qRT-PCR showed that inhibition of MyD88 can inhibit the expression of inflammatory factors and significantly reduce the upregulation of interleukin (IL)-1α (**o**), IL-1β (**p**), and tumor necrosis factor (TNF)-α (**q**) by E2F2. The effect of inhibitors of PI3K/AKT/NF-κB pathways (LY294002 and PDTC) on E2F2; qRT-PCR was used to detect the effect of inhibitors on expression of IL-1α (**r,u**), IL-1β (**s,v**), and TNF-α (**t,w**) in response to LPS. The results shown are means ± SEM of three independent experiments performed in triplicate. **P < 0.01, ***P < 0.001, versus the control. Ad-GFP adenovirus encoding green fluorescent protein, NC knockdown scramble control, si small interfering, WT wild-type

were knocked-down by siRNA with or without overexpression of E2F2 under stimulation with LPS (10 μg/mL). qRT-PCR showed that inhibition of both MyD88 and STAT1 could significantly attenuate the E2F2-stimulated expression of IL-1α (Fig. 6e), IL-1β (Fig. 6f), and TNF-α (Fig. 6g).

Discussion

Hyperplasia and excessive production of inflammatory factors in RASFs leads to joint damage, and RASFs play a central role in RA pathogenesis [26]. Previous studies have shown that inhibition of E2Fs by oligodeoxynucleotides can prevent cartilage destruction by inhibition of synovial cell proliferation [8, 28]. Our previous microarray assay and the following studies showed that E2F2 expression is significantly higher in RA synovial tissue than in osteoarthritis (OA), and that E2F2 is associated with the pathological progression of RA and can exacerbate inflammatory phenotypes in RASFs, such as proliferation, invasion, and cytokine production in vitro [7]. In the present study, we investigated the mechanism of E2F2 in RA inflammation.

We developed *E2f2*$^{-/-}$ mice to test the role of E2F2 in promoting inflammation. As previously reported by Murga et al. [11], *E2f2*$^{-/-}$ mice survive to adulthood, are fertile, produce normal offspring, and have normal gross and microscopic organ morphology at 4- to 8-weeks of age. However, only 27% of the E2F2-deficient animals survive to 15 months. When developing our CIA models, 8-week-old mice were used. We did not observe any significant differences in the blood routine index in WT and *E2f2*$^{-/-}$ mice. In *E2f2*$^{-/-}$ mice, IL-1α, IL-1β, and TNF-α expression in MEFs and secretion in the serum were significantly decreased. CIA was induced following traditional methods. After 2 months, *E2f2*$^{-/-}$ mice had significantly reduced progression of CIA, both in

incidence, severity, and cartilage destruction. We also aimed to uncover the mechanism by which E2F2 acts in RA inflammation. Indeed, we found that E2F2 can regulate the expression of STAT1 and activation of the PI3K/AKT/NF-κB pathway.

STAT1 is a member of the STAT family of transcription factors. STAT1 expression was reported to be significantly higher in RA synovial tissue than in OA and mandatory spondylitis [3]. In addition, functionalized STAT1 siRNA nanoparticles can regress CIA in a mouse model [29]. Notably, STAT1 regulates the expression of IL-1α, IL-1β, and TNF-α in THP-1 cells and RAW 264.7 cells [16, 30]. We tested whether STAT1 can also regulate the expression of these three cytokines in RASFs and MEFs. To investigate how E2F2 regulates STAT1, we performed co-IP and luciferase reporter assays. We found that E2F2 can bind to the promoter of STAT1 and regulate its expression. Expression of E2F2 significantly induced translocation of STAT1 into the nucleus and subsequently regulated the expression of IL-1α, IL-1β, and TNF-α. To further verify this, we knocked-down STAT1 in normal or E2F2-overexpressing RASFs and found that, in normal RASFs, siSTAT1 reduced the LPS-stimulated inflammatory cytokines by 25% while, in E2F2-overexpressing RASFs, siSTAT1 reduced the LPS-stimulated inflammatory cytokines by 50%. On the other hand, E2F2 knockdown can result in decreased STAT1 and LPS-stimulated inflammatory cytokines. Recovery of STAT1 prevented the inhibition of cytokine expression by siE2F2 and in *E2f2*$^{-/-}$ MEFs. Thus, it is important to explain how E2F2 regulates the expression of inflammatory cytokines. We inferred that E2F2 may play a role in regulation of RA inflammation through the STAT1 pathway. However, inhibition of STAT1 activity does not completely reverse the upregulation of IL-1α, IL-1β, and TNF-α by E2F2, suggesting that E2F2

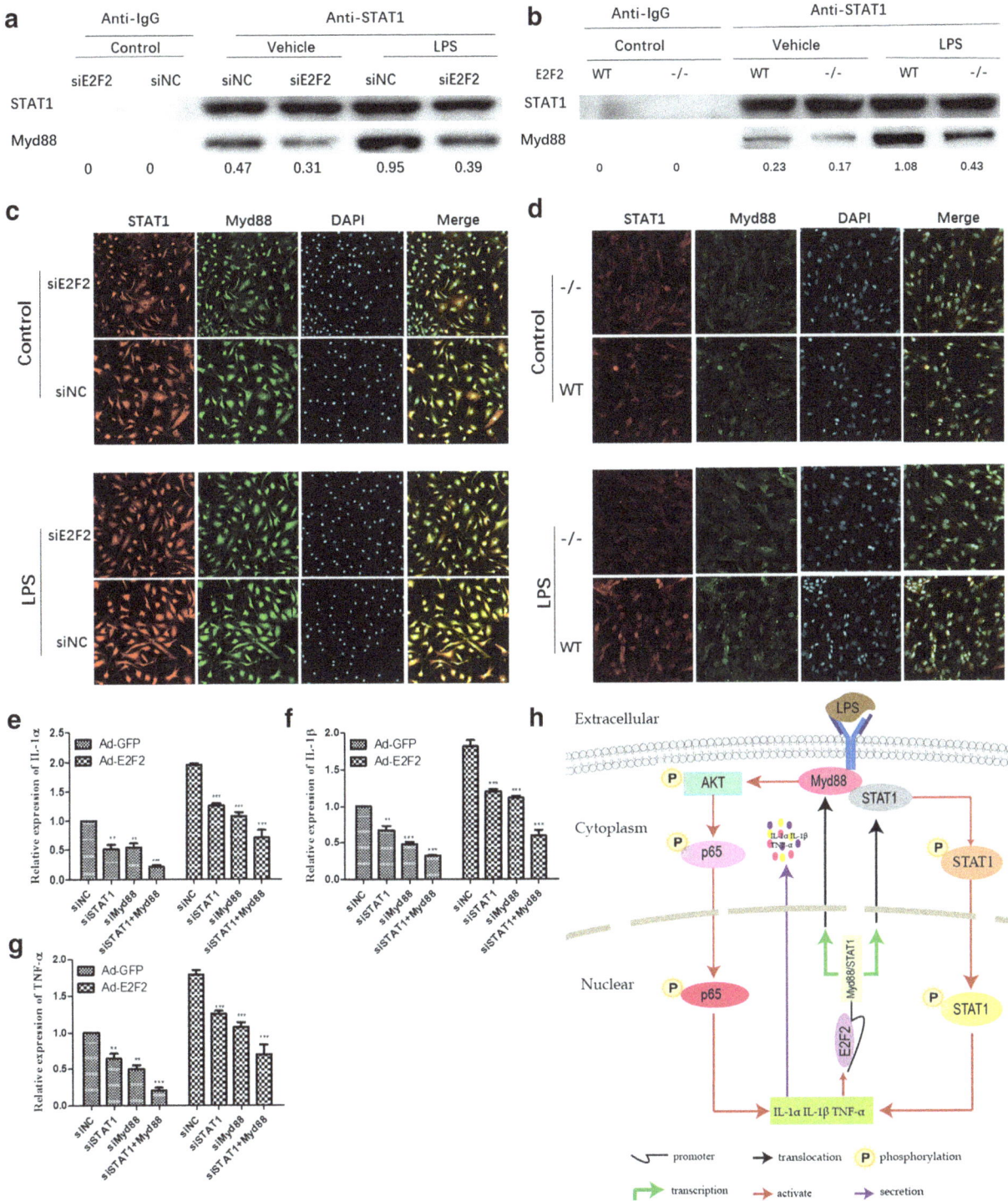

Fig. 6 STAT1/MyD88 complexes mediate E2F2 regulation of inflammatory cytokines. **a–d** STAT1/MyD88 complex is found in RASFs and MEFs. E2F2-silenced RASFs and *E2f2*$^{-/-}$ MEFs were cultured with or without lipopolysaccharide (LPS; 10 μg/mL). Co-IP (**a,b**) was performed to test the binding. Confocal immunofluorescence (**c,d**) was performed to confirm the result (magnification 10 × 40, MyD88 (green) and STAT1 (red)). **e–g** Effect of STAT1/MyD88 complexes on the expression of cytokines. qRT-PCR was performed to detect expression of interleukin (IL)-1α (**e**), IL-1β (**f**), and tumor necrosis factor (TNF)-α (**g**) in STAT1/MyD88 knockdown RASFs with or without E2F2 overexpression in the presence of LPS (10 μg/mL). The results shown are means ± SEM of three independent experiments performed in triplicate. ******$P < 0.01$, *******$P < 0.001$, versus the control. **h** Model depicting the role of E2F2 in RA pathogenesis. Ad-GFP adenovirus encoding green fluorescent protein, NC knockdown scramble control, si small interfering, WT wild-type

may have other pathogenic pathways. Therefore, we tried to find other pathways that participate in the effect of E2F2 in RA.

Using KEGG pathway analysis, we found that E2F2 had a significant effect on the PI3K/AKT/NF-κB pathway. The PI3K/AKT/NF-κB pathway regulates the immune response by provoking production of the cytokines IL-1α, IL-1β, and TNF-α in RASFs [21]. We demonstrated that E2F2 can significantly regulate the activation of the PI3K/AKT/NF-κB pathway and improve the translocation of p65 (a subunit of NF-κB) into the nucleus. We next tried to find a mediator between E2F2 and PI3K/AKT/NF-κB. From the literature, we found that MyD88, an adaptor protein for Toll-like receptor (TLR)4, can regulate expression of IL-1α, IL-1β, and TNF-α depending on activation of PI3K/AKT/NF-κB in RASFs [22, 31]. Notably, we further observed that E2F2 can bind to the promoter of the *MYD88* gene and directly regulate the expression of MyD88 both at the mRNA and protein level. Thus, MyD88 may be the mediator linking E2F2 to cytokines. To test this, we knocked-down MYD88 in RASFs, and found that inhibition of MYD88 may inactivate AKT and p65 and inhibit cytokine expression both in normal and E2F2-overexpressing RASFs. Specific inhibitors of PI3K/AKT and NF-κB were used to confirm the involvement of these pathways. Our results suggest that E2F2 can regulate expression of cytokines at the mRNA level via the PI3K/AKT/NF-κB pathway in RASFs. STAT1 can bind to MyD88 and the bond may affect activation of STAT1 [23]. Co-IP and immunofluorescence assays of RASFs and MEFs consistently confirmed the bond between STAT1 and MyD88. Furthermore, our data suggest that simultaneous knockdown of STAT1 and MyD88 could decrease the expression of inflammatory factors more significantly than inhibition of one of them alone, and the trend is more pronounced in E2F2-overexpressing RASFs. These results indicate that E2F2 can positively regulate the expression of STAT1/MyD88 in RASFs and MEFs, which in turn may play a role in mediating the expression of these proinflammatory cytokines. Therefore, there may be an E2F2-STAT1/MyD88-cytokine loop in the in vivo inflammatory microenvironment.

Conclusion

In summary, our study sheds light on the proinflammatory role of E2F2 in the pathogenesis of RA (Fig. 6h). E2F2 affects the formation of the STAT1/MYD88 complex by directly binding to the STAT1 and MYD88 promoters. This in turn influences the entry of STAT1 into the nucleus and activation of the PI3K/AKT/NF-KB pathway, ultimately regulating expression of inflammatory cytokines including IL-1α, IL-1β, and TNF-α. A better understanding of E2F2-mediated inflammatory pathways may lead to novel treatment strategies for RA.

Abbreviations

ChIP: Chromatin immunoprecipitation; CIA: Collagen-induced arthritis; Co-IP: Co-immunoprecipitation; E2F2: E2F transcription factor 2; ELISA: Enzyme-linked immunosorbent assay; IL: Interleukin; KO: Knockout; LPS: Lipopolysaccharide; MEF: Mouse embryonic fibroblast; Mut: Mutant; MyD88: Myeloid differentiation primary response 88; OA: Osteoarthritis; PBS: Phosphate-buffered saline; PCR: Polymerase chain reaction; qRT-PCR: Quantitative real-time polymerase chain reaction; RA: Rheumatoid arthritis; RASF: Rheumatoid arthritis synovial fibroblast; siRNA: Small interfering RNA; STAT1: Signal transducer and activator of transcription 1; TNF: Tumor necrosis factor; WT: Wild-type

Funding

This work was supported by grants from the National Natural Science Foundation of China (grant no. 81671624), the Key program of Shandong Province (grant no. 2017GSF218082), and the Innovation Project of Shandong Academy of Medical Sciences (2016–2018).

Authors' contributions

JP and LW designed the study and provided funding; SW and JP executed the study and prepared the manuscript; SW performed most of the experiments; LW analyzed the data. SS and CW preformed experiments and provided the samples. All authors read and approved the final manuscript.

Consent for publication

Not applicable.

Competing interests

The authors declare that they have no competing interests.

Author details

[1]Medical and Life Science College, University of Jinan, Jinan 250062, Shandong, China. [2]Shandong Medicinal Biotechnology Centre, Jingshi Road, Jinan 250000, Shandong, China. [3]Key Lab for Biotechnology Drugs of Ministry of Health, Jinan 250000, Shandong, China. [4]Key Lab for Rare & Uncommon Diseases, Jinan 250000, Shandong, China. [5]Shandong Provincial Hospital affiliated to Shandong University, Jinan 250000, Shandong, China.

References

1. Lafeber FP, Van der Laan WH. Progression of joint damage despite control of inflammation in rheumatoid arthritis: a role for cartilage damage driven synovial fibroblast activity. Ann Rheum Dis. 2012;71(6):793–5.
2. Andreas K, Lübke C, Häupl T, Dehne T, Morawietz L, Ringe J, et al. Key regulatory molecules of cartilage destruction in rheumatoid arthritis: an *in vitro* study. Arthritis Res Ther. 2008;10(1):R9.
3. Tomita T, Kunugiza V, Tomita N, Takano H, Morishita R, Kaneda V, et al. E2F decoy oligodeoxynucleotide ameliorates cartilage invasion by infiltrating synovium derived from rheumatoid arthritis. Int J Mol Med. 2006;18(2):257–65.
4. Cañete JD, Llena J, Collado A, Sanmartí R, Gayá A, Gratacós J, et al. Comparative cytokine gene expression in synovial tissue of early rheumatoid arthritis and seronegative spondyloarthropathies. Br J Rheumatol. 1997;36(1):38–42.
5. Brentano F, Kyburz D, Gay S. Toll-like receptors and rheumatoid arthritis. Springer Link. 2009;517(1):329–43.
6. Chang X, Yue L, Liu W, Wang Y, Wang L, Xu B, et al. CD38 and E2F transcription factor 2 have uniquely increased expression in rheumatoid arthritis synovial tissues. Clin Exp Immunol. 2014;176(2):222–31.
7. Zhang R, Wang L, Pan J, Han J. A critical role of E2F transcription factor 2 in proinflammatory cytokines-dependent proliferation and invasiveness of fibroblast-like synoviocytes in rheumatoid arthritis. Sci Rep. 2018;8(1):2623–33.
8. Farahat MN, Yanni G, Poston R, Panayi GS. Cytokine expression in synovial membranes of patients with rheumatoid arthritis and osteoarthritis. Ann Rheum Dis. 1993;52(12):870–5.

9. Nevins JR. Toward an understanding of the functional complexity of the E2F and retinoblastoma families. Cell Growth Differ. 2014;15(8):585–93.

10. Helmchen B, Weckauf H, Ehemann V, Berger I. Expression of cell cycle-related gene products in synovial stroma and synovial lining in active and quiescent stages of rheumatoid arthritis. Histol Histopathol. 2005; 20(2):365–72.

11. Murga M, Fernández-Capetillo O, Field SJ, Moreno B, Borlado LR, Fujiwara Y, et al. Mutation of E2F2 in mice causes enhanced T lymphocyte proliferation, leading to the development of autoimmunity. Immunity. 2001;15(6):959–70.

12. Wang ZJ, Zhang FM, Wang LS, Yao YW, Zhao Q, Gao X, et al. Lipopolysaccharides can protect mesenchymal stem cells (MSCs) from oxidative stress-induced apoptosis and enhance proliferation of MSCs via toll-like receptor (TLR)-4 and PI3K/Akt. Cell Biol Int. 2009;33(6):665–74.

13. Adámková L, Soucková K, Kovarík J. Transcription protein STAT1: biology and relation to cancer. Folia Biol. 2007;53(1):1.

14. Wang L, Song G, Zheng Y, Wang D, Dong H, Pan J, et al. miR-573 is a negative regulator in the pathogenesis of rheumatoid arthritis. Cell Mol Immunol. 2016;13(6):839–49.

15. Unlu S, Kumar A, Waterman WR, Tsukada J, Wang KZQ, Deborah L, et al. Phosphorylation of IRF8 in a pre-associated complex with Spi-1/PU.1 and non-phosphorylated Stat1 is critical for LPS induction of the IL1B gene. Mol Immunol. 2007;44(1):3364–79.

16. Wang H, Wang J, Xia Y. Defective suppressor of cytokine signaling 1 signaling contributes to the pathogenesis of systemic lupus erythematosus. Front Immunol. 2017;10(1):01292.

17. Zha L, Chen J, Sun S, Mao L, Chu X, Deng H, et al. Soyasaponins can blunt inflammation by inhibiting the reactive oxygen species-mediated activation of PI3K/Akt/NF-kB pathway. PLoS One. 2014;9(9):e107655.

18. Kim BH, Cho JY. Anti-inflammatory effect of honokiol is mediated by PI3K/Akt pathway suppression. Acta Pharm Sin. 2008;29(1):113–22.

19. Camps M, Ardissone V, Leroy D, Hirsch E. Blockade of PI3Kgamma suppresses joint inflammation and damage in mouse models of rheumatoid arthritis. Nat Med. 2005;11(9):936–43.

20. Weichhart T, MD S¨e. The PI3K/Akt/mTOR pathway in innate immune cells: emerging therapeutic applications. Ann Rheum Dis. 2008;67(9):iii70–4.

21. Xu H, He Y, Yang X, Liang L, Zhan Z, Ye Y, et al. Anti-malarial agent artesunate inhibits TNF-induced production of proinflammatory cytokines via inhibition of NF-kB and PI3 kinase/Akt signal pathway in human rheumatoid arthritis fibroblast-like synoviocytes. Rheumatology. 2007;46(6):920–6.

22. Lee JY, Ye J, Gao Z, Youn HS, Lee WH, et al. Reciprocal modulation of toll-like receptor-4 signaling pathways involving MyD88 and phosphatidylinositol 3-kinase/AKT by saturated and polyunsaturated fat acids. J Biol Chem. 2003;39(39):37041–51.

23. Ojaniemi M, Glumoff V, Harju K, Liljeroos M, Vuori K, Hallman M. Phosphatidylinositol 3-kinase is involved in toll-like receptor 4-mediated cytokine expression in mouse macrophages. Eur J Immunol. 2003;33(3):597–605.

24. Bauerfeld CP, Rastogi R, Pirockinaite G, Samavati L. TLR4-mediated AKT activation is MyD88/TRIF-dependent and critical for induction of OxPhos and mitochondrial transcription factor a in murine macrophages. J Immunol. 2012;188(6):2847–57.

25. de Hooge ASK, van de Loo FAJ, Koenders MI, Bennink MB, Arntz OJ, Kolbe T, et al. Local activation of STAT-1 and STAT-3 in the inflamed synovium during zymosan-induced arthritis: exacerbation of joint inflammation in STAT-1 gene-knockout mice. Arthritis Rheum. 2004;50(6):2014–23.

26. Laird MHW, Rhee SH, Perkins DJ, Medvedev AE, Piao W, Fenton MW, et al. TLR4/MyD88/PI3K interactions regulate TLR4 signaling. J Leukoc Biol. 2009; 85(6):966–77.

27. Jinghua W, Ma C, Wang H, Shuhui W, Xue G, Shi X. A MyD88–JAK1–STAT1 complex directly induces SOCS-1 expression in macrophages infected with group A streptococcus. Cell Mol Immunol. 2014;12(3):373–83.

28. Ospelt C, Kyburz D, Pierer M, Seibl R, Kurowska M, Distler O, et al. Toll-like receptors in rheumatoid arthritis joint destruction mediated by two distinct pathways. Ann Rheum Dis. 2004;63(Suppl 2):ii90–1.

29. Scheinman RI, Trivedi R, Vermillion S, Kompella UB, et al. Functionalized STAT1 siRNA nanoparticles regress rheumatoid arthritis in a mouse model. Nanomedicine. 2011;6(10):1669–82.

30. Boehm U, Klamp T, Groot M, Howard JC, et al. Cellular responses to interferon-gamma. Annu Rev Immunol. 1997;15(1):749–95.

31. Chi PL, Luo SF, Hsieh HL, Lee IT, Hsiao LD, Chen YL, et al. Cytosolic phospholipase A2 induction and prostaglandin E2 release by interleukin-1 via the myeloid differentiation factor 88-dependent pathway and cooperation of p300, Akt, and NF-kB activity in human rheumatoid arthritis synovial fibroblasts. Arthritis Rheum. 2011;63(10):2905–17.

Permissions

Contributors

Thijs Willem Swinnen
Division of Rheumatology, University Hospitals Leuven, Herestraat 49, 3000 Leuven, Belgium
Skeletal Biology and Engineering Research Center, Department of Development and Regeneration, KU Leuven, Herestraat 49 box 7003/13, 3000 Leuven, Belgium
Musculoskeletal Rehabilitation Research Unit, Department of Rehabilitation Sciences, KU Leuven, Tervuursevest 101 box 1501, 3001 Leuven, Belgium

René Westhovens and Kurt de Vlam
Division of Rheumatology, University Hospitals Leuven, Herestraat 49, 3000 Leuven, Belgium
Skeletal Biology and Engineering Research Center, Department of Development and Regeneration, KU Leuven, Herestraat 49 box 7003/13, 3000 Leuven, Belgium

Wim Dankaerts
Musculoskeletal Rehabilitation Research Unit, Department of Rehabilitation Sciences, KU Leuven, Tervuursevest 101 box 1501, 3001 Leuven, Belgium

Jasvinder A. Singh
Medicine Service, VA Medical Center, 510, 20th Street South, FOT 805B, Birmingham, AL 35233, USA
Department of Medicine at School of Medicine, University of Alabama at Birmingham, 20th Street South, FOT 805B, Birmingham, AL 35294-0022, USA

Division of Epidemiology at School of Public Health, University of Alabama at Birmingham, 1720 Second Avenue South, Birmingham, AL 35294-0022, USA
University of Alabama, Faculty Office Tower 805B, 510 20th Street South, Birmingham, AL 35294-0022, USA

John D. Cleveland
Department of Medicine at School of Medicine, University of Alabama at Birmingham, 20th Street South, FOT 805B, Birmingham, AL 35294-0022, USA

Timothy G. Brandon
Department of Pediatrics, Division of Rheumatology, Children's Hospital of Philadelphia, Philadelphia, PA, USA
Center for Pediatric Clinical Effectiveness (CPCE), Children's Hospital of Philadelphia, Philadelphia, PA, USA

Pamela F. Weiss
Department of Pediatrics, Division of Rheumatology, Children's Hospital of Philadelphia, Philadelphia, PA, USA
Center for Pediatric Clinical Effectiveness (CPCE), Children's Hospital of Philadelphia, Philadelphia, PA, USA
Center for Clinical Epidemiology and Biostatistics, Perelman School of Medicine at the University of Pennsylvania, Philadelphia, PA, USA
The Children's Hospital of Philadelphia, Roberts Center for Pediatric Research, 2716 South Street, Room 11121, Philadelphia, PA 19146, USA

David M. Biko and Nancy A. Chauvin
Department of Radiology, Children's Hospital of Philadelphia, Philadelphia, PA, USA

Rui Xiao
Center for Clinical Epidemiology and Biostatistics, Perelman School of Medicine at the University of Pennsylvania, Philadelphia, PA, USA

Walter P. Maksymowych
Department of Medicine, University of Alberta, Edmonton, AB, Canada
Canadian Research and Education (CaRE) Arthritis Organization, Edmonton, AB, Canada

Jacob L. Jaremko
Department of Radiology and Diagnostic Imaging, University of Alberta, Edmonton, AB, Canada

Robert G. Lambert
Department of Radiology and Diagnostic Imaging, University of Alberta, Edmonton, AB, Canada
Canadian Research and Education (CaRE) Arthritis Organization, Edmonton, AB, Canada

Eleni Kampylafka, Isabelle d'Oliveira, Christina Linz, Veronika Lerchen, Fabian Stemmler, David Simon, Matthias Englbrecht, Jürgen Rech, Arnd Kleyer, Georg Schett and Axel J. Hueber
Department of Internal Medicine 3 – Rheumatology and Immunology, Friedrich-Alexander-Universität Erlangen-Nürnberg (FAU) and Universitätsklinikum Erlangen, Ulmenweg 18, 91054 Erlangen, Germany

Michael Sticherling
Department of Dermatology, Friedrich-Alexander-Universität Erlangen-Nürnberg (FAU) and Universitätsklinikum Erlangen, Ulmenweg 18, 91054 Erlangen, Germany

Brigitte Michelsen, Stig Tengesdal and Inger Johanne Widding Hansen
Division of Rheumatology, Department of Medicine, Hospital of Southern Norway Trust, Servicebox 416, 4604 Kristiansand, Norway

Glenn Haugeberg
Division of Rheumatology, Department of Medicine, Hospital of Southern Norway Trust, Servicebox 416, 4604 Kristiansand, Norway
Department of Neuroscience, Division of Rheumatology, Norwegian University of Science and Technology, Trondheim, Norway

Andreas Diamantopoulos
Department of Rheumatology, Martina Hansens Hospital, Bærum, Norway

Arthur Kavanaugh
Division of Rheumatology, Allergy, and Immunology, School of Medicine, University of California, San Diego, USA

Cristina Rozo
1Hospital for Special Surgery, New York, NY 10021, USA.

Laura T. Donlin, Edd Ricker, Alessandra B. Pernis, Lionel B. Ivashkiv, Susan M. Goodman and Vivian P. Bykerk
Hospital for Special Surgery, New York, NY 10021, USA
Weill Cornell Medical College, New York, NY 10065, USA

Deepak A. Rao, Kevin Wei, Fumitaka Mizoguchi, Joshua Keegan, Adam Chicoine James A. Lederer, Soumya Raychaudhuri and Michael B. Brenner
Brigham and Women's Hospital, Harvard Medical School, Boston, MA 02115, USA

Kamil Slowikowski and Maria Gutierrez-Arcelus
Brigham and Women's Hospital,Harvard Medical School, Boston, MA 02115, USA
Broad Institute of MIT and Harvard University, Cambridge, MA 02142, USA

David J. Lieb, Thomas M. Eisenhaure, Shuqiang Li, Edward P. Browne, Danielle Sutherby, Akiko Noma and Chad Nusbaum
Broad Institute of MIT and Harvard University, Cambridge, MA 02142, USA

Nir Hacohen
Broad Institute of MIT and Harvard University, Cambridge, MA 02142, USA
Massachusetts General Hospital, Harvard Medical School, Boston, MA 02114, USA

Mandy J. McGeachy and Larry W. Moreland
University of Pittsburgh School of Medicine, Pittsburgh, PA 15261, USA

Jason D. Turner and Andrew Filer
University of Birmingham, Queen Elizabeth Hospital, B15 2WB, Birmingham, UK

Nida Meednu, Brendan F. Boyce and Jennifer H. Anolik
University of Rochester Medical Center, Rochester, NY 14642, USA

Kaylin Muskat, Gary S. Firestein, Joshua Hillman and David L. Boyle
University of California San Diego School of Medicine, La Jolla, CA 92093, USA

Stephen Kelly
Mile End Hospital, Barts Health NHS Trust, E1 1BB, London, UK

William H. Robinson and Paul J. Utz
Stanford University School of Medicine, Stanford, CA 94305, USA

Ellen M. Gravallese
University of Massachusetts Medical School, Worcester, MA 01605, USA
Massachusetts General Hospital, Harvard Medical School, Boston, MA 02114, USA

Costantino Pitzalis
Queen Mary University of London, E1 4NS, London, UK

Peter K. Gregersen
The Feinstein Institute for Medical Research, Manhasset, NY 11030, USA

V. Michael Holers
University of Colorado of Denver School of Medicine, Aurora, CO 80045, USA

John A. Reynolds, Ben Parker and Ian N. Bruce
Arthritis Research UK Centre for Epidemiology, Centre for Musculoskeletal Research, Manchester Academic Health Science Centre, University of Manchester, Manchester M13 9PT, UK
The Kellgren Centre for Rheumatology, NIHR Manchester Biomedical Research Centre, Manchester University Hospitals NHS Foundation Trust, Manchester Academic Health Science Centre, Manchester, UK

Pintip Ngamjanyaporn
Arthritis Research UK Centre for Epidemiology, Centre for Musculoskeletal Research, Manchester Academic Health Science Centre, University of Manchester, Manchester M13 9PT, UK
Division of Allergy, Immunology and Rheumatology, Department of Internal Medcine, Faculty of Medicine, Ramathibodi Hospital, Mahidol University, Bangkok, Thailand

Jamie C. Sergeant
Arthritis Research UK Centre for Epidemiology, Centre for Musculoskeletal Research, Manchester Academic Health Science Centre, University of Manchester, Manchester M13 9PT, UK
Centre for Biostatistics, Manchester Academic Health Science Centre, University of Manchester, Manchester, UK

Eoghan M. McCarthy
The Kellgren Centre for Rheumatology, NIHR Manchester Biomedical Research Centre, Manchester University Hospitals NHS Foundation Trust, Manchester Academic Health Science Centre, Manchester, UK

Sahena Haque
Rheumatology Department, Wythenshawe Hospital, Manchester University Hospitals NHS Foundation, Manchester, UK

Elaine Lee, Eileen Lee and Stephen A. Kilfeather
Aeirtec Ltd, The Smoke Houses Building, Clifford Fort, North Shields, Newcastle upon Tyne, UK

Yu-feng Liu and Feng-bin Liu
Guangzhou University of Chinese Medicine, Guangzhou, People's Republic of China

The First Affiliated Hospital of Guangzhou University of Chinese Medicine, The Lingnan Medicine Research Center, Guangzhou 510405,People's Republic of China

Kun-hai Zhuang, Bin Chen and Pei-wu Li
The First Affiliated Hospital of Guangzhou University of Chinese Medicine, The Lingnan Medicine Research Center, Guangzhou 510405, People's Republic of China

Xuan Zhou and Li-mei Zhong
Department of Laboratory Medicine, Guangdong Second Provincial General Hospital, Guangzhou 510317, People's Republic of China

Hua Jiang
Department of Hematology Oncology, Guangzhou Medical University, Guangzhou Women and Children's Medical Center, Guangzhou 510623, People's Republic of China

Tahzeeb Fatima, Cushla McKinney, Tanya J. Major and Tony R. Merriman
Department of Biochemistry, University of Otago, Dunedin, New Zealand

Lisa K. Stamp
Department of Medicine, University of Otago, Christchurch, New Zealand

Nicola Dalbeth
Department of Medicine, University of Auckland, Auckland, New Zealand

Cory Iverson
Medical Scientific Affairs, Ironwood Pharmaceuticals, Cambridge, MA, USA

Jeffrey N. Miner
Biology, Ardea Biosciences, Inc., San Diego, CA, USA

Jamie C. Sergeant
Centre for Biostatistics, Manchester Academic Health Science Centre, University of Manchester, Manchester, UK
Arthritis Research UK Centre for Epidemiology, Centre for Musculoskeletal Research, Manchester Academic Health Science Centre, University of Manchester, Manchester, UK

James Anderson, Kamilla Kopec-Harding, Holly F. Hope and Deborah P. M. Symmons
Arthritis Research UK Centre for Epidemiology, Centre for Musculoskeletal Research, Manchester Academic Health Science Centre, University of Manchester, Manchester, UK

Suzanne M. M. Verstappen and Kimme L. Hyrich
Arthritis Research UK Centre for Epidemiology, Centre for Musculoskeletal Research, Manchester Academic Health Science Centre, University of Manchester, Manchester, UK
NIHR Manchester Biomedical Research Centre, Central Manchester University Hospitals NHS Foundation Trust, Manchester Academic Health Science Centre, Manchester, UK

Anne Barton
NIHR Manchester Biomedical Research Centre, Central Manchester University Hospitals NHS Foundation Trust, Manchester Academic Health Science Centre, Manchester, UK

Arthritis Research UK Centre for Genetics and Genomics, Centre for Musculoskeletal Research, Manchester Academic Health Science Centre, University of Manchester, Manchester, UK

Roberta Goncalves Marangoni and Gabriel Lord
Northwestern Scleroderma Program, Division of Rheumatology, Northwestern University Feinberg School of Medicine, Chicago, IL, USA

Benjamin Korman
Northwestern Scleroderma Program, Division of Rheumatology, Northwestern University Feinberg School of Medicine, Chicago, IL, USA
Division of Allergy, Immunology and Rheumatology, University of Rochester Medical Center, Rochester, NY, USA

John Varga
Northwestern Scleroderma Program, Division of Rheumatology, Northwestern University Feinberg School of Medicine, Chicago, IL, USA
Department of Dermatology, Northwestern University Feinberg School of Medicine, Chicago, IL, USA

Jerrold Olefsky
Division of Endocrinology, University of California, San Diego, La Jolla, CA, USA

Warren Tourtellotte
Department of Pathology, Cedars Sinai Medical Center, Los Angeles, CA, USA

Joshua L. Lee
Sydney Medical School, University of Sydney, Sydney, Australia

Premarani Sinnathurai and Lyn March
Sydney Medical School, University of Sydney, Sydney, Australia
Institute of Bone and Joint Research, Kolling Institute, Northern Sydney Local Health District, St Leonards, NSW, Australia
Department of Rheumatology, Royal North Shore Hospital, Reserve Road, St Leonards, NSW 2065, Australia

Rachelle Buchbinder
Monash Department of Clinical Epidemiology, Cabrini Institute, Melbourne, VIC, Australia.
Centre of Cardiovascular Research and Education in Therapeutics, School of Public Health and Preventive Medicine, Monash University, Melbourne, VIC, Australia

Catherine Hill
Department of Rheumatology, The Queen Elizabeth Hospital, Adelaide, SA, Australia
University of Adelaide, Adelaide, SA, Australia

Marissa Lassere
School of Public Health and Community Medicine, University of New South Wales, Sydney, NSW, Australia
Rheumatology Department, St George Hospital, Sydney, NSW, Australia

Hana Hulejová and Ivana Půtová
Institute of Rheumatology, Prague, Czech Republic

Olga Kryštůfková, Heřman F. Mann and Jiří Vencovský
Institute of Rheumatology, Prague, Czech Republic
Department of Rheumatology, First Faculty of Medicine, Charles University, Prague, Czech Republic

Ondřej Pecha
Technology Centre ASCR, Prague, Czech Republic

Louise Ekholm and Ingrid E. Lundberg
Division of Rheumatology, Department of Medicine, Karolinska University Hospital, Solna, Karolinska Institutet, Stockholm, Sweden

Maria Karolina Jonsson and Bjørg-Tilde Svanes Fevang
Department of Rheumatology, Haukeland University Hospital, Pb 1400, NO-5021 Bergen, Norway
Department of Clinical Science, University of Bergen, Bergen, Norway

Aase Haj Hensvold, Monika Hansson and Anca Irinel Catrina
Center for Molecular Medicine, Karolinska University Hospital, Stockholm, Sweden

Martin Cornillet
Center for Molecular Medicine, Karolinska University Hospital, Stockholm, Sweden
Epithelial Differentation and Rheumatoid Autoimmunity Unit, UMRS 1056 Inserm University of Toulouse, Toulouse, France

Anna-Birgitte Aga, Joseph Sexton and Siri Lillegraven
Department of Rheumatology, Diakonhjemmet Hospital, Oslo, Norway

Espen Andre Haavardsholm
Department of Rheumatology, Diakonhjemmet Hospital, Oslo, Norway
Department of Health and Society, Oslo University Hospital, Oslo, Norway

Linda Mathsson-Alm
Thermo-Fisher Scientific, Uppsala, Sweden

Guy Serre
Epithelial Differentation and Rheumatoid Autoimmunity Unit, UMRS 1056 Inserm University of Toulouse, Toulouse, France

Raini Dutta, Jennifer L. Auger and Bryce A. Binstadt
Department of Pediatrics and Center for Immunology, University of Minnesota, 2-114 Wallin Medical Biosciences Building, 2101 6th Street SE, Minneapolis, MN 55414, USA
Department of Medicinal Chemistry, College of Pharmacy, University of Minnesota, Minneapolis, MN, USA

Yilun Wang, Shuang Chen, Sunyi Chen, Juan Du, Jinran Lin, Haihong Qin, Jun Liang and Jinhua Xu
Department of Dermatology, Huashan Hospital, Fudan University, 12 Wulumuqi Zhong Road, Shanghai 200040, People's Republic of China

Jie Wang
Department of Human Anatomy and Histoembryology, School of Basic Medical Science, Fudan University, Shanghai, People's Republic of China

Miranda van Lunteren, Désirée van der Heijde and Floris van Gaalen
Department of Rheumatology, Leiden University Medical Center, P.O. Box 9600, 2300 RC Leiden, the Netherlands

Alexandre Sepriano
Department of Rheumatology, Leiden University Medical Center, P.O. Box 9600, 2300 RC Leiden, the Netherlands

NOVA Medical School, Universidade Nova de Lisboa, Lisbon, Portugal

Robert Landewé
Department of Rheumatology, Amsterdam Rheumatology and Immunology Center, Amsterdam, the Netherlands
Department of Rheumatology, Zuyderland Hospital, Heerlen, the Netherlands

Joachim Sieper
Department of Rheumatology, Charité Campus Benjamin Franklin, Berlin, Germany.
German Rheumatism Research Centre, Berlin, Germany

Martin Rudwaleit
Department of Rheumatology, Charité Campus Benjamin Franklin, Berlin, Germany
Department of Internal Medicine and Rheumatology, Klinikum Bielefeld Rosenhöhe, Bielefeld, Germany

Le-meng Zhang
Thoracic Medicine Department, Hunan Cancer Hospital, Changsha 410013, People's Republic of China

Jing-Jing Zhou
Thoracic Medicine Department, Hunan Cancer Hospital, Changsha 410013, People's Republic of China
Department of Rheumatology, Navy General Hospital, Beijing 100048, People's Republic of China

Chun-lei Luo
Department of Nephrology, Ningbo First Hospital, Ningbo 3150102, People's Republic of China

Lisa M. Rice, Julio C. Mantero, Eric A. Stratton, Robert W. Simms and Harrison W. Farber
Boston University School of Medicine, E5 Arthritis Center, 72 E Concord Street, Boston, MA 0211, USA

Rod Warburton, Kari Roberts and Nicholas Hill
Tufts University, Boston, MA, USA

Robyn Domsic and Robert Layfatis
University of Pittsburgh Medical Center, Pittsburgh, PA, USA

Makiko Yashiro Furuya, Tomoyuki Asano, Yuya Sumichika, Shuzo Sato, Hiroko Kobayashi, Hiroshi Watanabe and Kiyoshi Migita
Department of Rheumatology, Fukushima Medical University School of Medicine, 1 Hikarigaoka, Fukushima, Fukushima 960-1295, Japan

Eiji Suzuki
Department of Rheumatology, Ohta Nishinouchi General Hospital Foundation, 2-5-20 Nishinouchi, Koriyama, Fukushima 963-8558, Japan

Hideko Kozuru and Hiroshi Yatsuhashi
Clinical Research Center, NHO Nagasaki Medical Center, Kubara 2-1001-1 Omura, Nagasaki 856-8562, Japan

Tomohiro Koga and Atsushi Kawakami
Department of Immunology and Rheumatology, Unit of Translational Medicine, Graduate School of Biomedical Sciences, Nagasaki University, Sakamoto1-7-1, Nagasaki 852-8501, Japan

Hiromasa Ohira
Department of Gastroenterology, Fukushima Medical University School of Medicine, 1 Hikarigaoka, Fukushima, Fukushima 960-1295, Japan

Hideharu Sekine
Department of Immunology, Fukushima Medical University School of Medicine, 1 Hikarigaoka, Fukushima, Fukushima 960-1295, Japan

Paola Di Benedetto, Vasiliki Liakouli, Piero Ruscitti, Onorina Berardicurti, Francesco Carubbi, Noemi Panzera, Salvatore Di Bartolomeo, Paola Cipriani and Roberto Giacomelli
Department of Biotechnological and Applied Clinical Sciences, Rheumatology Unit, School of Medicine, University of L'Aquila, Delta 6 Building, Via dell'Ospedale, 67100 L'Aquila, Italy

Giuliana Guggino, Francesco Ciccia and Giovanni Triolo
Department of Internal Medicine, Division of Rheumatology, University of Palermo, Piazza delle Cliniche 2, 90127 Palermo, Italy

Motomu Hashimoto and Masao Tanaka
Department of Advanced Medicine for Rheumatic Diseases, Graduate School of Medicine, Kyoto University, 53 Kawaharacho, Shogoin, Sakyo-ku, Kyoto 606-8507, Japan

Hiromu Ito
Department of Advanced Medicine for Rheumatic Diseases, Graduate School of Medicine, Kyoto University, 53 Kawaharacho, Shogoin, Sakyo-ku, Kyoto 606-8507, Japan

Department of Orthopedic Surgery, Graduate School of Medicine, Kyoto University, Kyoto, Japan

Wararu Yamamoto
Department of Advanced Medicine for Rheumatic Diseases, Graduate School of Medicine, Kyoto University, 53 Kawaharacho, Shogoin, Sakyo-ku, Kyoto 606-8507, Japan
Department of Health Information Management, Kurashiki Sweet Hospital, Kurashiki, Japan

Moritoshi Furu
Department of Orthopedic Surgery, Graduate School of Medicine, Kyoto University, Kyoto, Japan
Department of Health Information Management, Kurashiki Sweet Hospital, Kurashiki, Japan

Takanori Fujimura and Ryota Hara
The Center for Rheumatic Diseases, Nara Medical University, Nara, Japan

Masaki Katayama
Department of Rheumatology, Osaka Red Cross Hospital, Osaka, Japan

Akira Ohnishi and Kengo Akashi
Department of Rheumatology and Clinical Immunology, Kobe University Graduate School of Medicine, Kobe, Japan

Shuzo Yoshida and Koji Nagai
Department of Internal Medicine (IV), Osaka Medical College, Osaka, Japan

Yonsu Son and Hideki Amuro
First Department of Internal Medicine, Kansai Medical University, Osaka, Japan

Toru Hirano
Department of Respiratory Medicine, Allergy and Rheumatic Disease, Graduate School of Medicine, Osaka University, Osaka, Japan

Kosuke Ebina
Department of Orthopaedic Surgery, Osaka University, Graduate School of Medicine, Osaka, Japan

Ryuji Uozumi
Department of Biomedical Statistics and Bioinformatics, Graduate School of Medicine, Kyoto University, Kyoto, Japan

Koichiro Ohmura and Tsuneyo Mimori
Department of Rheumatology and Clinical Immunology, Graduate School of Medicine, Kyoto University, Kyoto, Japan

Takao Fujii
Department of Rheumatology and Clinical Immunology, Wakayama Medical University, Wakayama, Japan

Pan Liao, Yi He, Fangyuan Yang, Guihu Luo, Jian Zhuang, Zeqing Zhai, Lili Zhuang and Erwei Sun
Department of Rheumatology and Immunology, The Third Affiliated Hospital, Southern Medical University, No. 183, Zhongshan Avenue West, Tianhe District, Guangzhou 510630, China
Institute of Clinical Immunology, Academy of Orthopedics Guangdong Province, Guangzhou, China

Zhuomiao Lin and Jiehuang Zheng
School of Pharmaceutical Science, Southern Medical University, Guangzhou, China

Shiguan Wang
Medical and Life Science College, University of Jinan, Jinan 250062,Shandong, China
Shandong Medicinal Biotechnology Centre, Jingshi Road, Jinan 250000, Shandong, China
Key Lab for Biotechnology Drugs of Ministry of Health, Jinan 250000, Shandong, China

Lin Wang and Ji-hong Pan
Shandong Medicinal Biotechnology Centre, Jingshi Road, Jinan 250000, Shandong, China
Key Lab for Biotechnology Drugs of Ministry of Health, Jinan 250000, Shandong, China
Key Lab for Rare and Uncommon Diseases, Jinan 250000, Shandong, China

Changshun Wu and Shui Sun
Shandong Provincial Hospital affiliated to Shandong University, Jinan 250000, Shandong, China

Index